DUE DATE:

11 / 27 / 12

MRI and CT of the Cardiovascular System

Second Edition

MRI and CT of the Cardiovascular System
Second Edition

Charles B. Higgins, MD
Professor
Department of Radiology
University of California, San Francisco
San Francisco, California

Albert de Roos, MD
Professor and Vice Chairman
Department of Radiology
Leiden University Medical Center
Leiden, The Netherlands

LIPPINCOTT WILLIAMS & WILKINS
A **Wolters Kluwer** Company
Philadelphia • Baltimore • New York • London
Buenos Aires • Hong Kong • Sydney • Tokyo

Acquisitions Editor: *Lisa McAllister*
Managing Editor: *Kerry Barrett*
Marketing Manager: *Angela Panetta*
Project Manager: *Nicole Walz*
Senior Manufacturing Manager: *Ben Rivera*
Design Coordinator: *Terry Mallon*
Cover Design: *Joseph DePinho*
Production Services: *Maryland Composition Inc*
Printer: *Edwards Brothers*

Printed in the United States of America

Library of Congress Cataloging-in-Publication Data

MRI and CT of the cardiovascular system / [edited by] Charles B. Higgins and Albert de Roos.—2nd ed.
    p. ; cm
  Rev. ed. of: Cardiovascular MRI and MRA. c2003.
  Includes bibliographical references and index.
  ISBN 0-7817-6271-5
  1. Cardiovascular system—Magnetic resonance imaging. 2. Cardiovascular system—Diseases—Diagnosis. I. Higgins, Charles B. II. Roos, Albert de, 1953- III. Cardiovascular MRI and MRA.
  [DNLM: 1. Heart Diseases—diagnosis. 2. Magnetic Resonance Imaging. 3. Tomography, X-Ray Computed. 4. Vascular Diseases—diagnosis. WG 141.5.M2 M939 2006]
RC670.5.M33C375 2006
616.1'07548—dc22
                              2005014962

To purchase additional copies of this book, call our customer service department at (800) 639-3030 or fax orders to (301) 824-7390. International customers should call (301) 714-2324.

Visit Lippincott Williams & Wilkins on the Internet: http://www.lww.com. Lippincott Williams & Wilkins customer service representatives are available from 8:30 am to 6:30 pm, EST.

Dedication

To our residents and fellows whose work has contributed to progress in cardiovascular MRI and CT

PREFACE

The first edition of this book was published at a time when MR was becoming an important imaging technique for the diagnosis of cardiovascular diseases. Since that time, CT has also been recognized as an important technology for the evaluation of the cardiovascular system. Although the first images of the beating heart using CT were produced in the late 1970s and the first images of the heart using MR around 1982, both techniques remained immature and unfamiliar for cardiovascular diagnosis for two decades or more. Technological advances in the past several years have rendered both techniques highly effective and for some applications, unique in the evaluation of the cardiovascular system. These techniques can provide precise depiction of cardiovascular morphology and quantification of physiology.

The first edition was published in 2003. This second edition appears after a relatively short interval. This approach was dictated by rapid technological advances and increased recognition of clinical applications of cardiovascular MR.

Furthermore, during this interval, multi-detector CT has emerged as an important diagnostic modality, especially for the evaluation of ischemic heart disease.

Our goal in preparing this book is to provide fully updated information on the use of MR and CT for the assessment of cardiac and vascular diseases. Similar to the first edition, we recognized the rapid advance in both MR and CT technology and the constantly evolving concepts on their clinical use. Consequently, we again embarked upon a schedule for writing this book that spanned less than a year from conception to completion of the manuscript.

The authors include basic scientists, cardiologists, and radiologists from around the world. These experts have had a long involvement in fostering the development of cardiovascular MR and CT.

Charles B. Higgins, MD
Albert de Roos, MD

CONTRIBUTING AUTHORS

Charles M. Anderson, MD, PhD
Clinical Professor of Radiology
University of California, San Francisco
San Francisco, California

Evan Appelbaum, MD
Instructor in Medicine
Harvard Medical School
Department of Cardiology
Beth Israel Deaconess Medical Center
Boston, Massachusetts

Philip A. Araoz, MD
Assistant Professor of Radiology
Mayo Clinic
Rochester, Minnesota

Håkan Arheden, MD, PhD
Associate Professor and Vice Chairman of Radiology
   and Clinical Physiology
Lund University Hospital
Lund, Switzerland

Sonya V. Babu-Narayan, BSc, MRCP
Clinical Fellow in Adult Congenital Heart Disease
   and Cardiovascular Magnetic Resonance
Royal Brompton Hospital and Imperial College
London, United Kingdom

Frank M. Baer, PhD, MBA
Professor of Cardiology
MBA Public Health
Clinic for Internal Medicine
University of Köln
Köln, Germany

Jeroen J. Bax, MD
Department of Cardiology
Leiden University Medical Center
Leiden, The Netherlands

Christoph R. Becker, MD
Associate Professor
Section Chief Body CT
University Hospital Munich
Munich, Germany

Jan Bogaert, MD, PhD
Professor of Radiology
University Hospitals
Catholic University of Leuven
Leuven, Belgium

René Botnar, PhD
Cardiovascular Division
Beth Israel Deaconess Medical Center
Boston, Massachusetts

Jens Bremerich, MD, PhD
Department of Radiology
University Hospital Basel
Basel, Switzerland

Arno Bücker, MD, MSc
Associate Professor of Diagnostic Radiology
University Hospital Aachen
Aachen, Germany

Peter T. Buser, MD
Professor and Vice Chairman of Cardiology
University Hospital Basel
Basel, Switzerland

Filippo Cademartiri, MD, PhD
Department of Radiology
Erasmus Medical Center
Rotterdam, The Netherlands

Pierson Chiou, MD
Assistant Clinical Professor of Radiology
University of California, San Francisco
San Francisco, California

Albert de Roos, MD
Professor and Vice Chairman of Radiology
Leiden University Medical Center
Leiden, The Netherlands

Pim J. de Feyter, MD, PhD
Radiologist
Cardiologist, Thorax Center
Erasmus Medical Center
Rotterdam, The Netherlands

Joost Doornbos, MD
Department of Radiology
Leiden University Medical Center
Leiden, The Netherlands

Steven Dymarkowski, MD, PhD
Associate Professor in Radiology
University Hospitals K.U. Leuven
Leuven, Belgium

Michael D. Elliott, MD
Assistant Professor of Medicine
Attending Physician
Duke University Medical Center
Durham, North Carolina

Peter Ewert, MD
Assistant Professor of Pediatrics
Cardiac Catheterization Laboratory
Department of Congenital Heart Diseases
German Heart Institute Berlin
Berlin, Germany

Rossella Fattori, PhD
Professor of Radiology
Cardiovascular Unit
University Hospital Sant'Orsola
Bologna, Italy

Zahi A. Fayad, PhD
Mount Sinai School of Medicine
Mount Sinai Hospital
Imaging Science Laboratories
New York, New York

Matthias G. Friedrich, MD, FESC
Associate Professor
Director, Stephenson CMR Centre at the Libin
    Cardiovascular Institute
University of Calgary
Calgary, Alberta, Canada

Jacob Geleijns, PhD
Medical Physicist
Department of Radiology
Leiden University Medical Center
Leiden, The Netherlands

Thomas M. Grist, MD
John Juhl Professor and Chair of Radiology
Clinical Sciences Center
Madison, Wisconsin

Heynric B. Grotenhuis, MD
Departments of Radiology and Cardiology
Leiden University Medical Center
Leiden, The Netherlands

Thomas H. Hauser, MD
Instructor in Medicine
Cardiovascular Division
Harvard University Medical School
Beth Israel Deaconess Medical Center
Boston, Massachusetts

Marie-Christine Herregods, MD, PhD
Professor of Cardiology
University Hospitals
Catholic University of Leuven
Leuven, Belgium

Charles B. Higgins, MD
Professor of Radiology
University of California, San Francisco
San Francisco, California

Robert M. Judd, PhD
Associate Professor of Medicine and Radiology
Co-Director, Duke Cardiovascular-Magnetic Resonance
    Center
Duke University Medical Center
Durham, North Carolina

J. Wouter Jukema, MD
Department of Cardiology
Leiden University Medical Center
Leiden, The Netherlands

Dagmar I. Keller, MD
Division of Cardiology
University Hospital Basel
Basel, Switzerland

Philip J. Kilner, MD, PhD
Consultant and Reader in Cardiovascular Magnetic
    Resonance
Royal Brompton Hospital and Imperial College
London, United Kingdom

Raymond J. Kim, MD
Associate Professor of Medicine and Radiology
Co-Director, Duke Cardiovascular Magnetic-Resonance
    Center
Duke University Medical Center
Durham, North Carolina

Sebastian Kozerke, PhD
University of Zurich and Swiss Federal Institute of
    Technology (ETH)
Institute for Biomedical Engineering
Zurich, Switzerland

Dara L. Kraitchman, VMD, PhD
Associate Professor of Radiology
Russell H. Morgan Division of MRI Research
Johns Hopkins University
Baltimore, Maryland

Gabriel P. Krestin, MD, PhD
Professor and Head of Department of Radiology
University Hospital Rotterdam
Rotterdam, The Netherlands

Lucia J.M. Kroft, MD, PhD
Department of Radiology
Leiden University Medical Center
Leiden, The Netherlands

Gabriele A. Krombach, MD, PhD
Department of Diagnostic Radiology
University Hospital RWTH-Aachen
Aachen, Germany

Titus Kuehne, MD
Pediatric Cardiologist
Department of Congenital Heart Disease/Pediatric
  Cardiology
German Heart Institute Berlin
Berlin, Germany

Hildo J. Lamb, MD, MSc, PhD
Senior Scientist
Radiology Resident
Leiden University Medical Center
Leiden, The Netherlands

Boudewijn P.F. Lelieveldt, PhD
Assistant Professor of Radiology
Division of Image Processing
Leiden University Medical Center
Leiden, The Netherlands

Michael J. Lipinski, BS
Third Year Medical Student
Virginia Commonwealth University School of Medicine
Richmond, Virginia

Venkatesh Mani, PhD
Post Doctoral Fellow of Radiology
Mount Sinai School of Medicine
New York, New York

Warren J. Manning, MD
Professor of Medicine and Radiology
Harvard Medical School
Section Chief, Non-invasive Cardiac Imaging
Beth Israel Deaconess Medical Center
Boston, Massachusetts

Nico R. Mollet, MD
Departments of Radiology and Cardiology
Erasmus Medical Center
Rotterdam, The Netherlands

Eike Nagel, MD
Department of Cardiology
Germany Heart Institute Berlin
Berlin, Germany

Karen G. Ordovás, MD
Research Fellow in Cardiovascular Imaging
University of California, San Francisco
San Francisco, California

Jaap Ottenkamp, MD, PhD, FESC
Department of Pediatric Cardiology
Leiden University Medical Center
Leiden, The Netherlands
Emma Children's Hospital
Amsterdam, The Netherlands

Harald H. Quick, PhD
Senior Physicist
Department of Diagnostic and Interventional Radiology
Section Biomedical Imaging
University Hospital, Essen
Essen, Germany

Frank E. Rademakers, MD, PhD
Professor of Cardiology
Univeristy Hospitals Leuven
Catholic University Leuven
Leuven, Belgium

**Reza Razaavi, MBBS, MD, MRCP (UK),
MRCHPCH**
Professor of Pediatric Cardiovascular Science
Deputy Chair
Division of Imaging Sciences
King's College
Director of Cardiac Magnetic Resonance Imaging
Guy's and St. Thomas' NHS Trust
London, United Kingdom

Gautham P. Reddy, MD, PhD
Associate Professor of Radiology
Director, Diagnostic Radiology Residency Program
Chief, Cardiac Imaging
University of California, San Francisco
San Francisco, California

Johan H.C. Reiber, PhD
Professor of Radiology
Division of Image Processing
Leiden University Medical Center
Leiden, The Netherlands

Vincenzo Russo, MD
Department of Radiology
Cardiovascular Unit
University Hospital Sant'Orsola
Bologna, Italy

Maythem Saeed, DVM, PhD
Professor of Radiology
University of California, San Francisco
San Francisco, California

Hajime Sakuma, MD
Associate Professor and Vice Chairman
Department of Diagnostic Radiology
Mie University Hospital
Tsu, Mie, Japan

Liesbeth P. Salm, MD
Department of Cardiology
Leiden University Medical Center
Leiden, The Netherlands

David A. Saloner, PhD
Professor of Radiology
University of California, San Francisco
San Francisco, California

Matthias Schmidt, Priv.-Doz, MD
Clinic and Health Center for Nuclear Medicine
University of Köln
Köln, Germany

Joanne D. Schuijf, MD
Department of Cardiology
Leiden University Medical Center
Leiden, The Netherlands

Juerg Schwitter, MD
Co-Director Cardiac MR Unit
Department of Cardiology and Internal Medicine
University Hospital Zurich
Zurich, Switzerland

Marc Sirol, MD
Assistant Professor of Cardiology
Hôpital Lariboisière
Paris, France
Cardiovascular Institute
Mount Sinai School of Medicine
New York, New York

Freddy Ståhlberg
Professor of Medical Radiation Physics
Lund University
Lund, Sweden

William Stanford, MD
Professor of Radiology
Cardiovascular and Chest Division
Lucille A. & Roy J. Carver University of Iowa College of
    Medicine
Iowa City, Iowa

Matthias Stuber, PhD
Associate Professor of Radiology
Russel H. Morgan Division of MRI Research
Departments of Cardiology and Electrical and Computer
    Engineering
Johns Hopkins University
Baltimore, Maryland

**Andrew M. Taylor, BA (Hons.), BM BCh, MD,
MRCP (UK), FRCR**
Senior Clinical Lecturer in Cardiovascular Imaging
Institute of Child Health
Univerisity College London
Great Ormond Street Hospital for Children
London, United Kingdom

Brad H. Thompson, MD
Associate Professor of Radiology
Director of General Radiology
Roy J. and Lucille A. Carver College of Medicine
University of Iowa Hospitals and Clinics
Iowa City, Iowa

Frank J. Thornton, MD
Assistant Professor of Radiology
Clinical Sciences Center
Madison, Wisconsin

Rob J. van der Geest, MSc
Assistant Professor of Radiology
Division of Image Processing
Leiden University Medical Center
Leiden, The Netherlands

Edwin van der Linden, MD
Department of Radiology
Leiden University Medical Center
Leiden, The Netherlands

Ernst E. van der Wall, MD
Department of Cardiology
Leiden University Medical Center
Leiden, The Netherlands

Hubert W. Vliegen, MD, PhD, FESC
Department of Cardiology
Leiden University Medical Center
Leiden, The Netherlands

Martin N. Wasser, MD
Department of Radiology
Leiden University Medical Center
Leiden, The Netherlands

Ralf Wassmuth, MD
Franz-Volhard-Clinic
Helios Klinikum Berlin
Charité University Berlin
Berlin, Germany

Norbert Watzinger, MD
Associate Professor of Cardiology
Medical University Graz
Graz, Austria

Oliver Weber, PhD
Assistant Adjunct Professor of Radiology
University of California, San Francisco
San Francisco, California

François E.J.A. Willemssen, MD
Department of Radiology
Leiden University Medical Center
Leiden, The Netherlands

Susan B. Yeon, MD, JD
Assistant Professor of Medicine
Cardiovascular Division
Harvard Medical School
Beth Israel Deaconess Medical Center
Boston, Massachusetts

CONTENTS

xiv   Contents

1

Clinical Approach to Cardiovascular Magnetic Resonance Techniques

Hildo J. Lamb, Sebastian Kozerke, Joost Doornbos, Jeroen J. Bax, and Albert de Roos

Cardiovascular magnetic resonance (CVMR) techniques are changing rapidly, and CVMR is currently in an exciting and crucial phase for its final clinical acceptance. The main technical limitations are overcome by development of improved scanner hardware, software, and image processing tools. In this chapter, basic and advanced CVMR techniques will be discussed in the context of clinical application. Based on a virtual patient examination, relevant techniques will be discussed. The focus will be on techniques for functional evaluation of heart disease. Special attention is given to reduced data acquisition methods, because these techniques are causing a revolution within the field of CVMR. MR techniques for perfusion imaging, visualization of delayed enhancement, coronary artery MR angiography, and vessel wall imaging will be discussed in more detail in other chapters and will be briefly discussed here.

COILS

Clinical cardiac exams can be performed using the standard body coil, although image quality is suboptimal. The main problem is the limited in-plane spatial resolution of around 3 mm^2. High spatial resolution is especially important for accurate assessment of wall motion abnormalities due to, for example, myocardial infarction. In the past, reliable images were obtained using the body coil for assessment of global and regional myocardial wall motion (Fig. 1.1). When an imaging center is particularly interested in CVMR, using a standard surface coil is useful, such as a single circular coil with a diameter of approximately 14 cm, which improves substantially image quality and spatial resolution. The best alternative is a dedicated cardiac phased array coil constructed of multiple elements. This type of coil is now commercially available from most scanner manufacturers (Fig. 1.1). The main advantage is the further improved image qual-

1

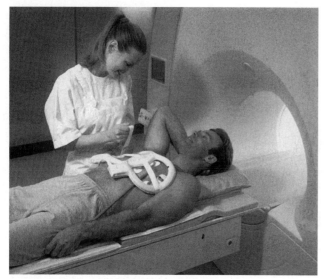

Figure 1.1. Practical setup of a dedicated cardiac phased array coil and vector ECG. The standard body coil is integrated with the magnet bore. (Courtesy of Philips Medical Systems, Best, The Netherlands.)

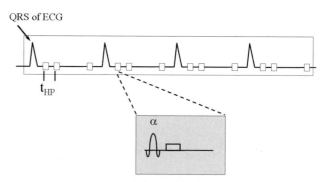

Figure 1.2. Schematic diagram of the basic principle of a gradient echo MR sequence [GRE, or fast-field echo (FFE)] in relation to the timing within the cardiac cycle. After each radio frequency (rf) excitation pulse (α), one line in k-space is acquired (gray area). In total, four heart beats are shown, resulting in an image of 4 k-lines. Suppose an image of 120 k-lines is required, the procedure needs to be repeated 30 times, leading to a total of heart beats of 120. With a heart rate of 60 beats-per-minute, the acquisition can be completed during continuous breathing within 2 minutes. White squares indicate heart phase image segments; t_{HP}, time between each heart phase (temporal resolution).

ity, spatial resolution, and the larger field of view. An additional advantage is that phased array coils allow application of the SENSE technique (1). SENSE represents a revolutionizing technology in CVMR; its principle is based on parallel imaging with use of all coil elements. Each coil has a different sensitivity profile, which can be exploited to unfold undersampled acquisitions and to reduce the density of the acquired k-space data, thus speeding up scan time (see later for details). Using SENSE, currently, a twofold increase in imaging speed can be obtained as standard; in an experimental setting higher factors were reached. In general, SENSE contributes significantly to the clinical acceptance of CVMR, because it reduces MR scan time, making it comparable to ultrasound or computed tomographic (CT) examinations.

CARDIAC MOTION COMPENSATION

Cardiac motion compensation is performed by synchronizing the image acquisition to the electrocardiogram (ECG) signal. Image formation in MR is based on filling "k-space" during data acquisition (see Appendix); this concept will not be explained further in this context, because many thorough and comprehensive publications are available on this topic (2–6). ECG-triggering is aimed at filling k-space in multiple steps, based on the timing within the cardiac cycle (Figs. 1.2 to 1.6). For example, to construct a movie of a cardiac slice, approximately 20 cardiac phases (time frames) are needed to obtain a sufficiently high temporal resolution. In general, a time resolution of less than 40 milliseconds per cardiac phase image is needed to enable selection of the end-systolic time frame, for calculation of, for example, the end-systolic volume and ejection fraction. For high resolution, clinical imaging, these 20 cardiac images per slice cannot be obtained at once. Therefore, ECG-triggering was devel-

oped, to synchronize the partial k-space filling to the cardiac cycle. Suppose we need 128 k-lines for the first cardiac phase image, but we can only acquire 12 k-lines for that image per heart beat, then 11 heart beats are needed to complete k-space filling for that image. This would take a breath-hold of approximately 11 seconds at a heart rate of 60 beats per minute. Of course, all 20 cardiac phases are acquired at once, so within 11 seconds a full movie of a cardiac slice can be obtained.

Currently, two types of ECG triggering methods are available. The first is prospective triggering, meaning that image

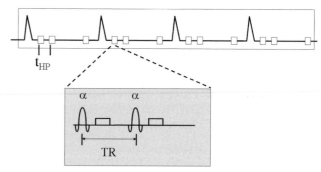

Figure 1.3. Schematic diagram of the basic principle of a turbo-field echo (TFE) MR sequence in relation to the timing within the cardiac cycle. After each rf excitation pulse (α), one line in k-space is acquired, which is repeated two times in this case (turbo-factor 2), leading to a total of two acquired k-lines per heart phase image segment per cardiac cycle (gray area). In total, four heart beats are shown, resulting in an image of 8 k-lines. Suppose an image of 120 k-lines is required, the procedure needs to be repeated 15 times, leading to a total of heart beats of 60. With a heart rate of 60 beats-per-minute, the acquisition can be completed during continuous breathing within 60 seconds. White squares indicate heart phase image segments; t_{HP}, time between each heart phase (temporal resolution); TR, repetition time between rf excitations.

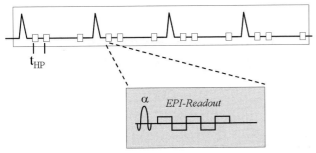

Figure 1.4. Schematic diagram of the basic principle of an echo-planar MR sequence (EPI) in relation to the timing within the cardiac cycle. After each rf excitation pulse (α), in this example five lines in k-space are acquired (EPI factor 5), leading to a total of five acquired k-lines per heart phase image segment per cardiac cycle (gray area). In total, 4 heart beats are shown, resulting in an image of 20 k-lines. Suppose an image of 120 k-lines is required, the procedure needs to be repeated six times, leading to a total of heart beats of 24. With a heart rate of 60 beats-per-minute, this can be performed during a breath-hold of 24 seconds. White squares indicate heart phase image segments; t_{HP}, time between each heart phase (temporal resolution).

acquisition starts at a fixed delay after the QRS-complex of the ECG and stops around 80% of the cardiac cycle. Consequently, the 20 cardiac phases are distributed during this 80% of time. The last 20% of the cardiac cycle is not imaged. This technique is suitable to image systolic heart function. When one is interested in the last part of the cardiac cycle to evaluate diastolic heart function, a different method can be applied. Retrospective ECG gating acquires image data irrespective of the ECG, while the ECG is recorded in parallel. Once the MR acquisition is finished, the computer calcu-

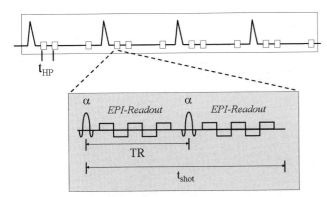

Figure 1.5. Schematic diagram of the basic principle of a turbo field echo-planar MR sequence (TFEPI) in relation to the timing within the cardiac cycle. After each rf excitation pulse (α), in this case five lines in k-space are acquired (EPI factor 5), which is repeated two times per shot (turbo-factor 2), leading to a total of 10 acquired k-lines per heart phase image segment per cardiac cycle (gray area). In total, 4 heart beats are shown, resulting in an image of 40 k-lines. Suppose an image of 120 k-lines is required, the procedure needs to be repeated three times, leading to a total of heart beats of 12. With a heart rate of 60 beats-per-minute, this can be performed during a breath-hold of 12 seconds. White squares indicate heart phase image segments; t_{HP}, time between each heart phase (temporal resolution); TR, repetition time; t_{shot}, shot duration.

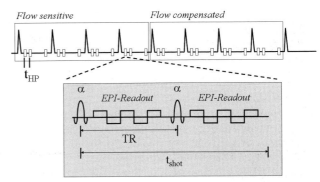

Figure 1.6. Schematic diagram of the basic principle of a turbo field echo-planar MR flow sequence (TFEPI flow) in relation to the timing within the cardiac cycle. After each rf excitation pulse (α), in this case five lines in k-space are acquired (EPI factor 5), which is repeated two times (turbo-factor 2), leading to a total of 10 acquired k-lines per heart phase image segment per cardiac cycle (gray area). In total, 4 heart beats are shown for the flow sensitive image, as well as 4 heart beats for the flow compensated image, resulting in images of 40 k-lines for each image type. Suppose the images require 120 k-lines for a sufficiently high spatial resolution, the procedure needs to be repeated three times, leading to a total of heart beats of 24. With a heart rate of 60 beats-per-minute, this can be performed during a breath-hold of 24 seconds. White squares indicate heart phase image segments; t_{HP}, time between each heart phase (temporal resolution); TR, repetition time; t_{shot}, shot duration.

lates afterward (retrospectively) the appropriate cardiac phases, based on the stored ECG and k-space data. The last part of the cardiac cycle can also be imaged. This technique has been applied clinically, mostly in conjunction with MR flow mapping (see later), because it allows estimation of, for example, diastolic filling pattern or regurgitation volume in patients with mitral valve insufficiency. Recently, retrospective gating became available in combination with faster scan techniques, such as echo-planar imaging and balanced gradient echo acquisitions (see later), so now the standard is retrospective ECG triggering for most CVMR imaging purposes.

A major problem for clinical application of cardiac CVMR is the practical worry of obtaining a reliable ECG signal from a patient inside the MR scanner. In about 2% to 5% of clinical cases no reliable ECG signal may be obtained. The electrical ECG signal is distorted by the interaction of the magnetic field and the pulsating blood flow through the aortic arch (magneto hemodynamic effect). Recently, a new approach was launched to correct this problem. The vector ECG (VCG) is based on the three-dimensional orientation of the QRS complex and T wave of the ECG and the distorting component (7). The MR acquisition can be triggered by the QRS-complex only and not by mistake by the T-wave or ECG distortions or by the signal induced by gradient switching. The VCG, in conjunction with the dedicated cardiac synergy surface coil and SENSE, has revolutionized clinical application of CVMR (Fig. 1.1). Today no practical limitation for CVMR exists, except for the conventional MR exclusion criteria, such as unstable or sensitive, implanted metal objects or pregnancy.

RESPIRATORY MOTION COMPENSATION

A second source of image distortion is respiratory motion. A decade ago, MR acquisitions were so time-consuming that it was impossible to perform breath-hold imaging. At that time, an inventive technique was introduced called ROPE (respiratory ordered phase encoding) (8) or PEAR (phase encoding artifact reduction), which was based on a special k-line reordering technique, combined with a respiratory tracking device around the abdomen. By positioning acquired k-lines during breathing in the periphery of k-space (the part that is less sensitive to motion), breathing artifacts were decreased. This type of artifact reduction improved image quality but was not yet optimal because of the indirect relation between abdominal movement and the actual heart motion.

Due to development of faster MR imaging techniques, such as echo-planar imaging and turbo-field echo imaging, it became possible to acquire image data during a short breath-hold of around 15 seconds. The general disadvantage of breath-hold acquisitions is that the reproducibility of the breath-hold level is not optimal. In a multislice, multiple breath-hold acquisition this may introduce errors in, for example, the summed end-diastolic volume of different slices that were acquired during different breath-holds. Without proper patient instruction, this can lead to high variability in the measurements or, even worse, to inaccurate clinical data. So when using breath-hold acquisitions, carefully instructing the patient to hold his breath in expiration is necessary, which minimizes the previously mentioned problem of breath-hold level reproducibility.

Some high-resolution MR acquisitions require longer acquisition times than possible during a breath-hold. For example, coronary artery MR angiography can be performed during a short breath-hold, but the optimal quality can be

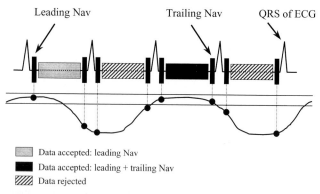

Figure 1.8. The MR acquisition is gated to a predefined acceptance window (*two solid horizontal lines*) based on the traced respiratory signal (*curved solid line*) around end-expiration. K-space data are acquired continuously, but only data are stored that fulfill the requirement that (a) before data acquisition, the navigator was within the acceptance window (leading navigator); or that (b) before and after data acquisition, the navigator was within the acceptance window (leading and trailing navigator). Other acquired image data are deleted. This is the principle of a real-time prospective respiratory navigator.

obtained by using the respiratory navigator technique only (9,10). Respiratory navigation is based on a one-dimensional image positioned at the interface between lung and liver, and the motion of the diaphragm can be tracked. Usually, the navigator beam is positioned on the right hemidiaphragm (Fig. 1.7) and is acquired before and after every MR data acquisition block (Fig. 1.8), with an acquisition duration of only 30 milliseconds. The acquisition is then gated to the automatically traced breathing signal derived from the respiratory navigator. A window around the end-expiration position of the diaphragm is defined, determining the positions in which MR data is accepted. For example, a 3-mm acceptance window means that in end-expiration a 3-mm motion is accepted. Respiratory navigators can also be used for slice

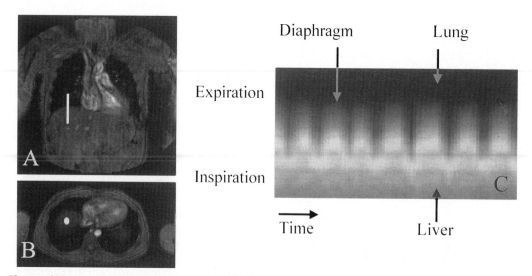

Figure 1.7. The respiratory navigator pencil beam (*A, white line; B, white dot*) is positioned on the right hemidiaphragm at the interface between lung and liver, based on a survey image in the coronal **(A)** and sagittal **(B)** planes. The one-dimensional navigator image is acquired repeatedly over time, thereby constructing an image of diaphragmatic motion **(C)**. The edge between lung and liver is traced automatically, yielding a breathing curve similar to that represented in the diagram of Figure 1.8.

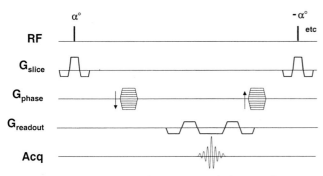

Figure 1.9. Balanced FFE pulse sequences belong to the group of "Steady State Free Precession" techniques. Time-balanced gradients are applied for all gradient directions: slice selection, phase encoding, and frequency readout. In combination with the alternating phase of the excitation pulse, this enables acquisition of both FID and Echo signal. The sequence produces a high image intensity for tissues with a high T2/T1 ratio, independent of the repetition time TR. Balanced FFE images are obtained after field shimming, because field homogeneity is very important.

tracking, which means that the slice position is adjusted respective to the breathing changes detected by the navigator. The acquisition is not gated to a certain predefined acceptance window but acquires all scanned data. The combination of these two techniques seems, currently, the best solution. Within the acceptance window, of, for instance, 3 mm, the remaining respiratory motion is compensated by using the tracking technique. This technique showed good results for coronary MRA (11).

Recent technical advances made it possible to acquire a stack of 12 slices, with around 25 cardiac phases each, in a single breath-hold of up to 20 seconds. These ultrafast techniques are combinations of turbo-field echo, echo-planar, or spiral k-space acquisition. The first application is the assessment of cardiac function, because the single breath-hold eliminates the previously mentioned problem of slice-level reproducibility in multiple breath-hold approaches. However, the image spatial resolution of this technique is still quite low, allowing only evaluation of ventricular volume changes and some rough estimation of wall motion abnormalities. In the future, combination of the ultrafast acquisition schemes with SENSE may allow higher resolu-

tion imaging. A promising technique for ultrafast whole heart functional imaging in a single breath-hold is the so-called *k-t BLAST* technique (see later).

Another promising development is real-time imaging of the heart. Real-time cardiac imaging was introduced in the early days of MR (12). Recently, data has been presented showing full ventricular coverage in real-time without the need for ECG-triggering or breath-holding (13,14). In these preliminary studies, accurate quantification was shown for ventricular function. In combination with future real-time image analysis, this may revolutionize the way we look at cardiovascular MR.

SURVEY

The first step for the cardiovascular MR examination is the acquisition of a localizer to determine general anatomy, which forms the basis for further acquisitions. The purpose of this first scan is to image the cardiac region in three basic orientations: coronal, transverse, and sagittal planes, using 15 slices of 10 mm each for every orientation. A decade ago, these "scout" images were obtained by using a multi-slice spin-echo technique, sometimes in combination with turbo spin-echo. This technique can still be used, if local MR scanner does not support faster imaging techniques. A faster technique for acquiring survey images is, for example, a turbo-field-echo or turbo-field-echo-planar MR sequence.

Recently, balanced gradient echo (bFFE, bTFE, true-FISP) techniques became available, yielding images with high contrast between blood and myocardium (Figs. 1.9 and 1.10). Survey images can be acquired during continuous breathing, using the respiratory navigator or during a breath-hold. Currently, excellent images can be obtained using balanced-FFE without respiratory motion compensation, with an acquisition time of only 15 seconds.

PLANSCAN

Based on survey images, further MR scans can be planned. This can be performed by hand, using the planning tools available in the standard scanner software. Since the begin-

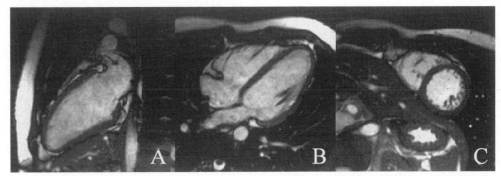

Figure 1.10. Example of balanced FFE images acquired in the two-chamber view **(A)**, four-chamber view **(B)**, and short-axis view **(C)**. Each image consists of 25 cardiac time frames, which were acquired during a breath-hold of 12 seconds for each view separately. Images are shown in the end-diastolic time frame. Note the excellent contrast between blood and myocardium, as compared to the echo-planar images in the other figures of this chapter.

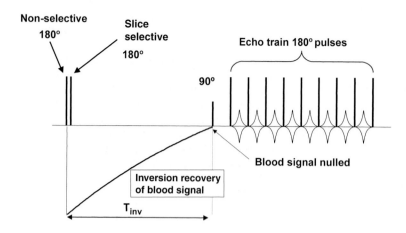

Figure 1.11. Schematic diagram of a black blood pulse sequence. A nonselective 180° pulse inverts all signal. Subsequently, a slice-selective 180° pulse resets signal of the studied slice. Blood with inverted signal flows into the slice plane. After a delay (T_{inv}, inversion time) the blood signal is nulled, and data acquisition is performed with a fast spin-echo pulse train. The image is obtained in a breath-hold. Note that T_{inv} is dependent on the heart rate.

ning of the new millennium, planning can be performed in real-time, even in combination with balanced-TFE. With a real-time planning tool, manual changes in imaging plane are executed immediately by the free-running MR acquisition, and the optimal imaging plane can be found within seconds. Once the desired imaging plane is reached, the geometry settings can be stored for later use during the cardiovascular MR exam. The time efficiency increases substantially by using this real-time planning tool, allowing routine application of cardiovascular MR.

Another approach is to use the survey images as input for an algorithm, which plans automatically the desired imaging planes (15). Its principle is that the software package finds automatically the position of the heart in the survey images and uses this information for planning of the other acquisitions. This operator-independent, automatic planscan method yields reliable quantification of, for example, end-diastolic volume and ejection fraction and reduces substantially interexamination variability. Therefore, this method is, ultimately, suitable for patient follow-up to evaluate therapy effects of, for example, antihypertensive or lipid-lowering drugs. However, the automatic planscan procedure is currently available only off-line as a research tool, and the time-efficiency of the real-time planning alternative seems to be higher.

ANATOMY

Today, the main patient category with a clinical referral for CVMR is congenital heart disease. The primary interest of the referring physician is usually evaluation of global cardiovascular anatomy. The purpose of these MR scans is to image the heart in three dimensions. In this way, complex, congenital cardiac deformations can be diagnosed and followed over time to evaluate surgical correction of the anomalies. In the past, the time-consuming (turbo) spin-echo was the technique of choice. The major disadvantage of this technique was the presence of major breathing artifacts, hampering routine evaluation of cardiac anatomy.

Today, several alternatives are available. The latest technique is a multiple breath-hold, dual inversion black blood turbo spin-echo technique (Figs. 1.11 and 1.12), which yields excellent image quality (16). Disadvantage of this approach is that each slice has to be imaged during a separate breath-hold, with, again, the problem of breath-hold level reproducibility. The expectation is that, in the future, this technique will be further optimized, for example, by combining it with SENSE, allowing single breath-hold or respiratory navigator gated acquisitions.

FUNCTION

The second stepping stone in cardiovascular MR is evaluation of cardiac function. The second most frequent indication for cardiac MR is evaluation of myocardial wall motion abnormalities in patients with suspected myocardial ischemia.

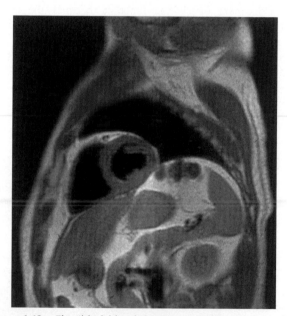

Figure 1.12. The "black blood" image was obtained using a dual inversion fast spin-echo technique, in combination with SENSE (factor 2). Echo spacing 4.3 ms, FOV 350 × 350 mm, matrix 192 × 146, slice thickness 8 mm. Scan time was 6 seconds. (Courtesy of Philips Medical Systems, Best, The Netherlands.)

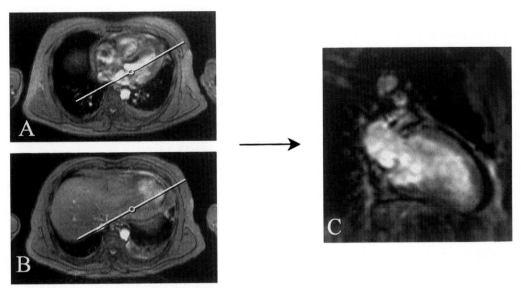

Figure 1.13. The vertical long-axis, or two-chamber view, is planned in the following way. Based on a transverse survey image at the level of the mitral valve **(A)**, the center of the slice is positioned approximately in the middle of the mitral valve and angulated in such a way that the slice intersects with the left ventricular apex on a lower transverse survey image **(B)**. An end-diastolic two-chamber image is shown here, acquired during a 12-second breath-hold in expiration using echo-planar MR **(C)**.

Most of these patients are referred by the echocardiography lab, because some patients are hard to image using ultrasound. Usually, these patients are obese or have lung emphysema. The expectation is that, due to the experience cardiologists are obtaining with MR through the aforementioned patient group, there will be an increasing demand for MR analysis of cardiac function.

Similar to echocardiography, the short-axis view of the left ventricle is the working horse view in cardiovascular MR. To be able to acquire the short-axis view, first two long-axis views need to be acquired, which can yield diagnostic information itself, especially concerning the apical wall motion pattern of both ventricles and valvular function. First, the vertical long-axis, or two-chamber view, needs to be acquired (Fig. 1.13). Based on a transverse survey image at the level of the mitral valve, the center of the slice is posi-

tioned approximately in the middle of the mitral valve and angulated in such a way that the slice cuts through the left ventricular apex on a lower transverse survey image. For selection of the end-systolic cardiac time frame, the two-chamber view needs to be acquired, using a dynamic gradient echo technique. This can be performed, using a conventional gradient-echo technique during continuous breathing, but better results can be obtained when using an ultrafast breath-hold technique, such as echo-planar imaging (17). Currently, the optimal option is the use of a balanced-TFE sequence, because the contrast between blood and myocardium is excellent.

Next, the horizontal long-axis, or four-chamber view, needs to be acquired (Fig. 1.14). Planning of the four-chamber view is based on the diastolic and systolic images of the two-chamber view. First, the center of the slice has to be

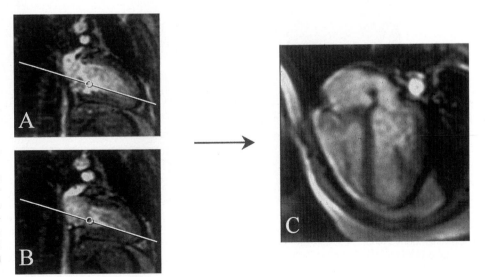

Figure 1.14. The horizontal long-axis, or four-chamber view, is planned in the following way. The center of the slice has to be positioned at one third of the lower part of the mitral valve on the end-systolic two-chamber image **(B)**; hereafter, the slice needs to be angulated through the apex **(A,B)**. After this, check the position of the slice in the diastolic two-chamber image **(A)** to ensure that the atrium is imaged properly. An end-diastolic four-chamber image is shown here, acquired during a 12-second breath-hold in expiration using echo-planar MR **(C)**.

positioned at one third of the lower part of the mitral valve on the end-systolic two-chamber image; hereafter, the slice needs to be angulated through the apex. Afterward, the position of the slice in the diastolic two-chamber image needs to be checked to ensure that the atrium is imaged properly. The four-chamber image also needs to be acquired, using a dynamic imaging technique, preferably balanced-TFE. The two- and four-chamber views yield some important clinical information, mainly concerning ventricular anatomy and dimensions, presence of hypertrophy or valve insufficiencies, and the like.

The final step for evaluation of ventricular function is the planning of the short-axis view itself (Fig. 1.15). Position a stack of 10 to 12 slices of 8- to 10-mm thickness each perpendicular to the long axis of the left ventricle, as defined from the mid-mitral point to the left ventricular apex, based on the systolic and diastolic images of the four-chamber view and the systolic two-chamber view. Be sure to include the entire ventricle in end-diastole, which can be checked on the end-diastolic images. The latter is important for calculation of the end-diastolic volume, stroke volume, ejection fraction, and other derived functional parameters.

The short-axis scan with 10 to 12 slices covering the entire ventricles can be acquired, using a conventional gradient-echo sequence during continuous breathing, which is very time-consuming. A better alternative is a breath-hold acquisition using echo-planar imaging, but, again, the best technique available today is the balanced-TFE MR sequence (Fig. 1.10). Today, these scans are performed using multiple breath-holds in expiration, with the associated problems as pointed out before. In the near future, it is expected that the entire short-axis stack of slices can be acquired within a single breath-hold for up to 15 seconds, using balanced-TFE k-t SENSE (see later). One step further into the future may lead to real-time imaging of the short-axis stack, although this poses several problems on the off-line image processing.

Real-time imaging of the short-axis view, currently, seems perfectly suitable for cardiac stress imaging during continuous increasing dobutamine dosage and for imaging of the heart in the presence of arrhythmias.

PERFUSION

Myocardial perfusion of the ischemic heart may be studied with MR (18). Most perfusion analysis approaches make use of intravenously injected gadolinium-based MR contrast agents. This type of contrast medium temporarily reduces the T1-relaxation time and, thereby, relatively increases the MR-signal intensity of well-perfused tissues. After contrast injection, ischemic myocardial regions show up as areas with no or little signal intensity change as compared to well-perfused myocardium. To visualize the myocardial passage of the injected contrast, fast T1-weighted MR-techniques should be used. The first reports on visualization of perfusion defects in human patients described the acquisition of a single slice level (19). Currently, perfusion studies apply fast gradient echo pulse sequences (magnetization prepared turbo-field echo/EPI/FLASH) that enable the repetitive registration of three or more anatomic levels at every heart beat, or, alternatively, six levels with a temporal resolution of every other heart beat (20). A very promising technique for myocardial perfusion imaging is k-t BLAST perfusion (see later). The training data are acquired and interleaved with undersampling data, thereby dynamically correcting for contrast changes during myocardial passage. It is expected that k-t BLAST will allow full cardiac coverage cardiovascular magnetic resonance (CMR) perfusion imaging during first pass of contrast.

Quantitative image analysis yields parameters to characterize the bolus passage immediately after administration of

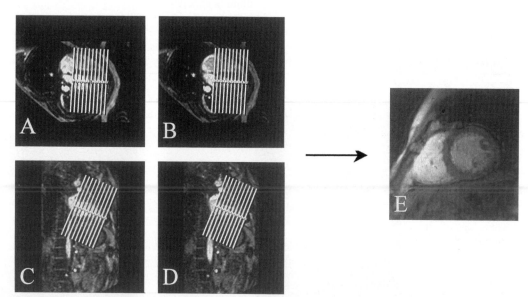

Figure 1.15. The short-axis view is planned in the following way. Position a stack of slices perpendicular to the long-axis of the left ventricle, as defined from the mid-mitral point to the left ventricular apex, based on the diastolic **(A)** and systolic **(B)** images of the four-chamber view, and the diastolic **(C)** and systolic **(D)** two-chamber view. Be sure to include the entire ventricle in end-diastole, as can be checked on the end-diastolic images **(A,C)**. An end-diastolic short-axis image is shown here, acquired during a 12-second breath-hold in expiration using echo-planar MR **(E)**.

the contrast agent. Parameters obtained from the image series describing this first-pass are rate and level of enhancement, time-to-peak, and mean transit time. These characteristic parameters may be obtained for each image pixel and can be graphically displayed in so-called parametric images visualizing the anatomic location of abnormalities (21).

DELAYED ENHANCEMENT

After injection of a low molecular weight contrast agent, its plasma concentration will reach a maximum value and rapidly decrease due to diffusion to the interstitial space and renal washout. Contrast agents that diffused to the interstitial space will be resorbed into the capillary bed and undergo renal excretion. However, when the tissue is damaged, for example, due to infarction, the resorption rate of contrast agent will be diminished. At 15 to 30 minutes after contrast injection, washout will be complete in normal myocardium in contrast to infarcted or edematous tissue. This phenomenon is the basis of "delayed enhancement imaging." Various authors (22,23) have described the relation between myocardial viability and the size of the area displaying delayed enhancement. In MR images the presence of contrast agent can be detected as a bright area on images acquired with T1-weighted MR pulse sequences ranging from basic spin-echo methods to more sophisticated gradient echo sequences, using an inversion or saturation prepulse. Currently, the principle "bright is dead," indicating that bright areas on a delayed MR-image after contrast injection correspond with nonviable myocardium, is subject to lively debate (24–26). The additional value of delayed enhancement to rest-stress wall motion imaging to determine myocardial viability is questionable. Delayed enhancement CVMR, in combination with first-pass perfusion and wall motion imaging at rest, has an important clinical value when stress CVMR cannot be performed.

FLOW

One of the advantages of MR in cardiovascular diagnosis is the possibility of this technique to measure flow velocity (cm/sec) and flow volume (mL/sec). MR flow measurement is based on the principle of "spin phase" (27). Usually, MR images use only the absolute value of the MR signal arising from the slice under investigation. However, the acquired data also contain information on a property called *spin phase*. MR data acquisition and postprocessing can be set up in such a way that two images of each slice are produced: an image with gray values representing spatial localization of the protons, and an image with gray values representing the velocity of the protons present in each image element. The latter image is called the *velocity map* (Fig. 1.16). In a velocity map, pixels of static tissue will be displayed with intensity zero, whereas pixels of, for example, moving blood will have a positive or negative value, dependent on the direction of flow. The use of additional magnetic field gradients in the imaging pulse sequence is the basis of velocity mapping. These field gradients may be applied "in-plane" or "through-plane," thus encoding different components of the flow direction. In most instances, the imaging slice is positioned to measure through-plane flow, but to quantify flow in all three dimensions by adding additional data acquisitions is also feasible.

To obtain useful data on blood flow, measuring flow in a vessel or valve of interest at many instances during the cardiac cycle is necessary. For example, the measurement of flow velocity, taken from a region of interest at many time frames, will result in a flow-velocity versus time curve (see later), which gives information on flow-velocity changes during the cardiac cycle. In such a flow-velocity curve the area under the curve is computed to obtain the

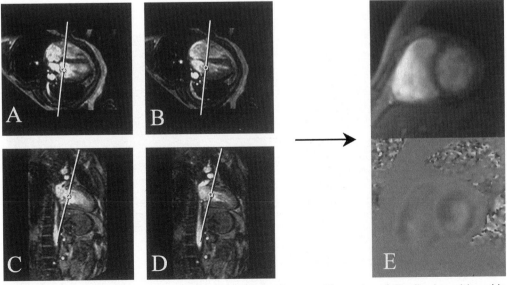

Figure 1.16. The mitral valve flow acquisition is planned in the following way. The center of the slice is positioned in the middle of the mitral valve on the end-systolic two- **(D)** and four-chamber **(B)** images and angulated parallel to the mitral valve, also based on the end-diastolic two- **(C)** and four-chamber **(A)** images. An end-diastolic image of the mitral valve is shown here **(E)**, the upper image shows the normal, or modulus image, and the lower image shows the velocity-encoded image (velocity map).

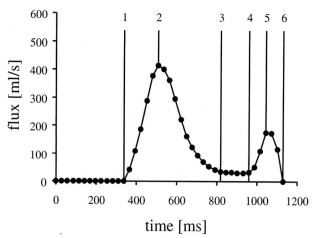

Figure 1.17. Typical mitral valve flow curve obtained after tracing the orifice of the valve in all cardiac time frames on the velocity encoded images. The integration of velocity data over time for all pixels enclosed in the traced area results in a volume flow (flux) curve. The early peak filling rate (2) is a result of the pressure difference between the left atrium and left ventricle, and is a passive process. The atrial peak filling rate (5) is a result of left atrial contraction and is an active process. Another functional parameter that can be derived from the curve is the fastest change in flux between, for example 2 and 3, the so-called "early deceleration" peak. Note the diastase between 3 and 4.

stroke volume, that is, the amount of blood passing through the region of interest during a cardiac cycle. Other valuable hemodynamic aspects related to cardiac contraction and relaxation may also be gleaned from the flow-velocity curve (28).

Flow encoding MR scans are based on gradient-echo pulse sequences, in combination with prospective-triggering or retrospective ECG-gating. For evaluation of diastolic ventricular function, retrospective ECG-gating is required, because prospective ECG-triggering images only the first 80% of the cardiac cycle, and the atrial contribution of ventricular filling occurs in the last 10% to 20% of the cardiac cycle. Currently, a standard flow measurement technique has a duration of 2 to 3 minutes, and the result will represent the average flow during the acquisition period. Recent developments in scanner hardware and software have enabled realization of real-time flow measurement (29) in a clinical setting (30), thus allowing phenomena with fast changes in flow to be investigated with MR. The k-t BLAST technique can also be used in combination with flow encoding. Currently, not much experience with this technique exists, but it is expected that k-t BLAST flow will allow ultrafast flow imaging.

The clinically, most feasible cardiac flow acquisitions are through the mitral valve, tricuspid valve, ascending aorta, and pulmonary artery:

The mitral valve flow acquisition is planned on the two- and four-chamber view in end-systole (Fig. 1.16). The center of the slice is positioned in the middle of the mitral valve, on the end-systolic two- and four-chamber images and angulated parallel to the mitral valve. A typical example of a mitral valve flow curve is given in Figure 1.17.

The tricuspid valve flow is based on an extra survey image—the right ventricular two-chamber view (Fig. 1.18). This view is planned on the end-systolic four-chamber view. The center of the slice is positioned in the middle of the tricuspid valve and angulated through the apex of the right ventricle. The tricuspid valve flow acquisition is first planned on the end-systolic four-chamber view (Fig. 1.19). The center of the slice is positioned on the center of the

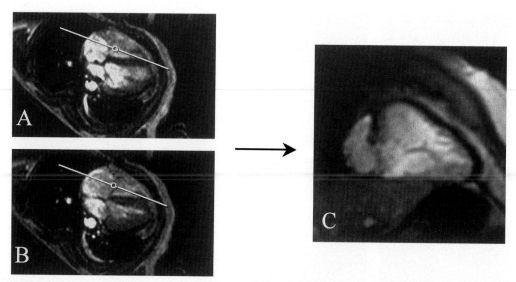

Figure 1.18. The tricuspid valve flow is based on an additional survey image; the right ventricular two-chamber view. The right ventricular two-chamber view is planned on the end-systolic four-chamber view **(B)**. The center of the slice is positioned in the middle of the tricuspid valve and angulated through the apex of the right ventricle based on the end-diastolic **(A)** and end-systolic images **(B)**. An end-diastolic right ventricular two-chamber image is shown here, acquired during a 12-second breath-hold in expiration using echo-planar MR **(C)**.

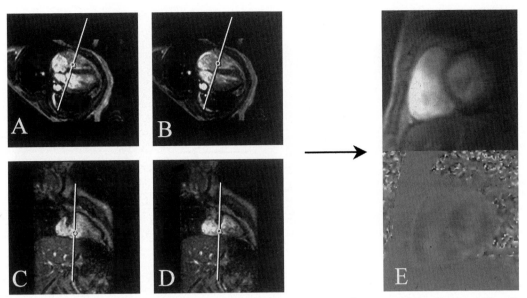

Figure 1.19.   The tricuspid valve flow acquisition is planned in the following way. The center of the slice is positioned on the center of the tricuspid valve on the end-systolic four-chamber view **(B)** and angulated parallel to the tricuspid valve, based on the end-diastolic four-chamber view **(A)**. Thereafter, the slice is angulated on the end-diastolic **(C)** and end-systolic **(D)** right ventricular two-chamber view parallel to the tricuspid valve. An end-diastolic image of the tricuspid valve is shown here **(E)**, the upper image shows the normal, or modulus image, and the lower image shows the velocity-encoded image.

tricuspid valve and angulated parallel to the tricuspid valve. Thereafter, the slice is angulated on the right ventricular two-chamber view parallel to the tricuspid valve. A typical example of a tricuspid valve flow curve is given in Figure 1.20.

The acquisition to measure blood flow velocities and volume through the ascending aorta is planned on the original survey images in the coronal and sagittal view (Fig. 1.21). An inangulated slice is positioned perpendicularly to the ascending aorta on a coronal image, usually at the level of the bifurcation of the pulmonary artery. On a sagittal image of the original survey, the angulation can be adjusted, if necessary, which is usually not the case. A typical example of a flow curve through the ascending aorta is given in Figure 1.22.

The acquisition to measure blood flow through the pulmonary artery is planned on some original survey images in the coronal and transverse views (Fig. 1.23). First, another survey image needs to be acquired of one to three slices in the center of and parallel to the pulmonary artery, based on an original sagittal image. Then, the pulmonary artery flow acquisition can be planned perpendicular to the pulmonary artery, based on the angulated survey image, as was described just before, and on the original sagittal survey image (Fig. 1.23). In addition, the slice position in caudo-cranial direction has to be positioned just before the bifurcation of the pulmonary artery on a transverse image of the original survey. A typical example of a flow curve through the pulmonary artery is given in Figure 1.24.

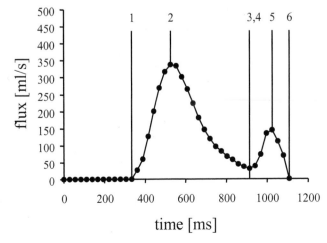

Figure 1.20.   Typical tricuspid valve flow curve obtained after tracing the orifice of the valve in all cardiac time frames on the velocity encoded images. The early peak filling rate (2) is a result of the pressure difference between the right atrium and right ventricle and is a passive process. The atrial peak filling rate (5) is a result of left atrial contraction and is an active process. Another possible functional parameter that can be derived from the curve is the fastest change in flux between, for example, 1 and 2, the so-called "early acceleration" peak.

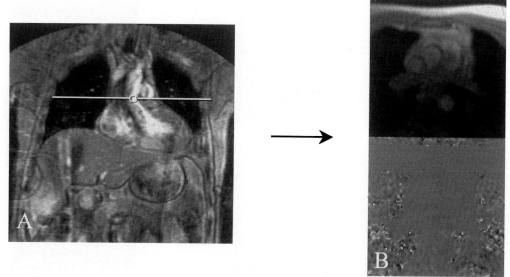

Figure 1.21. The flow acquisition through the ascending aorta is planned in the following way. An inangulated slice is positioned perpendicular to the ascending aorta on a coronal survey image **(A)**; usually, this is at the level of the bifurcation of the pulmonary artery. On a sagittal image of the original survey, the angulation can be adjusted, if necessary, although this is not usually the case (not shown). An end-diastolic image of the ascending aorta is shown here **(B)**, the upper image shows the normal, or modulus image, and the lower image shows the velocity-encoded image.

CORONARY MAGNETIC RESONANCE ANGIOGRAPHY

In this chapter, coronary MRA will not be discussed in great detail, and the reader is referred to later chapters for in depth explanation of the techniques and procedures. The only practical point for now is to realize that three major points of concern for coronary MRA exist. The first is the cardiac motion itself, limiting the shot length of image acquisition to below 100 milliseconds, and the second is respiratory motion, which can be corrected by using respiratory navigators with residual respiratory motion of up to 3 mm. Cur-

rently, the in-plane image resolution is limited to 0.7 mm because of the 100-millisecond shot duration; in this period some cardiac motion still occurs, causing blurring of the image. In theory, an in-plane resolution of around 0.3 mm can be reached, but this is currently hampered by the long shot duration of around 100 milliseconds. With improvement of scanner hardware and software, it is expected that isotropic resolution of 250 μm can be reached in the near future, possibly by performing coronary MRA at 3 tesla instead of the standard clinical field strength of 1.5 tesla. All major MR machine manufacturers now have 3-tesla MR scanners available. Initial results at 3 tesla, using SENSE, are very promising (31).

The third point is the way image contrast between the coronary vessel and surrounding tissue is optimized.

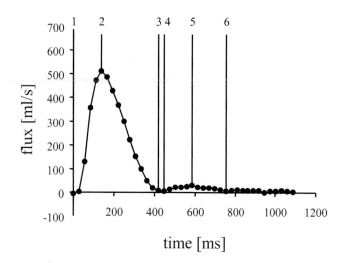

Figure 1.22. Typical flow curve through the ascending aorta obtained after tracing the contour of the ascending aorta in all cardiac time frames on the velocity encoded images. The peak ejection rate (2) is a result of left ventricular contraction. The area under the curve between 1 and 3 is the left ventricular stroke volume. Another interesting functional parameter that can be derived from the curve is the fastest change in flux between, for example, 1 and 2, the so-called "aortic acceleration" peak.

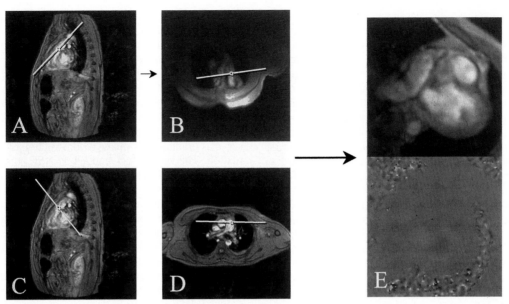

Figure 1.23. The flow acquisition through the pulmonary artery is planned in the following way. First, another survey image needs to be acquired of 1 to 3 slices in the center of and parallel to the pulmonary artery, based on an original sagittal survey image **(A)**. Then, the pulmonary artery flow acquisition can be planned perpendicular to the pulmonary artery, based on the angulated survey image **(B)**, and on the original sagittal survey image **(C)**. In addition, the slice position in caudo-cranial direction has to be positioned just before the bifurcation of the pulmonary artery on a transverse image of the original survey **(D)**. An end-diastolic image of the pulmonary artery is shown here **(E)**, the upper image shows the normal, or modulus image, and the lower image shows the velocity-encoded image.

Roughly, two alternatives are used—the T2-preparation technique, and, second, the use of a contrast agent combined with spiral k-space filling. Perfectly suppressing signal from surrounding tissue is more important than enhancing the signal inside the coronary arteries. Application of spiral acquisitions and the balanced-TFE technique showed a substantial increase in image quality (32) and is expected to have advantage of acquisition at 3 tesla.

VESSEL WALL IMAGING

In this chapter, vessel wall imaging will not be discussed in detail; see later chapters for an in-depth explanation of the techniques and procedures. In general, vessel wall imaging is an important feature of CVMR, which, currently, cannot be accomplished noninvasively with other imaging modalities. Therefore, much effort is now being undertaken to develop MR techniques capable of, for example, imaging of the coronary vessel wall (33). Again, a switch to a field strength of 3 tesla may improve earlier results in this area. One of the future prospects of vessel wall imaging is to determine the composition and stability of atherosclerotic plaque. In the future, vessel wall imaging may be combined with interventional CVMR and interventional MR procedures, such as dottering and stenting under MR guidance.

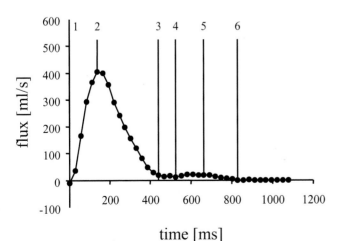

Figure 1.24. Typical flow curve through the pulmonary artery obtained after tracing the contour of the pulmonary artery in all cardiac time frames on the velocity encoded images. The peak ejection rate (2) is a result of right ventricular contraction. The area under the curve between 1 and 3, is the right ventricular stroke volume. Another interesting functional parameter that can be derived from the curve is the fastest change in flux between, for example, 2 and 3, the so-called "pulmonary deceleration" peak.

CARDIOVASCULAR MAGNETIC RESONANCE IMAGE PROCESSING

One of the main obstructions for routine clinical application of CVMR is the relatively underdeveloped state of cardiac image analysis. Currently, the only option to obtain reliable measurements is to manually perform image analysis. The drawing of, for example, endocardial and epicardial contours is a very time-consuming part of the cardiac exam. Several software packages are available to assist in this tedious task, such as the MASS and FLOW software (34,35). Recently, a new technique was developed to detect fully automatically myocardial borders, without any user interaction. This approach uses the "active appearance model" algorithm, based on a statistical description of the shape myocardial contours can have in four dimensions (36). The method showed excellent first results; therefore, this technique may, for the first time, allow accurate, fully automated evaluation of cardiac function. This technique can also be applied in the future on perfusion and delayed enhancement images.

Future developments in image processing are aimed at developing a single software package for evaluation of function, perfusion, delayed enhancement, as well as for coronary MRA images. In analogy to the development of a single, comprehensive cardiac acquisition scheme, the concept of one-stop-shop cardiac image processing is now within reach. A step further will be the analysis of CVMR images in real-time, so that clinical evaluation based on quantification can be performed while the patient is still in the MR scanner, allowing online quality control of the previous acquisitions. In the ideal world, real-time CVMR image acquisition and real-time image analysis are combined—the latter being not completely unrealistic on the time scale of a decennium.

REDUCED DATA ACQUISITION METHODS

In cardiac imaging, data acquisition speed is crucial not only because scans are run typically during breath-holding of the subject, but also because cardiac bulk motion limits the data acquisition period during the cardiac cycle. The limited data acquisition window available frequently requires trade-offs in spatial and/or temporal resolutions. Increasing imaging speed has been related mainly to stronger magnetic field gradients. Ever faster gradient systems have, however, led to potential risks, including peripheral nerve stimulation. Accordingly, further progress by mere engineering may be limited. The advent of parallel imaging has made available alternative means for speeding up data acquisition by exploiting the characteristics of antenna arrays for signal reception. Among all the different parallel imaging techniques presented so far, SENSE (1) and GRAPPA (generalized autocalibrating partially parallel acquisitions) (37) have been most successful and are now widely available on commercial MR systems. In parallel imaging, only a subset of the data required to reconstruct a full image is encoded by magnetic gradient action. The missing information is repopulated, based on differences in perception of the object signal by multiple receiver antennas placed around the object. Typical speed-up factors achievable in cardiac imaging with standard cardiac coil arrays range from two to four. Beyond this range, images are increasingly compromised by local noise amplification.

A different approach to faster imaging of dynamic objects is based on the observation of considerable correlation of image information in space and time. This becomes apparent, if, for example, a cine image series of the heart is considered. Large regions of the image remain static or move in a coherent fashion. Accordingly, an optimized acquisition scheme would need only to update highly dynamic information at a high rate, whereas less dynamic or static information can be acquired at a much lower rate. Among such techniques, k-t BLAST and k-t SENSE (38), have received widespread attention. In k-t BLAST and k-t SENSE the image content is estimated based on so-called training data that serve as guidance for image reconstruction of missing information. The k-t BLAST and k-t SENSE techniques permit typically fivefold to eightfold accelerations in cardiac imaging.

In MR imaging, the information necessary to reconstruct an image is sampled sequentially, typically line-by-line in the spatial frequency or k-space domain. The distance between the lines in k-space is inversely proportional to the size of the field-of-view that encloses the object (see Appendix). To reconstruct an image from the sampled data the Fourier transform is applied. Faster scanning by means of reduced data acquisition schemes implies less dense sampling, with a resultant reduction of the field-of-view. If the field-of-view becomes smaller than the actual object, aliasing occurs in the image, which manifests as backfolding artifacts of image portions. Deliberate reduction of k-space sampling density for faster data acquisition is referred to as *undersampling,* hereafter. Reduced data acquisition schemes, as outlined previously, may be classified into methods operating on a cardiac frame-by-frame basis, such as SENSE and GRAPPA, and into methods taking into account the temporal dimension. Examples for the latter kind are k-t BLAST and k-t SENSE. Although SENSE and GRAPPA can operate with all available scan protocols, k-t BLAST and k-t SENSE are possible only if time-resolved or cine data are acquired.

SENSE

Figure 1.25 illustrates the principle of parallel imaging. In this exemplary illustration, twofold faster data acquisition is achieved by sampling only every other line in k-space, which results in two-times backfolding artifacts in the reconstructed image. For example, the image intensity seen at point P as indicated in Figure 1.25 is the superposition of the original signal at that point and the signal folded in from position P′, which is at P plus the field-of-view divided by the reduction factor, which is, in this example, equal to two. To unfold the signal received at point P, additional information is required, because two unknowns exist with just the superposition thereof known. This additional information is derived from the difference of signal reception of multiple receive coils placed around the object. In the example, at least two receive coils, which "see" point P and the point P′ folded upon it with different intensity (and phase), are required to unfold the folded image pixel. By calculating the difference in sensitivity of coil no. 1 and coil no. 2 for all image points, all folded image pixels can be reassigned successively.

k-t BLAST AND k-t SENSE

In k-t BLAST and k-t SENSE, acquisition speed is increased in a similar fashion to parallel imaging, except that under-

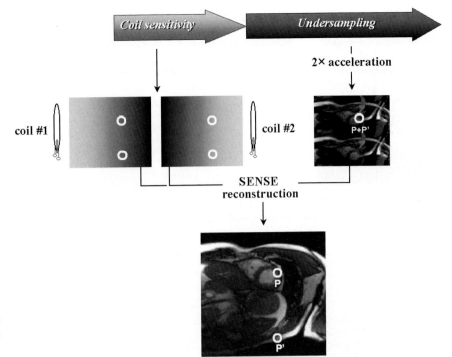

Figure 1.25. Principle of parallel imaging. Data acquisition is accelerated by skipping data lines in k-space, resulting in aliasing artifacts in the image (for example, point P contains signal from two points in the original). The folded image pixel can be resolved by exploiting differences in coil sensitivity of antenna elements (e.g., coil no. 1 and coil no. 2) placed around the object (i.e., point P and the point P′ folded upon it are "seen" differently by coil no. 1 and coil no. 2). For further explanation, see text.

sampling is not only applied along spatial axes but also along the time axis. Accordingly, k-t BLAST and k-t SENSE allow for higher reductions in scan time relative to methods operating on a frame-by-frame basis. On the other hand, the methods are possible for only dynamic or cine imaging protocols.

The undersampling pattern applied in the k-t BLAST and k-t SENSE method can be judiciously designed to take into account the characteristics of dynamic objects typically imaged. This, in particular, refers to, for example, that the chest wall, liver, and other structures surrounding the heart are relatively immobile or move slowly compared to the beating heart. Furthermore, if one knows information about the dynamics of one image point, considerable information about the spatiotemporal behavior of its neighboring points can be inferred. This enables to acquire very quickly an estimation of the object in a so-called training stage. In the training stage, images are acquired at very low spatial but at full temporal resolution. These data may be obtained either in a separate scan or in an interleaved fashion during the actual acquisition (39). During the undersampling stage, very sparse sampling is applied along space and time, resulting in, for example, eightfold scan time reduction. At the same time, eightfold aliasing is generated due to undersampling, as illustrated in Figure 1.26. To obtain a high-resolution, unaliased image series, the prior knowledge, as derived from the training data, is used to unfold the image, as outlined in Figure 1.26. In parlance of image reconstruction, the training data determine a filter that suppresses folding artifacts as a result of undersampled data. In a more general view, k-t BLAST and k-t SENSE may be compared to data compression, as used on personal computers to reduce file sizes on a hard disk. By identifying redundant information, such as the recurrence of certain patterns of numbers, an index for the pattern is saved instead of all individual numbers. In a similar sense, the training data in k-t BLAST/k-t SENSE

identify the pattern and allow decoding of the compressed information, as sampled in the undersampling stage.

Although data acquisition is identical for both k-t BLAST and k-t SENSE, image reconstruction differs. In k-t BLAST, image reconstruction is done separately for each receive coil. In case multiple coils are used, images from the individual coils are combined after reconstruction. In contrast, with k-t SENSE coil information is incorporated in the reconstruction process similar to conventional SENSE reconstruction to improve the accuracy of the reconstruction result.

Both SENSE and k-t BLAST/k-t SENSE can facilitate cardiac applications by shortening acquisition times or, alternately, providing higher spatial and/or temporal resolutions. In practice, SENSE has allowed reduction factors between two and three with current cardiac coil arrays, whereas k-t BLAST/k-t SENSE have already been shown to provide reduction factors of up to eight. This has, for instance, enabled acquisition of time-resolved three-dimensional volumetric data sets of the heart at high spatial and temporal resolutions in a single breath-hold, which has been impossible until now. Cine three-dimensional k-t BLAST at a reduction factor of five has been applied successfully to cardiac patients during interventional procedures. An exemplary case is given in Figure 1.27. The increased scan efficiency allowed the acquisition of volumetric data sets at high spatial ($2 \times 2 \times 5$ mm^3) and temporal (28–35 ms) resolution in a single breath-hold lasting 20 to 22 seconds, with the acquisition strategy well tolerated by the patients. Not only do k-t BLAST/k-t SENSE allow significant acceleration of cine imaging of periodic object motion, but also they can be used to accelerate dynamic imaging of nonperiodic processes, such as contrast agent passage in perfusion studies. The time saved during the CVMR exam by using k-t BLAST/k-t SENSE can be used for additional functional

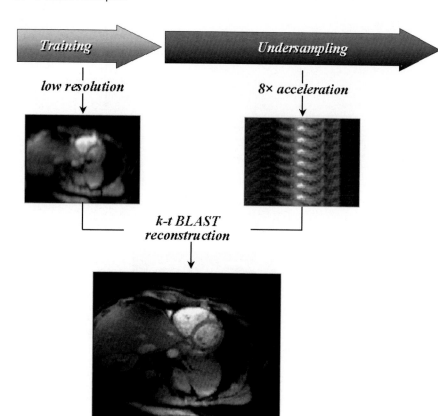

Figure 1.26. Outline of the k-t BLAST method. A low-resolution scan precedes the actual acquisition stage. Based on this training data, an estimate of the expected signal intensities of the moving object is obtained. In the actual acquisition stage, undersampling is applied, resulting in multiple foldover in the images. Using both training and acquisition data, unfolded high-resolution images can be reconstructed. For further explanation, see text.

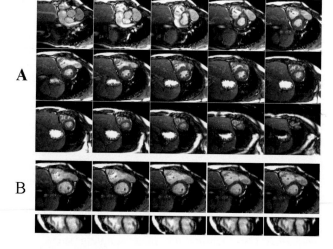

Figure 1.27. Example of cine three-dimensional balanced SSFP single breath-hold imaging with 5× k-t BLAST in a patient with repaired Tetrology of Fallot and pulmonary regurgitation causing right ventricular dilation. The upper 15 slices **(A)** are shown from base to apex of the heart (from left-to-right and from top-to-bottom) at end-systole. Selected time frames showing both short-axis and reformatted four-chamber view planes **(B)**. (Courtesy of R. Razaavi, Guy's Hospital, London.)

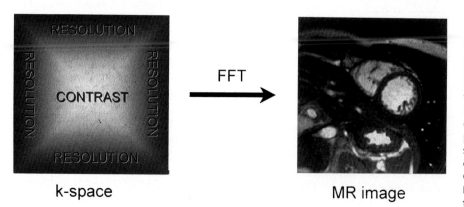

Figure 1.28. Schematic diagram of the relation between k-space and the MR image. The center of k-space contains relatively more information on contrast, whereas the periphery contains more information on resolution. Note that each point in k-space is related to each point in the MR image. The image shown was acquired using balanced FFE during a breath-hold of 15 seconds. CONTRAST, gray values in larger areas; RESOLUTION, visibility of small structures; FFT, fast Fourier transform.

and flow acquisitions or to allow inclusion of coronary MRA in the same CVMR examination.

APPENDIX: CALCULATIONS ON k-SPACE

Image formation in MR is based on filling "k-space" during data acquisition; this concept will not be explained further in this context, because many thorough and comprehensive publications are available on this topic (2–6). One of the main aspects of k-space needed for practical understanding of MR is to calculate the number of k-lines to be acquired and determine the spatial resolution of cardiac images.

The number of k-lines in the phase encoding (= Y) direction can be calculated by applying the formula:

Number of k-lines = acquisition matrix × rectangular FOV × symmetric reduction × asymmetric reduction,

where FOV = field of view, symmetric reduction factor = scan percentage, and asymmetric reduction factor = half-scan (Figs. 1.28 and 1.29). For example, with an acquisition matrix of 256, a rectangular FOV factor of 0.6, a symmetric reduction factor of 0.8, and an asymmetric reduction factor of 1 (meaning no half-scan), the number of k-lines equals:

$$256 \times 0.6 \times 0.8 \times 1 = 122.$$

The image pixel resolution can be calculated according to the formulas:

X-resolution (echo readout direction) = FOV/acquisition matrix
Y-resolution (phase encoding direction) = FOV/acquisition matrix × symmetric reduction,

For example, with a FOV of 300 mm, an acquisition matrix of 256, and a symmetric reduction factor of 0.8, X-resolution will be: 300/256 = 1.2 mm, and the Y-resolution will be: 300/(256 × 0.8) = 1.5 mm. Reconstructed to a 256 × 256 matrix, meaning the Y-resolution is interpolated to the X-resolution (in this case, 1.2 mm), resulting in an apparent in plane image resolution of 1.2 mm × 1.2 mm, and with a slice thickness of 8 mm, a final resolution of 1.2 × 1.2 × 8 mm³, displayed as a FOV of: 300 × 180 (= 300 × 0.6) mm².

REFERENCES

1. Pruessmann KP, Weiger M, Scheidegger MB, et al. SENSE: sensitivity encoding for fast MRI. *Magn Reson Med* 1999; 42(5):952–962.
2. Boxerman JL, Mosher TJ, McVeigh ER, et al. Advanced MR imaging techniques for evaluation of the heart and great vessels. *Radiographics* 1998;18(3):543–564.
3. Boxt LM. Primer on cardiac magnetic resonance imaging: how to perform the examination. *Top Magn Reson Imaging* 2000; 11(6):331–347.
4. Duerk JL. Principles of MR image formation and reconstruction. *Magn Reson Imaging Clin N Am* 1999;7(4):629–659.

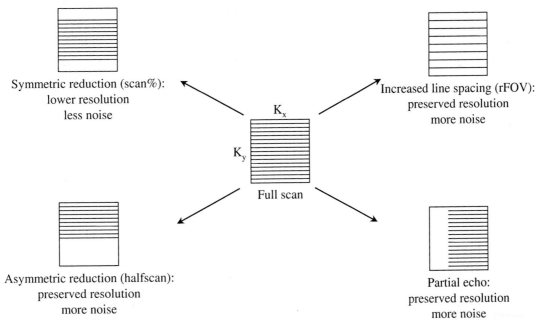

Figure 1.29. MR imaging can be performed faster by acquiring fewer k-lines per MR image. Symmetric reduction and increased line spacing are the most frequently used techniques to reduce the number of k-lines. Symmetric reduction means that on both the extreme edges of k-space in the Y- or phase encoding direction, the part that determines image resolution (see Fig. 1.25), k-lines are not acquired. This results in an image with fewer k-lines, but the trade-off is a reduction in plane spatial resolution. Increased line spacing decreases the density of k-lines in k-space, whereas still the entire k-space is traversed. The image resolution remains the same, the image noise increases, and the FOV is rectangular. Another way of reducing the number of k-lines is to acquire only, for example, five-eighths part of k-space with the same k-line density; this asymmetric reduction results in more image noise. Another way to speed up the MR acquisition is to not reduce the number of k-lines and instead to reduce the part of the generated echo that is sampled; this procedure increases image noise because less image data are acquired.

5. Reeder SB, Faranesh AZ. Ultrafast pulse sequence techniques for cardiac magnetic resonance imaging. *Top Magn Reson Imaging* 2000;11(6):312–330.

6. Sakuma H, Takeda K, Higgins CB. Fast magnetic resonance imaging of the heart. *Eur J Radiol* 1999;29(2):101–113.

7. Chia JM, Fischer SE, Wickline SA, Lorenz CH. Performance of QRS detection for cardiac magnetic resonance imaging with a novel vectorcardiographic triggering method. *J Magn Reson Imaging* 2000;12(5):678–688.

8. Bailes DR, Gilderdale DJ, Bydder GM, et al. Respiratory ordered phase encoding (ROPE): a method for reducing respiratory motion artifacts in MR imaging. *J Comput Assist Tomogr* 1985;9(4):835–838.

9. Wang Y, Rossman PJ, Grimm RC, et al. Navigator-echo-based real-time respiratory gating and triggering for reduction of respiration effects in three-dimensional coronary MR angiography. *Radiology* 1996;198(1):55–60.

10. Danias PG, McConnell MV, Khasgiwala VC, et al. Prospective navigator correction of image position for coronary MR angiography. *Radiology* 1997;203(3):733–736.

11. Stuber M, Botnar RM, Danias PG, et al. Submillimeter three-dimensional coronary MR angiography with real-time navigator correction: comparison of navigator locations. *Radiology* 1999;212(2):579–587.

12. Chapman B, Turner R, Ordidge RJ, et al. Real-time movie imaging from a single cardiac cycle by NMR. *Magn Reson Med* 1987;5(3):246–254.

13. Weber OM, Eggers H, Spiegel MA, et al. Real-time interactive magnetic resonance imaging with multiple coils for the assessment of left ventricular function. *J Magn Reson Imaging* 1999;10(5):826–832.

14. Yang PC, Kerr AB, Liu AC, et al. New real-time interactive cardiac magnetic resonance imaging system complements echocardiography. *J Am Coll Cardiol* 1998;32(7):2049–2056.

15. Lelieveldt BP, van der Geest RJ, Lamb HJ, et al. Automated observer-independent acquisition of cardiac short-axis MR images: a pilot study. *Radiology* 2001;221:537–542.

16. Simonetti OP, Finn JP, White RD, et al. "Black blood" T2-weighted inversion-recovery MR imaging of the heart. *Radiology.* 1996;199(1):49–57.

17. Lamb HJ, Doornbos J, van der Velde EA, et al. Echo planar MRI of the heart on a standard system: validation of measurements of left ventricular function and mass. *J Comput Assist Tomogr* 1996;20(6):942–949.

18. Wilke N, Jerosch-Herold M, Stillman AE, et al. Concepts of myocardial perfusion imaging in magnetic resonance imaging. *Magn Reson Q* 1994;10(4):249–286.

19. Cullen JH, Horsfield MA, Reek CR, et al. A myocardial perfusion reserve index in humans using first-pass contrast-enhanced magnetic resonance imaging. *J Am Coll Cardiol* 1999;33(5):1386–1394.

20. Lauerma K, Virtanen KS, Sipila LM, et al. Multislice MRI in assessment of myocardial perfusion in patients with single-vessel proximal left anterior descending coronary artery disease before and after revascularization. *Circulation* 1997;96(9):2859–2867.

21. Dromigny-Badin A, Zhu YM, Magnin I, et al. Fusion of cine magnetic resonance and contrast-enhanced first-pass magnetic resonance data in patients with coronary artery disease: a feasibility study. *Invest Radiol* 1998;33(1):12–21.

22. Gerber KH, Higgins CB. Quantitation of size of myocardial infarctions by computerized transmission tomography. Comparison with hot-spot and cold-spot radionuclide scans. *Invest Radiol* 1983;18(3):238–244.

23. de Roos A, Doornbos J, van der Wall EE, et al. MR imaging of acute myocardial infarction: value of Gd-DTPA. *Am J Roentgenol* 1988;150(3):531–534.

24. Kim RJ, Fieno DS, Parrish TB, et al. Relationship of MRI delayed contrast enhancement to irreversible injury, infarct age, and contractile function. *Circulation* 1999;100(19): 1992–2002.

25. Kim RJ, Wu E, Rafael A, et al. The use of contrast-enhanced magnetic resonance imaging to identify reversible myocardial dysfunction. *N Engl J Med* 2000;343(20):1445–1453.

26. Gerber BL, Rochitte CE, Melin JA, et al. Microvascular obstruction and left ventricular remodeling early after acute myocardial infarction. *Circulation* 2000;101(23):2734–2741.

27. van Dijk P. Direct cardiac NMR imaging of heart wall and blood flow velocity. *J Comput Assist Tomogr* 1984;8(3): 429–436.

28. Lamb HJ, Beyerbacht HP, van der LA, et al. Diastolic dysfunction in hypertensive heart disease is associated with altered myocardial metabolism. *Circulation* 1999;99(17):2261–2267.

29. Guilfoyle DN, Gibbs P, Ordidge RJ, et al. Real-time flow measurements using echo-planar imaging. *Magn Reson Med* 1991; 18(1):1–8.

30. Klein C, Schalla S, Schnackenburg B, et al. Magnetic resonance flow measurements in real time: comparison with a standard gradient-echo technique. *J Magn Reson Imaging* 2001; 14(3):306–310.

31. Huber ME, Kozerke S, Pruessmann KP, et al. Sensitivity-encoded coronary MRA at 3T. *Magn Reson Med* 2004;52(2): 221–227.

32. Maintz D, Aepfelbacher FC, Kissinger KV, et al. Coronary MR angiography: comparison of quantitative and qualitative data from four techniques. *AJR Am J Roentgenol* 2004;182(2): 515–521.

33. Botnar RM, Stuber M, Kissinger KV, et al. Noninvasive coronary vessel wall and plaque imaging with magnetic resonance imaging. *Circulation* 2000;102(21):2582–2587.

34. van der Geest RJ, Buller VG, Jansen E, et al. Comparison between manual and semiautomated analysis of left ventricular volume parameters from short-axis MR images. *J Comput Assist Tomogr* 1997;21(5):756–765.

35. van der Geest RJ, Niezen RA, van der Wall EE, et al. Automated measurement of volume flow in the ascending aorta using MR velocity maps: evaluation of inter- and intraobserver variability in healthy volunteers. *J Comput Assist Tomogr* 1998;22(6):904–911.

36. Mitchell SC, Lelieveldt BP, van der Geest RJ, et al. Multistage hybrid active appearance model matching: segmentation of left and right ventricles in cardiac MR images. *IEEE Trans Med Imaging* 2001;20(5):415–423.

37. Griswold MA, Jakob PM, Heidemann RM, et al. Generalized autocalibrating partially parallel acquisitions (GRAPPA). *Magn Reson Med* 2002;47(6):1202–1210.

38. Tsao J, Boesiger P, Pruessmann KP. k-t BLAST and k-t SENSE: dynamic MRI with high frame rate exploiting spatio-temporal correlations. *Magn Reson Med* 2003;50(5): 1031–1042.

39. Kozerke S, Tsao J, Razavi R, Boesiger P. Accelerating cardiac cine 3D imaging using k-t BLAST. *Magn Reson Med* 2004; 52(1):19–26.

2

Magnetic Resonance Angiography Techniques

David A. Saloner

Magnetic resonance (MR) imaging is well suited as a modality for evaluating vascular disease. The principal strengths of MR are that it can provide coverage of an extended vascular territory with information at all points in three-dimensional space while remaining non-invasive or, as in the case of venous-injected contrast-enhanced imaging, only minimally invasive. The three-dimensional data sets obtained permit display of the vessels in various formats, including contiguous slices that can be oriented in any obliquity or using a projection format. The major interest in MR angiography (MRA) has been in obtaining images of the vascular lumen, although there is an increased interest in delineating the disease process itself by imaging the vessel wall. Obtaining data on flow dynamics, similar to that obtained in catheter-injected x-ray angiography, is also of increasing interest.

As in other MR methods, MR angiography is least successful when there is substantial gross motion that occurs during the acquisition of the data. This can arise from poor patient compliance or because of physiologic motion, such as cardiac motion while imaging the coronaries or breathing motion for the visceral vessels. Also, blood flow itself can degrade the quality of the depiction of the vascular lumen when that flow is either extremely low, extremely high, or disordered.

Techniques for obtaining high quality MR angiograms have evolved with improvements in MR instrumentation. As new performance capabilities become available, new techniques become feasible, and this trend can be expected to continue. In this chapter, a number of different methods for obtaining MR angiograms will be discussed. Methods for displaying the data will also be presented.

FLOW DYNAMICS

The signal intensity that is measured in MRA studies of flowing blood depends on blood flow velocities (both magnitude and direction) and the variation of those quantities (e.g., from cardiac pulsatility) over the time that data are acquired. The design and implementation of imaging strategies and the choice of imaging parameters therefore require careful consideration of the anticipated hemodynamics in the vessels, in both the normal and the diseased conditions. Setting aside the problem of gross motion for the moment, MRA methods provide accurate images of the lumen when the image resolution is sufficiently high, to provide several pixels across the diameter of the lumen; where flow is sufficiently high that blood traveling through the imaging volume receives only a small number of radiofrequency excitations; and where the flow patterns remain regular and reproducible throughout the cardiac cycle. Deviations from these flow conditions can occur in both healthy and diseased vessels (1–3).

Variations in flow conditions can result from large differences in systolic and diastolic flow. This can be particularly pronounced, for example, in the arteries of the lower extremities where a pronounced interval of rapid antegrade flow is followed by a short, smaller retrograde component, which is, in turn, followed by an extended diastolic interval where the flow velocities are extremely low. In vivo flow patterns are also profoundly impacted by variations in geometry. Even in healthy individuals, blood vessels are curved with numerous branches and bifurcations. These geometric variations can substantially impact the velocity fields resulting in features, such as flattened profiles across the vascular lumen at the entrance to branch vessels or helical flow patterns in curved vessels, such as the aortic arch. However, in the absence of disease, flow is generally laminar and reproducible from cycle to cycle. In regions of atherosclerosis the vascular wall can be irregular, with a residual lumen that is highly asymmetric and that has rapid changes in diameter. These geometric variations can create regions of disturbed flow, such as velocity jets emanating from a tight stenosis accompanied by the shedding of flow vortices representing turbulent flow that varies from one cycle to the next.

PRIMARY MAGNETIC RESONANCE ANGIOGRAPHY METHODS

All MR angiographic techniques aim to create high contrast between spins that are moving and those that are stationary

(4–9). MR imaging methods are capable of measuring both the magnitude of the transverse magnetization and the orientation of that magnetization in space (the phase). Methods have therefore been devised that are designed to create large differences in either the magnitude or the phase of the magnetization between spins that are stationary and spins that are moving (5,7). MR sequences that rely on blood flow to transport fully magnetized blood into the imaging volume and thereby create a substantial difference between the magnetization of flowing and stationary spins are generally referred to as time-of-flight (TOF) methods, which display the magnitude of the transverse magnetization (4). Sequences that rely on the presence of contrast agents injected into the bloodstream to enhance vascular signal are referred to as *contrast-enhanced* MRA, and they create images that display the magnitude of the transverse magnetization (10). Images that display the phase of the magnetization are referred to as *phase contrast* (PC) images (11). These methods rely on the motion of spins, with respect to the imaging gradients for vessel-to-stationary tissue contrast.

FLOW COMPENSATION

Accurate spatial localization, providing images with a high signal-to-noise ratio (SNR), is accomplished by ensuring that in the center of the readout interval, an echo is formed where the orientation of the transverse magnetization of all excited material is the same (rephased). In general, when imaging gradients are applied, spins will accumulate a phase shift. Conventional imaging gradients that are designed to generate a signal echo from stationary material do not account for the motion of flowing spins and, at the center of the echo, moving spins accumulate a phase that depends on their motion between radiofrequency (RF) excitation and the time the echo is collected. In a voxel containing blood spins moving with a spread of velocities, various phases occur. The mean magnetization in the voxel is the sum of the individual vectors, and, because of the spread of phases, a drop in signal strength, referred to as *intravoxel phase dispersion*, takes place. For many MR angiographic sequences it is important to implement gradient waveforms such that the magnetization of moving blood is also rephased at the center of the echo (12,13). These are referred to as *motion compensation gradients* (14). Whereas conventional gradient echo (GRE) sequences use gradient waveforms consisting of two lobes of gradient field strength applied with opposite polarity, flow compensation gradients require additional lobes of applied gradients. In principle, flow compensation could be pursued to include all orders of motion (15). In practice, however, the added gradient lobes needed for higher order motion compensation require additional time to play out, thus lengthening the echo time. If motion compensation is used, the most effective method for improving signal retention from moving spins, even in disturbed flow that contains high-order motion terms, is to rephase constant velocity terms only (16–19).

Most MRA sequences incorporate velocity compensation gradients along the directions of the slice selection and frequency encoding gradients. The phase encoding direction is not compensated; the short duration of the phase encoding gradients minimizes the effects of motion during the application of those gradients.

TIME-OF-FLIGHT METHODS

The contrast obtained in an MRA study is closely related to the strength of the longitudinal magnetization in flowing blood relative to that in stationary tissue (6,20,21). In a GRE sequence (flip angle <90°), the strength of the longitudinal magnetization of spins subjected to a series of RF pulses decreases with each excitation. The longitudinal magnetization of spins will continue to decrease with increasing number of RF excitations received, a process referred to as *saturation,* until it reaches a steady state value that is determined by the flip angle, the repetition time, and the T1 relaxation time for that tissue. Stationary material remains in the imaging volume throughout data acquisition and, therefore, the magnetization strength of stationary spins decreases to the steady state value. In blood vessels, the longitudinal magnetization of spins at any given location depends on how many RF excitations those spins have received between entering the imaging volume and reaching that location. Fast moving blood may receive only a few RF pulses, thus retaining substantial magnetization strength. Slowly moving spins may receive a large number of pulses, and for those spins, their longitudinal magnetization, like stationary spins, may also drop to the steady state value. In magnitude images, spins that have received many RF pulses and are strongly saturated will appear dark, whereas spins that retain substantial magnetization strength will appear bright.

TWO-DIMENSIONAL TIME-OF-FLIGHT METHODS

The technique of engendering strong contrast between the longitudinal magnetization of flowing and stationary spins and then using flow compensated gradients to correctly encode the transverse magnetization has been used to good effect in thin slice strategies, also called *sequential two-dimensional time-of-flight (2D TOF)* (22,23). In the thin slice strategy, a single slice perpendicular to the blood vessel is acquired using a flow compensated gradient sequence (Fig. 2.1). By making the slice very thin, it is ensured that the slice will be replenished with relaxed blood and that it does not become saturated, even if moderately large flip angles are applied. Each single slice acquisition requires of the order of 8 seconds. The sequence can be repeated multiple times, each time shifting the position of the slice to permit the acquisition of a large set of consecutive slices in a reasonable imaging time. Note that unlike standard multislice imaging in which the images are collected simultaneously, images are collected sequentially so that blood is not saturated by one slice before entering another. High signal contrast is attained between blood vessels and the stationary surround. This procedure provides a full three-dimensional (3D) data

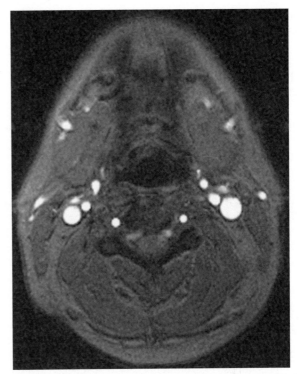

Figure 2.1. A 2D GRE sequence slice through the neck. Arteries and veins are shown with high contrast relative to stationary tissue (TR/TE/flip angle = 35/9/30°).

set, and the single slices can then be reformatted by stacking them and calculating the desired plane of projection.

Shortcomings of Two-dimensional Time-of-flight

Sequential 2D TOF techniques provide strong inflow enhancement when the slices are perpendicular to the vessels. When vessels run in the same plane as the slice, or reenter the slice, the blood becomes saturated, and contrast is progressively lost. This effect is more pronounced when the slices are thick. In addition, in examinations like an axial carotid artery study, a superior presaturation slab is applied, which is close to and moves along with the current slice. This removes venous structures. Vascular loops are sometimes found, especially in the cervical vertebral arteries of older patients. If the loop is large enough, inferiorly moving arterial blood may also be presaturated and yield no signal. For this reason, the method is most effective when the vessel runs in a straight course.

Slices collected perpendicular to the vessel result in projected images in which the plane of viewing, that is, along the length of the vessel, corresponds to the axis with poorest resolution. Resolution will improve, if thin slices are acquired, but this may not be practical because the total imaging time depends on the number of slices collected. In addition, thinner slices have a lower signal-to-noise ratio and require longer echo times.

In many cases, particularly in the abdomen, reduced resolution in the projection view can be successfully addressed by acquiring slices in the same plane as the desired projection. In-plane saturation of the inferior vena cava (IVC) while acquiring coronal slices may be reduced by use of small flip angles at the expense of contrast.

THREE-DIMENSIONAL TIME-OF-FLIGHT METHODS

The major shortcoming of the thin slice strategy is the limited resolution that can currently be achieved in the slice-selection direction. In 2D techniques using flow compensation gradients, slice thicknesses of 2 mm or greater are typically used. The use of 3D techniques permits the acquisition of a full 3D data set with isotropic voxels of less than 1 mm^3 (4,7,24). High-resolution voxels are critical for the visualization of small branch vessels, which might, otherwise, be obscured by partial voluming. They also provide clear depiction of tortuous vessels with equal fidelity in each spatial dimension.

Three-dimensional methods further permit the acquisition of data sets with echo times that are shorter than those achieved with 2D methods. In acquiring data from a 3D volume, the excitation volume in the "slice select" direction is chosen to be a slab that is of the order of 40 mm thick. Compared to 2D methods, an additional cycle of phase encoding is imposed to permit the data to be reduced to a set of partitions. The use of 3D acquisitions requires substantially greater acquisition times than do 2D methods but provide advantages in increased SNR. In 3D acquisition, blood flowing through the excitation volume receives more excitation pulses than is the case for 2D imaging. To avoid excessive saturation effects, the flip angle must be reduced (<30°). Like other MRI methods, TOF MRA benefits from the increased SNR that is available at high field. This permits the acquisition of images with reduced voxel sizes (Fig. 2.2).

PRESATURATION

In many cases, evaluating an arterial structure is confusing when it is obscured by an overlying vein and vice versa. To eliminate the signal from these vessels, a presaturation band with a flip angle ≥90° can be placed adjacent to the imaging slice or volume so that blood is saturated before it enters the slice (Fig. 2.3) (25,26). For example, to remove IVC signal from a renal artery origin study, one could place a transverse presaturation band across the abdomen inferior to the kidneys. Despite their usefulness, the application of presaturation pulses needs careful attention because their existence in a given acquisition is often not directly noted in the resultant images, if they are placed outside the imaging volume. Care must be taken to ensure that the vessel is not similarly presaturated.

PARAMETER CHOICES

In generating an MR angiogram, parameter choices are often made that optimize one feature of the angiogram at the expense of others. In choosing optimum pulse sequence parameters, one needs to take into account the expected flow velocity, the thickness of the imaging volume that must be traversed, and the acceptable level of contrast between flowing and stationary material.

REPETITION TIME (TR)

The selection of the most suitable repetition time is a compromise. The shorter the TR the more saturated the signal

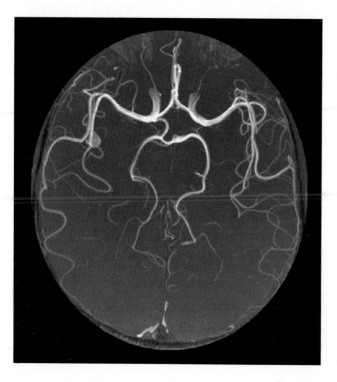

Figure 2.2. MIP from a 1024 matrix time of flight acquisition at 3.0 T with a voxel size of 0.13 mm^3 true resolution. The high resolution MRA is of a patient with a symptomatic right MCA aneurysm at the level of the M3 segment. In addition, perforating arteries and the ophthalmic arteries are clearly visible. (Courtesy of Dr. Winfried Willinek, University of Bonn, Germany.)

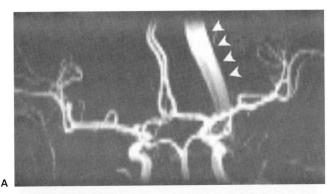

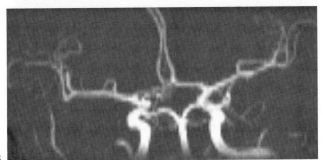

Figure 2.3. An MIP on the coronal plane of a 3D time-of-flight acquisition through the circle of Willis. **(A)** With no presaturation, the sagittal sinus is clearly depicted (*arrowheads*) and overlays the arterial signal. **(B)** A superior axial saturation band eliminates signal from venous blood.

from stationary material. However, as TR decreases, blood will receive more RF excitations in traversing the same distance than it would with a larger TR. Figure 2.4 illustrates this, which is a transverse 3D acquisition through the carotid bifurcation from a normal volunteer. The most suitable TR will depend on the rate at which blood transits a slice and will, therefore, vary from vessel to vessel and, for a given vessel, be somewhat patient-dependent. One should also note that an increased TR will dictate a larger total study time and, hence, an increased possibility of patient motions, which can substantially degrade image quality.

FLIP ANGLE

The choice of flip angle, α, is similarly a compromise with increasing α more heavily suppressing stationary signal but more rapidly saturating signal from blood that receives multiple excitations (Fig. 2.5). Again, there is an interaction between the choice of this variable and flow dynamics. For steady flow, the distribution of magnetization strength across the excited region will reflect the flip angle, and the variation will be larger with increasing flip angle.

As vessels pass through a volume of excitation, blood in the more distal portions becomes increasingly saturated. This tendency can be counteracted by designing a radiofrequency excitation pulse, a TONE pulse, with a flip angle that is relatively small on the proximal side of the slab but that becomes progressively larger across the slab. Spins entering the slab retain their signal strength for a greater distance.

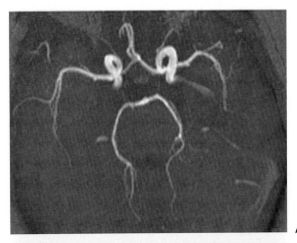

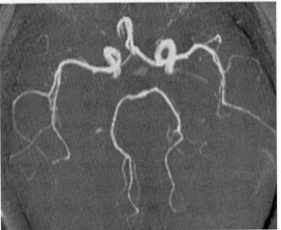

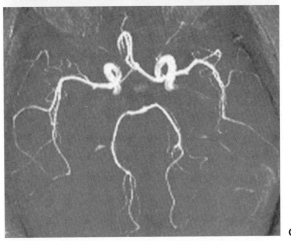

Figure 2.4. Time-of-flight acquisitions through the circle of Willis varying the repetition time, TR. With increasing TR there is less saturation of the stationary tissue and retention of more distal arterial signal. TR/TE/flip angle were **(A)** 25/7/10°, **(B)** 35/7/25°, and **(C)** 45/7/40°.

DISORDERED BLOOD FLOW

Laminar flow becomes unstable at high flow velocities and breaks down into turbulent flow. In regions where true turbu-

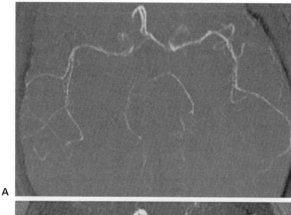

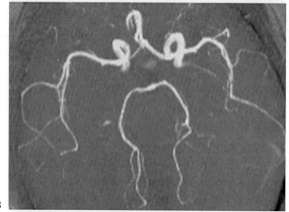

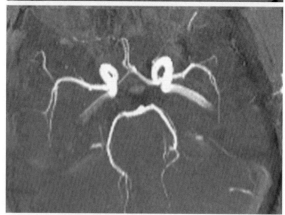

Figure 2.5. Time-of-flight acquisitions through the circle of Willis varying the flip angle. With increasing flip angle there is increasing saturation of the stationary tissue and reduction of more distal arterial signal. TR/TE/flip angle were **(A)** 35/7/10°, **(B)** 35/7/25°, and **(C)** 35/7/40°.

lence exists, such as immediately distal to a critical stenosis, the flow patterns are complicated because some regions will have laminar flow, other regions will have turbulent flow, and intermittent regions exist in which the flow randomly fluctuates between these two conditions. In this case, the different phase encoding steps needed to build up the MRA image will be collected with different signal distribution. These fluctuations will result in inconsistent data and image degradation (27,28). In addition, disturbed flow implies that between RF excitation and signal readout, protons will move through complicated trajectories, described not only by constant velocity terms but high-order motion terms that are

not rephased by constant velocity compensation. At time of readout there will be voxels that contain protons with a range of motion histories and a corresponding range of accumulated phases. Such voxels will have a reduced net transverse magnetization strength and will appear in the MR image with reduced signal intensity. The artifactual loss of signal associated with disturbed flow can mimic the appearance of vessel stenosis in vessels of normal caliber and can lead to the overestimation of the degree and extent of stenosis in diseased vessels.

ALTERNATIVE MAGNETIC RESONANCE ANGIOGRAPHY METHODS

Although significant progress has been made using conventional TOF methods, a series of innovative strategies have been pursued to further improve MRA. Specialized sequences have been proposed to reduce the well-known loss of signal noted at sites of disturbed flow. Other approaches have been pursued to enhance the contrast between flowing spins and stationary spins either by more effectively suppressing the signal from stationary spins or by retaining flow signal in the more distal portions of the vessels.

FLOW INDEPENDENT MAGNETIC RESONANCE ANGIOGRAPHY

Conventional MR imaging methods exploit differences in relaxation properties to obtain images with high contrast between different tissue types. It is similarly possible to create images with suitable timing values that exploit the specific T1 and T2 properties of flowing blood and chemical shift differences in surrounding tissue to provide good contrast between blood in the vascular lumen and surrounding tissue (Fig. 2.6). This type of approach obviates the need for contrast injection and is insensitive to many of the conditions that must be met by MRA methods that are dependent on specific flow properties of intraluminal blood. They do, however, require the careful implementation of a number of advanced methods, such as specialized water-fat suppression methods, and face the challenge of separating arterial from venous signal, which is more easily accomplished at higher field strengths.

SHORT ECHO SEQUENCES

In general, the effects of disturbed flow that result in intravoxel phase dispersion, can be reduced by shortening the duration of the encoding gradients (17,19,29–32). The extent to which this can be pursued is limited by the rate at which the magnetic field gradients can be altered (the slew rate) and the maximum achievable gradient strength. Further, acquiring data with a strong frequency encoding gradient results in a reduced signal-to-noise ratio. Nevertheless, great progress in MRA quality has been achieved with the development of higher performance gradients.

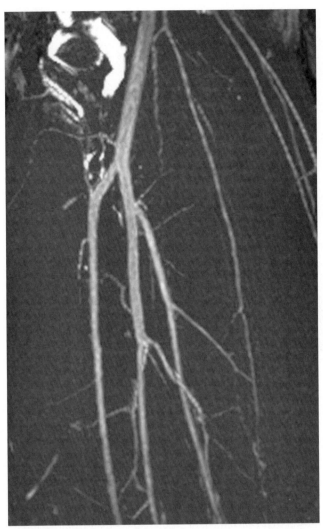

Figure 2.6. Flow-independent MR angiography. Image of popliteal trifurcation in a healthy volunteer obtained at 3 T. TR/TE/flip angle = 8/4/50°; resolution = 0.9 × 0.9 × 1 mm³. (Courtesy of Dr. Jean Brittain, General Electric Medical Systems.)

An important consideration in selecting the echo time of time-of-flight MRA sequences is the dependence of the background signal on the echo time. In voxels where there are significant contributions from protons attached to fat and protons attached to water, the signal strength depends on the phase relationship between these two components. The phase relationship is determined by the slight difference in precessional frequencies of protons in the two different environments. At 1.5 tesla (T), this translates to the fat and water signal being out of phase at odd multiples of 2.3 milliseconds and in phase at even multiples of 2.3 milliseconds. As such, images acquired with an echo time of 7 milliseconds will have more effective background suppression than will images acquired at 5 milliseconds (33). Nevertheless, the benefits of short echo time MRA are still apparent in regions where there is little fat contribution, such as the brain.

Reduced echo time sequences can also be achieved by relaxing the requirement that the full echo be placed symmetrically in the data acquisition window. Conventional MRA sequences sacrifice a fraction of the echo and place the echo

closer to the excitation pulse to reduce the echo time. The slight loss in resolution that results by dropping the high-order frequency components is compensated by the reduced sensitivity to flow disturbance (34,35). This strategy can be further pursued by using partial Fourier techniques where highly asymmetric echoes are acquired. In this case, the loss in resolution is unacceptable, and additional postprocessing steps must be taken, using the inherent symmetry of the Fourier data to reconstruct the missing information.

SEQUENTIAL THREE-DIMENSIONAL METHODS

Distal saturation of blood flow that occurs in 3D time-of-flight sequences can also be reduced by reducing the thickness of the excitation slab and by using multiple 3D volumes to cover the region of interest. This method has been termed *multiple overlapping thin slab acquisition* or MOTSA (36). In this approach, the 3D slabs are placed orthogonal to the principal direction of flow (e.g., axial slabs for studies of the extracranial carotids). To avoid bands of signal loss where the RF profiles trail off at the slab edges, substantial overlap of consecutive slabs is provided. This comes with a penalty of increased total acquisition time. Patient motion between acquisition of consecutive slabs will be seen (as in sequential 2D studies) as a sharp discontinuity of the lumen edge. The reduced slab thickness limits the duration that spins remain in the excited volume, resulting in better retention of signal in the distal vessels (Fig. 2.7). This method provides the high resolution capabilities of 3D sequences (37).

SPIRAL SCAN

An artifact that was recognized in early clinical studies is the so-called misregistration artifact (38,39). In this case, signal from spins—that move obliquely with respect to the phase and frequency encoding axes—appear at a different spatial location in the image than the lumen of the vessel. This can be noted as a bright vessel running diagonally and parallel to a dark lumen. This artifact occurs because in conventional 2D Fourier encoding, phase encoding occurs at an earlier time than does frequency encoding. Consequently, the location of flowing spins in the image is mismapped. One approach to correcting this problem is to replace the phase encoding gradient lobe with a bipolar lobe designed to encode spins moving with constant velocity with the phase appropriate to their location, when the center of the frequency encoding axis occurs (40). Although helpful, this approach, again, corrects for only spins moving with constant velocity, and there remain displacement artifacts for spins moving with higher order motion.

A more fundamental approach to correcting displacement artifact is to use pulse sequences, such as spiral scan where spatial information along both axes is acquired simultaneously. Spiral scan methods build up k-space by designing gradient trajectories that start in the center of k-space and spiral out to the edge (41,42). In the case of flow, spiral scan methods have the attraction that the two dimensions of spatial encoding occur simultaneously in time; therefore, there is little or no misregistration artifact. They are attrac-

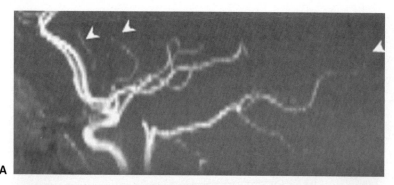

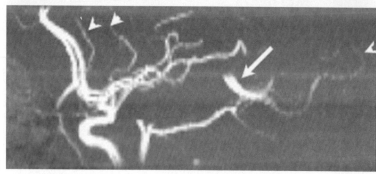

Figure 2.7. A comparison of a single slab excitation through the circle of Willis with a two-slab MOTSA acquisition. The MOTSA acquisition retains signal in the distal small arteries (*arrowheads*) and also shows signal in the lower slab from venous signal (*arrow*) entering from above (no presaturation). **(A)** Single slab TR/TE = 35/7. **(B)** Two-slab MOTSA; TR/TE/flip angle = 35/7/25°.

tive also because they effectively have greatly reduced echo times, particularly for the low spatial frequency information in the center of k-space, providing added insensitivity to disturbed flow.

BLACK BLOOD

Conventional bright blood MR angiography methods are limited in their ability to clearly define the lumen edge at locations of disturbed flow. They are also poor at delineating the soft tissue signal of disease processes in the vessel wall, such as atheroma or mural thrombus. Black blood angiography can reduce the overestimation of stenotic disease (43–47) and provide excellent information on the vessel wall (Fig. 2.8).

Black blood methods use typically spin-echo sequences where flowing blood appears as a signal void. Spin-echo sequences can be further modified to more fully obliterate signal from moving spins while retaining signal from stationary spins. This is accomplished by adding presaturation pulses to selectively saturate spins prior to their entering the vessel segment. Further, flow compensation is removed, and the gradient lobes can be designed to accentuate intravoxel phase dispersion. Increased echo times also increase the likelihood that flowing spins will leave the selected slice between the 90° and 180° pulses, thereby preventing echo formation for these spins.

Finally, so-called double inversion methods can be used to retain signal from stationary tissue but provide a condition where any blood that enters the slice yields no net signal.

When using a black blood sequence, caution must be exercised to ensure that regions of low signal strength are the patent lumen and not regions of inherently low signal, such as calcification or air that is close to the vessel. The other potential problem is that slow or recirculating blood may not appear black.

RADIOFREQUENCY EXCITATION PULSES

Much of the progress in the development of MRA has come from improved methods of manipulating the magnetic field gradients. The other key ingredient that the pulse programmer can use for modifying signal characteristics is the use of tailored radiofrequency pulses. Although the TONE pulses referred to previously are designed to more effectively retain signal from flowing blood, alternative pulses have been proposed that can selectively reduce the signal from stationary tissue while leaving the signal from flowing spins unaffected.

One such RF pulse is a fat saturation pulse that is designed to selectively excite protons attached to lipids (48,49). This method uses the property that protons attached to lipids see a slightly different chemical environment than do protons attached to free water and, therefore, have different precessional frequencies. A saturating pulse (90°) can therefore be delivered at the resonant frequency of fat protons, leaving the magnetization of flowing blood unchanged but effectively eliminating the fat signal from the MR image providing improved background suppression.

A mediating mechanism can also be used that exploits the different relaxation properties of protons that are attached to free water compared to protons that are bound to membranes and other macromolecules. Bound protons have a very short T2 relaxation time and have a broad spectrum of precessional frequencies. They can therefore be excited with pulses that are far from the resonance of mobile protons and their magnetization strength thereby saturated. This, in turn, reduces the signal strength of mobile protons in the tissue parenchyma, which undergo a rapid exchange with the bound protons. Moving spins do not participate in this mechanism, and the magnetization of flowing blood is largely unaffected by these off-resonance excitation pulses (Fig. 2.9). This approach is termed *magnetization transfer satura-*

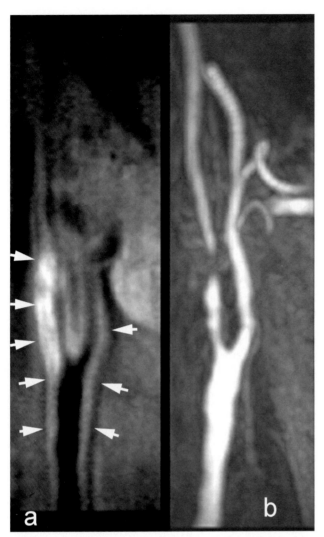

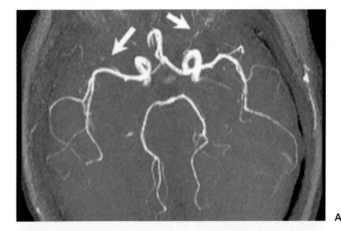

A

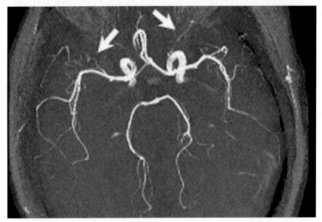

B

Figure 2.8. A comparison of a black-blood image with a reformatted contrast-enhanced image in the longitudinal plane through the carotid bifurcation. **(A)** A T1-weighted double inversion recovery, fat saturated, spin-echo sequence shows a black patent lumen and atheroma in the wall (*arrow*). **(B)** An MIP from a 3D contrast-enhanced study in the same plane shows the patent lumen as bright.

Figure 2.9. Comparison of MIP projections of 3D time-of-flight images acquired through the circle of Willis with and without magnetization transfer saturation. **(A)** Without magnetization transfer saturation, small vessels (*arrow*) are hard to see because of the low contrast with respect to stationary tissue. **(B)** With magnetization transfer saturation. Increased signal saturation of the parenchyma occurs and improved delineation of the smaller vessels (*arrow*).

tion (50–52). Both magnetization transfer saturation pulses and fat saturation pulses impose additional time requirements on pulse sequences and lengthen the minimum possible repetition time.

PHASE DIFFERENCE METHODS

The contrast provided by *longitudinal* amplitude methods described previously depends on the difference in longitudinal magnetization strength that exists between material that has received few prior excitation pulses and stationary material that has received numerous excitations at the time that the RF acquisition pulse is applied. A different approach to angiographic contrast is to modulate the phase of the *trans-*

verse magnetization between the time of RF excitation and the time of signal acquisition (11,53).

In this approach the phase of moving spins is purposely altered by appropriate gradient waveforms. An additional phase modulating gradient is added to a sequence that is, otherwise, flow compensated. This gradient produces a phase accumulation for a moving spin that is proportional to the spin's velocity. A second image is acquired, with the sense of the phase modulation gradient reversed. In this case, the magnitude of the transverse magnetization is identical for both images, but the phase of the transverse magnetization is proportional to the flow velocity and to the duration and magnitude of the phase modulation gradients. Provided that the gradients are not too great, an image can be constructed from the raw data of the two images by subtracting their magnetization vectors. Stationary tissue magnitude and phase are identical in both data sets and, therefore, no signal from the stationary tissue is present in the subtraction image.

The gradient strength should be selected in proportion to the velocity of blood in the vessel under investigation. With strong gradients the method can be tailored to provide high sensitivity to slow blood flow, such as that in veins. The signal-to-noise ratio in a phase contrast image increases as the phase difference of the magnetization of flowing spins increases, which is what is represented in the subtracted images. However, if the combination of blood velocity and gradient strength is too high, there will be a phase aliasing artifact that results in areas of the vasculature having signal dropout in regions of high flow velocities.

Like time-of-flight methods, phase contrast angiograms can be obtained of 2D or 3D volumes. However, in phase contrast, because of the excellent suppression of stationary tissue signal, 2D slabs can be acquired in which the slab thickness can be several centimeters thick, while retaining projection views of the vasculature with good contrast properties. Two-dimensional cine phase contrast studies are capable of giving informative displays of flow dynamics as they vary over the cardiac cycle.

Because the signal intensity is proportional to the velocity of flow, the phase contrast method can be used to determine flow velocities. Flow components can lie along any of three orthogonal directions, and repeating the measurements for all three spatial directions is necessary to acquire a total flow map. The total time can be reduced by acquiring one reference image and three encoded images, although the total acquisition time is still long relative to the time-of-flight method, and it is susceptible to machine imperfections, such as eddy currents. Nevertheless, because of the relative insensitivity of this method to flow saturation effects and the strong suppression of signal from stationary tissue, it remains an attractive technique for slow flow situations.

CONTRAST ENHANCED MAGNETIC RESONANCE ANGIOGRAPHY (CE-MRA)

Signal contrast in MRA is determined predominantly by blood flow patterns as opposed to conventional MRI, where Tl and T2 values are critically important. Contrast agents have been used to advantage in MRA studies exploiting the short Tl properties that these agents produce (54,55) (Fig. 2.10). The use of contrast agents requires much of the same analysis that is used in other angiographic methods, such as spiral computed tomography (CT) angiography, where the initiation and duration of the injection of the contrast bolus relative to the interval of data acquisition must be carefully timed.

T1 SHORTENING

At the dosages applied in MRA studies, contrast agents act to reduce the T1 relaxation time of intraluminal blood. The T1 relaxation time of blood is 1.2 seconds at field strengths of 1.5 T, the field strength of a high-field magnet. When gadolinium contrast agents are used at sufficiently high concentrations, the T1 relaxation time of blood is reduced to less than 150 milliseconds, well below the T1 of all tissue material. This means that contrast-enhanced blood will rapidly recover magnetization and will have high signal strength, even for short values of the repetition time.

The acquisition of MR angiograms when using contrast agents requires a different approach than standard MRA.

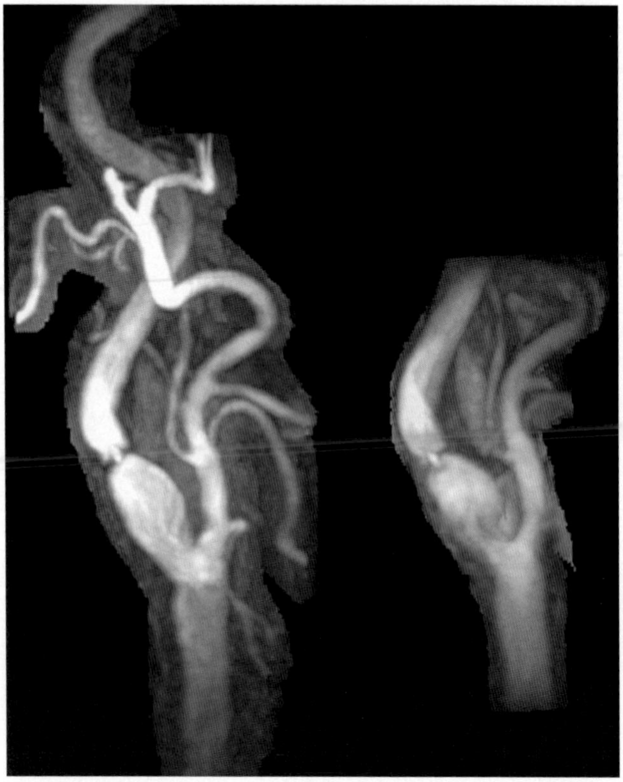

Figure 2.10. Comparison of contrast-enhanced MRA and MOTSA time-of-flight through the carotid bifurcation of a patient with a dilated internal carotid artery proximal to a tight stenosis. The CE-MRA image has crisper edges because of the reduced total acquisition time and the reduced signal saturation in blood recirculating within the dilatation. **(A)** MIP from a longitudinal slab acquired in 25 seconds with a pixel size of 0.5 mm × 1.0 mm × 1.5 mm; TR/TE/flip angle = 6/2.2/25°. **(B)** MIP from a two-slab MOTSA acquired in 4 minutes, 30 seconds with a pixel size of 0.7 mm × 0.7 mm × 1 mm; TR/TE/flip angle = 35/7/25°.

With a bolus injection of the contrast agent, a short interval exists, during which the agent will be in the arterial phase (56,57). Timing the MR data acquisition is important so that it coincides with the period during which there is peak arterial signal. After reaching a peak, the arterial signal strength drops, and the venous signal starts to increase. In conventional MRA studies of arteries, presaturation pulses are applied superior or inferior to the volume to eliminate signal from the veins. In CE-MRA, the application of presaturation pulses is not a viable strategy for eliminating venous signal. Most contrast-enhanced studies rely on using parameters providing the shortest possible data acquisition time, and the addition of a presaturation pulse substantially increases that time. Presaturation has limited use because the reduced T1 values of the blood rapidly restores saturated magnetization strength.

In certain applications, to be able to acquire a 3D study in a short time is important. This includes the extracranial carotids, where there is a short interval when the first pass of the bolus provides maximal intra-arterial signal and when the venous enhancement, which occurs shortly after the arterial phase because of the blood-brain barrier, has not yet occurred. Similarly, short acquisition times are desirable for the vessels of the abdomen, so that studies can be obtained within a breath-hold. The use of current high performance gradient systems permits the echo time, TE, to be reduced to less than 2 milliseconds, and the repetition time, TR, to be 5 milliseconds. This short TR value permits acquisition of 3D studies from 10 to 20 seconds. Conventional TOF MRA methods rely on spins with full magnetization strength flowing into the imaging volume between one excitation pulse and the next. With short repetition times very little inflow enhancement takes place. The signal strength in contrast-enhanced studies, therefore, depends heavily on the T1 relaxation time of the material in the volume.

PHASE ENCODING CONSIDERATIONS

To achieve a rapid acquisition time, choosing a small number of phase encoding lines is desirable. However, one is limited by the need to achieve adequate resolution—the pixel size varying as (*field of view*) / (*number of phase encoding lines*). The field of view (FOV) along the phase encoding axis must also be chosen large enough to accommodate the anatomy along that axis. Failure to choose a large enough FOV will result in misinterpretation of signal and the appearance of "wrap-around" artifact. In cases where the vessels of interest are in the center of the anatomy, this edge artifact can be tolerated.

The overall contrast in an MR image is largely dictated by the signal measured at the center of k-space, whereas much of the high resolution detail is determined by the periphery of k-space. Because of the time course of the intravascular magnetization strength following contrast injection, the use of linear phase encoding can result either in large portions of k-space being measured before the magnetization enhancement occurs or in the center of k-space being sampled well after the peak enhancement is over.

A wide range of alternative methods can be used for sampling the k-space data points needed to create an image. Particularly relevant to CE-MRA methods are techniques that permit the center of k-space to be measured when there is peak magnetization strength. One such method is centric phase encoding. For 2D this consists of first collecting the echo with zero y-phase encoding strength, and then moving out from the center of k-space to the periphery, collecting echoes with alternately positive and negative values of phase encoding strength. This can be extended to 3D, where both z-phase encoding and y-phase encoding values can be varied so that the center of k-space is collected at the beginning of the data acquisition, and the edges of k-space are collected later. This has been referred to as *elliptical centric phase encoding view order* (57).

CE-MRA methods are particularly well suited for parallel imaging methods, such as SENSE or SMASH. In these methods, coil arrays with coil elements of differing spatial sensitivity are used to acquire data from small fields of view (with concomitant savings in acquisition time). The wrap-around artifact that would normally result is resolved by the redundant information from the different coil elements. Provided that the signal-to-noise ratio is sufficiently high, these methods can be used to either reduce acquisition times or increase spatial resolution (Fig. 2.11).

ACQUISITION TIMING

As in other angiographic techniques that use a contrast agent, timing of image acquisition relative to the passage of the contrast agent is important for CE-MRA. In some applications, multiple injections of contrast material can be used. However, to reduce effects from venous enhancement, and to fully exploit the high magnetization strength that prevails immediately following injection of the contrast agent, timing of data acquisition remains important. Appropriate timing of data acquisition will depend on the specifics of the acquisition strategy (as discussed later) but can be achieved with several different approaches.

ACQUISITION TIMING: TEST BOLUS

A straightforward approach to sequence timing is the use of a test bolus (56,58). A small amount of contrast agent (e.g., 2 mL of gadolinium) is injected and immediately followed with a saline flush to ensure that the contrast agent does not remain in the injection tubing. A rapid imaging sequence is applied covering the anatomy, and images are collected at 1-second intervals for about 50 seconds. If the image acquisition is correctly prescribed, for example, a thick slab in the plane of the vessel or using saturation slabs, no temporally varying inflow enhancement effects will occur, and the arrival of contrast agent at the target area will be apparent. This provides a determination of the time interval between injection and peak magnetization enhancement in the region.

The full study is then performed using the knowledge of the time delay between injection and peak magnetization strength. The volume of gadolinium appropriate for the target vessels in question is injected, again followed by a saline flush, and, after a delay time, the CE-MRA sequence is initiated. Generally, the delay time in the CE-MRA sequence is chosen such that the center of k-space is collected when the magnetization strength reaches a peak. Because the center of k-space determines the overall contrast properties of the

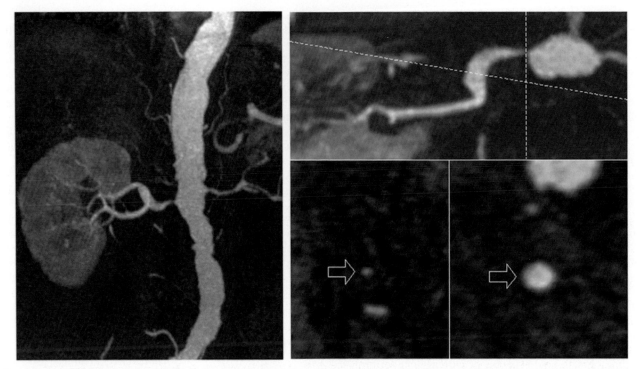

Figure 2.11. MIP from a contrast-enhanced MRA study of the aorta and renal arteries obtained in 23 seconds with a nearly isotropic spatial resolution of 0.9 mm × 0.8 mm × 0.9 mm. Parallel imaging methods are used with an acceleration factor of 2. Also shown are the location of two planes that are drawn transverse to the vessel at the level of the stenosis in the right renal artery and more distal, and the luminal cross sections at these levels. (Courtesy of Dr. Stefan Schonberg, Ludwig-Maximilians-University, Munich.)

image, this strategy ensures maximum contrast between blood and stationary material. With this approach, the high spatial frequency data are collected when there is less magnetization strength; although, this compromise, which results in edge blurring, is not readily apparent in CE-MRA images.

ACQUISITION TIMING: SIGNAL INITIATED ACQUISITION

An alternative approach to the test bolus technique is to use an automated method (57,59,60). A pulse sequence is initiated that samples the magnetization strength in the vessel or in a parent vessel. The sampling sequence is chosen to be a low resolution 2D study with rapid image acquisition time and with immediate reconstruction and display of images, a method referred to as *magnetic resonance fluoroscopy*, or using a line scan study where signal can be sampled as rapidly as every 20 milliseconds. After contrast injection, the sampling study is terminated as soon as signal enhancement exceeds a preset threshold, and the CE-MRA study is begun. This technique accounts for variations in transit time that might occur when a test bolus is used as compared to when a full dose is injected. Because the contrast agent has already begun its rapid enhancement phase when the leading edge is detected, the use of an imaging sequence that is constructed to acquire the central portion of k-space early on in the data acquisition period is important. For this purpose the centric or elliptic phase encoding strategies can be used.

ACQUISITION TIMING: DYNAMIC SUBTRACTION CONTRAST ENHANCED MAGNETIC RESONANCE ANGIOGRAPHY

The ideal solution to the problem of determining injection timing would simply be to collect 3D image sets continuously, beginning prior to injection and ending well after the agent has passed into the venous phase. If that were possible, it would no longer be necessary to synchronize data collection with the injection. Magnetization enhancement following a bolus injection occurs relatively rapidly (in 5 to 10 seconds); and to capture the phase of strong magnetization enhancement and to differentiate the arterial phase from the venous phase, collection of the k-space data for the full 3D volume in an interval of 5 seconds is desirable. Currently, 3D data sets require acquisition times that are generally 10 seconds.

This limitation can be addressed by constructing image data sets, neighboring in time and sharing k-space data (61,62). In this method, a desired temporal resolution is specified. Three-dimensional data sets can then be created within any desired temporal window, using the k-space data that are actually acquired in that window and k-space data that are created by interpolation from the measurements made before and after the desired time window that are closest in time to the specified interval. Many specific implementations of this strategy are possible, and a typical approach is to sample the blocks of k-space that cover the middle of k-space more frequently than the blocks that cover the periphery of k-space. This increases the likelihood that the important regions of k-space that determine the overall contrast to noise ratio are captured in the phase when there is high intravascular magnetization strength.

An alternative approach for acquiring time resolved CE-MR angiograms is simply to use an ultrashort repetition time (<2 milliseconds), to reduce the through-plane resolution to provide quasi-projection type angiograms, and to use parallel imaging methods to further reduce acquisition times (63). This combination can provide subsecond acquisitions of 3D data sets (albeit with resolution that is so poor that data can be viewed in the plane of acquisition only). This same strategy can then be extended to include view sharing as described previously, to provide images with high dynamic information content (Fig. 2.12).

ZERO-FILLED INTERPOLATION

Because of contrast passage considerations, CE-MRA acquisitions are designed to collect the necessary data in as short a time interval as possible. Apart from the time savings pro-

vided by the reduction in repetition time, scan time reduction is often accomplished by reducing the number of phase encoding steps used, particularly along the slab select direction. The slab volume often cannot be commensurately reduced because vessel coverage would otherwise be compromised, and, therefore, a loss in spatial resolution occurs. Image presentation then suffers, particularly when the data are viewed on a plane containing the reduced resolution dimension. Image appearance can be made more visually appealing by applying an interpolation algorithm. Zero-filled interpolation operates on the basic feature of MR imaging that MR data are acquired with a discrete matrix (64).

When an MR image is acquired, data are collected from the true underlying magnetization distribution of the object. This magnetization distribution is continuous. In the process of image acquisition, a finite matrix of data is collected for a given field of view, thus defining the image resolution. This process is the equivalent of convolving or "blurring" the continuous magnetization distribution with a point spread function that has a width equal to the acquisition resolution.

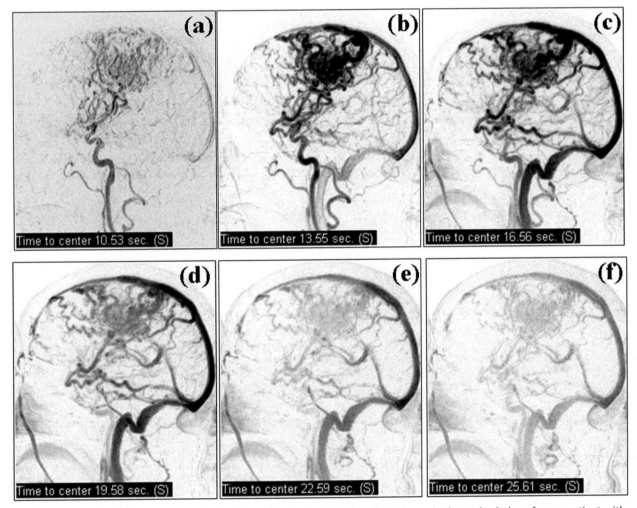

Figure 2.12. A series of MIP images acquired of the dynamic passage of contrast shown in the sagittal plane from a patient with an arteriovenous malformation. Images were acquired with a T1-weighted, spoiled, 3D gradient-echo pulse sequence on a 3-T system with an 8-channel head coil. Parallel imaging was implemented, and scan time was further reduced using partial Fourier acquisition on all three axes. Images were obtained at a frame rate of 3 seconds, with a voxel size of 1.04 mm × 0.78 mm × 2.0 mm; TR/TE/flip angle = 3.2 milliseconds/1.6 milliseconds/15°. Successive frames are shown beginning 10.5 seconds after injection. (Courtesy of Dr. Timothy Carroll, Northwestern University, Illinois.)

The blurred image is the closest that one can get to the underlying "true" magnetization distribution. However, it is standard for MR images to present the continuous data in a lower display format. For example, for a 256-mm FOV and a 256 data matrix, the image is formed by sampling the blurred signal intensity distribution at 1-mm spatial intervals and linearly interpolating the intensities between these points. The "raw" data (i.e., both the magnetization magnitude and phase) are collected in any event and contain all the information necessary to correctly construct the image intensity variations of the "blurred" image at arbitrarily small spatial intervals. This process of reconstructing the image at smaller spatial steps than simply that of the acquired resolution is termed *zero-filled interpolation.*

In practice, the process of zero-filled interpolation doubles the data file size with every successive order of interpolation, and it is unusual for zero-filled interpolation to be performed with other than a factor of two increase in image matrix size. Importantly, one should realize that even with infinitely small image reconstruction steps, the final reconstructed image will approach the "blurred" image only, and the image acquisition resolution simply remains the value obtained by dividing the FOV by the matrix. Another way of saying this is that zero-filled interpolation does not improve the inherent resolution of the acquired data; it restores some of the resolution that conventional MR image reconstruction loses through linear interpolation.

IMAGING PARAMETERS

The MR technologist can select several imaging parameters that affect the quality of the CE-MR angiogram. These include parameters, such as the flip angle, and timing parameters, such as TR and TE. Other parameters, such as the phase encode ordering schemes, are determined by the pulse sequence programmer. In conventional MRA, evaluation of the specific impact of parameter variations on image appearance is straightforward. To accomplish this in CE-MRA is difficult because the initial contrast bolus affects the image appearance of all subsequent injections. Parameter choices have been made by theoretic considerations, from phantom studies, and by limited human studies.

The choice of repetition time is dictated by the desirability of having short acquisition times that permit breath-hold studies and capture of the phase when contrast material reaches peak concentration in the arteries. The minimum value of TR that can be prescribed depends on the structure of the pulse sequence. This again is related to the need to apply gradients of magnetic field to encode the spatial location of the magnetization and, particularly, to form and measure the "echo." Increasing the strength of the applied gradient used while measuring the echo decreases the time needed to measure the signal. This, however, results in a decrease in SNR. The choice of the minimum TR is therefore a compromise between SNR and acquisition time.

In conventional time-of-flight MRA, the choice of flip angle is a sensitive determinant of the overall quality of the image. In particular, because the T1 of blood is longer than that of most tissue, choosing a flip angle greater than 30° in a 3D study typically results in saturation of signal in the distal territories of the vessels. In CE-MRA, the T1 of con-

trast enhanced blood is significantly shorter than the surrounding tissue, and these studies are more forgiving, with respect to the specific flip angle chosen. Flip angles between 30° and 60° are found to be satisfactory. The optimum flip angle depends somewhat on the repetition time chosen, and some saturation will occur for larger flip angles with very short TRs.

ADVANTAGES OF CONTRAST ENHANCED MAGNETIC RESONANCE ANGIOGRAPHY

Three main advantages to the use of contrast agents in MRA are described here. First, the total study time required to collect the data for a three-dimensional study is quite short, between 10 and 20 seconds. This means that gross patient motion can be substantially reduced. Studies of the visceral arteries can be performed in a single breath-hold (65–67). With TOF methods studies of the extracranial carotid arteries take up to 10 minutes to acquire, and patient motion, such as swallowing, snoring, and neck movement, can substantially degrade image quality. Short duration CE-MRA avoids these problems (Fig. 2.10). It also makes possible the study of rapid dynamic processes, such as flow through an arteriovenous malformation (68,69). The second major advantage is the increased coverage that is available with CE-MRA. Because TOF methods rely on inflow enhancement, signal strength in distal vessels is diminished, and the only way to ensure uniformly high vascular signal through a large volume is to use multiple overlapping subvolumes to cover the region. This results in long acquisition times, data inefficiencies because of overlap requirements, and the increased possibility of patient motion. Provided that contrast material fills the vessels, CE-MRA can be used to cover a very large volume with excellent contrast to noise properties (Fig. 2.13). The third major benefit of CE-MRA is that because of the signal strength, these sequences can be applied using a high bandwidth to give very short echo times, while still retaining an adequate signal-to-noise ratio. All MRA sequences benefit from reduced echo times because they restrict the extent of signal loss that is associated with disordered flow.

LIMITATIONS OF CONTRAST ENHANCED MAGNETIC RESONANCE ANGIOGRAPHY

Several disadvantages to the use of CE-MRA are described in the following. A principal disadvantage is the need to inject a contrast agent, despite the low-risk profile of side effects for the agents that are used (70). Although the actual data acquisition time is reduced, increased preparation time is required because of the need to place an intravenous line prior to placing the patient in the scanner. The administration of an injection requires the presence of additional personnel, which, together with the cost of the contrast agent, adds to the cost of the study. As noted previously, a major concern is the presence of venous signal that increases with increasing time following injection. This has proved to be a major obstacle in studies of the intracranial circulation, particularly for the Circle of Willis, where the venous signal in the cavernous sinus obscures a delineation of the arterial lumen and

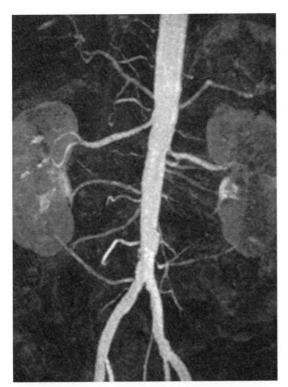

Figure 2.13. MIP from a contrast-enhanced MRA study of the aorta and renal arteries showing excellent signal retention through the aorta into the distal renal arteries and into the iliac arteries. TR/TE/flip angle = 4.6/1.8/25°; total acquisition time = 21 seconds.

in locations, such as the lower extremities, where the veins and arteries abut each other. An additional limitation of CE-MRA is the time constraints imposed by the need to capture the high intensity signal in the short interval that it is in the arterial phase. Even with the short repetition times used, 3D studies can be acquired only by compromising in terms of coverage and/or resolution.

The very strong suppression of signal from stationary material is advantageous for the visualization of vascular contours. Conventional MRA sequences also strongly suppress stationary material signal but still retain considerably more of that signal than do CE-MRA sequences. Stationary material signal can add valuable information to a study of vascular pathology. At regions of stenosis, conventional MRA sequences often show features of the atheromatous plaque that cannot be seen in CE-MRA. The extent of atheroma can be assessed, and the presence of features, such as high signal hematomas, is easily noted on TOF studies.

POSTPROCESSING AND DISPLAY

MR angiography studies cover a 3D volume either by acquiring multiple 2D slices or by an explicit 3D study of the volume of interest that produces a series of 2D partition images. Rarely, one may find that a substantial portion of the vessel lies within a single partition. More commonly, each slice will contain a small segment of the vessel. Overall

interpretation of the relationship of one vessel segment to another is difficult. The analysis of complex vascular anatomy, in particular, the tortuous 3D path followed by most vessels, is facilitated by postprocessing algorithms that provide a general overview of the anatomy. Several algorithms have been investigated that provide projection capability, and the one most commonly used is the maximum intensity projection (MIP) technique (71).

MAXIMUM INTENSITY PROJECTION (MIP) ALGORITHM

The MIP algorithm exploits the property of MRA sequences that signal from moving spins is high, whereas that from stationary spins is low. The MIP is a postprocessing algorithm—it can be implemented at any time after the data are collected. Processing of the data can be performed without additional acquisitions or increased scan time.

The algorithm operates by first specifying the desired viewing plane. Once the viewing plane is specified, an imaginary ray is projected perpendicular to a given pixel in that viewing plane through the 3D data set. The algorithm then searches through all voxels in the acquired 3D data set that lie along the specified ray and determines the signal strength of the voxel with the highest signal intensity. That intensity value is then assigned to the image pixel in the viewing plane that is being generated. This process is repeated for every pixel in the viewing plane, thereby creating a projection image. This approach should be compared with the projection image created in x-ray projection. In that case, the projection image represents a summation of all attenuation effects along the ray traversed by the x-ray. In MR angiography, stationary material typically has signal strength, albeit substantially smaller than that of the flow signal. If one were to perform a summation projection of an MR data set, the flow signal would be buried in the signal from the stationary background.

The MIP algorithm is attractive because it is not computationally intensive. The algorithm is easy to prescribe and helpful in providing access to the projection views. The MIP provides a road map to the overall vessel anatomy and can indicate sites of probable disease that must be more carefully evaluated on the source images.

LIMITATIONS OF MAXIMUM INTENSITY PROJECTION

Although the MIP algorithm is quick and easy to use, it is known to generate significant artifacts (72,73). A common problem is that low intravascular signal can appear in the base images with lower signal strength than stationary material (such as fat, hemorrhage, or when contrast agents have been administered). In this case, the stationary signal will be mapped to the projection image, and information will be lost. This can result in images with the appearance of clinically significant disease, such as stenosis or occlusion. One should keep in mind that the MIP is only a convenience and that the base images contain additional information that can be pivotal in correctly interpreting a study.

Because artifacts of the kind referred to previously are a function of the volume of data that is being processed (the probability of including high signal stationary material increases with increasing volume), an important consideration is to limit the postprocessing to as small a volume as possible to fully include the vessel but still exclude unwanted stationary signal. The probability of including a voxel from the stationary material of higher signal strength than a voxel from the flowing material increases as the thickness of stationary material included in the data set increases. The contrast in the MIP can therefore be improved by restricting the MIP to a volume that includes only the immediate vicinity of the vessels. This can be performed iteratively, using MIP images on three orthogonal planes as a guide in defining the volume to be included for postprocessing. Although fairly user intensive, the algorithms are sufficiently fast that the manipulation of these data sets can be performed in a few minutes, using high performance array processors. In addition, this technique can be used to eliminate overlapping vessels.

REFORMATTING

Viewing vascular contours in planes different from that of the native acquisition is often useful. A change in luminal cross section, for example, is often more readily identified from longitudinal views of the vessel than from slices transverse to the vessel (74). Because no overlapping background signal occurs in this case, which might obscure the vessel, this technique provides the strongest achievable contrast. Both 2D and 3D data sets covering a volume of interest can be reformatted to generate views with arbitrary orientation to the original data set. The presentation is particularly appealing for 3D data sets that have been acquired with isotropic voxels, that is, voxels that have the same length along all three axes. In this case, reformatted images can be created with comparable resolution in any obliquity. The disadvantage of this approach is its labor intensive quality. The appropriate planes must be interactively specified by the user and cannot be automated. Further, the resultant image can provide a depiction of the data through one plane only. Creating an MIP image of a small number of reformatted images is sometimes advantageous, thereby retaining good contrast, an overview of the vessels, and a desirable viewing plane.

Further processing can be invoked, which makes use of depth information. Volume rendering techniques can be used to provide spatial relationships between vessels and soft-tissue structures (75,76). Surface rendering can also be used with virtual light sources to provide images with intensity proportional to the surface gradients, providing information on the texture of vessels.

SUMMARY

MR methods provide a wide range of approaches that can be used to obtain images of blood vessels, with high contrast and good resolution. The ability to determine the course of the vessel through three-dimensional space and the relation of the vasculature to the surrounding soft tissue is valuable. Although a number of exciting new capabilities are in devel-

opment, and the true usefulness of others is still under evaluation, a core of reliable and dependable methods are available for clinical use.

REFERENCES

1. Milnor WR. *Hemodynamics.* Baltimore: Williams & Wilkins; 1989:xii, 419.
2. Strandness DE, Sumner DS. *Hemodynamics for Surgeons.* New York: Grune & Stratton; 1975:xi, 698.
3. Stroud JS, Berger SA, Saloner D. Influence of stenosis morphology on flow through severely stenotic vessels: implications for plaque rupture. *J Biomech* 2000;33(4):443–455.
4. Dumoulin CL, Cline HE, Souza SP, et al. Three-dimensional time-of-flight magnetic resonance angiography using spin saturation. *Magn Reson Med* 1989;11(1):35–46.
5. Dumoulin CL, Souza SP, Walker MF, et al. Three-dimensional phase contrast angiography. *Magn Reson Med* 1989;9(1):139–149.
6. Haacke EM, Masaryk TJ. The salient features of MR angiography. *Radiology* 1989;173(3):611–612.
7. Laub GA, Kaiser WA. MR angiography with gradient motion refocusing. *J Comput Assist Tomogr* 1988;12(3):377–382.
8. Lenz GW, Haacke EM, Masaryk TJ, et al. In-plane vascular imaging: pulse sequence design and strategy. *Radiology* 1988;166(3):875–882.
9. Masaryk TJ, Tkach J, Glicklich M. Flow, radiofrequency pulse sequences, and gradient magnetic fields: basic interactions and adaptations to angiographic imaging. *Top Magn Reson Imaging* 1991;3(3):1–11.
10. Prince MR. Contrast-enhanced MR angiography: theory and optimization. *Magn Reson Imaging Clin N Am* 1998;6(2):257–267.
11. Moran PR. A flow velocity zeugmatographic interlace for NMR imaging in humans. *Magn Reson Imaging* 1982;1(4):197–203.
12. Constantinesco A, Mallet JJ, Bonmartin A, et al. Spatial or flow velocity phase encoding gradients in NMR imaging. *Magn Reson Imaging* 1984;2(4):335–340.
13. Pattany PM, Phillips JJ, Chiu LC, et al. Motion artifact suppression technique (MAST) for MR imaging. *J Comput Assist Tomogr* 1987;11(3):369–377.
14. Saloner D. Flow and motion. *Magn Reson Imaging Clin N Am* 1999;7(4):699–715.
15. Xiang QS, Nalcioglu O. Differential flow imaging by NMR. *Magn Reson Med* 1989;12(1):14–24.
16. Lee JN, Riederer SJ, Pelc NJ. Flow-compensated limited flip angle MR angiography. *Magn Reson Med* 1989;12(1):1–13.
17. Tkach JA, Lin W, Duda JJ Jr, et al. Optimizing three-dimensional time-of-flight MR angiography with variable repetition time. *Radiology* 1994;191(3):805–811.
18. Tkach JA, Ruggieri PM, Ross JS, et al. Pulse sequence strategies for vascular contrast in time-of-flight carotid MR angiography. *J Magn Reson Imaging* 1993;3(6):811–820.
19. Urchuk SN, Plewes DB. Mechanisms of flow-induced signal loss in MR angiography. *J Magn Reson Imaging* 1992;2(4):453462.
20. Gao JH, Holland SK, Gore JC. Nuclear magnetic resonance signal from flowing nuclei in rapid imaging using gradient echoes. *Med Phys* 1988;15(6):809–814.
21. Saloner D. Determinants of image appearance in contrast-enhanced magnetic resonance angiography. A review. *Invest Radiol* 1998;33(9):488–495.
22. Gullberg GT, Wehrli FW, Shimakawa A, et al. MR vascular imaging with a fast gradient refocusing pulse sequence and reformatted images from transaxial sections. *Radiology* 1987;165(1):241–246.

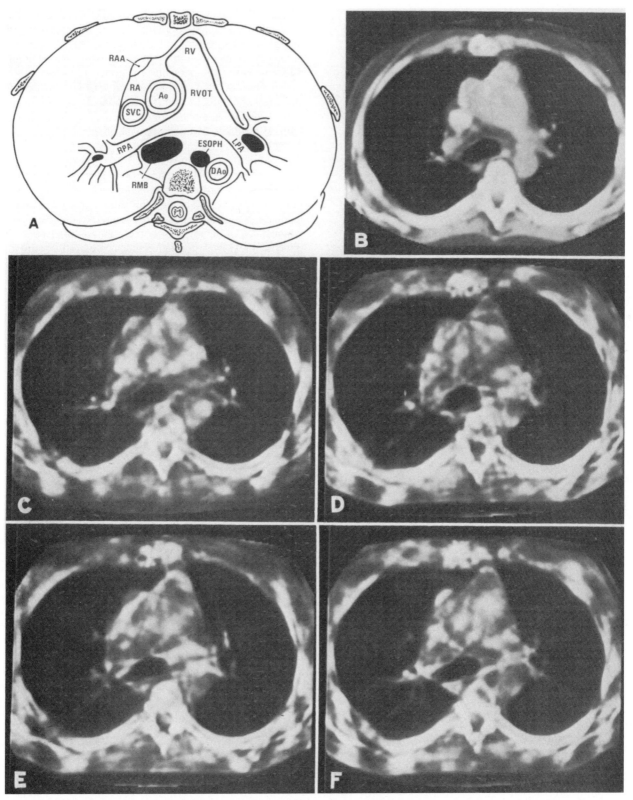

Figure 3.1. CT cardiovascular "stop action" images at five phases of the cardiac cycle obtained in 1976, using 6-second rotation time and 12-second acquisition time. A retrospective segmented sinogram space reconstruction was performed. (From Harell GS, Guthaner DF, Breiman RS, et al. Stop-action cardiac computed tomography. *Radiology* 1977;123(2):515–517, with permission.)

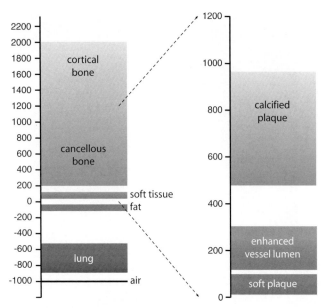

Figure 3.2. Range of Hounsfield units for several tissues and for plaque and enhanced lumen of the coronary arteries.

typical acquisition configuration for a 64-section scanner is, for example, 64 × 0.5 mm for coronary artery imaging.

Rotation time is the duration in milliseconds of a 360-degree rotation of the x-ray tube. The higher the rotation speed, the faster data acquisition and the shorter the rotation time. In helical CT, to achieve coverage of the entire volume of interest, the rotation of the x-ray tube is coupled with a continuous linear translation of the patient through the gantry

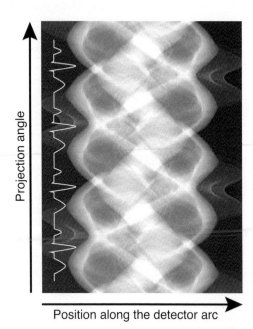

Figure 3.3. Cardiac CT involves simultaneous registration of transmission profiles and an ECG. Each horizontal line in sinogram space represents one transmission profile, at a certain acquisition angle and is associated with the registered ECG signal. Multisection CT yields multiple sinogram space, that is, each acquisition channel generates its own sinogram space.

of the CT scanner. The gantry contains the rotating x-ray tube and the detector assembly. The pitch factor is the ratio of patient displacement in the horizontal direction per 360-degree rotation of the x-ray tube divided by the total nominal thickness of all simultaneously acquired sections.

Selection of rotation time and pitch factor must comply strict requirements to achieve the optimal acquisition window. Acquisition window, or temporal resolution, is the time interval available for measurement of transmission profiles under successive projection angles at any location within the volume under investigation. The acquisition window in cardiac CT can be estimated by dividing rotation time by the pitch factor. In cardiac CT, the acquisition window should be long enough to catch at least the entire cardiac cycle at any level along the entire volume. A relatively long acquisition window can be achieved by a long rotation time and a small pitch factor. However, rotation time is preferably maintained short to avoid motion artifacts. Therefore, cardiac CT can be characterized by the application of an exceptionally small pitch factor. A small pitch factor implies temporal oversampling of the volume, and it provides a sinogram space covering not only the entire volume of interest but also the entire cardiac cycle. To achieve a short reconstruction window, most reconstruction algorithms for cardiac CT are now capable to include, for each reconstructed section, transmission data acquired during more than just one cardiac cycle. These reconstruction algorithms require, consequently, a further reduction of the pitch factor down to 0.2 or even lower at the cost of radiation exposure (Fig. 3.4).

IMAGE RECONSTRUCTION

Essential in cardiac CT reconstructions is retrospective phase selection, generally referred to as *retrospective gated reconstruction,* that is, the synchronization of the recorded transmission profiles with the cardiac cycle prior to image reconstruction. The main challenge of cardiac CT reconstructions is to minimize blurring as a result of motion. This can be achieved by minimizing the reconstruction window or, in other words, by minimizing the period of time, relative to the cardiac cycle, that is required for coverage of sufficient sinogram space to provide one complete reconstructed section.

To facilitate retrospective synchronization of transmission profiles, cardiac CT scanners are equipped with a device for recording an electrocardiogram (ECG). Data acquisition in cardiac MSCT thus consists of simultaneous registration of transmission profiles together with the associated ECG signal. The first cardiac MSCT scanners provided 4 acquisition channels; with subsequent models 16, 32, and 64 channels became available. In cardiac CT, each acquisition channel generates its own sinogram space; each line in sinogram space represents one transmission profile, its acquisition angle, and the registered ECG signal. Retrospective reconstruction algorithms provide the synchronization of transmission profiles with the ECG signal, sometimes referred to as four-dimensional (4-D) imaging. To achieve this, all R waves in the ECG have to be identified. In retrospective gated cardiac CT, any cardiac phase point can be selected relative to the R wave. These phase points define a recon-

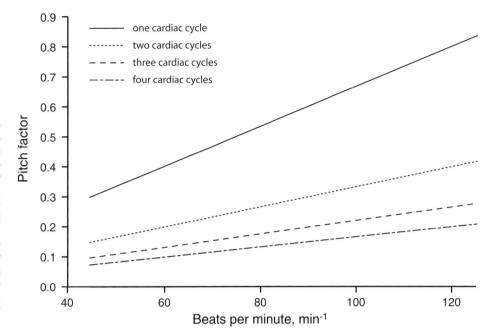

Figure 3.4. Temporal oversampling of the entire volume is required to achieve a sufficient long acquisition time for the registration of one, two, three, or four cardiac cycles and, consequently, a low pitch factor. The lower the heart rate the lower the required pitch factor to "catch" enough cardiac cycles. At an x-ray tube rotation time of 0.4 seconds, for including three or more cardiac cycles in the segmented reconstruction at heart rates lower than 90 beats per minute, a pitch factor lower than 0.2 is needed.

struction window within the cardiac cycle. The reconstruction window either follows or precedes the R wave, and the trigger for the reconstruction window is generally defined by either a delay or reverse delay relative to the R waves. This delay may either be relative or absolute, meaning that the start of the reconstruction window is determined by either a fixed moment after, or before, each R-peak or a certain percentage relative to the RR interval. These techniques assume a linear relationship between the ECG and the actual contraction and relaxation of the heart chambers, which might be a good assumption, if the heart rate does not vary too much; however, artifacts occur even in a case of mild sinus arrhythmia.

In general, in noncardiovascular applications of CT, the reconstruction window of any reconstructed section simply equals the rotation time of the x-ray tube. In this case, each reconstructed section is derived from a 360-degree sinogram space. Rotation times of modern scanners are well below 1 second, and a reconstruction window of this magnitude is sufficiently low for most applications of CT but not for cardiac CT. In CT, opposing projections yield identical transmission profiles, meaning that 360-degree sinogram space contains redundant information. The minimal requirements for the reconstruction of any section by filtered backprojection are achieved by excluding all redundant transmission profiles from sinogram space. This yields a 180-degree sinogram space corresponding to a reconstruction window of approximately 50% of the rotation time. For typical rotation times of 0.4, 0.5, and 0.6 seconds, the reconstruction window for acquiring a 180-degree sinogram space would be approximately 200, 250, and 300 milliseconds, respectively. However, this yield is still not sufficient for most applications in cardiovascular MSCT because a reconstruction window of 100 milliseconds or shorter is required.

To achieve a sufficient, short reconstruction window, manufacturers generally apply the method for "stop-action" cardiac computed tomography that was described in 1977 by Harell et al (8). This method is based on a relatively long acquisition window and thus on recording transmission profiles during more than one heart cycle throughout the entire volume. The reconstructed sections can be derived from a so-called 180-degree segmented sinogram space, where small, complementary subsegments of sinogram space are derived from successive heart beats, together yielding the 180-degree segmented sinogram space (Fig. 3.5). The reconstruction window that can be achieved theoretically with this technique is shown in Figure 3.6. The figure applies to a reconstruction algorithm that allows for including all available subsegments in sinogram space. Note that the reconstruction window is independent of rotation time and thus explains the feasibility of cardiac CT by Harell et al, even at a CT scanner with a rotation time of 6 seconds (8). To achieve the optimal curves in Figure 3-6, rotation time is presumably adapted accurately to the heart rate. In general practice, the theoretically achievable lowest reconstruction window cannot be realized, because optimal adaptation of rotation time to the actual heart rate cannot be achieved because of the fixed values of rotation time and variations in heart rate during the CT scan.

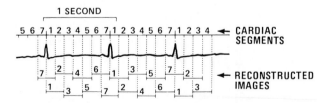

Figure 3.5. Three of the acquired 13 1/2 cardiac cycles. The RR interval for each cycle was subdivided into seven cardiac segments representing different phases. In reconstructing seven images, the angular projections from two successive segments in each of the 13 1/2 beats were merged. For example, reconstructed image 1 consisted of the merged angular projection from cardiac segments one and two in beats 1, 2, 3,..., 13 1/2. (From Harell GS, Guthaner DF, Breiman RS, et al. Stop-action cardiac computed tomography. *Radiology* 1977;123(2):515–517, with permission.)

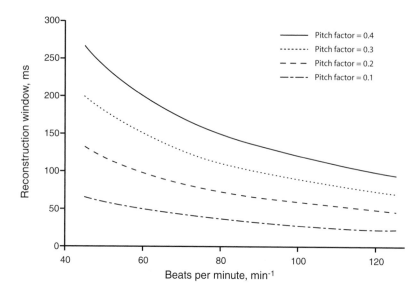

Figure 3.6. Theoretic reconstruction window as a function of heart rate and pitch factor. The graphs are calculated, assuming optimal segmentation of sinogram space and thus optimal adaptation of rotation time to the heart rate. Note that the acquisition window is strongly dependent on the pitch factor; a sufficiently short temporal window requires a low pitch factor, especially at low heart rates.

Volume rendering of two scans of the same patient (Fig. 3.7) illustrates the difference in image quality obtained with a retrospectively gated 180-degree segmented sinogram space reconstruction (ECG synchronized) versus a regular 360-degree sinogram space reconstruction (nonsynchronized). The volume rendering of the synchronized images shows the heart in the retrospectively selected diastolic phase. All different phases of the cardiac cycle express, in the nonsynchronized images, as smooth deformations of the heart. The long reconstruction window leads to blurring of the coronary arteries in the nonsynchronized images, whereas the short reconstruction window of the synchronized retrospectively gated segmented sinogram space reconstruction enables visualization of the coronary arteries.

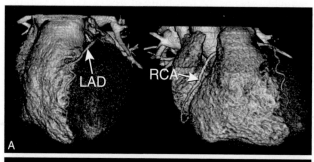

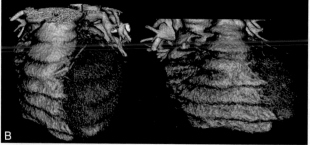

Figure 3.7. Volume rendering of two scans of the same patient illustrates the difference in image quality obtained with a retrospectively gated 180-degree segmented sinogram space reconstruction (ECG synchronized) **(A)** versus a regular 360-degree sinogram space reconstruction (nonsynchronized) **(B)**.

MULTISECTION COMPUTED TOMOGRAPHY IMAGING REQUIREMENTS

Imaging requirements for MSCT image acquisition in heart disease depend on the clinical problem, including spatial resolution, temporal resolution and low-contrast resolution, intravascular contrast enhancement, and scan time.

SPATIAL RESOLUTION

Spatial resolution, or high-contrast resolution, is the ability to observe the contours of small objects within the scanned volume. Small objects can be resolved only when they provide a rather large difference in signal (Hounsfield units) compared to the direct environment. Spatial resolution plays an important role in the visualization of contrast-enhanced distal segments of coronary arteries, calcifications, or stents (Fig. 3.8). In CT, spatial resolution is, in essence, limited by the acquisition geometry of a particular CT scanner, that is, the dimensions of the detector elements, smallest available section thickness, focus size and focus to detector distance, and also on the reconstruction filter and the reconstructed slice thickness.

The acquisition of small, isotropic voxels facilitates advanced postprocessing and 3D image viewing and is, particularly, advantageous for review of cardiac CT images. The actual diameters of the lumen of normal coronary artery segments range from 5 mm in the proximal segments to less than 1 mm in the distal segments. Bypass grafts typically range from 4 to 6 mm (Table 3.1). This means that a voxel size of 1.0 mm^3 in all three dimensions should be sufficient for imaging of the coronary arteries, except for distal segments that would require a spatial resolution of at least 0.5 mm^3. A spatial resolution of 2 mm^3 might be sufficient for imaging the lumen of bypass grafts, but for imaging of structures within the coronary arteries, such as atherosclerotic plaque and stents, excellent spatial resolution better than 0.5 mm^3 might be required. The requirements for spatial

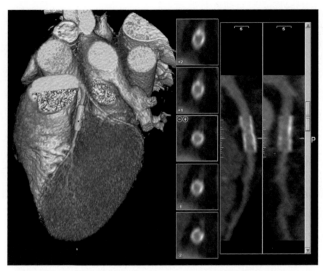

Figure 3.8. Stent imaging requires good spatial resolution. The volume rendering shows the heart of a 38-year-old male patient. Stent with fine struts in the left anterior descending coronary artery can be observed as open on the multiplanar reconstructions.

resolution are less demanding for imaging larger structures, such as large thrombi or heart chambers.

TEMPORAL RESOLUTION

Temporal resolution is the ability to resolve fast moving objects in the displayed CT image. Principally, this can be achieved by a short reconstruction window providing a snapshot relative to the cardiac cycle that can provide all the transmission profiles needed for the reconstruction of one section. Temporal resolution plays an essential role in the visualization of a beating heart and its coronary arteries. A good temporal resolution in cardiac CT is realized by fast data acquisition (fast rotation of the x-ray tube) and, more important, by a dedicated 180-degree sinogram space recon-

TABLE 3-1 | Lumen Diameter of Normal Coronary Artery Segments and Bypass Vein Grafts

First segment (mm)	Last segment (mm)
Coronary arteries	
LM 4.3 (3.5–5.1)	–
LAD 3.5 (2.9–4.2)	0.8 (0.5–1.2)
LCX 3.2 (2.4–3.9)	1.3 (0.6–1.8)
RCA 3.7 (2.7–4.6)	1.8 (1.2–2.5)
Bypass grafts	6.0 (4.0–8.0)

LM, left main; LAD, left anterior descending; LCX, left circumflex; RCA, right coronary artery.
From Dodge JT Jr, Brown BG, Bolson EL, et al. Lumen diameter of normal human coronary arteries. Influence of age, sex, anatomic variation, and left ventricular hypertrophy or dilation. *Circulation* 1992;86(1):232–246, with permission.

struction algorithm. This avoids degradation of both low-contrast resolution and spatial resolution in the image, generally referred to as *blurring* of the image, as a result of movement of the cardiac wall and coronary arteries. Actual in-plane velocities of human coronary arteries have been measured at different moments during the cardiac cycle by means of imaging techniques that allow for a short reconstruction window, that is, gradient-echo MRI (14) and prospectively triggered electron beam tomography (EBT) (15). With these techniques a temporal resolution as low as 15 milliseconds (MRI) and 50 milliseconds (EBT) was achieved. In these publications, the conclusion showed that the reconstruction window should be lower than 100 milliseconds for coronary angiography in middiastole at 62 ± 10 beats per minute (BPM) (16), and that a 100-millisecond reconstruction window is relatively optimal for most patients at heart rates up to 90 BPM (15). A reconstruction window of 100 milliseconds is probably not sufficient at heart rates higher than 80 to 90 BPM. These considerations assume imaging at the cardiac phase point that is associated with least motion, for example, reconstruction window starting between 60% and 80% of the interval between two consecutive R-waves. More strict criteria for the reconstruction window apply, if the heart should be assessed at more than one cardiac phase point, including those that are associated with rapid movement of the heart wall, for example, for studying the dynamics of the myocardium. Alfidi et al (17) already concluded in 1976 that for imaging the dynamics of the heart with CT, such as the detection of akinetic and dyskinetic myocardium, achieving a reconstruction window smaller than 50 milliseconds should become possible. Although the reconstruction window with current techniques is generally longer than 50 milliseconds, successful evaluations of cardiac function by CT have been reported (18).

LOW-CONTRAST RESOLUTION

Low-contrast resolution is the ability to detect structures that express only a small difference in signal (Hounsfield units) compared to their direct environment. For the detection of low contrasts in CT images, the lesions must be fairly large in size. In x-ray computed tomography, native tissue contrasts are, in general, not sufficient to differentiate between structures, such as the vessel wall, its unenhanced lumen, and the myocardium, or to distinguish pathology within the myocardium. Contrast enhancement is thus mandatory for visualizing the lumen of the coronary arteries, the heart chambers, and the myocardium. However, even with proper enhancement using iodinated contrast media, the contrast between normal, ischemic, and infarcted myocardium remains rather low (Fig. 3.9). Image noise is the main limitation for CT when imaging structures exhibit low contrast. Image noise may be decreased by either raising tube current (mA) at the cost of patient exposure or increasing the reconstructed slice thickness, at the cost of spatial resolution. In addition, low-contrast resolution depends on tube voltage, beam filtration, and the reconstruction filter.

SCAN TIME

Scan time is the time interval between the start and the end of an acquisition of the entire volume. To avoid breathing

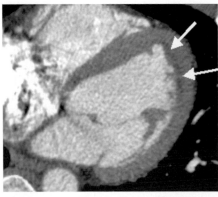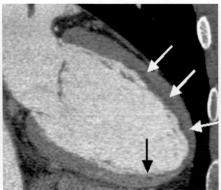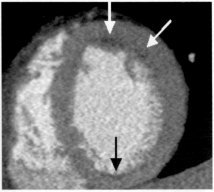

A,B

C

Figure 3.9. Imaging of a perfusion defect requires good low-contrast resolution. ECG-synchronized CT in a 38-year-old male patient after left ventricular anterior wall infarction. Axial plane **(A)** and parasagittal **(B)** and left ventricular short axis **(C)** reformats. A subendocardial perfusion defect is shown in the left ventricular anterior wall (*white arrows*). Also, a small subendocardial perfusion defect can be observed at the posterior wall (*black arrow*, **B, C**).

artifacts and to limit the amount of contrast material, scan time should remain at least below 30 seconds but preferably below 20 seconds. The extent of the target volume and acquisition parameters, such as rotation time, pitch factor, section thickness, and number of simultaneously acquired sections, define scan time.

PATIENT PREPARATION

Contraindications for cardiovascular MSCT include severe arrhythmias and allergy for iodinated intravenous contrast media. Good fixation of the ECG wires is essential. The ECG signal should be clear and specifically yield a clear demarcation between the R-peaks and the rest of the signal. It should be avoided that lines may drop as a result of motion of the table or movements of the patient during the scan because they may cause signal distortion on the ECG. No image postprocessing can solve this problem with ECG misregistration.

Beta blockers may be useful to reduce the heart rate to a lower range, for example, 50 to 60 BPM. The resulting performance is more predictable and shows more consistent quality when using medication. Special algorithms for the reconstruction pose an alternative to the use of medication. The so-called segmented 180-degree sinogram reconstruction yields good quality even at higher heart rates. The less variation in heart rate that occurs during the scan, the better the result. Also, when total scanning time is short, for example, below 15 seconds, the quality of the scan improves because of the reduction of total amount of heart beats in the scan and less variation in the heart rate. Furthermore, the patient should be positioned supine with the heart at the center of rotation and the arms outside the region. Moreover, providing a good explanation to the patient about the scan procedure is important in patient preparation. A patient should respond adequately on breathing instructions and practicing prior to scanning is advised. The patient should be informed about the breath-holding time and should be instructed that the breath-hold should be at the same depth. Hyperventilation and administration of oxygen prior to breath-holding may be used to support breath-holding, par-

ticularly at scan times of approximately 20 seconds scanning time or longer.

Scanograms should be sufficient in length, which is much larger than the required range for coverage of the volume. In cardiac CT it can be difficult to exactly set the scanning range from the scanogram. Therefore, a low dose axial orientation scan may be useful. Areas difficult to recognize in the scanogram are the bottom of the heart, the origin of the coronary arteries, and the origin of bypass grafts. If exact positions cannot be found on the scanogram, and an orientation scan is not performed, longer scanning ranges are set to avoid the risk of not scanning the total target volume at the cost of elevated radiation exposure. Scanning directions are to be set according to total breath-holding time and according to scan volume. Standard cranio-caudal scanning is used for coronary artery scans. If the superior mediastinum is included, for visualization of the aorta or bypass grafts, a caudo-cranial direction is preferred.

SPECIAL APPLICATIONS

MSCT provides special opportunities for cardiovascular CT, in addition to imaging of the coronary arteries, coronary bypass grafts, and the myocardium. These options include assessment of left ventricular (LV) and right ventricular (RV) function, assessment of a coronary calcification score, and assessment of the anatomy of pulmonary veins in patients with atrial fibrillation. Each of these applications can be characterized by its specific techniques for acquisition and reconstruction.

ASSESSMENT OF VENTRICULAR FUNCTION

Any contrast-enhanced MSCT examination of the entire heart that allows for a retrospective gated 180-degree segmented sinogram space reconstruction is suitable for assessment of ventricular function (18). Assessment of ventricular function can thus be performed without the need for acquiring extra scans after MSCT coronary angiography. It requires only reconstruction of the entire ventricle at 10 to 20 cardiac phase points.

Global ventricular function is generally measured as the end-systolic volume and end-diastolic volume (ESV, EDV). Subsequently, stroke volume (SV) and ejection fraction (EF) can be derived easily from ESV and EDV. Semiautomatic software may be used for ventricular cavity contour detection and for the calculation of global ventricular function. Figure 3.10 shows semiautomatic software for the assessment of LV function.

Regional LV wall motion can be assessed by visual scoring of cinematic loops of well-described myocardial segments (19). Each segment is assigned a wall motion score of 1 to 4, ranging from normal, hypokinetic, akinetic to dyskinetic myocardium (19).

Integrated CT assessment of the coronary arteries and regional myocardial function allows more complete evaluation of the functional consequences of a coronary artery stenosis. The usefulness of this combined approach has been reported in patients with hypertension and diabetes mellitus (20,21). From the same data set global function and left ventricular mass can also be determined, which has clinical relevance for prognosis and guidance of therapy.

The temporal resolution of current MSCT scanners that offer segmented 180-degree sinogram space reconstructions now approaches the criterion of 50 milliseconds for the reconstruction window published by Alfidi in 1976. At longer reconstruction windows, underestimation of ESV and EDV is likely to occur owing to blurring of the wall of the LV cavity as a result of contraction and relaxation (22).

Not only left ventricular function, but also right ventricular function can be measured by dynamic CT. Contrast-enhanced CT is now routinely used as a first-line imaging tool in patients with suspected pulmonary embolism. Right ventricular enlargement on chest computed tomography has been shown to be a predictor of early death in patients with acute pulmonary embolism (23,24). Even the dimensions of the right ventricle on nondynamic routine CT images may be predictive for mortality in this setting. Further study is required to assess the additional value of dynamic CT of the right ventricle for prognostication and guiding therapy in patients with acute pulmonary embolism.

CORONARY ARTERY CALCIFICATION SCORE

Coronary artery calcification is a manifestation of atherosclerosis in the vessel wall, which becomes more extensive in advanced lesions. Coronary artery calcification is strongly correlated to coronary events. CT provides a noninvasive method for detecting and quantifying coronary artery calcification (25). This may contribute to improved sensitivity in the stratification of high-risk, asymptomatic individuals.

Coronary calcification is best detected and measured in a plain MSCT acquisition without contrast enhancement.

Prospective ECG triggering is generally used to avoid motion artifacts. This means that the acquisition of nonsegmented 180-degree sinogram space is ECG-triggered at a prospectively selected delay after the R peak (diastolic phase). Translation of the patient through the gantry of the CT scanner is achieved between successive acquisitions. In general, four to eight acquisitions are sufficient for coverage of the entire volume, depending on the acquisition configuration and the size of the heart. In prospective ECG-triggered acquisitions, the patient is exposed within only the 200- to 250-millisecond acquisition window at diastole, and radiation exposure is therefore significantly less compared to retrospective gated cardiovascular examinations. Note that in prospectively triggered acquisitions, the reconstruction window equals the acquisition window.

However, a lack of standardization of the MSCT techniques exists, with regard to image acquisition as well as to the methodologies for quantitative coronary calcification scoring. The development of standardized and reproducible algorithms for measurements are a technical prerequisite for the use of coronary calcification scoring to become a useful clinical tool. In addition, the coronary calcification score will have to be established as an independent predictor of existing risk factors for cardiovascular disease (26).

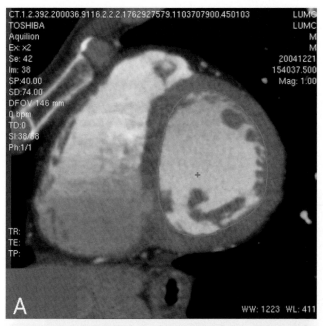

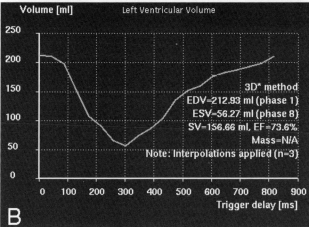

Figure 3.10. Semiautomatic software may be used for ventricular cavity contour detection **(A)** and calculation of global function **(B)**. (Courtesy of CT-MASS, LKEB, Leiden, The Netherlands.)

ASSESSMENT OF PULMONARY VEINS

Atrial arrhythmias often originate in the pulmonary veins and can be treated with percutaneous radiofrequency catheter ablation. With this technique, the arrhythmic foci are electrically disconnected from the left atrium by means of catheters placed in the left atrium (27). Preprocedural multi-detector-row computed tomography (MDCT) examination is helpful to depict the anatomy of the pulmonary veins and left atrium and, particularly, to demonstrate additional pulmonary veins (e.g., middle lobe vein), which is important for planning the interventional procedure. Variations in pulmonary venous anatomy are common and comprise variation in the number of veins as well as the occurrence of common ostia and early branching (28). Three-dimensional surface rendering reconstructions provide a quick overview of the pulmonary venous anatomy, but cross-sectional reconstruction in coronal, sagittal, and transverse orientations are necessary for full appreciation of the morphology of the pulmonary veins (29). MSCT allows visualization of pulmonary vein anatomy, providing the cardiologist with a road map prior to ablation in patients with atrial fibrillation (29). Postprocedural MSCT also offers an opportunity for follow-up of the pulmonary vein after ablation (30).

MSCT pulmonary venography requires a contrast-enhanced helical acquisition. To avoid motion artifacts, a 180-degree sinogram space reconstruction is generally performed, yielding a reconstruction window of 200 to 250 milliseconds, which, in general, is sufficient for imaging the large pulmonary veins with diameters well above 10 mm. In contrast to other applications of cardiovascular MSCT described in this chapter, pulmonary venography does not require synchronization of transmission profiles with the ECG because cardiac phase selection is not essential in the evaluation of the pulmonary veins. This means that a regular MSCT acquisition, with a high pitch factor and resulting low patient dose, can be performed. However, for assessment of complications related to the ablation procedure, such as pulmonary venous stenoses, ECG-synchronized MSCT may be preferred for better visualization of details (Fig. 3.11).

MULTISECTION COMPUTED TOMOGRAPHY ARTIFACTS

Computed tomography is sensitive for the occurrence of image artifacts. Well-known CT artifacts occur as a result of the partial volume effect, beam hardening, and motion. Typical artifacts, in general multisection CT, are helical artifacts (31), "windmill," and "cone-beam" artifacts (32). Cardiac CT is particularly susceptible to artifacts, including both general CT artifacts as well as artifacts that are introduced by the dedicated reconstruction algorithms that are used in cardiac CT.

HIGH-CONTRAST ARTIFACTS

High-contrast artifacts are caused by high attenuating objects, either metal objects—such as stents and surgical clips—calcifications, or a high concentration of iodinated contrast material. The high-contrast artifacts are caused by the partial volume effect, beam hardening, and a relatively low detector signal leading a nonlinear response of the detector and its elec-

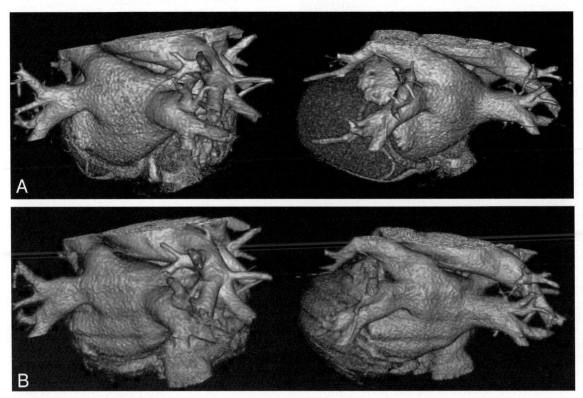

Figure 3.11. Volume rendering of the pulmonary veins and the left atrium. ECG-synchronized CT with segmented reconstruction **(A)** and nonsynchronized images **(B)**.

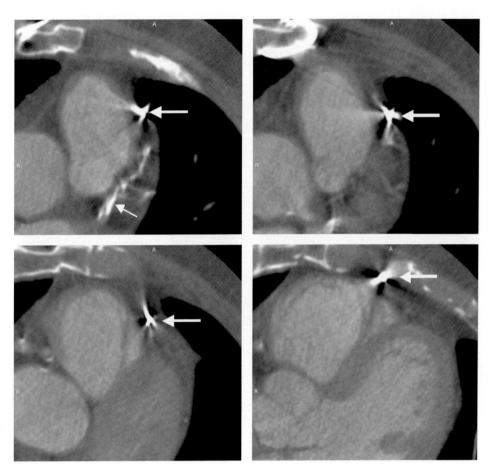

Figure 3.12. Surgical vascular clip artifacts. A 67-year-old male patient after coronary bypass operation. Coronary calcifications (**A**, *small arrow*) and metal clip artifacts in the course of the left anterior descending coronary artery (LAD) (**A–C**, *arrow*) after left internal mammarian artery (LIMA) to LAD bypass. Left parasternal vascular clip artifact in the previous LIMA-location (**D**). Because of these artifacts, the coronary artery cannot be evaluated properly.

tronics. In the CT images this leads to blooming and streaks (Fig. 3.12). Blooming artifacts caused by calcifications, stents, or clips may seriously affect the evaluation of the lumen of coronary arteries or bypasses. Streaks caused by high concentrations of iodinated contrast material or clips extend throughout a relatively large part of the image and may obscure structures. The effect of high contrast artifacts, especially blooming, was most prominent at 4-section scanners and decreased with 16- and 64-section CT scanners that allow for scanning the heart at a smaller section thickness.

CARDIAC MOTION

Cardiac motion leads to blurring of the coronary arteries and the myocardium and may affect visualization of relevant structures (Fig. 3.13). Motion-related artifacts are most severe for the right coronary artery (RCA) because it moves at the highest velocity and least for the left anterior descending (LAD) artery (15). Most consistent image quality is generally observed at middiastole. Breath-holding also influences the heart rate, because during the breath-hold, heart rate initially decreases then gradually increases (33). Cardiac motion particularly complicates the evaluation of small distal segments of coronary arteries and, in particular, the anastomoses of bypass grafts to the distal coronary arteries.

Countermeasures for cardiac motion artifacts are heart rate reducing medication (beta blockers) in the case of a high heart rate, especially warranted in case of nonsegmented

180-degree sinogram reconstructions and by optimal selection of acquisition parameters, especially a low pitch factor and short rotation time.

RESPIRATORY MOTION

Respiratory motion leads to deformations in the reconstructed images that can be easily recognized in multiplanar reformat (MPR) or 3D reconstructions. Four-section CT scanners are particularly susceptible to breathing artifacts because the small number of simultaneously acquired sections results in a rather long scan time and, consequently, a

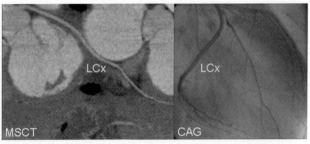

Figure 3.13. Although temporal resolution of MSCT has improved, blurring of the vessel wall still occurs. Compare, for example, MSCT coronary angiography (curved MPR) with selective coronary angiography. The latter technique is superior to cardiovascular MSCT, with regard to temporal resolution.

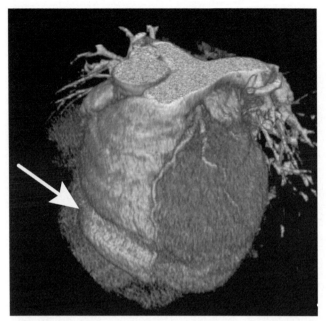

Figure 3.14. Motion artifact: the smooth deformation of the cardiac wall as a result of breathing during the scan can be recognized easily in the 3D reconstruction (*arrow*).

long breath-hold. Figure 3.14 shows a typical breathing artifact, as a smooth deformation of the heart wall. Countermeasures for respiratory motion artifacts include proper patient preparation and instruction and hyperventilation just before the acquisition.

TECHNICAL ERRORS

Cardiac CT is also prone to technical errors. Incomplete coverage of the volume might occur in the case of inaccurate planning of the scan range. Erroneous timing of the start of the scan relative to contrast administration might cause poor contrast enhancement. Synchronization artifacts may occur in the case of a spurious ECG signal, leading to misregistrations of the R peaks, or they may occur in the case of serious arrhythmias (Fig. 3.15). Selection of a pitch factor that is

too high, or a rotation time that is too long in relation to the heart rate of the patient, will result in missing one or more slices within the reconstructed volume.

PATIENT DOSE IN MULTISECTION COMPUTED TOMOGRAPHY

Radiation protection of patients is based on the principles of justification and optimization. Justification implies that the benefit for the patient, for example, exclusion of pathology, diagnosis of disease, or follow-up of treatment, outweighs the risk of radiation exposure. Generic justification requires that CT imaging will usually improve the diagnosis or treatment of a well-described clinical problem and patient population. Individual justification means that the cardiac CT scan is expected to do more good than harm to the individual patient. Once justified, incorporating measures that tend to lower radiation doses should optimize the CT examination. Patient dose assessment is thus required for balancing harm and benefit of the CT examination and to assess the effect of measures for optimization of cardiac CT. Note that neither dose constraints nor dose limits apply to patients. Today most CT scanners provide the user with an indication of patient dose.

A general consensus exists concerning the dose descriptors to be used in computed tomography. These are the Computed Tomography Dose Index (CTDI), originally proposed by the Food and Drug Administration (FDA) in the United States (34); and two derivates of the CTDI, that is, the weighted CTDI (CTDI$_w$), originally proposed under the name practical CTDI (35), and the volume CTDI (CTDI$_{vol}$) introduced by the International Electrotechnical Commission (IEC) (36). In addition, the dose length product (DLP), as proposed by the European CT Working Group (37), is derived from the CTDI and is available at most CT scanners. Today CT dosimetry is, in general, based on the quantities CTDI$_{vol}$ and DLP.

The CTDI$_{vol}$ is a measure of the local, absorbed dose. The CTDI$_{vol}$ (mGy) depends primarily on technical acquisition parameters, such as tube current, rotation time, tube voltage,

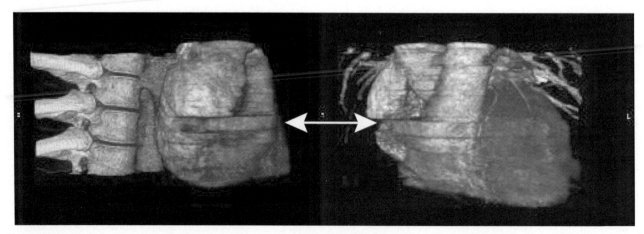

Figure 3.15. Technical error, synchronization artifact: wrongly identified R-waves, for example, as a result of a bad ECG signal, result in synchronization errors during the reconstruction leading to abrupt deformations that can be recognized easily in a 3D reconstruction.

beam filtration, pitch factor, and geometric efficiency. The $CTDI_{vol}$ for scans of the body is derived from measurements in a 32-cm diameter cylindrical polymethyl methacrylate (PMMA) CT dosimetry phantom representing the adult body. The $CTDI_{vol}$ is particularly suitable for comparison of different acquisition protocols irrespective of the type of MSCT scanner. In addition, a quantity is required that expresses patient exposure from the complete MSCT examination. Such a quantity should take into account the extent of the exposed range and the exposures during all sequences of the examination. A dosimetric quantity that fulfills these conditions is the dose length product (DLP, mGy cm). Dose length product is the $CTDI_{vol}$ multiplied by the length of the exposed range for each sequence.

Assessment of the effective dose (38) for cardiac CT is sometimes needed to allow comparison with other types of radiologic examination, such as selective coronary angiography or risk assessment. The effective dose for a particular cardiac CT scanning protocol can be estimated from the $CTDI_{vol}$ and the acquisition protocol by using dedicated software (39,40).

Alternatively, broad estimates of effective dose (E) may be derived from the DLP that is available for the operator at all modern CT scanners by multiplying DLP with the normalized effective dose coefficient of 0.02 mSv/mGy cm; this value is valid for a typical cardiac CT acquisition at a tube voltage of 120 kVp. Table 3-2 provides typical values for the radiation exposure for patients and workers and, for comparison, some dose limits and natural radiation levels.

Effective dose from cardiac CT is relatively high, mainly because of the need to catch all cardiac phases at any level of the scan and the resulting slow moving table and low pitch factor. This is particularly true for segmented sinogram-space reconstruction, requiring a higher dose (30%) compared to nonsegmented sinogram-space reconstructions (41). Concern about radiation exposure stimulates the development of methods for dose reduction in cardiac CT, including small field scanning and ECG-triggered modulation of dose. The field of view in cardiac CT is small and, therefore, radiation exposure of tissue outside this field of view can be limited by means of a special "small field" beam-shaping filter. Another method for dose reduction is to reduce x-ray output during the systolic phases that are expected to be of less interest for the evaluation of the coronary arteries. Pitfalls of small-field scanning are the occurrence of artifacts and reduced image quality. A pitfall of tube modulation is reduced image quality at certain relevant phases of cardiac cycle, for example, as a result of an irregular heart rate.

FUTURE PERSPECTIVE

Cardiac CT has developed into a reliable, operator independent and minimally invasive clinical technique. Further developments in the field of MSCT technology and reconstruction algorithms are expected to contribute to a further improvement of the quality of the cardiovascular MSCT scans. Compared to other 3D imaging modalities, MSCT offers excellent spatial resolution but still at a long reconstruction window, typically exceeding 100 milliseconds

(Table 3.3). Best in-plane resolution and temporal resolution can still be achieved with 2D selective coronary angiography.

With regard to CT scanner engineering, a further reduction of the rotation time is expected to contribute to improvement of temporal resolution. Detector technology is expected to improve, mainly by a further increase of the number of sections that can be registered simultaneously (13). This may finally lead to the implementation of detectors that have enough detector rows to measure simultaneously transmission profiles through the entire region, resulting in shorter scan times.

Reconstruction algorithms based on the generation of an 180-degree segmented sinogram space, which are required to achieve adequate temporal resolution, are now available for most users of cardiac CT scanners. With these algorithms the necessity for routine use of beta blockers to reduce heart rate might be reduced or avoided. Image artifacts introduced by linear models for the synchronization of transmission profiles, particularly in the case of arrhythmias, might be reduced by the application of nonlinear models. Such models are expected to be advantageous because it is well known that the relationship between the recording of electrical activity, that is, the ECG, and the actual physiologic phase of the heart is not linear (42). Alternatively, algorithms that are based on self-gated synchronization of the motion of the heart and the acquired transmission profiles are being developed (kymogram), thus rendering the recording of an ECG superfluous (43). In this case, synchronization is derived from the sinogram itself, that is, from the same raw data that are used for image reconstruction.

Alternatives for the CT reconstruction technique of filtered backprojection might provide specific benefits in cardiac applications, for example, the technique of statistical reconstruction. Statistical reconstruction provides possibly advantages over analytic algorithms, such as filtered backprojection in terms of flexibility, resolution, contrast, and image noise. However, statistical reconstructed images may be affected by some artifacts that are not present in filtered backprojection images, for example, as aliasing patterns and severe overshoots in the areas of sharp intensity transitions. Potential benefits of using statistical reconstruction methods include the removal of streak artifacts when fewer projections are used, contrast enhancement, and better noise properties in low-dose studies (44).

Cardiac CT was initially developed using electron beam CT scanners (EBCT) (45,46). EBCT appeared to be particularly successful for the quantitative application of coronary calcification scoring. EBCT provides a short reconstruction window compared to MSCT and is performed at a low, effective dose. Nevertheless, the potential of EBCT for coronary angiography is seriously affected by its poor low-contrast performance (as a result of a low signal-to-noise ratio) and poor spatial resolution (as a result of large slice thickness) of EBCT compared to cardiovascular MSCT.

The technique of rotational coronary angiography with C-arm mounted flat detectors has the potential to provide additional functionality within the cathlab during x-ray guided interventions (10). However, rotational coronary angiography is not expected to provide the same diagnostic quality of coronary MSCT angiography because of the limi-

TABLE 3-2 Typical Effective Doses (mSv) for Chest Examinations of Patients (mSv per examination), Regulatory Dose Limits (mSv per year), and Natural Background (mSv per year)

X-ray examinations

Chest radiographs (PA & LAT)	0.1–0.3 mSv
Selective coronary angiography	2–10 mSv
Cardiac MSCT angiography[a]	8–12 mSv
MSCT coronary calcification score[b]	2–4 mSv
MSCT angiography, pulmonary embolism[c]	4–8 mSv
MSCT angiography, pulmonary veins[d]	1–2 mSv

PET

Heart ^{18}F-fluorodeoxyglucose (185 MBq)	3.5 mSv

SPECT

Heart ^{99m}Tc-sestamibi (400 MBq, at rest)	4 mSv
Heart ^{99m}Tc-sestamibi (400 MBq, at stress)	3 mSv

Lung scintigraphy

Lung Perfusion ^{99m}Tc-MAA (100 MBq)	1 mSv

Regulatory dose limits (38)

General public	1 mSv/y
Radiation worker	20 mSv/y

Natural background (49)

The Netherlands	2 mSv/y
The World	2.5–3 mSv/y
Kerala and Madras (India)[e]	15 mSv/y
Certain locations in Kerala (India)[f]	70 mSv/y (50)

[a] Cardiac MSCT angiography, contrast-enhanced study of the heart, enabling assessment and diagnosis of the myocardium, coronary arteries, bypass grafts, and cardiac function; retrospective gated, segmented 180-degree sinogram space reconstruction.
[b] MSCT calcium scoring, native study of the heart, enabling assessment of the calcium load of the coronary arteries for risk stratification; prospective triggering of the acquisition, 180-degree nonsegmented sinogram space reconstruction.
[c] Whole chest MSCT, contrast-enhanced study of the entire chest, enabling assessment and diagnosis of the lungs (tumors), aorta and pulmonary arteries (pulmonary embolism); nontriggered acquisition, nongated reconstruction, 360-degree nonsegmented sinogram space reconstruction.
[d] MSCT of pulmonary veins (range from truncus pulmonalis to apex LV); contrast-enhanced study; nontriggered acquisition, nongated reconstruction, 360-degree nonsegmented sinogram space reconstruction.
[e–f] No evidence of increased cancers or other health problems arising from these high, natural radiation levels.
LAT, lateral; MBq, megabecquerel; MSCT, multisection computed tomography; mSv, millisievert; PA, posteranterior; PET, positron emission tomography; SPECT, single photon emission computed tomography; y, year.
From ICRP Publication 60. *1990 Recommendations of the International Commission on Radiological Protection.* Oxford, UK: Pergamon Press; 1991, with permission; United Nations Scientific Committee on the Effects of Atomic Radiation. Sources and effects of ionizing radiation, volume 1. Vienna, Austria: Sources, 2000, with permission; and Nair MK, Nambi KS, Amma NS, et al. Population study in the high natural background radiation area in Kerala, India. *Radiat Res* 1999;152(6 Suppl):S145–S148, with permission.

tation of the flat detector, with regard to its dynamic range and response time.

In addition to coronary MSCT angiography, MSCT can provide information about myocardial perfusion and function. Using MSCT, myocardial perfusion defects can be ob-

served in the early phase of the contrast bolus phase (early defect). In the late phase, residual defects and late enhancement can be observed. The clinical significance of MSCT imaging of myocardial perfusion has still to be established (3).

	TABLE 3-3	Comparison of Techniques for Coronary Angiography		

Technique	In-plane (mm × mm)	Thickness (mm)	Temporal window (ms)
MSCT (3D volume acquisition)	0.4 × 0.4	0.5	50–200[a]
EBT (2D tomographic acquisition)	0.8 × 0.8	3.0	100
MRI (3D volume acquisition)	1.2 × 1.2	3.0	40–100[b]
Selective (2D projection)	0.15 × 0.15	–[c]	10–20

[a–c] The good temporal resolution is obtained by combining raw data acquired during successive heart beats.
EBT, electron beam tomography; mm, millimeter; MRI, magnetic resonance imaging; ms, milliseconds; MSCT, multisection computed tomography.

Coronary plaque imaging may be important to improve risk stratification and to monitor progression of coronary atherosclerosis. Contrast-enhanced MSCT permits identification of coronary plaques, and CT density values measured within plaques reflect plaque composition (47). However, the performance of cardiovascular MSCT plaque imaging is seriously limited by the current technical performance of MSCT, especially with regard to its spatial resolution and, even more, its temporal resolution resulting in considerable blurring of small plaques.

REFERENCES

1. Achenbach S, Giesler T, Ropers D, et al. Detection of coronary artery stenoses by contrast-enhanced, retrospectively electrocardiographically-gated, multislice spiral computed tomography. *Circulation* 2001;103(21):2535–2538.
2. Nieman K, Oudkerk M, Rensing BJ, et al. Coronary angiography with multi-slice computed tomography. *Lancet* 2001; 357(9256):599–603.
3. Koyama Y, Mochizuki T, Higaki J. Computed tomography assessment of myocardial perfusion, viability, and function. *J Magn Reson Imaging* 2004;19(6):800–815.
4. de Feyter PJ, Nieman K. Noninvasive multi-slice computed tomography coronary angiography: an emerging clinical modality. *J Am Coll Cardiol* 2004;44(6):1238–1240.
5. Adams DF, Hessel SJ, Judy PF, et al. Computed tomography of the normal and infarcted myocardium. *Am J Roentgenol* 1976;126(4):786–791.
6. Higgins CB, Siemers PT, Schmidt W, et al. Evaluation of myocardial ischemic damage of various ages by computerized transmission tomography. Time-dependent effects of contrast material. *Circulation* 1979;60(2):284–291.
7. Ter Pogossian MM, Weiss ES, Coleman RE, et al. Computed tomography of the heart. *Am J Roentgenol* 1976;127(1):79–90.
8. Harell GS, Guthaner DF, Breiman RS, et al. Stop-action cardiac computed tomography. *Radiology* 1977;123(2):515–517.
9. McCollough CH, Morin RL. The technical design and performance of ultrafast computed tomography. *Radiol Clin North Am* 1994;32(3):521–536.
10. Raman SV, Morford R, Neff M, et al. Rotational x-ray coronary angiography. *Catheter Cardiovasc Interv* 2004;63(2): 201–207.
11. Kalender WA, Vock P, Polacin A, et al. [Spiral-CT: a new technique for volumetric scans. I. Basic principles and methodology.] *Rontgenpraxis* 1990;43(9):323–330.
12. Klingenbeck-Regn K, Schaller S, Flohr T, et al. Subsecond multislice computed tomography: basics and applications. *Eur J Radiol* 1999;31(2):110–124.
13. Mori S, Endo M, Tsunoo T, et al. Physical performance evaluation of a 256-slice CT-scanner for four-dimensional imaging. *Med Phys* 2004;31(6):1348–1356.
14. Hofman MB, Wickline SA, Lorenz CH. Quantification of in-plane motion of the coronary arteries during the cardiac cycle: implications for acquisition window duration for MR flow quantification. *J Magn Reson Imaging* 1998;8(3):568–576.
15. Lu B, Mao SS, Zhuang N, et al. Coronary artery motion during the cardiac cycle and optimal ECG triggering for coronary artery imaging. *Invest Radiol* 2001;36(5):250–256.
16. Hoffmann MH, Shi H, Manzke R, et al. Noninvasive coronary angiography with 16-detector row CT: effect of heart rate. *Radiology* 2005;234(1):86–97.
17. Alfidi RJ, MacIntyre WJ, Haaga JR. The effects of biological motion on CT resolution. *Am J Roentgenol* 1976;127(1): 11–15.
18. Dirksen MS, Bax JJ, de Roos A, et al. Usefulness of dynamic multislice computed tomography of left ventricular function in unstable angina pectoris and comparison with echocardiography. *Am J Cardiol* 2002;90(10):1157–1160.
19. Cerqueira MD, Weissman NJ, Dilsizian V, et al. Standardized myocardial segmentation and nomenclature for tomographic imaging of the heart: a statement for healthcare professionals from the Cardiac Imaging Committee of the Council on Clinical Cardiology of the American Heart Association. *Circulation* 2002;105(4):539–542.
20. Schuijf JD, Bax JJ, Jukema JW, et al. Noninvasive evaluation of the coronary arteries with multislice computed tomography in hypertensive patients. *Hypertension* 2005;45(2):227–232.
21. Schuijf JD, Bax JJ, Jukema JW, et al. Noninvasive angiography and assessment of left ventricular function using multislice computed tomography in patients with type 2 diabetes. *Diabetes Care* 2004;27(12):2905–2910.
22. Koch K, Oellig F, Kunz P, et al. [Assessment of global and regional left ventricular function with a 16-slice spiral-CT using two different software tools for quantitative functional analysis and qualitative evaluation of wall motion changes in comparison with magnetic resonance imaging.] *Rofo* 2004; 176(12):1786–1793.
23. Schoepf UJ, Kucher N, Kipfmueller F, et al. Right ventricular enlargement on chest computed tomography: a predictor of early death in acute pulmonary embolism. *Circulation* 2004; 110(20):3276–3280.
24. van der Meer RW, Pattynama PM, van Strijen MJ, et al. Right ventricular dysfunction and pulmonary obstruction index at helical CT: prediction of clinical outcome during 3-month fol-

low-up in patients with acute pulmonary embolism. *Radiology* 2005. In press.

25. Girshman J, Wolff SD. Techniques for quantifying coronary artery calcification. *Semin Ultrasound CT MR* 2003;24(1): 33–38.

26. Thompson GR, Partridge J. Coronary calcification score: the coronary-risk impact factor. *Lancet* 2004;363(9408):557–559.

27. Pappone C, Rosanio S, Oreto G, et al. Circumferential radiofrequency ablation of pulmonary vein ostia: a new anatomic approach for curing atrial fibrillation. *Circulation* 2000;102(21): 2619–2628.

28. Ghaye B, Szapiro D, Dacher JN, et al. Percutaneous ablation for atrial fibrillation: the role of cross-sectional imaging. *Radiographics* 2003;23:S19–S33.

29. Jongbloed MR, Dirksen MS, Bax JJ, et al. Multislice computed tomography to evaluate pulmonary vein anatomy prior to radiofrequency catheter ablation of atrial fibrillation. *Radiology* 2005;45(3):343–350.

30. Maksimovic R, Cademartiri F, Scholten M, et al. Sixteen-row multislice computed tomography in the assessment of pulmonary veins prior to ablative treatment: validation vs conventional pulmonary venography and study of reproducibility. *Eur Radiol* 2004;14(3):369–374.

31. Wilting JE, Timmer J. Artifacts in spiral-CT images and their relation to pitch and subject morphology. *Eur Radiol* 1999; 9(2):316–322.

32. Manzke R, Grass M, Hawkes D. Artifact analysis and reconstruction improvement in helical cardiac cone beam CT. *IEEE Trans Med Imaging* 2004;23(9):1150–1164.

33. Nieman K, Rensing BJ, Van Geuns RJ, et al. Noninvasive coronary angiography with multislice spiral computed tomography: impact of heart rate. *Heart* 2002;88(5):470–474.

34. Shope TB, Gagne RM, Johnson GC. A method for describing the doses delivered by transmission x-ray computed tomography. *Med Phys* 1981;8(4):488–495.

35. Leitz W, Axelsson B, Szendro G. Computed tomography dose assessment: a practical approach. *Radiat Prot Dosimetry* 1995; 57(1–4):377–380.

36. IEC. 60601-2-44 Ed 2 Amendment 1: Medical Electrical Equipment—Part 2-44: Particular requirements for the safety of x-ray equipment for computed tomography. International standard of IEC, 2003.

37. Bongartz G, Golding SJ, Jurik A, et al. Quality criteria for computed tomography. The European Commission's Study Group on Development of Quality Criteria for Computed Tomography. EUR 16262 2000.

38. ICRP Publication 60. *1990 Recommendations of the International Commission on Radiological Protection.* Oxford, UK: Pergamon Press; 1991.

39. Shrimpton PC, Edyvean S. CT scanner dosimetry. *Br J Radiol* 1998;71(841):1–3.

40. Schmidt B, Kalender WA. A fast voxel-based Monte Carlo method for scanner- and patient-specific dose calculations in computed tomography. *Phys Med* 2002;18(2):43–53.

41. Dewey M, Schnapauff D, Laule M, et al. Multislice CT coronary angiography: evaluation of an automatic vessel detection tool. *Rofo* 2004;176(4):478–483.

42. Vembar M, Garcia MJ, Heuscher DJ, et al. A dynamic approach to identifying desired physiological phases for cardiac imaging using multislice spiral CT. *Med Phys* 2003;30(7): 1683–1693.

43. Kachelriess M, Sennst DA, Maxlmoser W, et al. Kymogram detection and kymogram-correlated image reconstruction from subsecond spiral computed tomography scans of the heart. *Med Phys* 2002;29(7):1489–1503.

44. Zbijewski W, Beekman FJ. Characterization and suppression of edge and aliasing artifacts in iterative x-ray CT reconstruction. *Phys Med Biol* 2004;49(1):145–157.

45. Agatston AS, Janowitz WR, Hildner FJ, et al. Quantification of coronary artery calcium using ultrafast computed tomography. *J Am Coll Cardiol* 1990;15(4):827–832.

46. Callister TQ, Cooil B, Raya SP, et al. Coronary artery disease: improved reproducibility of calcium scoring with an electron-beam CT volumetric method. *Radiology* 1998;208(3):807–814.

47. Leber AW, Knez A, Becker A, et al. Accuracy of multidetector spiral computed tomography in identifying and differentiating the composition of coronary atherosclerotic plaques: a comparative study with intracoronary ultrasound. *J Am Coll Cardiol* 2004;43(7):1241–1247.

48. Dodge JT Jr, Brown BG, Bolson EL, et al. Lumen diameter of normal human coronary arteries. Influence of age, sex, anatomic variation, and left ventricular hypertrophy or dilation. *Circulation* 1992;86(1):232–246.

49. United Nations Scientific Committee on the Effects of Atomic Radiation. Sources and effects of ionizing radiation, volume 1. Vienna, Austria: Sources, 2000.

50. Nair MK, Nambi KS, Amma NS, et al. Population study in the high natural background radiation area in Kerala, India. *Radiat Res* 1999;152(6 Suppl):S145–S148.

4

Cardiac Anatomy and Physiology: Imaging Aspects

Frank E. Rademakers

The technical capabilities of cardiovascular magnetic resonance (CMR) and, consequently, the clinical indications in which it can contribute to better patient management, continue to expand. For some indications it has become the gold standard, whereas for others it is the preferred alternative when echo-Doppler fails. However, to be able to translate these superior imaging capabilities into improved patient care requires a good understanding of cardiovascular physiology and pathophysiology.

The purpose of this chapter is to reintroduce some of the general concepts of cardiovascular physiology that can be useful in the interpretation of CMR still images, perfusion and flow curves, and cine loops.

From the early days of Galen (about 200 AD) and through the times of Servetus (1511), Vesalius (1514), Harvey (1578), Frank (1895), Starling (1918), and many others, the anatomy and function of the heart have fascinated scientists all over the world (Fig. 4.1). Even today, not all of the anatomic and functional aspects of the heart are fully understood. The fiber organization in bundles, lamina, and sheets remains a topic of discussion, and the famous Frank-Starling law cannot be fully explained by present knowledge. Experimental techniques using molecular technology are rapidly adding to our understanding of some of the basic mechanisms, but a noninvasive method like CMR—with the ability to provide a comprehensive evaluation of morphology, regional and global function, flow, and perfusion—is needed to shed new light on the function of the human heart in vivo.

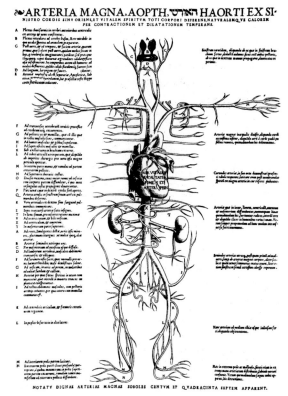

Figure 4.1. Andreas Vesalius (1514–1564) Tabulae Anatomicae: schematic of the circulation.

Cardiovascular disease remains the most important killer in the Western world, so a technique that provides comprehensive information noninvasively and repetitively in the aging population is valuable.

Because of the need for a combination of advanced technical skills and a good knowledge of anatomy, physiology, pathophysiology, and patient management, a close cooperation between all disciplines involved will be required for the successful application of this technology.

FUNCTIONAL ANATOMY

GENERAL ANATOMY

The heart, as a muscle and pump, consists of two serial systems joined in one organ enveloped by the pericardium. It weighs between 250 and 350 gm and is located in the mediastinum. It extends obliquely from the second rib to the fifth intercostal space and spans about 13 cm.

The heart rests on the superior surface of the diaphragm and is flanked and partially covered by the lungs. Its broad base is directed toward the right shoulder, and the apex points inferiorly toward the left hip. It has four chambers, two inferiorly located ventricles and two superiorly located atria. The heart is divided longitudinally by the fibrous interatrial and the muscular interventricular septum. The right ventricle is the most anterior part of the heart, and the pulmonary trunk is the most anterior vessel. The left ventricle (LV) forms the inferoposterior part of the heart and the apex.

Several grooves (usually filled with epicardial fat) are visible on the surface of the heart, delineating the different cavities and carrying the blood vessels supplying the myocardium. The atrioventricular groove, or coronary sulcus, encircles the junction between the atria and ventricles and contains the right coronary artery, the circumflex coronary artery, and the coronary sinus. The anterior interventricular groove lies at the anterior junction of right and left ventricles and contains the anterior descending coronary artery and the great cardiac vein. The posterior interventricular sulcus marks the same junction on the inferoposterior surface of the heart and contains the posterior descending artery, which can originate from the circumflex or right coronary artery and the middle cardiac vein. The small cardiac vein runs along the right inferior margin of the heart and empties in the coronary sinus, just before the latter opens into the right atrium (RA).

DEFINING REGIONS AND SURFACES

Defining several surfaces and regions of the heart differ depending on the imaging technique, so that a great deal of confusion can arise when results from echocardiographic, nuclear, angiographic, and CMR studies are compared. Part of the confusion derives from the reference point used and part from the changing position of the heart in the thoracic cavity that is associated mainly with aging but also with disease. At a younger age, the heart is more vertically positioned, with a smaller "diaphragmatic" part and a larger "posterior" part.

With aging and in pulmonary disease, the heart assumes a more horizontal position, and the apex is more laterally located; as a result, the contact area with the diaphragm is larger, and the "posterior" face of the heart is more "inferior." Clearly, the confusion in nomenclature stems from definitions, which are based on either external references, body anatomy, or cardiac anatomy. A good example is a comparison of echo with angiography. Echo adapts the acoustic window to obtain a standard view of the heart and from there defines the different regions; angio uses a standard external positioning of the x-ray tubes and defines regions from the projection boundaries thus obtained.

CMR provides an unlimited choice of image planes; one can therefore choose standardized two-dimensional (2D) slices of the heart (e.g., two-chamber, four-chamber, short axis slices) and use intrinsic cardiac anatomy (insertion of right ventricle, papillary muscles) as the reference for naming the different regions. When standard transversal, sagittal, or frontal views are used, the same problems encountered with angio arise, and one has to be aware of the impact of differing positions of the heart in the thorax on naming the surfaces and regions.

On the other hand, because of its large field of view, CMR is extremely well suited to depict the relationship of the heart to the surrounding structures and to define masses (i.e., tumors) extending from the surrounding area into the heart or vice versa.

CIRCULATION

The right side of the heart accepts desaturated blood from the body through the inferior and superior vena cava and from the heart itself through the coronary sinus and pumps it through the pulmonary circulation. The left side of the heart receives oxygenated blood from the four pulmonary veins and pumps it into the aorta, from where it is distributed through the systemic circulation to the entire body.

ATRIA

Blood is continuously received in the thin-walled, muscular atria. During systole, when the atrioventricular valves are closed, the atria have a reservoir function and, during fast-filling and diastasis, they function as conduits. Only during atrial contraction do they have an active, boosting function, optimizing ventricular filling. Because no valves are present at the entrance of the veins into the atria, some retrograde blood flow occurs at the time of atrial contraction.

Only the inflow regions of the atria are smooth; the auricula and the anterior wall are muscular and have muscle bundles called the *pectinate muscles*. Several other structures can be recognized, mainly in the right atrium. The origin of the inferior vena cava (IVC) is delineated by the Eustachian valve, which is intended to direct the blood from the IVC toward the interatrial septum, where it crossed the foramen ovale in the prenatal circulation. After birth (and the subsequent normal closure of the foramen ovale, which remains as a depression on the interatrial septum) this flow deviation persists, often with some acceleration and turbulence. Higher in the atrium, but continuous with the Eustachian valve, the Chiari network spans the atrium with small chords that can be mistaken for thrombi or vegetations. On the posterior surface of the atrium, the *crista terminalis* delineates the smooth inlet portion of the right atrium from the highly trabecular auriculam and can sometimes be very prominent and mistaken for an abnormal structure.

The left atrium (LA) receives the four pulmonary veins and has an appendage with a smaller orifice than that in the RA. The LA appendage may contain thrombi, as in the case of atrial fibrillation, and can be the origin of thrombotic cerebral or peripheral disease.

CMR can accurately identify the veins emptying in the atria and abnormal pulmonary right venous return to the RA or to the superior vena cava. Stenosis of the pulmonary veins (after ablation for atrial fibrillation) is common and can be quantified, both morphologically and by flow measurements. Flow in the pulmonary veins, used to analyze diastolic function, can be easily obtained, but optimal temporal resolution is required. Abnormal structures or masses seen or suspected on echocardiography can be identified as normal anatomic variants or true thrombi or tumors.

VALVES

During diastole, blood flows from the atria into the ventricles through the mitral and tricuspid valves: the mitral valve, resembling a bishop's miter, has a larger anterior and smaller posterior leaflet; each leaflet is a flexible, thin sheath of connective tissue that is firmly attached to the mitral valve annulus. This annulus has the shape of a horseshoe, is flexible, does not lie in one plane, and changes shape during the cardiac cycle. On the right side, the tricuspid valve has three leaflets (anterior, posterior, and septal) that differ in size and shape; therefore, this valve is difficult to evaluate morpho-

logically because it can never be captured in one plane. The mitral and tricuspid valves are suspended in the ventricle by the *chordae tendineae*. These are thin, tendinous structures, connecting the free edges but also some neighboring parts of the valves to the papillary muscles, which are elongated protrusions of the muscular wall of the ventricles. Contraction of the papillary muscles during systole prevents the atrioventricular valves from prolapsing into the atria as pressure rises in the ventricles.

During systole, blood is expelled from the ventricles through the aortic and pulmonary semilunar valves into the aorta and pulmonary artery, respectively. Both the aortic valve and the pulmonary valve are tricuspid, consisting of three pocketlike cusps that are freely suspended in the valve ring.

With regular CMR, it is difficult to image the thin, fast-moving valve structures, but newer techniques, also involving valve tracking, provide an accurate visualization of valve leaflets and openings and permit the direct quantification of a stenotic valve area. However, structures with fast, irregular, or erratic movements, such as endocarditis lesions, can be missed by the average CMR images.

VENTRICLES

The major difference between the left and right sides of the heart is the difference in load level: the pulmonary circulation is a short, low-pressure system that works at a peak of 25 mm Hg, whereas the left side of the heart operates at a level of up to 125 mm Hg and drives a longer circuit. This difference has major structural consequences; the wall of the right side of the heart is thinner than that of the left side (2 to 3 mm versus 9 mm). The purpose of this difference is to normalize wall tension and the tension on the myocardial fibers in the wall (Fig. 4.2).

Tension is difficult to measure or calculate, but it is roughly directly proportional to the pressure in the cavity and the diameter of the cavity and inversely proportional to the thickness of the wall. Other factors, such as the shape of the ventricle and the curvature, also play a role: the more curved, the lower the tension; the flatter the surface, the higher the tension.

A major consequence of the structural difference between the ventricles is the way in which they eject blood. The left

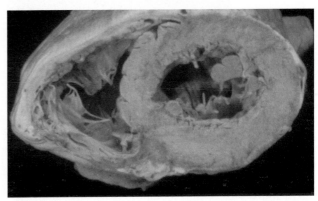

Figure 4.2. Transverse section through the left and right ventricles.

ventricle must overcome a larger afterload, and pressure in the cavity must increase to aortic pressure before ejection can start; the former is accomplished mainly by the contraction of fibers running circumferentially (in the midportion of the wall) and the latter by contraction of more obliquely oriented fibers, which leads to thickening, longitudinal shortening, and inward motion of the endocardium and ejection. On the right side, the pressure that must be overcome is lower; therefore, ejection starts earlier (the pulmonary valve opens before the aortic valve) and is mainly accomplished by segmental shortening (mostly in the long axis) of the crescent shaped ventricle rather than by wall thickening. Because the resistance to ejection is lower, the contraction continues for a longer time, and the pulmonary valve closes after the aortic valve.

CMR can image both ventricles in detail, and the steady-state free precession (SSFP) sequences show the marked intraventricular trabeculation. Because the entire ventricle can be imaged with a stack of short-axis slices, ventricular mass and volume can be derived from the epicardial and endocardial contours. For mass calculations, the trabeculation and papillary muscles are included in the myocardial volume; for functional measurements (wall thickening), they are excluded. Volume and mass measurements are accurate and reproducible and can be used for the follow-up of individual patients. When both end-diastolic and end-systolic images are acquired, wall thickening, stroke volume, cardiac output, and ejection fraction can be calculated. Some difficulties arise at the ventricular apex and base as a result of tapering of the wall and the erroneous inclusion of some atrial volume secondary to long-axis shortening during ejection; this can be avoided by combining short- with long-axis images.

MYOFIBER STRUCTURE

As alluded to earlier, the myofiber structure in the wall of the ventricles is intricate. Although some layers can be recognized in the right ventricle, they are most prominent in the left ventricle. The midlayer is mostly circumferential (circular in short-axis views), whereas the more epicardial and endocardial layers are obliquely oriented but in an oppo-

site sense: when the ventricle is viewed with the base at the top, the epicardial fibers run from base left to apex right, the endocardial fibers in just the opposite direction and, at the cavity surface, several bundles run completely along the long axis of the ventricle (Fig. 4.3).

The consequence of this changing fiber orientation is that fibers at the epicardium and endocardium are at nearly right angles to each other and will show an interaction or tethering; also, when the oblique fibers contract, the ventricle exhibits a twisting motion or torsion, which contributes to the efficiency of ejection. A physical effect of LV torsion is elevation and motion of the apex toward the chest wall, which can be felt as the apical impulse or apex beat; finally, long-axis shortening during systole, produced by oblique and longitudinal fibers, causes the base to move toward the apex, which is nearly stationary because of the fixation of the pericardium to the diaphragm (this fixation is partially lost after the pericardium has been opened, i.e., after cardiac surgery). As a result, when a short-axis slice of the left ventricle is imaged near the base, different parts of myocardium are visualized at end-diastole versus end-systole so that erroneous calculations of segmental shortening and thickening of the wall are possible.

Although diffusion imaging can identify local fiber orientation, in vivo is difficult because of the concomitant overall motion of the heart. On normal CMR images, the ventricular wall is seen as a solid, homogeneous structure. To visualize the different components of myocardial deformation, which ensue from the variable fiber orientation (i.e., circumferential, radial, and longitudinal deformation as well as shearing or twisting), a marking or tagging technique must be used.

COLLAGEN MATRIX

The myocardium also has a "scaffold" structure, the fibrous skeleton, consisting of a network of collagen and elastin fibers. This fibrous skeleton supports the myofibers and transmits force throughout the myocardium. Some regions are thicker, i.e., at the valvular rings and where the myocardium attaches to the great vessels. Because the fibrous skeleton is not electrically excitable, the ring plane, joining the

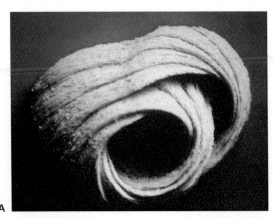
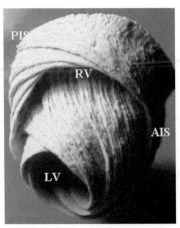

Figure 4.3. Dissection of myofiber layers (Torrent-Guasp). AIS, anterior insertion septum; LV, left ventricle; PIS, posterior insertion septum; RV, right ventricle.

atrioventricular valves, provides a barrier to electrical conduction, which can be passed only at the atrioventricular node.

Because of its specific MR characteristics, the collagen skeleton at the valve plane can be easily identified.

PERICARDIUM

The pericardium is a thin, fibrous structure that surrounds the entire heart, except at the entry and exit of the great vessels. It consists of two layers, one adhering to the outer surface of the heart, and another in contact with lungs and other surrounding tissues. The former, the visceral serous layer, is an integral part of the heart wall. The latter consists of a fibrous part and the parietal serous layer. The fibrous part is made of tough, dense connective tissue and anchors the heart to surrounding structures, i.e., the diaphragm and the great vessels. Although the pericardium is stretchable, it resists large, sudden increases in cardiac volume; when the volume increase is slow, the pericardium will grow to accommodate the enlarged content.

The parietal serous layer lines the internal surface of the fibrous pericardium and is continuous with the visceral layer as it folds over where the pericardium is attached to the great vessels. The two serous layers are separated by a small amount of lubricating fluid, which accommodates the twisting and shortening movements of the heart during contraction and relaxation. Epicardial and pericardial fat are present in differing amounts, depending on an individual's constitution. It is found mostly in the atrioventricular and interventricular grooves, containing the epicardial vessels.

Increased amounts of epicardial fat are often mistaken for a pericardial effusion on echocardiography, which is readily recognized on CMR. Pericardial thickening (>4 mm) can cause constrictive pericarditis, a clinical entity difficult to diagnose. CMR can easily measure this pericardial thickness; this needs to be done at various locations because thickening and constriction can be confined to one ventricle; on the other, a normal pericardial thickness does not exclude constriction because a thin pericardium can also be excessively stiff.

INTERVENTRICULAR DEPENDENCE

Because of the presence of the constraining pericardium and the fact that they share the interventricular and interatrial septum, the right and left sides of the heart show a great deal of interdependence in pathologic circumstances but also in cases of (sudden) ventricular enlargement and in healthy persons. The lower pressure and thinner wall of the right side of the heart make it more vulnerable to compressive forces, but the interdependence between the ventricles works both ways. When filling increases on the right side, as during inspiration, less filling occurs on the left side; in addition, pooling of blood in the pulmonary circulation decreases, filling pressures in the left side of the heart. The reverse occurs during expiration, further augmented by the increase in intrathoracic pressure, increasing LV afterload. Interdependence is increased when ventricular volumes are in-

creased (dilated cardiomyopathies) or when the pericardium is more resistant to stretch (stiffer pericardium of constrictive pericarditis or increased intrapericardial pressure of pericardial effusion and tamponade). Pressures in the cavity should always be referred to the pressure in the pericardium which, in normal circumstances, is about the same as pleural pressure (0 to 2 mm Hg) and becomes negative during inspiration. In pathologic conditions, however, intracavitary pressure can be significantly increased by elevated intrapericardial pressure or effective pericardial resistance. Because this extra pressure is "felt" inside the heart only and not in the supplying veins, there is a resistance to filling; also, during some phases of the cardiac cycle when the pressure drops in the atria and in the (right) ventricle, pericardial pressure can become higher than intracavitary pressure, so that collapse of the cavity ensues.

Another example of the major impact of the pericardium on interventricular dependence is the change in regional motion that occurs after cardiac surgery, in which the pericardium was opened. The motion of the interventricular septum can be changed for months afterward, although thickening and intrinsic contractility are unhampered. This is a consequence of the changed interaction between the left and right ventricles after removal of the constraints of an otherwise normal pericardium, whereby the left ventricle shows a more eccentric contraction, and the interventricular septum is nearly immobile in an external reference system. If one were to reposition the images to fix the center of the left ventricle on the screen, contraction would look more normal, but the right ventricle would tend to move outward.

The abnormal motion of the pericardium with respiration, which is a discerning sign in the differential diagnosis between restrictive cardiomyopathy and constrictive pericarditis, can be well observed and quantified with CMR. The newer, fast imaging techniques allow the identification of the typical morphologic and flow (velocity encoding) changes with the different phases of the respiration. The specific causes of pericardial constriction, such as pericardial thickening, accumulation of fluid, blood, tumor material, or thrombi in the pericardium, can be identified.

ENDOCARDIUM

The endocardium covers the entire inner surface of the heart and valves and has a large surface area because of the extensive trabeculation in both ventricles. Only the subaortic septal region of the LV is completely smooth. The function of the endocardium is still under investigation, but alterations mainly to the relaxation phase have been shown. The endocardium also covers the valves and is continuous with the endothelial lining of the blood vessels as they enter or leave the heart.

Thickening of the endocardium, as in endomyocardial fibrosis, can be well visualized.

CONDUCTION SYSTEM

The conduction system of the heart consists of specialized, spontaneously active cells and a conduction system. The trigger cells are concentrated in specific areas (the sinoatrial node and the atrioventricular node), but impulses can originate along the conduction system; the intrinsic frequency of these cells, however, decreases from the sinoatrial node to the atrioventricular (AV) node to the His bundle and further in the subendocardial Purkinje system. In normal circumstances, the sinoatrial node is the driving pacemaker of the heart at an average pace of 60 to 70 beats per minute. This cardiac frequency is the result of a balance between parasympathetic and orthosympathetic tone which, at rest, is shifted toward parasympathetic (the intrinsic rate of the sinoatrial node is about 100 beats per minute).

The sinoatrial node is located in the posterior wall of the right atrium just inferior to the entrance of the superior vena cava. From the sinoatrial node, the impulses spread through the gap junctions between myocytes over both atria, activating atrial muscle and initiating atrial contraction. The impulse then reaches the AV node, in the inferior part of the interatrial septum, where it slows for optimal timing and coordination between atrial and ventricular contraction (atrioventricular time delay is about 150 milliseconds). From there, the impulse runs through the His bundle and is conducted to the left and right ventricles over the bundle branches and, finally, the Purkinje fibers. Because the course of the latter is subendocardially, the impulse must spread through the thick, left ventricular wall; it does so preferentially along the fiber bundles, which have an inward trajectory or imbrication angle and ultimately reach the subepicardial myocardial layers. The time between the onset of activation at the sinoatrial node and the activation of the last ventricular myocyte takes about 220 milliseconds in the normal heart. The cells that are activated last have the shortest action potential and are therefore inactivated first. The activation front, therefore, runs from endocardium to epicardium and the inactivation front from epicardium to endocardium, so that a T wave has the same orientation as the QRS complex on the surface electrocardiogram (ECG). Consequently, contraction starts at the endocardium and moves to the epicardium, but the epicardium relaxes first. In addition to this local inhomogeneity of activation and inactivation, the spread of the impulse over the ventricle—reaching the septum first, traveling toward the apex and free wall, and arriving at the basal parts latest—causes an inhomogeneity in contraction and relaxation, with respect to both timing and extent. This comes on top of the regional inhomogeneity of contraction because of differences in local loading, secondary to variations in wall thickness and curvature.

A fairly high degree of temporal and spatial resolutions is required to fully appreciate this inhomogeneity, but it should not be mistaken for abnormalities of conduction (bundle branch block) or contraction (caused by ischemia, hypertrophy, or loading).

Knowledge of the microscopic and macroscopic anatomy of the heart is important to understand the mechanics of the heart. A technique like CMR can contribute to a better characterization of cardiac anatomy by providing in vivo images with a high level of spatial resolution and nearly "pathologic" characterization. Imaging of the cavity and wall provides detailed information on volumes, mass, and global and regional deformation; it also provides quantitative information on shape and curvature, which make possible a better evaluation of local loading conditions. This knowledge of loading is needed to derive intrinsic contractility or true systolic function from measurements of deformation.

CONTRACTION AND RELAXATION

INTRODUCTION

Like skeletal muscle, cardiac muscle is striated, and the sliding of the myofilaments generates force and shortening. In contrast to the long, multinucleate fibers of skeletal muscle, the cardiac cells are short, wide, branched, and interconnected with one or two nuclei. A loose, connective tissue or endomysium surrounding the cells connects them to one another and to the fibrous skeleton of the heart. Whereas skeletal muscle fibers are structurally and functionally independent, cardiac cells are interlocked by intercalated disks, containing desmosomes and gap junctions; the cells are firmly attached to one another, and electrical impulses can be easily transmitted from one cell to adjacent cells. Once stimulated, the heart contracts as a unit, although in sequence, as the electrical impulse is spread through the conduction system and along the myocytes. The entire myocardium thus behaves as a large functional syncytium, structured in bundles and sheets and wrapped around the ventricles in a figure-eight configuration; a bundle originating at the mitral valve ring can be followed at the epicardium as it runs obliquely over the heart and penetrates the wall to turn on itself at the apical dimple, and it returns as an endocardial bundle, running again obliquely but at about 90 degrees to the epicardial part of its trajectory, and finally inserts again at the valve ring. Some investigators believe that the entire heart, including left and right ventricles, can be unwrapped in a single continuous bundle, which is single-coiled for the right ventricle and double-coiled for the left ventricle.

MYOCYTES

Large mitochondria are abundantly present in the myocardial cells because these cells must operate aerobically nearly exclusively. On the other hand, cardiac myocytes can switch readily from burning carbohydrates to fats and even lactic acid; lack of oxygen, not lack of nutrients, is therefore the main cause of problems.

The myofilaments are typically organized in sarcomeres. They consist of thin actin filaments and thick myosin filaments. The head region of the myosin filament can attach to the actin and generate shortening of the sarcomere (Fig. 4.4). Calcium is needed for this contraction.

Calcium homeostasis is governed by sarcolemmal and sarcoplasmic reticular transport (Fig. 4.5). Because of the long, absolute refractory period, which is nearly as long as the contraction itself, cardiac myocytes cannot be tetanized.

CARDIAC CYCLE

As a result of the cyclic increase and decrease in intracellular calcium, the myocytes and the myocardial syncytium exhibit a cycle of contraction and relaxation. The cardiac cycle can be described in terms of changes in blood volume and pressure and is divided into phases related to the opening and closing of the valves (Fig. 4.6).

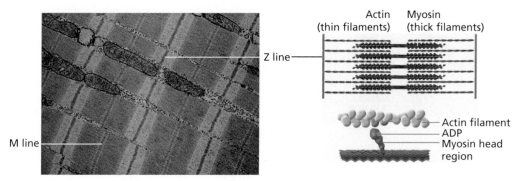

Figure 4.4. Sarcomeres and their actin and myosin components.

With the onset of ventricular contraction, pressure increases in the cavity, and the atrioventricular valves are forced to close. Because the impulse through the Purkinje system is transmitted to the papillary muscles before the wall itself, these papillary muscles contract first and prevent the atrioventricular valves from bulging under the rising ventricular pressure. During the subsequent isovolumic contraction phase, in which both the atrioventricular and ventriculoarterial, semilunar valves are closed, pressure in the ventricular cavities rises to equal that in the aorta and pulmonary artery. Parts of the ventricles contract and shorten during this phase, thereby changing the shape of the ventricle and displacing blood in the cavity, mainly from the apical region toward the outflow tract in preparation for the subsequent ejection. As soon as the pressure in the cavity exceeds the one in the connecting artery, the semilunar valve opens, and blood is accelerated and ejected. Although the ventricles start to relax after about 100 milliseconds (i.e., after one third to one half

of the ejection phase has elapsed), flow is maintained because of inertia and compliance of the aorta (Windkessel effect). Relaxation of the ventricle is accompanied by a decrease of ventricular pressure to below aortic pressure. Pressure in the ventricle drops further, and flow reverses briefly; consequently, the semilunar valve closes, and the isovolumic relaxation phase starts. Again, this phase is characterized not only by a decrease in pressure but also by specific mechanical events: untwisting of the left ventricle occurs for the largest part during this phase, together with some longitudinal lengthening. Consequently, the mitral ring starts to move upward, engulfing blood of the left atrium. The mitral valve, which was flattened toward the atrium during the high-pressure phase, returns to a more pointed configuration, and blood is shifted from the inflow region toward the apex. These phenomena prepare the ventricle for an efficient subsequent filling. As soon as the ventricle, through its active relaxation and the release of restoring forces, lowers its pres-

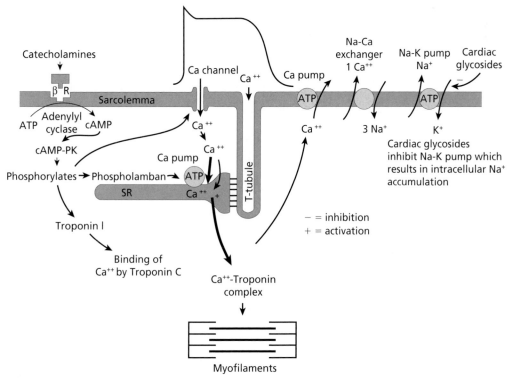

Figure 4.5. Schematic of calcium homeostasis.

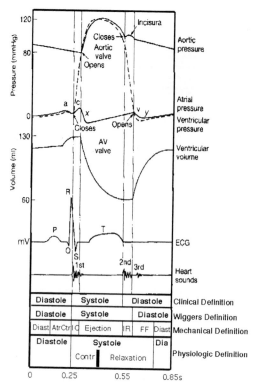

Figure 4.6. The cardiac cycle, divided in phases, according to different definitions.

sure below the level of atrial pressure, the atrioventricular valves open, and fast, active filling follows. The "active" character of early filling is proven by the continuous drop of ventricular pressure, even while the ventricle starts to fill, which is incompatible with a passive filling phenomenon. After relaxation is completed, filling continues, but ventricular pressure now concomitantly rises. Flow is dependent on inertia during this passive diastasis period. Upon electrical activation of the atria, they contract and further optimize ventricular filling by adding a final blood volume.

In normal resting conditions at a heart rate of 60 beats per minute, the cardiac cycle takes 1,000 milliseconds. Isovolumic contraction takes about 30 milliseconds; ejection, 260 milliseconds; isovolumic relaxation, 60 milliseconds; and filling the remaining, 650 milliseconds. When the heart rate and contractility increase, mainly the filling period is shortened; therefore, in normal circumstances, the diastolic or filling function is more stressed during dynamic exercise than the systolic function.

CMR is especially appropriate to evaluate the global and regional changes in shape and morphology of the ventricles during systole and early diastole. When combined with tagging, quantifying these deformations and studying the underlying mechanisms of ejection and filling is possible. Because long-axis shortening is an important component of the efficient ejection of blood, obtaining this parameter should be a routine measurement in the evaluation of systolic function.

HEART SOUNDS

Closure of the atrioventricular and semilunar valves is audible through the chest wall on auscultation. The first heart

sound is caused by the nearly simultaneous closure of the atrioventricular valves. The second heart sound represents closure of the semilunar valves, with aortic valve closure preceding pulmonary valve closure. With respiration and because of ventricular interdependence, an audible difference occurs in the separation between the aortic and pulmonary components of the second heart sound: During inspiration, increased filling of the right side of the heart, prolonged ejection, and delayed pulmonary closure result in a wider splitting of the second heart sound. The third heart sound is caused by sudden deceleration of the inflowing blood during early filling, either by a very fast inflow (young, healthy individuals) or by a decreased compliance of the left ventricle (pathologic S3). The fourth heart sound occurs during atrial contraction on the same basis in cases of a decreased compliance. Finally, an opening snap refers to the abbreviated opening of a stenotic mitral (or tricuspid) valve.

Heart sounds have been used extensively to identify the different periods of the cardiac cycle. As an alternative, CMR can register valve openings and closures to obtain the same information, provided that the temporal resolution is high enough (minimally 25 milliseconds).

LOADING AND CONTRACTILITY AS DETERMINANTS OF SYSTOLIC AND DIASTOLIC FUNCTION

All imaging techniques attempt to optimally characterize motion and deformation of the heart. To move from motion to function or performance, several factors must be taken into account.

INTRINSIC DEFORMATION

Whole body motion of the myocardium (i.e., swinging or rotation) in the thoracic cavity must be "subtracted" to obtain intrinsic motion or deformation. In other words, myocardial deformation must be measured in a cardiac coordinate system (Fig. 4.7). When motion and deformation are referenced to the heart itself—that is, when markers or references are

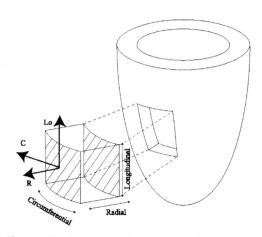

Figure 4.7. Definition of cardiac coordinate system.

used that are part of the cardiac structure itself—these whole body motions are excluded. Similarly, when deformation of the myocardial wall must be quantified, a local cardiac coordinate system must be adopted: usually, a perpendicular coordinate system is used, in which one axis points outward, perpendicular to the surface of the heart (radial axis R), one is aligned to the short axis or circumference (circumferential axis C), and the last one is perpendicular to the other two axes and is aligned to the long axis of the ventricle (longitudinal axis L). At each site of the left ventricle, such a coordinate system would have other orientations when viewed from the outside; for example, it would point a little downward near the apex to account for the tapering of the wall in this region.

Radial deformation will then quantify everywhere true three-dimensional (3D) thickening and can be compared from region to region. If thickening is calculated from a simple short axis, this would give falsely high values near the apex as a result of the oblique cut through the wall. Although in most instances, simple calculations of deformation will suffice for a given clinical indication, the limitations of not using true, oblique cuts and real 3D calculations of deformation must be remembered. Only by using a marker system (i.e., myocardial tagging) can all deformation components (normal and shear strains) be quantified in such a local cardiac coordinate system. One of these shear strains is the torsion motion of the ventricle, which has an important function in equalizing fiber load and optimizing LV performance, transforming 18% of fiber shortening into an ejection fraction of 70%. This can be accomplished, possibly, with only an amplification mechanism in which the different layers of the LV myocardium work together and influence each other to enhance thickening in the endocardial part of the wall (endocardial thickening can exceed 70%, whereas epicardial thickening is only 20%).

CMR is the only imaging technique capable of true 3D imaging of the heart in clinical routine. With a combination of short- and long-axis information, a reliable and accurate evaluation of global and regional parameters is feasible. Full 3D visualization is not usually required in clinical routine, but the parameters can be extracted, if needed. Further evolution of automated contouring, segmentation, and reconstruction could bring this into the clinical realm and provide further useful information for the evaluation and follow-up of individual patients in several cardiac conditions, i.e., ischemic heart disease, valvular, and dilated cardiomyopathies. Multislice CT has similar capabilities but involves contrast and radiation. Three-dimensional echocardiography has recently undergone some major technical advances, but image quality remains suboptimal in a significant proportion of patients.

LOADING

Whichever technique is used, still only deformation is quantified, and whatever the level of sophistication, deformation is only half of the contractility equation. The other part is load. The higher the load, the lower the deformation will be for a given degree of contractility. Conversely, a small deformation (low ejection fraction or thickening) can be caused by decreased contractility or high loading conditions

or both. In most cases, we are interested in intrinsic contractility to make decisions on therapy and revascularization procedures. Thus, to be able to at least judge and qualitatively evaluate the loading conditions is important, because quantifying them has proved very difficult.

Load is usually divided into preload and afterload, although the muscle feels only one load at each instant (Fig. 4.8). Load has several components, dependent on the size and shape of the ventricle. Although muscle load is what we are really interested in, tension at the myofiber level is difficult to obtain. We therefore try to infer tension in the wall from a simplification of Laplace's law: tension in the wall increases with a larger cavity size and a thinner wall for a given pressure.

Load during ejection is mainly dependent on the level of blood pressure. Aortic stenotic disease is another obvious cause of increased systolic load. Another is dilatation without adequate compensatory hypertrophy or wall thinning, as in nontransmural myocardial infarction. Changes in the shape of the ventricle can also increase wall tension: a rounder ventricle, in comparison with a more ellipsoidal normal ventricle, will have a higher load at the same pressure. In physiologic circumstances (intermittent volume or pressure load), an increase of the cavity size (endurance athletes) is compensated for by an adequate hypertrophy, which consists of myofiber hypertrophy. In contrast to this is pathologic enlargement, where hypertrophy is inadequate and/or consists of both myofiber hypertrophy (to a smaller extent) and hypertrophy of the collagen matrix with fibrosis. Fewer muscle fibers must carry an increased load that leads to a negative, vicious circle with further dilatation and, ultimately, cardiac failure.

CMR is uniquely appropriate to measure the different components of loading: cavity size, wall thickness, shape, and wall curvature. Although no absolute wall tension can be calculated, CMR thus far provides the best approximation that can be obtained.

During filling, the load is determined by the pressure difference between atrium and ventricle, but resistance to flow by the mitral valve (including the subvalvular apparatus, mitral ring, and so forth) and resistance to filling by the left ventricle also determine the ultimate filling dynamics. The resistance to filling by the LV depends on the rate of myocar-

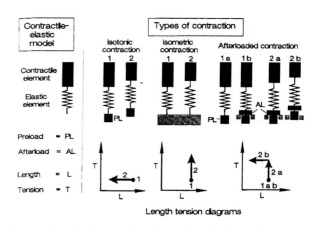

Figure 4.8. Definition of preloaded and afterloaded contractions.

dial relaxation and on the stiffness of the myocardium. The less compliant the myocardium, the more difficult it is to fill the ventricle, the higher the filling pressures, and the lower the filling volume.

Filling dynamics can be addressed by measuring the duration of isovolumic relaxation, the mitral inflow pattern, the pulmonary vein flow, and the dimensions of atrium and ventricle, beside color M-mode propagation and myocardial velocity imaging (Fig. 4.9). In healthy, young individuals, LV compliance is high and relaxation is fast, so that a large, early filling volume and velocity and a smaller volume and velocity on atrial contraction are seen. With aging, filling pressures may drop, and/or relaxation may slow, so that isovolumic relaxation is prolonged and early filling volume and velocity are lower; in compensation atrial filling increases, which is possible because the compliance of the ventricle is still normal. With hypertrophy caused by systolic overload (hypertension, aortic valve disease), a similar pattern develops but mainly as a result of prolonged ejection with a subsequent slowed relaxation. When the changes in the myocardium lead to a decreased compliance (fibrosis), filling

pressures increase, thereby shortening the isovolumic relaxation time and increasing early filling velocity; because resistance to filling is higher at larger volumes (at atrial contraction after early filling), the volume/velocity on atrial contraction drops, and the pattern resembles the normal values. This is called "pseudo-normalization." In the early stages of disease, this pattern can be reversed to a "slowed relaxation, aging" pattern by decreasing the filling pressure, such as during a Valsalva maneuver. In the final stage of restrictive disease, such an intervention will not change the filling pattern any more, and this is designated as "irreversible," and treatment will have less effect.

Such a restrictive syndrome can be the final stage of various cardiac abnormalities, i.e., ischemic heart disease, dilated cardiomyopathy, and hypertrophic heart disease (hypertension). It also exists in primary restrictive cardiomyopathies that often involve some infiltrative abnormality (amyloidosis, metabolic abnormalities). The same pattern, finally, can be found in constrictive pericarditis, where the stiff pericardium does not allow any filling during the last phase of diastole (atrial contraction).

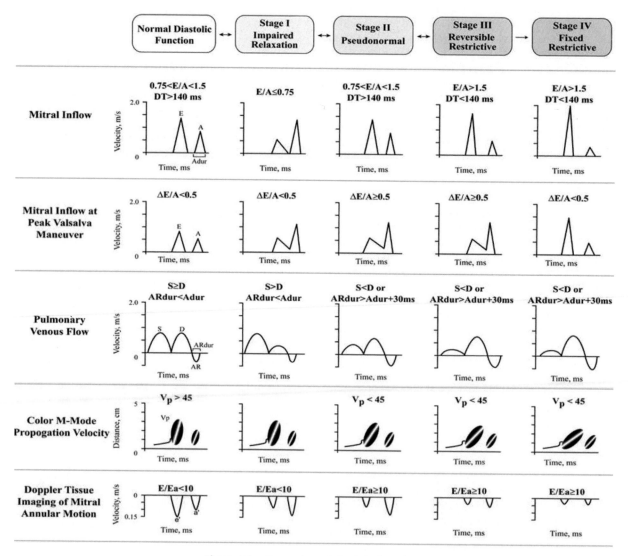

Figure 4.9. Parameters of diastolic function.

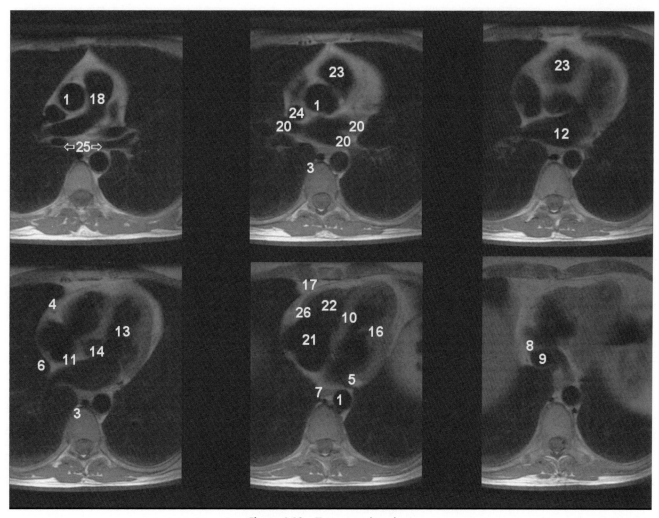

Figure 4.16. Transverse imaging.

vulnerability to ischemia. Similarly, after total coronary occlusion, infarcts expand in a wave front from the endocardium to the epicardium, with a greater expanse seen in the subendocardium.

CMR can visualize regional perfusion using first-pass techniques after contrast injection and provide qualitative and semiquantitative analyses. The high spatial resolution permits study of subendocardial versus subepicardial perfusion (this is impossible with SPECT imaging for the moment) and the ratio between both, which is a more sensitive parameter for ischemic problems. Like most other techniques (including nuclear), CMR does not really measure perfusion but rather contrast content of the tissue, and special algorithms are needed to obtain quantitative flow in milliliters per gram of tissue.

VENTRICULOARTERIAL COUPLING

The blood that is ejected by the left ventricle must be "accepted" by the aorta. Similarly, as the resistance to flow in the aorta is the afterload for the ventricle, the stroke volume is the input function for the vasculature. If a system is to be efficient, input and output must be optimally matched, that is, ventriculoarterial coupling must be fine-tuned, and an equilibrium situation must be reached. If not, performance of the system will be less than optimal, and more energy will be spent to obtain the same resulting combination of flow and pressure: cardiac output or stroke volume and blood pressure. Although these concepts are not widely used clinically, they can clarify ventricular dysfunction in some cases and also help to direct therapy (Fig. 4.15).

It is easiest to consider equilibrium as the point where two performance lines (of ventricle and aorta) cross on a diagram of pressure and LV stroke volume. For the ventricle, the relation is inverse. The higher the pressure (afterload), the lower the stroke volume; for the arterial system, the relation is direct: the more blood entering the aorta, the greater the rise in pressure. Depending on ventricular performance and arterial compliance, the lines can be more or less steep, but equilibrium is where they cross. At that point, the transmission of energy is most efficient.

VALVULAR FUNCTION

The function of the valves is to direct the blood flow through the circulation. They can be found in the heart and veins,

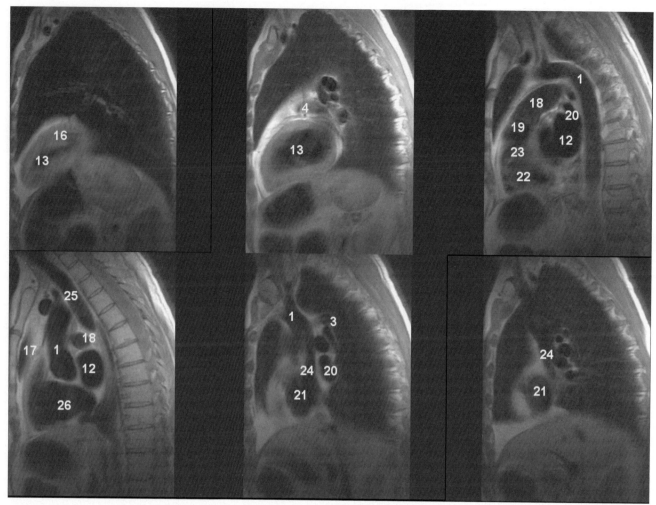

Figure 4.17. Sagittal imaging.

and dysfunction is a major cause of symptoms and disease. In the heart, the atrioventricular and the semilunar valves are quite different in structure, but they both must resist a high-pressure gradient in closed position, while allowing opening and high-volume flow in low-gradient conditions. Problems can be caused by an increased resistance to flow (stenosis) or a leakage (insufficiency). Quantification of these disorders is quite difficult, but very important when decisions must be made regarding prognosis, therapy, and timing of intervention.

STENOSIS

An evaluation of the severity of stenosis can be based on the stenotic area, gradient across the valve, or resistance to flow. A stenotic area can be measured directly with an imaging technique that is capable of choosing an image plane, perpendicular to the valve, and tracking valvular through-plane motion. *CMR has such capabilities and is the most reliable technique to perform such direct measurements.* The stenotic area can also be derived from gradient measurements and the continuity equation. In echo-Doppler, this technique is commonly used. The velocity at one site is measured together with the area at that same site, as well as the

velocity at the stenotic site. Because the velocity integral times the area equals flow volume, and the flow at two sites of a continuous circuit must be the same, the one unknown—which is the stenotic area—can be computed. With echo-Doppler, the peak stenotic velocity is measured with continuous-wave Doppler that captures the highest velocities along the trajectory, wherever they occur. This point, also called the *vena contracta,* is usually situated a little beyond the physically smallest opening because the flow lines of a stenotic lesion continue to converge after passing this smallest area. *With CMR, velocity can be measured in-plane and through-plane, but choosing the location where the highest velocity can be obtained is not always easy. Using the void created by dephasing on cine imaging effectively detects the presence of a stenotic lesion but cannot quantify it.*

INSUFFICIENCY

If quantifying stenosis is difficult, this case is even more true for insufficiency. Many techniques have been used in echo-Doppler to quantify insufficiency, but all have significant disadvantages. Regurgitant orifice, fraction, and volume, in addition to semiquantitative grading on color mapping, are all being used. *CMR velocity mapping, especially*

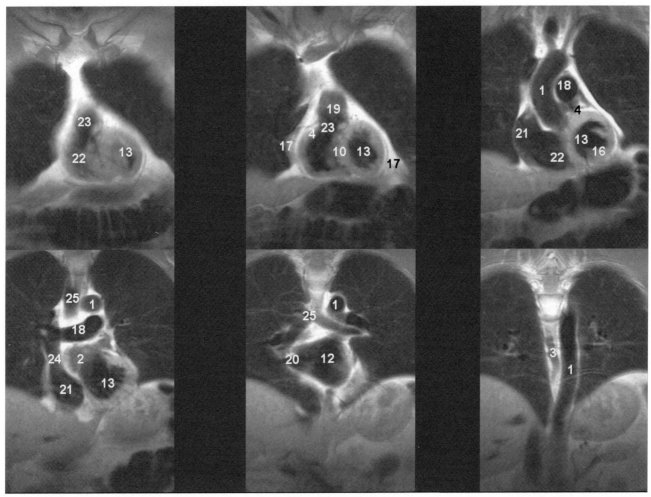

Figure 4.18. Frontal imaging.

when combined with valve tracking, effectively measures antegrade and retrograde flow over the valve, from which the regurgitant fraction can be readily calculated. To find the regurgitant orifice, the maximal gradient velocity must also be measured, and this entails the same difficulties as for a stenotic valve. Overall, CMR is underused for quantification of regurgitant lesions, and even without valve tracking it performs at least as well, if not better, than most echo techniques. Furthermore, the effect of valvular insufficiency on chamber dimensions (atrial and ventricular dilatation in cases of AV valve insufficiency) can be reliably and reproducibly documented, making CMR the technique of choice for individual follow-up of these patients.

FUTURE PERSPECTIVE

Although the insights into physiology and pathophysiology do not develop as fast as CMR itself, the data obtained with this technique have enhanced our understanding in numerous areas, and this positive interaction will continue in the future.

A major aspect where pathophysiology could impact on the clinical use of CMR is the paradigm of ischemic heart disease. At the moment, cardiology focuses on the presence of luminal narrowing of the coronary tree, and treatment is aimed at relief of the stenosis, often irrespective of the impact on flow or flow reserve. It might be more appropriate to first evaluate the presence of impaired flow/flow reserve and to go to noninvasive coronary imaging only in cases where such an abnormality is present. This would require studies looking at prognosis of asymptomatic patients with intermediate coronary lesions but without abnormal flow reserve (as performed for nuclear techniques). The noninvasive, nonradiation character of CMR could position the technique as the optimal tool for evaluation of patients with ischemic heart disease.

APPENDIX: CARDIOVASCULAR MAGNETIC RESONANCE ANATOMY

LIST OF STRUCTURES

Aorta   1
  Aortic valve   2
  Azygos vein   3
  Coronary artery   4

Coronary sinus 5
Crista terminalis 6
Esophagus 7
Eustachian valve 8
Inferior vena cava 9
Interventricular septum 10
Interatrial septum 11
Left atrium 12
Left ventricle 13
Left ventricular outflow tract 14
Mitral valve 15
Papillary muscle 16
Pericardium 17
Pulmonary artery 18
Pulmonary valve 19
Pulmonary vein 20
Right atrium 21
Right ventricle 22
Right ventricular outflow tract 23
Superior vena cava 24

Trachea (branches) 25
Tricuspid valve 26
Transverse imaging (Fig. 4.16)
Sagittal imaging (Fig. 4.17)
Frontal imaging (Fig. 4.18)

SUGGESTED READING

Berne RM, Levy MN. *Cardiovascular Physiology*. 8th ed. St. Louis: Mosby; 2001.

Bers DM. *Excitation-Contraction Coupling and Cardiac Contractile Force*. Boston: Kluwer Academic Publishers; 2001.

Boron WF, Boelpaep EL. *Medical Physiology*. 1st ed. Philadelphia: Saunders; 2003.

Braunwald EM, Zipes DP. *Heart Diseases*. 2nd ed. Philadelphia: Current Medicine; 2001.

McManus BM, ed. *Atlas of cardiovascular pathology*. Philadelphia: Current Science; 2001.

Page E, Fozzard HA, Solaro RJ, eds. *The heart*. New York: Oxford University Press; 2002.

5

Blood Flow Measurements

Håkan Arheden and Freddy Ståhlberg

BACKGROUND

Blood flow is a central physiologic parameter that can be measured, using magnetic resonance (MR) velocity mapping with high accuracy and precision, noninvasively, without ionizing radiation, in any part of the body and at any angle. Under normal physiologic conditions, blood flows with minimal resistance in conducting vessels. Disturbances to normal physiology, such as decreased pumping energy in heart failure, regurgitation in valve disease, increased resistance in stenosis, or rerouting of blood in shunting, can thus be quantified.

HISTORICAL OVERVIEW OF FLOW MEASUREMENTS WITH MAGNETIC RESONANCE IMAGING

Shortly after the first essential discoveries regarding the nuclear magnetic resonance (NMR) phenomenon (1,2), the effect of motion on the NMR signal was described, and the possible use of NMR for motion detection was investigated. Among the pioneers in this field were Suryan (3), who demonstrated a signal-enhancing inflow effect from water flowing through an NMR probe; Bowman and Kudravcev (4), who proposed a method for the construction of an NMR blood flow meter where this phenomenon was used; Singer (5), who proposed a motion induced signal enhancement effect for measurements of blood flow; and Hahn (6), who developed a method for the detection of the motion of seawater using phase dispersion effects. In 1960, Grover and Singer (7) proposed a spin-echo-based method for the measurement of in-vivo blood velocity distributions, while NMR flow meters for the measurement of flow in the extremities using magnetic tagging of protons were developed by Battocletti et al (8). Washout effects, creating an apparent T2 shorter than that for stationary spins were also used early for velocity measurements (9).

After the revolutionary introduction of NMR as an imaging modality (10), a large number of potential methods for the in vivo visualization and quantification of blood flow using magnetic resonance imaging (MRI) emerged. Flow effects were theoretically, as well as experimentally examined, and flow measurement methods with varying degrees of complexity were presented, ranging from straightforward methods, using standard sequences for the visualization of flow-induced signal voids, to quantitative methods requiring specially designed pulse sequences. Among the first to explore the field were Herfkens et al (11), who stated that the information in a conventional MR image was flow-dependent; Grant and Back (12), who showed washout effects in tubes; and Crooks et al (13), who published a signal versus velocity curve obtained with a spin-echo sequence. The possibility of using MRI for studies of obstructions in vessels was pointed out by, among others, Kaufman et al (14) while Singer and Crooks (15), as well as Wehrli (16), who proposed quantitative methods for velocity measurements in vessels, based on wash-in/washout effects. Magnetic tagging methods, often known as bolus tracking or time-of-flight methods, were early proposed for use in MRI by, e.g., Shimizu (17). With respect to flow-induced phase effects on motion, the attenuation in modulus images as a result of phase spread or loss of phase coherence, within the voxel, was investigated by Waluch and Bradley (18), and the so-called even echo rephasing effect was pointed out. Development along another line uses more directly the phase altering properties of motion. Here, the theoretic framework was made by Moran (19), who proposed a method for the creation of velocity images by the addition of flow-sensitive or flow-encoding gradients to a standard pulse sequence. Several quantification methods using this basic idea were rapidly suggested (20,21) and led into clinical application.

As a result of the work outlined above, quantitative flow measurement sequences and evaluation tools have become available on standard MRI scanners, providing the possibility not only to measure velocity and flow, but also to evaluate important physiologic parameters, such as wall shear stress and compliance. Furthermore, increased knowledge concerning flow effects in MR imaging has led to improved image quality in standard imaging because flow-induced image artifacts have been effectively reduced by the use of techniques, such as flow refocusing, respiratory gating, retrospective/prospective ECG-triggering and presaturation.

FLOW MEASUREMENT TECHNIQUES

In general, MR signal acquisition and image reconstruction mathematically requires so-called complex or vectorial treatment. After Fourier transformation in two dimensions of the spatially encoded signal, the reconstructed volume element (voxel) magnetization M_{xy} is obtained as a vector in the transverse (or x, y) plane. M_{xy} can be decomposed into real and imaginary parts according to Figure 5.1. MR images are normally displayed in absolute (modulus) mode; that is, the picture element (pixel) intensity is proportional to the length of the vector. This vector length is dependent on the object

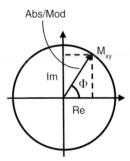

Figure 5.1. Illustration of different types of information in an MR image: The modulus or absolute value is the length of the signal vector, which creates a phase angle φ with the real axis. Components (*Re*) and (*Im*) are the projections of the modulus vector on the real and imaginary axis, respectively.

parameters (e.g., relaxation, flow, diffusion) as well as on acquisition parameters (echo time [TE], repetition time [TR], inversion time [TI], and so forth) and may hence be used for flow estimation.

Also possible is to reconstruct images where the intensity is proportional to the real or imaginary part of the vector or simply to the phase angle φ between M_{xy} and the real axis. The latter type of image is referred to as a *phase image* and can, in principle, be reconstructed after acquisition of all types of pulse sequences. The phase angle is ideally independent of relaxation parameters and is zero in the absence of macroscopic motion. Presence of such motion will give rise to a flow-dependent phase angle, but caution should be taken regarding confounding phase effects introduced by, e.g., nonlinear gradients, eddy currents, and concomitant gradients.

On the basis of the type of image representation that is used, MRI flow measurement techniques are often divided into modulus-based and phase-sensitive techniques, respectively.

MODULUS-BASED TECHNIQUES

Slice-selective pulse sequences using two or more spatially selective RF pulses prior to the sampling of the echo are sensitive to the transport of spins into and out of the excited slice. If the flow has components perpendicular to the imaging slice, the signal will decrease owing to the outflow of spins during the time between RF pulses (washout). On the other hand, for sequences that require repetition, the inflow of nonsaturated spins during the repetition time will increase the magnetization compared with the static, saturated, spins and thus give an increase in signal (wash-in). In a conventional spin-echo sequence, these competing mechanisms make the modulus signal behavior versus velocity biphasic and, possibly, difficult to interpret, although, with a rough knowledge of the velocities involved, the experimental parameters could be adjusted so that one mechanism is dominant. If, however, only one RF pulse is used prior to the sampling of the echo, as in basic gradient-echo sequences, the signal decrease due to washout will not occur, and wash-in effects may give prominent increase of vessel signal. For repeated sequences including multiple RF pulses—such as inversion recovery, fast spin-echo, and fast inversion recovery, as well as in multislice imaging—a complicated relation between velocity and signal is to be expected.

Washout and wash-in effects are predominantly used for qualitative evaluation of flow phenomena, and several clinically useful techniques have been proposed for this purpose. In cardiac applications, "black-blood imaging" based on combined effects of washout phenomena and spin dephasing is used to visualize vessel walls in triggered multislice spin-echo imaging, whereas the inflow effect in gradient-echo imaging forms the contrast basis in time-of-flight MR angiography, as well as in rapid cine imaging of the heart.

Quantifying flow from transport effects reflected in modulus images is possible, if suitable models describing the signal-versus-velocity behavior are applied (16,22–24). However, signal-versus-velocity relations obtained using modulus images are generally nonlinear and influenced by relaxation times, which are difficult to determine accurately in vivo (25). In spite of such methodologic drawbacks, several quantitative methods of flow measurement on the basis of information from modulus images have been proposed. As an example, Matthaei (26) proposed the use of a gradient-echo sequence, assuming a linear signal increase with flow in combination with a calibration made, using an external reference image at a place and time where the velocity was known, e.g., in the aorta at diastole.

An alternative modulus-based method uses so-called bolus tracking (17). Here, a bolus is first labeled or tagged with an RF pulse at a specific position and then observed downstream using a second RF pulse. Bolus tracking, which can be performed as a through-plane as well as an in-plane flow measurement method, is rapid and does not use relaxation time information, although methodologic drawbacks are, e.g., that a minimum velocity is required, that the obtained information is generally not two-dimensional (2D) and that the method is best suited for nonpulsating flow.

PHASE-SENSITIVE TECHNIQUES

Background

As mentioned earlier, reconstruction of images is possible, where the intensity is proportional to the phase angle that the M_{xy} vector describes with the real axis. In MRI, the phase angle is used in the spatial encoding procedure. After the Fourier decoding, ideally the phase information has been translated into position information, and no phase information remains. However, objects that move in a varying magnetic field (e.g., a pulsed gradient field) change their precession frequency and therefore obtain an offset phase angle not removed by the decoding procedure (19). The exact phase behavior for different types of gradients and motion patterns can be calculated, and a very simple linear relationship between constant velocity (so-called first-order motion) and phase angle is predicted by theory as well as confirmed in

experiments. This relationship forms the basis for most of the clinically used flow measurement techniques in MRI. In its most frequent 2D form, the method is known as velocity mapping, phase mapping, or phase contrast technique.

Theory

The Larmour equation states that the precession frequency f of a proton is proportional to the external magnetic field B, where the proportionality constant for protons in the hydrogen nuclei of water is 42.6 MHz/T. Because accumulated phase (ϕ) is proportional to the time integral of frequency, a proton will accumulate a phase shift proportional to the time integral of the magnitude of the magnetic field in each position.

In presence of a linear magnetic field gradient along a direction x, the magnetic field at a position x can be described as $B(x) = B_0 + G_x(t) \times x$, where B_0 is the main magnetic field (T) and $G_x(t)$ is the time-dependent gradient (T/m) along the direction x (m). Hence, the additional phase shift introduced by the gradient can be calculated as

$$\text{Equation 1: } \phi \sim \int G_x(t) \times x(t) \, dt$$

Consequently, application of a gradient will result in an additional phase shift according to the location along this gradient. Now consider application of two consecutive gradients with same duration and magnitude but with opposite sign (Fig. 5.2).

When the first gradient is applied, all stationary protons will accumulate a phase shift determined by their location x according to equation 1. Immediately after the first gradient, the second gradient is applied and, again according to equation 1, all the stationary protons lose their accumulated phase shift and obtain a net phase shift of zero. This procedure is known as refocusing and is used in MRI to prevent gradient-induced signal dephasing along the slice-encoding and the frequency-encoding gradient. However, a proton

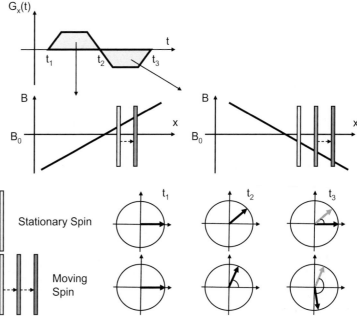

Figure 5.2. Application of two consecutive magnetic gradients with same duration and magnitude but with opposite sign. When the first magnetic gradient is applied, all stationary protons will accumulate a phase shift determined by their location in the magnetic gradient field. Immediately after the first gradient, the second magnetic gradient is applied, and all of the stationary protons lose their accumulated phase shift and obtain a net phase shift of zero. A proton moving along the magnetic field gradients during their execution will experience unequal positive and negative magnetic gradients and, consequently, accumulates a net phase shift ϕ according to the motion.

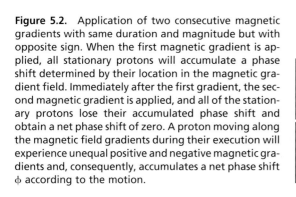

moving along the magnetic field gradients during their execution will experience unequal positive and negative magnetic gradients and, consequently, accumulate a net phase shift φ. In the case of constant velocity v along x, the position of each proton can be written x(t) = v × t, and an additional velocity-dependent phase shift ϕ_v is obtained from equation 1:

$$\text{Equation 2: } \phi_v \sim v \times \int G_x(t) \times t \, dt$$

where the phase shift is proportional to the velocity along the magnetic gradient. Consequently, the phase image can be regarded as a *velocity map*, where the phase shift in each voxel is proportional to velocity with a proportionality constant depending on the time course of the applied gradient in the investigated direction. Theoretically, the phase shift in voxels with stationary tissue should be zero, but additional phase shifts may be caused by many other factors than motion—for example, main magnetic field inhomogeneities, eddy currents, concomitant gradient effects, and local magnetic field gradients induced by magnetic susceptibility variations—but also by specific acquisition strategies, such as asymmetric echo sampling. These problems may be partly overcome by creating an additional phase image using a different set of gradient amplitudes which, in turn, gives a different velocity sensitivity or often no velocity sensitivity at all but with similar nonmotion related phase shift behavior. Subtraction of these two phase images results in a velocity map, ideally showing φ = 0 for stationary voxels.

Basic Sequences and Postprocessing

Magnetic field gradients are present in all types of pulse sequences, and standard sequences usually exhibit some flow dependent phase behavior unless this is specifically prevented by using motion-compensated gradient patterns. However, if flow is to be carefully quantified, additional gradients are applied to maximize the sensitivity for a particular velocity range. Use of the full power of the gradient system to increase phase signal is theoretically possible, while phase noise depends on several factors, such as RF

transmit and receive coil performance and scales with the noise in the magnitude image (27).

Normally, velocity-sensitive and velocity-insensitive phase images are obtained in an interleaved way using two different pulse sequences, and complex voxel-wise subtraction of the two phase images will result in a net phase image where the phase shift is ideally determined only by motion.

Phase-sensitive flow MRI (henceforth denoted *velocity mapping*) is in its simplest form performed in single-slice mode, using two interleaved gradient-echo sequences with different flow sensitivity in one spatial direction (21,28), either through the imaging plane or in the imaging plane. If flow is determined in the through-plane direction, either the slice-selective gradient can be redesigned to create sufficient velocity sensitivity or a bipolar gradient can be added in the slice-selective direction, although at the cost of prolonged echo time. For in-plane measurements, either the frequency encoding or the phase encoding direction is used in a similar way for velocity sensitization.

An important prerequisite for MR velocity mapping of pulsatile motion is synchronization of the sequence execution to the time course of the flow pattern. Two strategies are commonly used for this purpose: prospective ECG-triggering and retrospective gating (29,30). In ECG triggered velocity mapping, sampling of each phase encoding line is triggered by the R-wave in the ECG (Fig. 5.3). The total number of image frames that can be obtained within an R-R interval depends upon the minimum sequence TR and the heart rate of the patient. Typical values for adults are 30 to 40 frames, but the number of frames will, as a rule, be lower in children as a result of a higher heart rate in children than in adults. ECG-triggering involves drawbacks related to an almost certain change of the patient's heart rate during the examination. Hence, it is difficult to obtain an image exactly at end-diastole during which atrial contraction occurs, unless the experiment is performed over two cardiac cycles. Furthermore, additional longitudinal relaxation in the delay time previous to each trigger pulse may lead to increased signal intensity and ghost artifacts in the first frames. These draw-

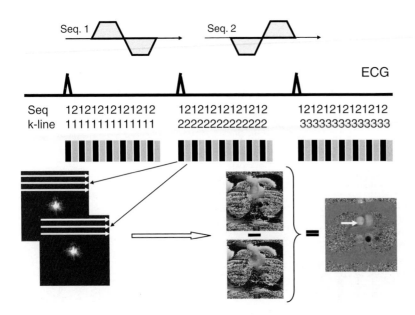

Figure 5.3. Prospectively ECG-triggered velocity mapping with interleaving of two differently velocity-encoded sequences 1 and 2. After collection of a sufficient number of k-space lines for each sequence, pairs of raw data images are obtained for a number of time frames (cardiac phases) in the cardiac cycle. After Fourier transform, the resulting phase image pairs are subtracted to give the final phase map. Note that if synchronization is performed on every heart beat, k-space sampling is stopped prior to the end of the cardiac cycle because the R-R interval can be expected to vary in vivo, and hence end-diastolic phase maps cannot be obtained.

backs can be overcome by using retrospective gating, where the MR signal is acquired continuously, asynchronously with the ECG. By postprocessing, the MR information is sorted and interpolated to fixed times in the cardiac cycle before reconstruction of the image frames. However, potential disadvantages in retrospective gating include signal manipulation, such as filtering and interpolation (31).

If the studied vessel also moves periodically in space because of respiratory motion, a second synchronization, with respect to the vessel motion in space, may be necessary. Another method to overcome this problem is to use the so-called segmented k-space technique, where the entire data acquisition can be made within a breath-hold by the sampling of several phase encoding lines within a limited time window during each heart cycle (32–34). Although early studies have pointed out that the long acquisition windows introduced by the segmentation technique may cause unacceptable blurring in vessels moving rapidly with the cardiac rhythm (35,36), the use of so-called view-sharing (37) and/or the use of powerful gradient systems can improve the temporal resolution.

Velocity mapping can be extended to all three spatial directions (38,39), although, for time-resolved measurements, at the cost of prolonged acquisition time or reduced temporal resolution, because in such a case at least four images (one reference image and three velocity-sensitized images in each geometrical direction) has to be obtained to create subtracted net phase images for each time point in the cardiac cycle.

The resulting velocity-induced phase shift in the subtracted images can (without additional phase unwrapping) only be unambiguously determined in the phase angle interval ($-180°$, $+180°$). The velocity corresponding to a phase angle of $180°$ is known as the velocity encoding (VENC). The VENC can be calculated for a specific velocity-sensitive sequence pair, using equation 2. Using the VENC concept, velocity is obtained from measured phase angle by:

Equation 3: $v = VENC \times \Phi_v / 180°$; $\Phi_v = [-180°, 180°]$

Basic parameters that can be determined from a velocity map with an adequately designed through-plane experiment are:

The (average) linear velocity in each voxel (cm/s): This basic parameter is obtained with direct use of equation 3. Mean velocity within a region of interest (ROI) is obtained by averaging linear velocities in each voxel within the ROI.

The cross-sectional flow area (cm²): An accurate way to obtain this parameter is to use the half-value of the maximum velocity ($v_{max}/2$) as threshold for pixels included in the orifice, giving a precision of over 90% for realistic orifice areas (40).

The volume flow (cm³/s): Adequately found by multiplying the entire flow area with the mean velocity within it. The net flow rate over a whole cardiac cycle can thereafter be determined by discrete summation of velocity points over the whole cardiac cycle (Fig. 5.4). Postprocessing and data analysis, although automated techniques have been proposed (41,42), may still be time-consuming and generally include a significant amount of manual operation in a standard clinical setting.

Potential Error Sources

By now, the basic velocity mapping technique, on the basis of a pair of conventional gradient echo sequences with differ-

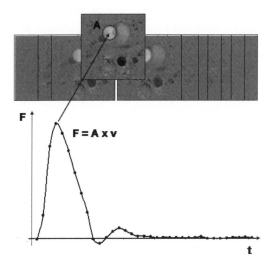

Figure 5.4. Calculation of a flow-versus-time curve from time-separated phase maps. Volume flow F is obtained using the relation $F = v*A$ for each phase map, where A is the area of the region of interest (ROI) encompassing the vessel and v is the average velocity measured in the ROI.

ent velocity sensitivity, has been thoroughly validated. For an overview of validation results, please see later section "Validation." Nevertheless, several sources of error might hamper the accuracy of a velocity mapping measurement, and such error sources are described in the next section.

Aliasing and Slice Misalignment

As stated previously, the net phase shift can only be unambiguously determined in the phase angle interval ($-180°$, $+180°$) and hence, velocities resulting in phase angles outside this interval will result in wrapped or *aliased* phase information. For example, with VENC = 20 cm/s, a velocity of 20 cm/s would give a phase angle of $180°$, whereas a velocity of 30 cm/s would give a phase angle of $270°$. Because the latter angle is outside of the interval ($-180°$, $+180°$), it will be interpreted as $-90°$ and, by equation 3, result in a velocity of -10 cm/s. To avoid aliasing, a certain a priori knowledge of expected velocities in the investigated vessel is useful. If average flow (F) and vessel area (A) can be estimated, average velocity (v) is easily calculated by $v = F/A$, and assuming laminar flow in the vessel, the highest expected velocity is $v_{max} = 2 \times v$. By setting VENC slightly higher than v_{max}, aliasing can be avoided. Methods to correct for aliasing (so-called unwrapping) have been proposed (43,44), but these techniques are rarely included in standard scanner software.

Misalignment between the direction of flow and the direction of the motion-encoding magnetic gradients may also lead to erroneous MR velocity measurements. The phenomena can be avoided in through-plane velocity mapping by careful adjustment of the imaging plane so that it is aligned perpendicular to the flow direction. However, if the angle ϕ of misalignment is known, then the true velocity value v_{true} can theoretically be calculated from the measured value v_{mea} using $v_{mea} = v_{true} \times \cos\phi$. In the absence of partial volume errors, a misalignment of as much as $20°$ will produce only a 6% error, whereas a more realistic misalignment of 5° causes an error <1% (45). Volume flow measurements are ideally unaffected by misalignment because the measured cross-sectional area increases proportionally to the decrease in v_{mea}; however, in practice partial-volume errors may result in overestimation of flow in the presence of misalignment (46).

Selection of Region-of-Interest (ROI)

A general, and perhaps slightly overseen, problem hampering accurate volume flow measurements using the velocity mapping technique, specifically in through-plane applications, is the selection of the size and shape of the ROI that encompass the vessel. Ideally, average flow can be calculated by the product between average velocity and ROI area; that is, $F = v*A_{ROI}$, provided that the ROI area is chosen equal to or larger than the cross-sectional vessel area, while selection of an area smaller than A_{ROI} will lead to flow underestimation. For larger vessels at normal resolution and signal-to-noise ratio (SNR) level, selection of an ROI slightly larger than A_{ROI} will give accurate values of F (47).

A different type of problem becomes important, if the number of pixels per vessel diameter (N_d) is low, a situation occurring for imaging of smaller vessels and cavities or even for intermediate vessel sizes at low spatial resolution. In this case, partial-volume effects at the edges of the vessel may become significant (48). The partial-volume effects originate from within a voxel where stationary and flowing tissue is mixed, and the modulus signal is a vector summation between signals from these two compartments. The net phase angle will correctly relate to average voxel velocity, only if magnitude signal components reflect the concentration relation between the two compartments. Normally, flowing liquid has higher magnitude than stationary tissue in a through-plane investigation as a result of inflow effects, and the net phase angle may therefore overestimate velocity if an ROI is chosen so that all edge pixels are included. Errors may reach over 10% if $N_d \leq 5$ (48). Several methods for reduction of the partial volume effect have been suggested, for example, selection of an ROI slightly smaller than the entire visible flow area by thresholding a number of pixels in the corresponding modulus image (38), empiric corrections based on phantom measurements (49), thresholding in combination with seed growing (50), magnitude-based corrections (51), corrections based on complex difference (CD) techniques (52), and automatic active contour models (53). In addition to the partial volume effect, it should also be noted that when the vessel size is small and the inflow effect gives high magnitude signal in the vessel, Gibbs ringing artifacts significantly influence modulus as well as phase signal, and a characteristic sinusoidal ringing pattern may be seen surrounding the vessel center.

In two recent phantom studies, it was shown that an ROI size equal to the nominal tube size was the best choice for accurate volume flow measurements in small vessels (46), and that the ringing pattern could be used to obtain a well-defined vessel segmentation which, after correction, provided accurate vessel radius and volume flow estimations (54).

Furthermore, regardless of vessel size, great care must be taken that A_{ROI} does not encompass areas with signal at or close to the noise level (e.g., air spaces), because in such areas the phase value will be random unless the phase image is postprocessed to give zero phase. Therefore, in evaluation tools for ROI delineation, the ability to draw the ROI in the corresponding modulus image and then transfer the ROI to the phase image may be helpful (55).

Background Correction

As described earlier, several factors may contribute to the net phase information in an MR phase image. The subtraction routine in velocity mapping outlined previously is intended to cancel all phase effects not related to encoding of motion, but residual effects are unavoidable and may cause significant errors, for example, when flow over a whole cardiac cycle is calculated by summation of flow data from a large number of time-resolved phase maps (56). Several reasons for nonzero phase background can be found.

First, the use of alternating magnetic gradient fields induces eddy currents in the conducting parts of the MR system (57). These eddy currents generate transient magnetic fields, which create phase offsets that vary linearly in space. Because different gradient patterns are used in the two sequences in a basic velocity mapping experiment, different phase effects can be expected, and a residual phase effect will appear in the subtracted image.

Second, when magnetic field gradients are applied for image formation and velocity encoding, concomitant magnetic fields are created in accordance with Maxwell's equations. These additional magnetic fields may create significant errors in velocity measurements (58) because, again, different gradient patterns are used in the two basic sequences, giving a net effect from concomitant gradients in the subtracted phase image. It should be noted that effects from concomitant gradients scale quadratically with gradient amplitude and distance from the magnet isocenter but inversely with magnetic field strength. The largest effects can be anticipated in measurements performed at positions significantly displaced from the isocenter with a combination of strong magnetic field gradients and low main magnetic field strength (59).

Third, nonlinearity in the applied magnetic field gradients can be caused by the finite size of the coils in the gradient system. In the images, gradient nonlinearities result in image distortion as a result of differences between the actual and expected magnetic field strengths. In the case of velocity mapping, nonlinear gradients will introduce differences between expected and actual velocity encoding and, similar to the Maxwell effects, these errors become more prominent the more distant the investigated voxels are from the isocenter of the magnet.

Although technical developments, e.g., the use of self-shielded gradient coils, may reduce the phase offset problem substantially other development lines, such as the use of increased gradient strengths act in the opposite direction, and the effects of background phase should not be neglected in precise velocity and volume flow measurements using velocity mapping. Consequently, several methods for background phase corrections have been proposed. Removal of linear phase effects can be done by modeling linear functions based on the measured velocities in the stationary regions in the image (60,61). Correction is then achieved by subtracting the position-dependent modeled background phase from measured phases in the vessel. A simplified version of linear correction is to select two ROIs on opposite sides of and at equal distances from the vessel, and subtract the average background phase value from the vessel data (62). However, selection of adequate background ROIs may be difficult, especially in the thoracic region. Other methods include combined noise reduction and semiautomatized background correction (63) as well as phase filtering.

The additional phase shift that is generated by the concomitant fields is nonlinear and can be analytically determined from knowledge of the pulse sequence and the positions relative to the isocenter. The erroneous phase shift as a result of concomitant fields can therefore be eliminated using postprocessing by first calculating expected phase effects from concomitant gradients and then subtracting these values from the phase images.

Furthermore, a reconstruction method has recently been proposed that corrects for errors in the velocity measurements caused by nonlinear gradient fields (64).

Phase Dispersion

In MR velocity mapping of flow, each voxel may contain a spectrum of velocities as well as higher order motion components, such as acceleration, jerk, and so forth. This inhomogeneity of motion components will give rise to a distribution of phase shifts within the voxel (phase dispersion). The net flow-induced phase shift within a voxel is obtained from a vectorial summation of all of the elementary phase contributions, and, when this vectorial summation is made, several situations can occur that will affect the phase-versus-velocity linearity. For example, errors in velocity estimated from average voxel phase may occur, if modulus signal differs within the voxel because of different degrees of inflow enhancement (65). Furthermore, phase dispersion inevitably leads to loss of magnitude signal and increased uncertainty in the corresponding phase information. In extreme cases phase information cannot be unambiguously determined, and the linearity between velocity and measured phase is lost.

In MR velocity mapping of laminar flow the phase-velocity relation is, however, generally preserved. When the Reynolds number (which is related to the ratio between velocity and viscosity of the liquid) is increased, the flow profile changes and at very high Reynolds numbers, a flat velocity profile, although randomly fluctuating in time at every position, is obtained (turbulent flow). However, even with this time-dependent random motion, there is a well-defined average velocity profile in the vessel, and the instantaneous velocity at a point is given by this average velocity plus the fluctuating velocity at that instant. Transition from laminar to turbulent flow in straight, smooth-walled vessels is not associated with a decreased modulus signal in gradient-echo imaging (66), and the phase-velocity relation in MR velocity mapping is not affected, owing to that the so-called turbulent intensity (the ratio between fluctuating velocity and average velocity) in a turbulent flow field is relatively low in such cases (67).

Another situation may occur in a constriction, where so-called separated or complex flow is at hand. It has been shown that if a constriction is present, turbulence intensity values may drastically increase (67). Although several other explanation models, such as influence of higher-order motion, has been proposed (68), fluctuations of velocity in time as well as in space might be the most important reason for reduction in modulus signal and breakdown of phase-versus-velocity linearity after a constriction. Systematic investigations using flow phantoms have revealed that several factors in relation to the complex flow patterns influence the phase-versus-velocity linearity (68). Thus, for a given volume flow, the breakdown in linearity becomes more pronounced as the cross-sectional area of the stenosis is reduced. Furthermore, for a certain constriction the phase-velocity relation is more likely to become nonlinear as the volume flow increased. Even though the phase-velocity relation is regained as the imaging plane for MR velocity mapping is moved downstream the constriction, disturbances may appear several centimeters distal to the tightest constrictions. Regardless of the correct explanation model for such findings, results from several groups show that a reduction of echo time, or, more formally, velocity encoding gradient duration, will reduce signal loss and regain unambiguous phase information (68–70).

Displacement

In MR imaging of flow, time differences between phase and frequency encoding may lead to a displacement artifact that is manifested as a distortion of the vessel lumen (71) and which can be prominent for rapid flow moving obliquely relative to these gradients. Alternative names for this phenomenon are *misregistration* and *oblique flow artifact*.

Furthermore, when the moving spins are subjected to acceleration and other higher orders of motion, the obtained phase shift no longer depends solely on velocity, and equation 2 does not hold (72). The induced phase shift in the presence of higher orders of motion has been identified as a potentially confounding factor in velocity measurements (73), but it can be further analyzed theoretically by so-called Taylor expansion of the expression for the position $x(t)$ of a spin as a function of time. According to such analysis, the total phase shift in a bipolar experiment can be regarded as a velocity measurement free from the influence of higher-order motion but spatially misplaced in the reconstructed velocity image owing to differences in time between true velocity encoding, occurring at the so-called moment center time or gravity center and spatial encoding (72,74,75).

Velocity measurement displacements, hence, occur in situations where the flow is oblique and/or contains higher-order motion components. The only type of flow that can be measured without being influenced by the displacement artifacts, therefore, is nonaccelerating flow parallel to one encoding direction.

Displacement errors can therefore be expected when measuring physiologic flows in the heart and great vessels with the phase-contrast technique. One way of reducing the oblique flow artifact is to reduce the time difference between phase and frequency encoding and, similarly, the displacement effects of higher-order motion components can be reduced by reduction of the time difference between the true velocity encoding time and the time for spatial encoding (76).

Calculation of Derived Parameters

Apart from blood flow measurements, there are many examples where the acquired velocity data can be used for extended visualization of flow patterns as well as for calculation of different physiologic parameters. From velocity mapping data, visualization of flow in 2D as well as in three dimensions (3D) can be made, e.g., using velocity vector mapping (77), streamline visualization (78), and particle traces (79) (Fig. 5.5A).

The transstenotic pressure gradient (in case of stenotic vessels), which gives information about the severity of constrictions in the vessels, can be estimated by inserting v_{max} (meters per second) in the stenotic jet in the modified Bernoulli equation $\Delta P = 4 \times v_{max}^2$ (80). However, the simplified Bernoulli equation is based on several assumptions, for example, that the velocity of blood is zero before the constriction. The measurement accuracy of this parameter can also be compromised by partial volume effects and malpositioning of the imaging slice (40).

A proposed marker for localization of areas where formation of atherosclerosis will appear is the wall shear stress (81). The calculation of the wall shear stress τ is given by $\tau = \mu^* \, dv/dr$, where the quotient *dv/dr* corresponds to the velocity gradient at the vessel wall and μ is the viscosity, which for the blood is 0.004 Ns/m^2. Several studies have shown the possibility of calculating the wall shear stress in vessels using MRI velocity data (82,83).

The elasticity of the greater blood vessels can be assessed by calculation of the vascular compliance. Compliance provides an estimate on the vessel conditions because low compliance is associated with a number of different cardiovascular diseases whereas large values correlate to overall fitness and youth. It has been shown feasible to calculate vascular compliance using time-resolved velocity data (84).

The contraction and relaxation of the pumping heart imply varying strains in different regions of the myocardial muscle. Quantification of strain and strain rate in the myocardium has been suggested as methods to identify ischemic areas in the heart, and velocity data in the myocardium can be used to calculate strain rate (85–87). In the case of velocity-mapping based strain and strain-rate calculations, no tracking of fictive markers has to be performed because the measured velocities provide enough information for the calculation of this parameter (Fig. 5.5B) (87).

Technical Extensions

Several methods for reduction of the acquisition time in MR flow quantification have been suggested. For example, strategies using reduction to one spatial dimension (88–90) give possibilities for either dynamic recording of flow in 1-D projections or full so-called Fourier velocity encoding within a reasonable acquisition time. Another approach is to use nontriggered measurements (91). Echo-planar imaging methods for flow quantification using the velocity mapping strategy have been proposed for 2D and 3D measurements in vessels and structures with a reasonably large area (92–94), and spiral imaging techniques (95) have been suggested and compared with conventional techniques (96).

Recently, the phase-contrast imaging method has also been combined with the balanced steady-state free precession (SSFP) pulse sequence (97,98). Because the SNR in

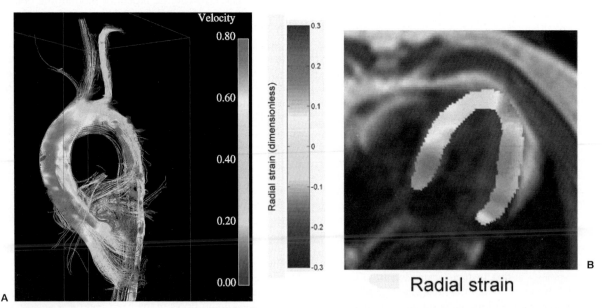

Figure 5.5. **(A)** Particle trace visualization of flow through the aorta of a healthy volunteer calculated, using velocity data from time-resolved 3D phase-contrast images. The traces are color coded according to velocity (m/s). (Courtesy of Lars Wigstöm and John-Peder Eskobar Kvitting, Linköping University, Linköping, Sweden.) **(B)** Radial strain at peak systole in a patient with an infarct in the apical septal region (superimposed on a conventional MR image of the corresponding area). The strain map is calculated from 2D phase contrast images where in-plane velocities in the myocardium are measured. By integrating these velocities with respect to time, a dense description of myocardial motion and strain is obtained. The strain map is color coded using an RGB scale showing expansion, no deformation and compression, respectively. (From Bergvall E, Cain P, Sparr G, et al. Very fast and highly automated method for myocardial motion analysis with phase contrast MRI. *J Cardiovasc Magn Reson* 2004;6:394A, with permission.)

ping is an accurate, noninvasive method of measuring collateral blood flow in coarctation and that collaterals develop within a few weeks (157).

PULMONARY VESSELS

MR velocity mapping can measure blood flow individually in the right and left pulmonary arteries (108) as well as in the four lung veins (123,131).

It has been shown that arterial switch repair after transposition may lead to temporary stenosis of the primary pulmonary arterial branches. The hemodynamic effects of these can be evaluated by MR velocity mapping but go undetected with other imaging modalities (158).

Blood flow distribution to the right and left lungs and the contribution to venous flow from the superior and inferior caval veins can be measured after total cavopulmonary connection (TCPC) (159,160).

MR velocity mapping has demonstrated 100% specificity and 100% sensitivity in detecting pulmonary venous obstruction in 7 pediatric patients with pulmonary obstruction and 27 controls, using Doppler echocardiography and catheterization as the gold standard (131).

Some studies have proposed that MR velocity mapping in the pulmonary trunk may be used to estimate pulmonary artery hypertension (161–163).

QUANTIFICATION OF SHUNTS

Quantification of shunt size may be performed to evaluate the need for surgery and to follow up the result postoperatively. Quantification of intracardiac shunt by MR velocity mapping is accomplished by measuring pulmonary to systemic flow (QP:QS) in the pulmonary trunk and in the aorta (Fig. 5.8). A specific feature of MR velocity mapping is that it, as opposed to other modalities, also quantifies right-to-left shunt. Shunted volume is the difference between the pulmonary and the aortic flow.

Extracardiac shunt size may prove more difficult to measure unless the complete nature of the shunting is known. In the case of anomalous veins, shunt size can be measured in the same way as intracardiac left-to-right shunt (cf. above) or by direct measurement of volume flow in the anomalous veins that may serve as an internal control.

Measurement of QP:QS ratio by MR velocity mapping has been extensively validated by comparison to results from flow phantoms (62,111) to planimetry of the left ventricle, in end-systole and end-diastole (118,121,134), to catheter-based oximetry (118,133–137) to radionuclide angiography (62), with convincing accuracy. Preliminary results using parallel imaging (101) and real-time MR imaging (102) to shorten acquisition time have been presented.

The usefulness of MR in assessment of shunt size (QP:QS) is considered "Class I = provides clinically relevant information and is frequently useful; may be used as first-line imaging technique; usually supported by substantial literature" (164).

VALVULAR OBSTRUCTION AND REGURGITATION

See "Valvular Heart Disease" in next section.

CONDUITS

Extracardiac ventriculopulmonary conduits have a tendency to develop both obstruction and regurgitation over time and are better examined by MR for both morphologic and functional evaluation compared to echocardiography (55,69,165).

ACQUIRED HEART DISEASE

Acquired heart disease encompasses derangements to normal anatomy and physiology that cause loss of pumping efficiency as a result of myocardial ischemia and failure, or loss of flow energy as a result of stenosis or valvular regurgitation. Situations in acquired heart disease, where MR velocity mapping provides important quantitative physiologic information are, therefore, heart failure, valvular disease, or coronary artery disease.

HEART FAILURE

Ventricular Function

Systolic ventricular function, at least under stress conditions, may be assessed by MR velocity mapping of ejected blood into the aorta. Peak flow acceleration has been shown to be a sensitive indicator of the effect of ischemia on global ventricular function (166).

Diastolic ventricular function can be assessed by MR velocity mapping of blood flow patterns over the mitral (77,167–173) and the tricuspid valve (122,174).

Cardiac Output

Cardiac output (CO) is the volume flow delivered from the left ventricle to the aorta. CO is often corrected for by body surface area to give cardiac index (CI). Cardiac index at resting conditions varies from about 4 L/min/m^2 for teenagers to about 2.5 L/min/m^2 in the eighth decade of life (175). Cardiac output has been measured by MR velocity mapping and compared to measurements by the Fick principle and thermodilution after cardiac catheterization, with high agreement (176).

Low cardiac output may be caused by myocardial infarction, severe valvular heart disease, myocarditis, cardiac tamponade, and certain cardiac metabolic derangements or by peripheral factors leading to decreased venous return, as in decreased blood volume or obstruction of large veins (175). When cardiac index decreases below a certain level, physiologic compensatory mechanisms come into play that serve a purpose in the short perspective, increasing preload and afterload to restore blood pressure, but worsen the situation in the long run by loading the failing heart. Measurement of cardiac index can therefore provide information on the degree of cardiac failure.

VALVULAR HEART DISEASE

Regurgitation

Valvular regurgitation leads to increased preload and thus a loss of pumping energy. The regurgitant volume can be quantified with high accuracy by magnetic resonance in two principally different ways: (a) directly by velocity mapping in the valvular plane (Fig. 5.9) or (b) as the difference between left ventricular stroke volume assessed by planimetry and ejected volume assessed by velocity mapping (see Chap. 12).

Direct measurements of valvular regurgitation can be achieved by measuring forward and backward flow at the level of the valve in aortic regurgitation (60,177,178), mitral regurgitation (60,179), and pulmonary regurgitation in congenital heart disease (119,180,181). This can be performed for all valves but is most reliable for the aortic and pulmonary valves. A complicating factor is through-plane motion of the valves, during the measurement, which may introduce errors. These errors can be minimized by placing the measurement plane as close as possible to the valve plane (182,183). A promising feature is "moving slice" velocity mapping (184,185). With this technique, the measurement plane follows the motion of the valve and thus minimizes errors caused by through-plane motion of valves.

Indirect measurement of valvular regurgitation is achieved by subtracting the net ejected volume (forward stroke volume) into the aorta or the pulmonary trunk from the planimetrically derived stroke volume of the ventricle (total stroke volume) (186–188). This method works better for the mitral and tricuspid valves in comparison to direct measurement of regurgitant volume by velocity mapping.

When both valves of a ventricle are regurgitant, each regurgitant volume can be measured as, for example, in aortic and mitral regurgitation (188). The aortic regurgitation is measured directly as backward flow in the valve plane assessed by velocity mapping. The mitral regurgitation is calculated indirectly, as previously mentioned, minus the regurgitant volume of the aortic valve.

The usefulness of MR in valvular regurgitation is considered "Class I = provides clinically relevant information and is frequently useful; may be used as first-line imaging technique; usually supported by substantial literature" (164).

Stenosis

Severity of valvular stenosis is derived essentially in the same way as for Doppler ultrasound, using the modified Bernoulli equation to estimate the pressure gradient across a stenotic lesion by measuring peak velocity in the lesion: $\Delta P = 4v^2$, where ΔP is the peak pressure gradient (mm Hg) across the lesion and v is the peak blood velocity (m/s). Shortcomings of derived pressure gradients are discussed previously in section "Calculation of Derived Parameters."

Assessment of the severity of stenosis can be achieved with good accuracy by MR velocity mapping compared to Doppler ultrasound in mitral (124,129) and aortic stenosis (124).

Prosthetic Valves

Prosthetic valves cause signal loss in the immediate vicinity of the metal parts. Despite this, MR velocity mapping has been shown to provide valuable information on velocity fields around prosthetic aortic valves (94,189–193).

CORONARY DISEASE

Coronary Flow Measurements

Coronary flow measurements using MR velocity mapping are sparsely used in clinical routine. The technique, however, is subject to development and great interest for research applications. Several in vitro and in vivo studies have validated MR velocity mapping for coronary flow measurements (see previous section, "Validation in Vivo"). The following section describes measurements in humans.

Global left ventricular perfusion and perfusion reserve can be estimated by measuring coronary sinus blood flow, which is an approximation of the amount of blood that has perfused the left ventricular myocardium, divided by left ventricular mass. This has been performed in healthy volunteers to estimate resting perfusion (194), as well as perfusion reserve, which has been shown to be in the range of 2.8 to 4.3 (149,151,195,196). The perfusion reserve is decreased in patients with hypertrophic obstructive cardiomyopathy (195), orthotopic heart transplant (149), ischemic heart disease (152), and chronic heart failure (196).

Measurement of blood flow velocity or volume flow is more difficult in the coronary arteries compared to the coronary sinus because of smaller dimensions and a higher degree of motion during the cardiac cycle. Flow velocity or flow volume and flow reserve have been investigated in the left anterior descending (LAD) and right coronary artery of healthy subjects, and flow velocities typically increased 3 to 5 times using pharmacologic stress (32,148,197,198)—the higher values usually obtained by adenosine stress and the lower by using dipyridamole. The same type of measurements has been undertaken in the LAD artery in patient populations and has showed high agreement with intravascular ultrasound for measurement of flow and flow reserve (141,142,144,199) and may be used to identify patients with significant coronary artery stenosis (145,199,200), restenosis after stent implantation (201,202), or to evaluate the physiologic status of venous grafts (203–205).

BASIC PHYSIOLOGY

Properties of flowing blood have been studied in the aorta (117,206–210), in the left ventricle (79,211,212), and in the left atrium (213), which has substantially increased the understanding of fundamental cardiovascular hemodynamics. Measurement of all in-flows and out-flows of the heart has been used to derive total heart volume change during a heart beat (123).

A promising feature of MR velocity mapping is derivation of intravascular and intracavitary pressure gradients from acceleration and deceleration of blood, using an algorithm based on the Navier-Stokes equations for incompressible Newtonian fluid (214–220).

Important to mention in this context is that MR velocity mapping can also be used to calculate strain rate in myocardium (85,221–223) and to track myocardial motion (87,224,225).

a comparison of phase-contrast MR imaging with positron emission tomography. *AJR Am J Roentgenol* 2001;177: 1161–1166.

153. Varaprasathan GA, Araoz PA, Higgins CB, et al. Quantification of flow dynamics in congenital heart disease: applications of velocity-encoded cine MR imaging. *Radiographics* 2002; 22:895–905; discussion 905–906.

154. Steffens JC, Bourne MW, Sakuma H, et al. Quantification of collateral blood flow in coarctation of the aorta by velocity encoded cine magnetic resonance imaging. *Circulation* 1994; 90:937–943.

155. Holmqvist C, Stahlberg F, Hanseus K, et al. Collateral flow in coarctation of the aorta with magnetic resonance velocity mapping: correlation to morphological imaging of collateral vessels. *J Magn Reson Imaging* 2002;15:39–46.

156. Araoz PA, Reddy GP, Tarnoff H, et al. MR findings of collateral circulation are more accurate measures of hemodynamic significance than arm-leg blood pressure gradient after repair of coarctation of the aorta. *J Magn Reson Imaging* 2003;17: 177–183.

157. Chernoff DM, Derugin N, Rajasinghe HA, et al. Measurement of collateral blood flow in a porcine model of aortic coarctation by velocity-encoded cine MRI. *J Magn Reson Imaging* 1997;7:557–563.

158. Gutberlet M, Boeckel T, Hosten N, et al. Arterial switch procedure for D-transposition of the great arteries: quantitative midterm evaluation of hemodynamic changes with cine MR imaging and phase-shift velocity mapping-initial experience. *Radiology* 2000;214:467–475.

159. Houlind K, Stenbog EV, Sorensen KE, et al. Pulmonary and caval flow dynamics after total cavopulmonary connection. *Heart* 1999;81:67–72.

160. Pedersen EM, Stenbog EV, Frund T, et al. Flow during exercise in the total cavopulmonary connection measured by magnetic resonance velocity mapping. *Heart* 2002;87:554–558.

161. Bogren HG, Klipstein RH, Mohiaddin RH, et al. Pulmonary artery distensibility and blood flow patterns: a magnetic resonance study of normal subjects and of patients with pulmonary arterial hypertension. *Am Heart J* 1989;118:990–999.

162. Laffon E, Laurent F, Bernard V, et al. Noninvasive assessment of pulmonary arterial hypertension by MR phase-mapping method. *J Appl Physiol* 2001;90:2197–2202.

163. Laffon E, Vallet C, Bernard V, et al. A computed method for noninvasive MRI assessment of pulmonary arterial hypertension. *J Appl Physiol* 2004;96:463–468.

164. Pennell DJ, Sechtem UP, Higgins CB, et al. Clinical indications for cardiovascular magnetic resonance (CMR): Consensus Panel report. *Eur Heart J* 2004;25:1940–1965.

165. Martinez JE, Mohiaddin RH, Kilner PJ, et al. Obstruction in extracardiac ventriculopulmonary conduits: value of nuclear magnetic resonance imaging with velocity mapping and Doppler echocardiography. *J Am Coll Cardiol* 1992;20: 338–344.

166. Pennell DJ, Firmin DN, Burger P, et al. Assessment of magnetic resonance velocity mapping of global ventricular function during dobutamine infusion in coronary artery disease. *Br Heart J* 1995;74:163–170.

167. Hartiala JJ, Mostbeck GH, Foster E, et al. Velocity-encoded cine MRI in the evaluation of left ventricular diastolic function: measurement of mitral valve and pulmonary vein flow velocities and flow volume across the mitral valve. *Am Heart J* 1993;125:1054–1066.

168. Engels G, Muller E, Reynen K, et al. Evaluation of left ventricular inflow and volume by MR. *Magn Reson Imaging* 1993;11:957–964.

169. Fujimoto S, Mohiaddin RH, Parker KH, et al. Magnetic resonance velocity mapping of normal human transmitral velocity profiles. *Heart Vessels* 1995;10:236–240.

170. Karwatowski SP, Brecker SJ, Yang GZ, et al. Mitral valve flow measured with cine MR velocity mapping in patients with ischemic heart disease: comparison with Doppler echocardiography. *J Magn Reson Imaging* 1995;5:89–92.

171. Milet SF, Mayberry JL, Ivarsen HR, et al. A semi-automated method to quantify left ventricular diastolic inflow propagation by magnetic resonance phase velocity mapping. *J Magn Reson Imaging* 1999;9:544–551.

172. Houlind K, Schroeder AP, Egeblad H, et al. Age-dependent changes in spatial and temporal blood velocity distribution of early left ventricular filling. *Magn Reson Imaging* 1999; 17:859–868.

173. Houlind K, Schroeder AP, Stodkilde-Jorgensen H, et al. Intraventricular dispersion and temporal delay of early left ventricular filling after acute myocardial infarction. Assessment by magnetic resonance velocity mapping. *Magn Reson Imaging* 2002;20:249–260.

174. Helbing WA, Niezen RA, Le Cessie S, et al. Right ventricular diastolic function in children with pulmonary regurgitation after repair of tetralogy of Fallot: volumetric evaluation by magnetic resonance velocity mapping. *J Am Coll Cardiol* 1996;28:1827–1835.

175. Guyton AC. *Textbook of Medical Physiology.* 5th ed. Philadelphia: WB Saunders; 1991.

176. Hundley WG, Li HF, Hillis LD, et al. Quantitation of cardiac output with velocity-encoded, phase-difference magnetic resonance imaging. *Am J Cardiol* 1995;75:1250–1255.

177. Sondergaard L, Lindvig K, Hildebrandt P, et al. Quantification of aortic regurgitation by magnetic resonance velocity mapping. *Am Heart J* 1993;125:1081–1090.

178. Honda N, Machida K, Hashimoto M, et al. Aortic regurgitation: quantitation with MR imaging velocity mapping. *Radiology* 1993;186:189–194.

179. Fujita N, Chazouilleres AF, Hartiala JJ, et al. Quantification of mitral regurgitation by velocity-encoded cine nuclear magnetic resonance imaging. *J Am Coll Cardiol* 1994;23: 951–958.

180. Roest AA, Helbing WA, Kunz P, et al. Exercise MR imaging in the assessment of pulmonary regurgitation and biventricular function in patients after tetralogy of Fallot repair. *Radiology* 2002;223:204–211.

181. Li W, Davlouros PA, Kilner PJ, et al. Doppler-echocardiographic assessment of pulmonary regurgitation in adults with repaired tetralogy of Fallot: comparison with cardiovascular magnetic resonance imaging. *Am Heart J* 2004;147:165–172.

182. Chatzimavroudis GP, Walker PG, Oshinski JN, et al. The importance of slice location on the accuracy of aortic regurgitation measurements with magnetic resonance phase velocity mapping. *Ann Biomed Eng* 1997;25:644–652.

183. Chatzimavroudis GP, Oshinski JN, Franch RH, et al. Quantification of the aortic regurgitant volume with magnetic resonance phase velocity mapping: a clinical investigation of the importance of imaging slice location. *J Heart Valve Dis* 1998; 7:94–101.

184. Kozerke S, Scheidegger MB, Pedersen EM, et al. Heart motion adapted cine phase-contrast flow measurements through the aortic valve. *Magn Reson Med* 1999;42:970–978.

185. Kozerke S, Schwitter J, Pedersen EM, et al. Aortic and mitral regurgitation: quantification using moving slice velocity mapping. *J Magn Reson Imaging* 2001;14:106–112.

186. Hundley WG, Li HF, Willard JE, et al. Magnetic resonance imaging assessment of the severity of mitral regurgitation. Comparison with invasive techniques. *Circulation* 1995;92: 1151–1158.

187. Kizilbash AM, Hundley WG, Willett DL, et al. Comparison of quantitative Doppler with magnetic resonance imaging for assessment of the severity of mitral regurgitation. *Am J Cardiol* 1998;81:792–795.

188. Kon MW, Myerson SG, Moat NE, et al. Quantification of regurgitant fraction in mitral regurgitation by cardiovascular magnetic resonance: comparison of techniques. *J Heart Valve Dis* 2004;13:600–607.

189. Houlind K, Eschen O, Pedersen EM, et al. Magnetic resonance imaging of blood velocity distribution around St. Jude medical aortic valves in patients. *J Heart Valve Dis* 1996;5:511–517.

190. Ringgaard S, Botnar RM, Djurhuus C, et al. High-resolution assessment of velocity fields and shear stresses distal to prosthetic heart valves using high-field magnetic resonance imaging. *J Heart Valve Dis* 1999;8:96–103.

191. Hasenkam JM, Ringgaard S, Houlind K, et al. Prosthetic heart valve evaluation by magnetic resonance imaging. *Eur J Cardiothorac Surg* 1999;16:300–305.

192. Botnar R, Nagel E, Scheidegger MB, et al. Assessment of prosthetic aortic valve performance by magnetic resonance velocity imaging. *Magma* 2000;10:18–26.

193. Kozerke S, Hasenkam JM, Nygaard H, et al. Heart motion-adapted MR velocity mapping of blood velocity distribution downstream of aortic valve prostheses: initial experience. *Radiology* 2001;218:548–555.

194. van Rossum AC, Visser FC, Hofman MB, et al. Global left ventricular perfusion: noninvasive measurement with cine MR imaging and phase velocity mapping of coronary venous outflow. *Radiology* 1992;182:685–691.

195. Kawada N, Sakuma H, Yamakado T, et al. Hypertrophic cardiomyopathy: MR measurement of coronary blood flow and vasodilator flow reserve in patients and healthy subjects. *Radiology* 1999;211:129–135.

196. Lund GK, Watzinger N, Saeed M, et al. Chronic heart failure: global left ventricular perfusion and coronary flow reserve with velocity-encoded cine MR imaging: initial results. *Radiology* 2003;227:209–215.

197. Davis CP, Liu PF, Hauser M, et al. Coronary flow and coronary flow reserve measurements in humans with breath-held magnetic resonance phase contrast velocity mapping. *Magn Reson Med* 1997;37:537–544.

198. Grist TM, Polzin JA, Bianco JA, et al. Measurement of coronary blood flow and flow reserve using magnetic resonance imaging. *Cardiology* 1997;88:80–89.

199. Hundley WG, Hamilton CA, Clarke GD, et al. Visualization and functional assessment of proximal and middle left anterior descending coronary stenoses in humans with magnetic resonance imaging. *Circulation* 1999;99:3248–3254.

200. Hundley WG, Hillis LD, Hamilton CA, et al. Assessment of coronary arterial restenosis with phase-contrast magnetic resonance imaging measurements of coronary flow reserve. *Circulation* 2000;101:2375–2381.

201. Saito Y, Sakuma H, Shibata M, et al. Assessment of coronary flow velocity reserve using fast velocity-encoded cine MRI for noninvasive detection of restenosis after coronary stent implantation. *J Cardiovasc Magn Reson* 2001;3:209–214.

202. Nagel E, Thouet T, Klein C, et al. Noninvasive determination of coronary blood flow velocity with cardiovascular magnetic resonance in patients after stent deployment. *Circulation* 2003;107:1738–1743.

203. Galjee MA, van Rossum AC, Doesburg T, et al. Quantification of coronary artery bypass graft flow by magnetic resonance phase velocity mapping. *Magn Reson Imaging* 1996;14:485–493.

204. Bedaux WL, Hofman MB, Vyt SL, et al. Assessment of coronary artery bypass graft disease using cardiovascular magnetic resonance determination of flow reserve. *J Am Coll Cardiol* 2002;40:1848–1855.

205. Salm LP, Langerak SE, Vliegen HW, et al. Blood flow in coronary artery bypass vein grafts: volume versus velocity at cardiovascular MR imaging. *Radiology* 2004;232:915–920.

206. Klipstein RH, Firmin DN, Underwood SR, et al. Blood flow patterns in the human aorta studied by magnetic resonance. *Br Heart J* 1987;58:316–323.

207. Kilner PJ, Yang GZ, Mohiaddin RH, et al. Helical and retrograde secondary flow patterns in the aortic arch studied by three-directional magnetic resonance velocity mapping. *Circulation* 1993;88:2235–2247.

208. Bogren HG, Buonocore MH. Blood flow measurements in the aorta and major arteries with MR velocity mapping. *J Magn Reson Imaging* 1994;4:119–130.

209. Bogren HG, Buonocore MH. 4D magnetic resonance velocity mapping of blood flow patterns in the aorta in young vs. elderly normal subjects. *J Magn Reson Imaging* 1999;10:861–869.

210. Markl M, Draney MT, Hope MD, et al. Time-resolved 3Dimensional velocity mapping in the thoracic aorta: visualization of 3Directional blood flow patterns in healthy volunteers and patients. *J Comput Assist Tomogr* 2004;28:459–468.

211. Kim WY, Walker PG, Pedersen EM, et al. Left ventricular blood flow patterns in normal subjects: a quantitative analysis by three-dimensional magnetic resonance velocity mapping. *J Am Coll Cardiol* 1995;26:224–238.

212. Kilner PJ, Yang GZ, Wilkes AJ, et al. Asymmetric redirection of flow through the heart. *Nature* 2000;404:759–761.

213. Fyrenius A, Wigstrom L, Ebbers T, et al. Three dimensional flow in the human left atrium. *Heart* 2001;86:448–455.

214. Urchuk SN, Plewes DB. MR measurements of pulsatile pressure gradients. *J Magn Reson Imaging* 1994;4:829–836.

215. Yang GZ, Kilner PJ, Wood NB, et al. Computation of flow pressure fields from magnetic resonance velocity mapping. *Magn Reson Med* 1996;36:520–526.

216. Urchuk SN, Fremes SE, Plewes DB. In vivo validation of MR pulse pressure measurement in an aortic flow model: preliminary results. *Magn Reson Med* 1997;38:215–223.

217. Tasu JP, Mousseaux E, Delouche A, et al. Estimation of pressure gradients in pulsatile flow from magnetic resonance acceleration measurements. *Magn Reson Med* 2000;44:66–72.

218. Tyszka JM, Laidlaw DH, Asa JW, et al. Three-dimensional, time-resolved (4D) relative pressure mapping using magnetic resonance imaging. *J Magn Reson Imaging* 2000;12:321–329.

219. Ebbers T, Wigstrom L, Bolger AF, et al. Estimation of relative cardiovascular pressures using time-resolved three-dimensional phase contrast MRI. *Magn Reson Med* 2001;45:872–879.

220. Thompson RB, McVeigh ER. Fast measurement of intracardiac pressure differences with 2D breath-hold phase-contrast MRI. *Magn Reson Med* 2003;49:1056–1066.

221. Robson MD, Constable RT. Three-dimensional strain-rate imaging. *Magn Reson Med* 1996;36:537–546.

222. Arai AE, Gaither CC III, Epstein FH, et al. Myocardial velocity gradient imaging by phase contrast MRI with application to regional function in myocardial ischemia. *Magn Reson Med* 1999;42:98–109.

223. Selskog P, Heiberg E, Ebbers T, et al. Kinematics of the heart: strain-rate imaging from time-resolved three-dimensional phase contrast MRI. *IEEE Trans Med Imaging* 2002;21:1105–1109.

224. Zhu Y, Drangova M, Pelc NJ. Fourier tracking of myocardial motion using cine-PC data. *Magn Reson Med* 1996;35:471–480.

225. Zhu Y, Drangova M, Pelc NJ. Estimation of deformation gradient and strain from cine-PC velocity data. *IEEE Trans Med Imaging* 1997;16:840–851.

6

Quantification in Cardiac Magnetic Resonance Imaging and Computed Tomography

Rob J. van der Geest, Boudewijn P.F. Lelieveldt, and Johan H.C. Reiber

Magnetic resonance imaging (MRI) and multislice computed tomography (MSCT) have become indispensable imaging modalities for evaluation of the cardiac system. MRI provides unique capabilities for studying many aspects of cardiac anatomy, function, perfusion, and viability in a single imaging session. Nevertheless, MSCT is rapidly gaining widespread clinical use for the evaluation of coronary anatomy and cardiac function. The recent technologic developments in MSCT have resulted in a tremendous improvement of image quality and high sensitivity and specificity for the detection of coronary stenosis.

Both MRI and MSCT are three-dimensional (3D) imaging modalities that are used for the evaluation of ventricular function. Volumetric measurement of the ventricular cavities and myocardium can be performed at high accuracy and precision as has been demonstrated in many experimental and clinical research studies. The 3D nature of these imaging modalities also provides detailed information of the cardiac system at a regional level. Among others, regional end-diastolic wall thickness and systolic wall thickening provide useful information for the assessment of the location, extent, and severity of ventricular abnormalities in ischemic heart disease. MRI can also be used to study blood flow and myocardial perfusion. Velocity-encoded cine MRI (VEC-MRI) is often used for the quantification of blood flow through the aortic and pulmonary valves and atrioventricular valve planes, which has shown to be clinically valuable in the evaluation of patients with complex congenital heart disease.

Typical cardiac MRI and MSCT examinations generate large data sets of images. To optimally and efficiently extract the relevant clinical information from these data sets, dedicated software solutions featuring automated image segmentation and optimal quantification and visualization methods are needed. Quantitative image analysis requires the definition of contours describing the inner and outer boundaries of the ventricles, which is a laborious and tedious task when based on manual contour tracing. Reliable automated or semiautomated image analysis software would be required to overcome these limitations. This chapter focuses on the state-of-the-art postprocessing techniques for quantitative assessment of global and regional ventricular function from cardiac MRI and MSCT.

QUANTIFICATION OF VENTRICULAR DIMENSIONS AND GLOBAL FUNCTION

ACCURACY AND REPRODUCIBILITY OF VOLUMETRIC MEASUREMENTS FROM MULTISLICE SHORT-AXIS ACQUISITIONS

MRI and MSCT allow imaging of anatomic objects in multiple parallel sections, enabling volumetric measurements using the Simpson's rule. According to Simpson's rule the volume of an object can be estimated by summation of the cross-sectional areas in each section multiplied by the section thickness. When there is a gap in between slices, this must be corrected for and the formula for volume becomes:

$$V = \Sigma \{Area_i * (Thickness + Gap)\},$$

where V is the volume of the 3D object and $Area_i$ the area of the cross section in section number i.

The short-axis orientation is the most commonly applied image orientation for the assessment of left ventricular chamber size and mass. Although MRI is capable of directly acquiring images in any orientation, MSCT images are always generated in the axial orientation and image reformatting is required to obtain short-axis images. The short-axis orientation has advantages over other slice orientations because it yields cross-sectional slices almost perpendicular to the myocardium for the largest part of the left ventricle (LV). This results in minimal partial volume effect at the myocardial boundaries and subsequently provides optimal depiction of the myocardial boundaries. However, the curvature of the LV at the apical level leads to significant partial volume averaging. The image voxels in this area simultaneously intersect with blood and myocardium yielding indistinct myocardial boundaries. By minimizing the slice thickness, while keeping sufficient signal to noise, this partial volume effect at the apex can be reduced. Given the relatively small cross-sectional area of the LV in the apical section, the error introduced because of the partial volume effect will be minimal. However, partial volume averaging at the basal level of the heart has a much greater impact because at this level the cross-sectional area of the LV is largest. The base of the LV exhibits a through-plane motion in the apical direction during systole on the order of 1.3 cm (1,2). Therefore, the significance of partial volume varies over the cardiac cycle. Additional long-axis views may prove helpful in determining more accurately how a basal short-axis slice intersects with the various anatomic regions.

IMPACT OF SLICE THICKNESS AND SLICE GAP

It is a prerequisite for the accurate assessment of the ventricular volumes that the stack of short-axis slices covers the complete ventricle from base to apex. With MRI, a section thickness between 6 and 10 mm is used, and the gap between slices varies from no gap (consecutive slices) to 4 mm. With MSCT, any value can be chosen for the slice thickness and gap when generating a short-axis data set by reformatting the original images. Typical parameters for MSCT are a slice thickness between 4 and 8 mm usually without any intersection gap. Quantification of volumes and mass requires the definition of contours in the images describing the endocardial and epicardial boundaries of the myocardium in several phases of the cardiac cycle. Although an image voxel may contain several tissues, because of the partial volume effect, it is assumed that the traced contours represent the geometry of the ventricle at the center of the imaged section. As shown in Figure 6.1, the partial volume effect may lead to both over- and underestimation in the assessment of ventricular volume.

With a simple experiment using synthetically created left ventricular shapes and short-axis cross sections it can be shown how the partial volume problem may affect measurement accuracy and reproducibility. For this purpose a computer-generated average left ventricular geometry with a fixed size was constructed and short-axis cross sections were automatically derived while varying the position of the ventricular geometry along the long-axis direction. The shape used and its dimensions are presented in Figure 6.2. In this experiment it is assumed that the contours in a short-axis slice will only be drawn in case more than 50% of the slice thickness intersects with myocardium. The results of the simulations as depicted in Figure 6.3 demonstrate that the measurement precision (or measurement variability) degrades with increasing distance between the slices. For typical imaging parameters (section thickness 6 mm, gap 4 mm) the measurement variability is between 4% and 5%. The measurement accuracy is not dependent on the slice thickness or slice gap used. A section thickness of 10 mm with no gap results in the same variability as a section thickness of 6 mm with a gap of 4 mm.

The result of this experiment has two important implications. First, variations between successive scans of the same patient may result in volumetric differences of up to 5%, which are inherent to the imaging technique used. Second, because the base of the heart has a significant through-plane motion component, the measurement variability of up to 5% will also be present over the cardiac cycle. Therefore, ejection fraction measurements will also be affected. By reducing the section thickness and the intersection gap, the variability in volumetric measurements can be reduced. For MSCT, in which short-axis reformats are derived from high-resolution near-isotropic volumetric data, it is useful to use small values for the slice thickness without applying any gap.

Overestimation

Underestimation

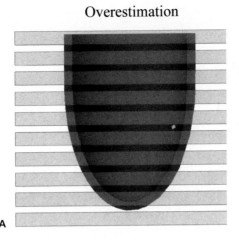
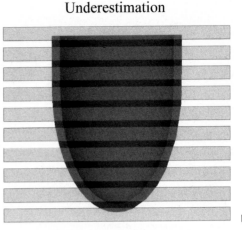

Figure 6.1. Left ventricular geometry intersected by multiple parallel short-axis sections. Given the same section thickness and intersection gap, both over- and underestimation of left ventricular volume can occur dependent on the position of the left ventricle (LV) with respect to the imaging slices. In situation **(A)** the most basal slice will be included in the volumetric assessment, whereas in **(B)**, the most basal slice will not be taken into account because it intersects by less than 50% with the left ventricular myocardium.   **A**   **B**

GLOBAL FUNCTION ASSESSMENT USING RADIAL LONG-AXIS VIEWS

The accuracy of volumetric measurements from multislice short-axis acquisitions is mainly determined by the accurate identification of the most basal slice level and the accurate definition of the endocardial and epicardial contours in this slice level. However, because of the relatively large section thickness used, this is often difficult. The origin of the problem is the highly anisotropic nature of a typical short-axis examination in which the resolution in the Z-direction is much worse than the in-pane resolution. To overcome this limitation, Bloomer et al (3) investigated the use of multiple radial long-axis views for quantification of left ventricular volumes and mass using a steady-state free precession (SSFP) MRI sequence. With a radial long-axis acquisition multiple long-axis views are acquired sharing a common axis of rotation (the LV long-axis) at equiangular intervals. This orientation has intrinsic advantages over short-axis imaging because it allows clear visualization of the mitral and aortic valve planes. In addition, long-axis views have less partial volume effect near the apex. After definition of the

ventricular contours, calculation of LV volume is performed by adding pie-shaped volume elements defined by the location of the axis of rotation, position of the contour, and angular interval between the image sections. Bloomer et al demonstrated a good agreement between multislice short-axis and radial long-axis acquisitions. As a result of the improved visualization of the myocardial boundaries and definition of the base, interobserver agreement was better using the radial long-axis method. Figure 6.4 illustrates examples of magnetic resonance images acquired using radial long-axis orientation. It clearly shows that the definition of the base and the contrast between blood and myocardium are excellent. Further research is needed to evaluate whether radial long-axis acquisitions also prove to be valuable for the assessment of regional function.

MYOCARDIAL MASS

The measurement of heart muscle weight is of clinical importance to properly diagnose and understand a patient's illness and condition, and to estimate the effects of treatment.

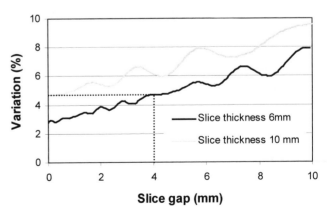

Figure 6.2. Left ventricular geometry used for the simulation experiments. The phantom consists of a half ellipsoid with a length of 70 mm and an outer diameter at the base of 60 mm; at the base the shape is extended with a cylinder with a diameter of 60 mm and a length of 30 mm. The thickness of the phantom was set to 5 mm. In the experiments the size of the object was varied between the dimensions shown and 80% of this size.

Figure 6.3. Results of volume calculation experiments using synthetically constructed left ventricular geometries. The variability of left ventricular volume estimates increases with increasing slice thickness and slice gap. For a setting of the imaging parameters, such as a thickness of 6 mm and a gap of 4 mm, the measurement variability is 5%.

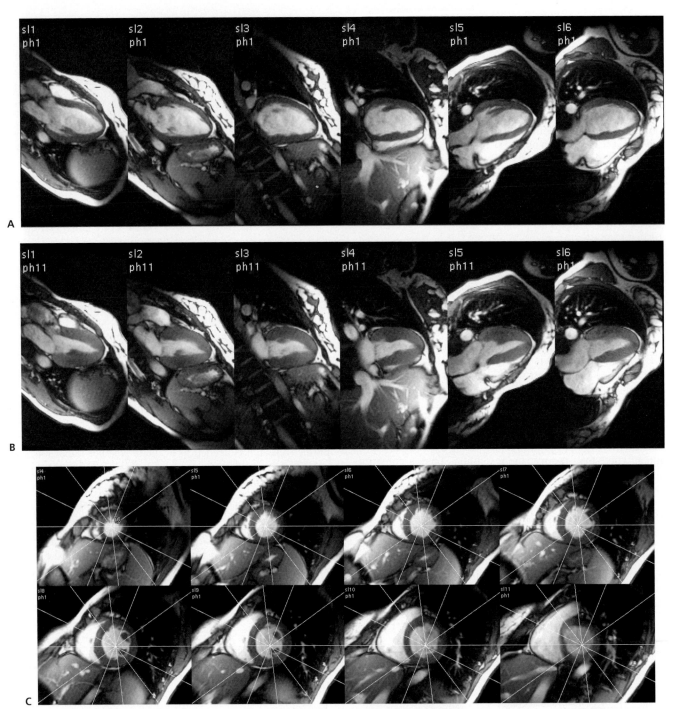

Figure 6.4. End-diastolic (*top*) and end-systolic (*middle*) magnetic resonance images acquired in radial long-axis views using steady-state free precession (SSFP) magnetic resonance imaging (MRI). Note the excellent conspicuity of the LV myocardial wall from base to apex. Orientation of the radial long-axis views (*white lines in short-axis images, bottom*). (Image data courtesy of M. Friedrich.)

To detect small changes in mass it is of paramount importance to use an accurate and reproducible measurement technique. Several validation studies have been performed comparing mass estimates as derived from MRI with postmortem mass measurements. In a study by Florentine et al (4) a stack of axial slices was used to quantify left ventricular mass using the Simpson rule. In this early study, they found good agreement ($r = 0.95$, standard error of estimate $= 13$ g). Maddahi et al (5) carried out extensive studies in a dog model comparing several slice orientations and measurement techniques for quantifying left ventricular mass. It was shown that in vivo estimates of left ventricular myocardial mass are most accurate when the images are obtained in the short-axis plane ($r = 0.98$, standard error of estimate $= 4.9$ g).

Left Ventricular Mass

For the LV it is generally believed and also supported by literature that the short-axis orientation is the most appropriate imaging plane. To obtain optimal accuracy and reproducibility it is important to cover the complete ventricle from apex to base with a sufficient number of slices. Quantification of mass requires the definition of contours in the images describing the endocardial and epicardial boundaries in the stack of images. The muscle volume is assessed from these contours by applying Simpson's rule. The myocardial mass is derived by multiplying the muscle volume with the specific density of myocardium (1.05 g/cm^3).

Typically, a section thickness between 6 and 10 mm is used with an intersection gap between 0 and 4 mm. At the apex and basal sections significant partial volume averaging will occur because of the section thickness used and tracing of the myocardial boundaries may not be trivial. Similarly, partial volume averaging will cause significant difficulties in interpreting sections with a highly trabeculated myocardial wall and papillary muscles (6). There is no general consensus on whether to include or exclude papillary muscles and trabeculae in the left ventricular mass. Although it is evident that inclusion of these structures would result in more accurate myocardial mass measurements, for regional wall thickening analysis it is important to exclude these structures to avoid artifacts in the quantification. Whether to use an end-diastolic or end-systolic time frame for the measurement is also a subject of ongoing debate. Most likely, optimal accuracy and reproducibility are obtained by averaging multiple time frames, but this will have practical objections in case the contours are derived by manual tracing.

Right Ventricular Mass

For the right ventricle (RV) and geometrically abnormally shaped LVs, multiple sections are required for an accurate volume assessment (7). MRI experiments with different slice orientations in phantoms and ventricular casts have shown that no significant difference can be observed in accuracy and reproducibility between slice orientations (8). However, in a clinical situation the choice of slice orientation also depends on the availability of a clear depiction of anatomic features that are needed to define the myocardial boundaries. Volumetric quantification of the RV may be better performed on the basis of axial views (9). This view shows improved anatomic detail and allows better differentiation between the right ventricular and atrial lumen. Nevertheless, for practical reasons, the right ventricular mass is often measured using a stack of short-axis slices, which is also used for measuring the left ventricular dimensions.

QUANTIFICATION OF VENTRICULAR VOLUMES AND GLOBAL FUNCTION

Assessment of global ventricular function requires volumetric measurement of the ventricular cavities in at least two points in the cardiac cycle: the end-diastolic and end-systolic phases. A vast amount of reports describe the applicability of MRI for accurate and reproducible quantification of left and right ventricular volumes using various MRI strategies

(4,10). Cardiac-gated MSCT also allows quantification of global function (11). Sufficient temporal resolution is required to properly capture the end-systolic phase. Generally a temporal resolution, or phase interval, on the order of 40 to 50 ms is assumed to be sufficient. Although MRI can provide such temporal resolution, the temporal resolution of MSCT does not yet fulfill this requirement. However, global function results obtained by MSCT are in good agreement with results derived from MRI (12,13). For geometrically normal LVs one could rely on geometric models to derive the volumes from one or two long-axis imaging sections. In a group of 10 patients with LV hypertrophy and 10 healthy subjects, Dulce et al (14) demonstrated a good agreement between biplane volumetric measurements using either the modified Simpson's rule of an ellipsoid model or true 3D volumetric measurements using a multislice MRI approach. In another study by Chuang et al (15), 25 patients with dilated cardiomyopathies were evaluated using both a biplane and a 3D multislice approach. They reported a poor correlation between the two measurement methods. At the present state, a single section with sufficient temporal resolution can be acquired within a single breath hold on most available MRI systems. The total duration of acquiring the 8 to 12 sections required to image the entire ventricular cavity is on the order of 5 minutes (16,17). All sections should be acquired at the same end-expiration or end-inspiration phase; otherwise reliable 3D-quantification of volumes from the obtained images is not possible. In MSCT, the complete volumetric data set is acquired during a single breath hold of 10 to 30 seconds.

Quantitative analysis starts with manual or (semi-) automated segmentation of the myocardium and blood pool in the images. Once contours have been defined in the stack of images describing the endocardial and epicardial boundaries of the myocardium, volumetric measurements including stroke volume and ejection fraction can be obtained by applying Simpson's rule. Normal values for global ventricular function and mass have been reported by several investigators for different populations and pulse sequences (18–20). It is important to note that normal values obtained using the newer SSFP-type sequences differ significantly from values obtained with previous techniques. The improved contrast between blood and myocardium in SSFP is associated with larger end-diastolic and end-systolic cavity volumes, smaller wall thickness values, and lower LV mass (20–22). In direct comparisons of SSFP with conventional fast gradient-echo techniques within the same individuals, differences in LV mass of up to 16.5% were reported (Fig. 6.5).

At the basal imaging sections, a clear visual separation between the LV and left atrium is often absent because the imaging section may contain both ventricular and atrial cavity and muscle. It is important to realize that while the imaging sections are fixed in space, the left ventricular annulus exhibits a motion in the apical direction on the order of 1.3 cm in normal hearts (1). Consequently, myocardium that is readily visible in an end-diastolic time frame may be replaced by left ventricular atrium in the end-systolic time frame. Additional long-axis views may be helpful to more reliably analyze the most basal and apical slice levels of a multislice short-axis study (2). Figure 6.6 displays end-diastolic and end-systolic time frames in a long-axis view and three basal short-axis sections obtained during a single

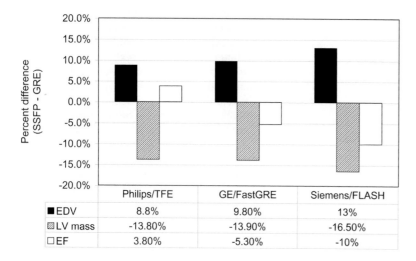

Figure 6.5. Comparison of LV dimensions measured with an SSFP sequence or segmented gradient-echo technique. (Data derived from Alfakih K, Plein S, Thiele H, et al. Normal human left and right ventricular dimensions for MRI as assessed by turbo gradient echo and steady-state free precession imaging sequences. *J Magn Reson Imaging* 2003;17(3):323–329; Lee VS, Resnick D, Bundy JM, et al. Cardiac function: MR evaluation in one breath hold with real-time True Fisp imaging with steady-state precession. *Radiology* 2002;222: 835–842; and Wei LI, Stern JS, Mai VM, et al. MR assessment of left ventricular function: quantitative comparison of fast imaging employing steady-state acquisition (FIESTA) with fast gradient echo cine technique. *J Magn Reson Imaging* 2002;16(5): 559–564, with permission.)

MRI examination. The white lines, indicating the intersection lines of the imaging planes, provide helpful additional information for interpreting the structures seen in the short-axis images.

QUANTIFICATION OF REGIONAL WALL MOTION AND WALL THICKENING USING THE CENTERLINE METHOD FROM DYNAMIC SHORT-AXIS IMAGES

The excellent depiction of the endocardial and epicardial boundaries of the left ventricular myocardium forms the basis of quantitative analysis of regional myocardial function. Quantitative analysis methods for endocardial wall motion are hampered by the presence of rigid body motion of the heart. A floating centroid, based on the center of gravity of the endocardial or epicardial contours, can be used to isolate the rigid body motion from the actual endocardial deformation. On the other hand, quantification of wall thickness and thickening does not have this disadvantage. It has been demonstrated that wall-thickening analysis is more sensitive in the detection of dysfunctional myocardium than wall-motion analysis (23,24). The optimal slice orientation for wall-thickness analysis of the LV is the short-axis plane because in this orientation the major part of the myocardial

End-diastole   End-systole

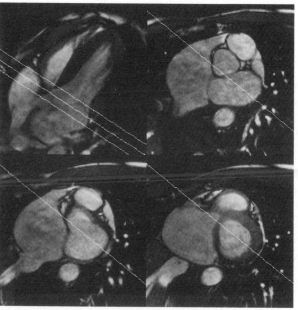

Figure 6.6. Four-chamber long-axis view and three basal level short-axis views acquired within the same examination. Short-axis and long-axis imaging planes intersect with each other (*white lines*). The movement of the base toward the apex in systole can easily be appreciated. Long-axis and short-axis planes intersecting may facilitate the interpretation of basal level short-axis images and may be valuable during tracing of the contours.

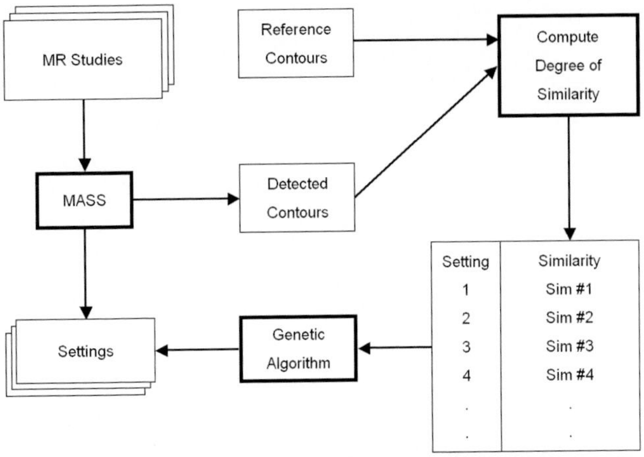

Figure 6.10. Automated optimization procedure to find the optimal contour detection settings for a specific pulse sequence. In an iterative procedure, MASS performs automated contour detection in a set of MRI studies using a number of different parameter settings. The detected contours are compared with manually defined reference contours, and the average degree of similarity is computed for each parameter setting. A genetic algorithm is used to generate new parameter settings based on the results of the parameter settings from the previous iteration.

a theoretic upper bound of 77%. The described optimization approach was evaluated on a set of 30 SSFP examinations from the three main magnetic resonance scanner vendors to assess the improvement in the performance of automated contour detection. In all 30 studies endocardial contours were carefully traced in the end-diastolic and end-systolic phases, which were used as reference. Automated contour detection was performed in all studies with and without optimized settings. The average degree of similarity was 49.5% when the unoptimized settings were used, which increased to 63.3% when the optimized settings were used.

NEW AUTOMATED SEGMENTATION METHODS

Reliable fully automated contour detection, not requiring any user interaction, would clearly be an important step to further improve the clinical utility of CMR. Despite a lot of research in this area, two major problems limit the success rate of many of the previously described contour detection strategies for cardiovascular structures. First, because of the presence of noise and image acquisition artifacts, image information can be ill defined, unreliable, or missing. In these cases a human observer is still capable of tracing the myocardial contours in the image data based on experience and prior knowledge, whereas many automated techniques fail. Second, a contour as drawn by an expert human observer may not always correspond to the location of the strongest local image evidence. In particular, in short-axis images the papillary muscles and trabeculae pose a problem. For example, many experts prefer to draw the left ventricular endocardial border as a convex hull around the blood pool, at a location somewhat "outside" of the strongest edge (53,54). A second example is the epicardial boundary, which may be embedded in fatty tissue, as a result of which the edge is strongest at the fat-air transitions. However, often the contour should be drawn on the inside of this fatty layer, an intensity transition that is marked by only a faint edge. Therefore, a decision about the exact location of the contour cannot always be made on the basis of the strongest image evidence but should be learned from the examples and preferences provided by expert observers.

To overcome these problems, prior knowledge about the image appearance, spatial organ embedding, and characteristic organ shape and its anatomic and pathologic shape variations should form an integral part of a contour detection approach. Moreover, it should be adaptive to accommodate the preferences of an observer and to easily adjust to image characteristics of various pulse sequences and magnetic resonance and MSCT systems.

Recently, Cootes et al (55) introduced the concept of active appearance models (AAMs), which are trainable mathematic models that can learn the shape and appearance of an imaged object from a set of example images. This method was originally developed for facial recognition and later optimized for the detection of the LV in CMR (56). An AAM consists of two components: a statistical model of the *shape* of an object and a statistical model of the *image appearance* of the object. The combined model is trained to learn the shape and image structure of an organ from a representative set of example images from different subjects. The AAM can be automatically matched to a new study image by minimizing an error function expressing the difference between the model and the underlying image evidence. During this matching process, the model is constrained to only resemble statistically plausible shapes and appearances. Consequently, AAMs are able to capture the association between observer preference and the underlying image evidence, making the AAMs highly suitable to model the expert observer's analysis behavior. Moreover, AAMs can model multiple objects (in our case the left and right cardiac ventricles) in their spatial embedding. In a study by Mitchell et al (57), this AAM technique showed excellent agreement with manually defined contours, both for the LV and RV simultaneously. Figure 6.11 shows examples of automatically detected contours for the LV and RV obtained by this new approach.

Van der Geest et al (58) investigated the value of incorporating image information of complete time series in an AAM-based contour detection method. The advantage of this approach lies in the fact that information from a complete time series is used during training and detection, which results in consistent time-continuous segmentation results, even in the presence of image frames with poor image quality.

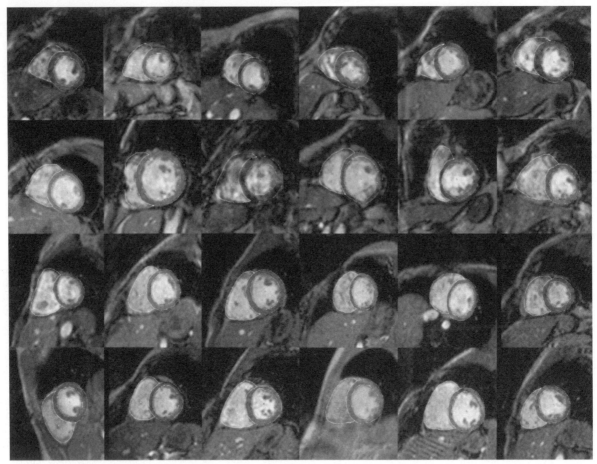

Figure 6.11. Detection results of left and right ventricular contours using the active appearance model (AAM) contour detection method.

MAGNETIC RESONANCE IMAGING FLOW QUANTIFICATION

VEC-MRI also plays an important role in the evaluation of global ventricular function. The accuracy of this imaging technique has been demonstrated in in vitro experiments using flow phantoms and comparison against other imaging techniques such as Doppler echocardiography and invasive oximetry (59,60).

Because flow measurements are obtained at high temporal resolution over the complete cardiac cycle, VEC-MRI is especially useful in the evaluation of left and right ventricular diastolic function parameters by measuring flow over the atrioventricular valves. Application of this technique to the proximal portion of the ascending aorta or pulmonary artery allows the assessment of left and right ventricular systolic function. After the cross section of a vessel is identified in the image by manual or automated contour detection, the instantaneous flow rate within the vessel cross section is obtained by multiplying the average velocity within the contour by its area. Ventricular stroke volume measurements are derived by integrating the flow over a complete cardiac cycle (61). The presence of aortic or pulmonary regurgitation can be easily identified and quantified from the derived flow curve. VEC-MRI has an established role in the evaluation of patients with congenital heart disease (62,63).

AUTOMATED QUANTIFICATION OF AORTIC FLOW

Application of VEC-MRI to the proximal portion of the ascending aorta allows the assessment of left ventricular systolic function by evaluating the flow over a complete cardiac cycle. Such a study requires a VEC-MRI acquisition in the transversal plane crossing the ascending aorta. The left ventricular stroke volume can be measured by integrating the flow over a complete cardiac cycle. For an accurate assessment of volume flow, contours describing the lumen of the vessels have to be obtained in the images. The in-plane motion of the greater vessels and changes in shape of the vessel cross section over the cardiac cycle would require the user to trace the luminal border of the vessel in each individual phase of the MRI examination. To overcome these practical limitations, an automated analysis method was developed in our department to automatically detect the required contours in each of the cardiac phases (64). This contour-detection algorithm was integrated in the FLOW software package.

The only user interaction required is the manual definition of an approximate center in one of the available images. In this first image an initial model contour is detected using gray value and edge information. The position of the same vessel at another time frame can be estimated by shifting the model contour in a limited region around the initial location and examining the edge values measured in the modulus image along the contour points. An algorithm was developed that finds the most likely contour position for each time frame, with the restriction that a contour is only allowed to displace 2 pixels (1.6 mm) from phase to phase, thereby imposing a temporal continuity of the motion. After the correct contour location was found, a final optimized contour was detected by allowing small deformations of the model contour such that it would follow the edges in the modulus image. For this purpose a 2D graph searching technique was used. The resulting contour was dilated by 1 pixel to be sure to encompass the complete region with flowing blood. The total contour detection process takes less than 10 seconds for a study with 30 cardiac phases.

Validation was performed on flow velocity maps from a study population of 12 healthy volunteers. Two independent observers performed manual and automated image analyses. The first observer repeated the automated and manual analyses after a 2-week interval to avoid learning effects. The time required for manual analysis was 5 to 10 minutes. During automated analysis the user had to identify the approximate location of the center of the aorta in one of the available images. The total analysis time for automated analysis was less than 10 seconds. Stroke volume measurements were obtained by integrating the flow over the complete cardiac cycle. The mean left ventricular stroke volume obtained by VEC-MRI in the group of 12 volunteers was 86.4 mL [standard deviation (SD): 13.6 mL]. No statistically significant differences were

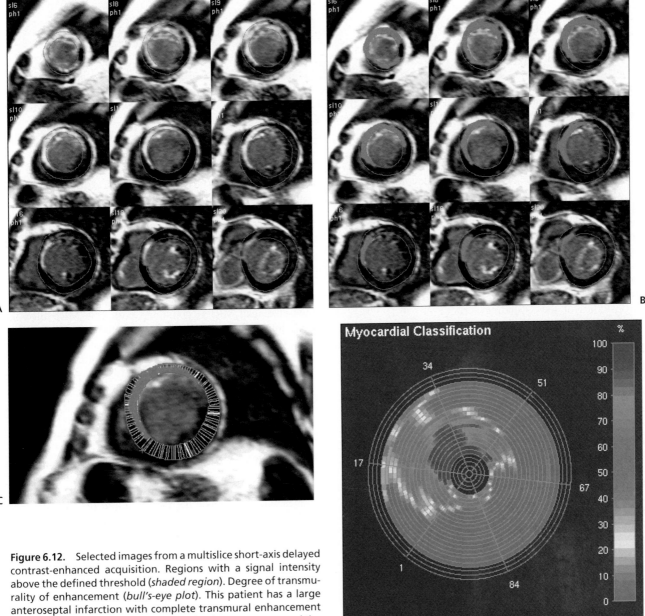

Figure 6.12. Selected images from a multislice short-axis delayed contrast-enhanced acquisition. Regions with a signal intensity above the defined threshold (*shaded region*). Degree of transmurality of enhancement (*bull's-eye plot*). This patient has a large anteroseptal infarction with complete transmural enhancement in the apical region and subendocardial enhancement toward the base.

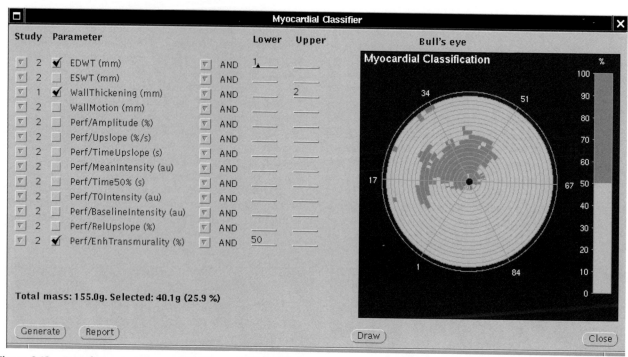

Figure 6.13. Data fusion between a multislice multiphase function scan and a delayed enhancement scan on the level of a bull's-eye display. Nonviable myocardium is defined as regions where the wall thickening in the function scan is less than 2 mm and the infarct transmurality is more than 50% in the delayed enhancement scan (*shaded region*).

found between the results of manual and automated analyses. The mean difference between automated and manually assessed stroke volume was 0.78 mL (SD: 1.99 mL). The intraobserver variability was 0.65 mL for manual analysis and 0.58 mL for automated analysis; the intraobserver variability was 0.99 mL for manual analysis and 0.90 mL for automated analysis. From this study, it can be concluded that the automated contour detection algorithm performs equally well as the manual method in the determination of left ventricular stroke volume derived from VEC-MRI studies of the ascending aorta.

DELAYED CONTRAST-ENHANCED MAGNETIC RESONANCE IMAGING

Delayed contrast-enhanced MRI has become part of a standard MRI examination because it is extremely valuable for the assessment of viable and nonviable myocardium in infarcted and poor contractile areas (65,66). The excellent resolution of MRI enables the depiction of both transmural and nontransmural regions of infarction. It was shown that the transmural extent of enhancement is inversely related to the likelihood of recovery of function after revascularization. Therefore, large nontransmural infarcts may have a better prognosis than relatively small transmural infarcts. Quantification of the size of the infarction involves defining a signal intensity threshold that separates normal myocardium from enhanced tissue. One approach to define this threshold is to assess the mean and SD of the signal intensity in a remote normal region and use a number of SDs above the mean as the threshold value (65,67). Although this method has shown to work in a specific setting,

it highly depends on the characteristics of the actual images. Schuijf et al (68) and Amado et al (69) propose to use a Full Width Half Maximum criterion to obtain a threshold value. Amado et al demonstrated in an animal experimental study that myocardial infarct size measurements using a Full Width Half Maximum criterion agreed very well with pathology. With the defined threshold, the enhanced regions within the myocardium are objectively defined and the regional degree of transmurality can be defined as illustrated in Figure 6.12. When delayed contrast-enhanced MRI is combined with cine MRI information, infarct transmurality can be related to the regions with poor contraction. This enables quantification of the location and size of regions of poor contraction that are still viable (Fig. 6.13).

SUMMARY

Cardiovascular MRI and MSCT are valuable techniques for noninvasive quantitative assessment of global and regional ventricular function. Computed tomography analysis techniques can help reduce the time required for quantification and interpretation of the many images. In this chapter, analytic methods for left ventricular function and vascular flow measurements based on automated contour detection approaches have been described. Validation studies of these methods have confirmed their accuracy, precision, robustness, and usefulness for clinical research studies. Fully automated contour detection methods that operate reliably in a routine clinical environment are needed and may become available in the near future.

REFERENCES

1. Rogers WJ Jr, Shapiro EP, Weiss JL, et al. Quantification and correction for left ventricular systolic long-axis shortening by magnetic resonance tissue tagging and slice isolation. *Circulation* 1991;84:721–731.
2. Marcus JT, Götte MJW, de Waal LK, et al. The influence of through-plane motion on left ventricular volumes measured by magnetic resonance imaging: implications for image acquisition and analysis. *J Cardiovasc Magn Res* 1998;1(1):1–6.
3. Bloomer TN, Plein S, Radjenovic A, et al. Cine MRI using steady state free precession in the radial long axis orientation is a fast accurate method for obtaining volumetric data of the left ventricle. *J Magn Reson Imaging* 2002;14(6):685–692.
4. Florentine MS, Grosskreutz CJ, Chang W, et al. Measurement of left ventricular mass in vivo using gated nuclear magnetic resonance imaging. *J Am Coll Cardiol* 1986;8:107–112.
5. Maddahi J, Crues J, Berman DS, et al. Noninvasive quantitation of left ventricular mass by gated proton magnetic resonance imaging. *J Am Coll Cardiol* 1987;10(3):682–692.
6. Matheijssen NAA, Baur LHB, Reiber JHC, et al. Assessment of left ventricular volume and mass by cine-magnetic resonance imaging in patients with anterior myocardial infarction intra-observer and inter-observer variability on contour detection. *Int J Card Imaging* 1996;12:11–19.
7. Niwa K, Uchishiba M, Aotsuka H, et al. Measurement of ventricular volumes by cine magnetic resonance imaging in complex congenital heart disease with morphologically abnormal ventricles. *Am Heart J* 1996;131:567–575.
8. Jauhiainen T, Järvinen VM, Hekali PE, et al. MR gradient echo volumetric analysis of the human cardiac casts: focus on the right ventricle. *J Comput Assist Tomogr* 1998;22(6):899–903.
9. Alfakih K, Thiele H, Plein S, et al. Comparison of right ventricular volume measurement between segmented k-space gradient-echo and steady-state free precession magnetic resonance imaging. *J Magn Reson Imaging* 2002;16(3):253–258.
10. Semelka RC, Tomei E, Wagner S, et al. Normal left ventricular dimensions and function: interstudy reproducibility of measurements with cine MR imaging. *Radiology* 1990;174:763–768.
11. Dirksen MS, Bax JJ, de Roos A, et al. Usefulness of dynamic multislice computed tomography of left ventricular function in unstable angina pectoris and comparison with echocardiography. *Am J Cardiol* 2002;90:1157–1160.
12. Mahnken AH, Spuentrup E, Niethammer M, et al. Quantitative and qualitative assessment of left ventricular volume with ECG-gated multislice spiral CT: value of different image reconstruction algorithms in comparison to MRI. *Acta Radiol* 2003;44(6):604–611.
13. Juergens KU, Grude M, Maintz D, et al. Multi-detector row CT of left ventricular function with dedicated analysis software versus MR imaging: initial experience. *Radiology* 2004;230:403–410.
14. Dulce MC, Mostbeck GH, Friese KK, et al. Quantification of left ventricular volumes and function with cine MR imaging: comparison of geometrical models with three-dimensional data. *Radiology* 1993;188:371–376.
15. Chuang ML, Hibberd MG, Salton CJ, et al. Importance of imaging method over imaging modality in noninvasive determination of left ventricular volumes and ejection fraction: assessment by two- and three-dimensional echocardiography and magnetic resonance imaging. *J Am Coll Cardiol* 2000;35(2):477–484.
16. Sakuma H, Fujita N, Foo TKF, et al. Evaluation of left ventricular volume and mass with breath-hold cine MR imaging. *Radiology* 1993;188:377–380.
17. Lamb HJ, Singleton RR, van der Geest RJ, et al. MR imaging of regional cardiac function: low-pass filtering of wall thickness curves. *Magn Res Med* 1995;34:498–502.
18. Lorenz CH, Walker ES, Morgan VL, et al. Normal human right and left ventricular mass, systolic function and gender differences by cine magnetic resonance imaging. *J Cardiovasc Magn Reson* 1999;1:7–21.
19. Rominger MB, Bachmann GF, Pabst W, et al. Right ventricular volumes and ejection fraction with fast cine MR imaging in breath-hold technique: applicability, normal values from 52 volunteers, and evaluation of 325 adult cardiac patients. *J Magn Reson Imaging* 1999;10(6):908–918.
20. Alfakih K, Plein S, Thiele H, et al. Normal human left and right ventricular dimensions for MRI as assessed by turbo gradient echo and Steady-State Free Precession imaging sequences. *J Magn Reson Imaging* 2003;17(3):323–329.
21. Lee VS, Resnick D, Bundy JM, et al. Cardiac function: MR evaluation in one breath hold with real-time True Fisp imaging with steady-state precession. *Radiology* 2002;222:835–842.
22. Wei LI, Stern JS, Mai VM, et al. MR assessment of left ventricular function: quantitative comparison of fast imaging employing steady-state acquisition (FIESTA) with fast gradient echo cine technique. *J Magn Reson Imaging* 2002;16(5):559–564.
23. Lieberman AN, Weiss JL, Jugdutt BI, et al. Two-dimensional echocardiography and infarct size: relationship of regional wall motion and thickening to the extent of myocardial infarction in the dog. *Circulation* 1981;63(4):739–746.
24. Azhari H, Sideman S, Weiss JL, et al. Three-dimensional mapping of acute ischemic regions using MRI: wall thickening versus motion analysis. *Am J Physiol* 1990;259:H1492–H1503.
25. van Rugge FP, van der Wall EE, Spanjersberg SJ, et al. Magnetic resonance imaging during dobutamine stress for detection of coronary artery disease; quantitative wall motion analysis using a modification of the centerline method. *Circulation* 1994;90:127–138.
26. Haag UJ, Maier SE, Jakob M, et al. Left ventricular wall thickness measurements by magnetic resonance: a validation study. *Int J Card Imaging* 1991;7:31–41.
27. Baer FM, Smolarz K, Theissen P, et al. Regional 99mTc-methoxyisobutyl-isonitrile-uptake at rest in patients with myocardial infarcts: comparison with morphological and functional parameters obtained from gradient-echo magnetic resonance imaging. *Eur Heart J* 1994;15:97–107.
28. Holman ER, Vliegen HW, van der Geest RJ, et al. Quantitative analysis of regional left ventricular function after myocardial infarction in the pig assessed with cine magnetic resonance imaging. *Magn Reson Med* 1995;34:161–169.
29. Sheehan FH, Bolson EL, Dodge HT, et al. Advantages and applications of the centerline method for characterizing regional ventricular function. *Circulation* 1986;74:293–305.
30. von Land CD, Rao SR, Reiber JHC. Development of an improved centerline wall motion model. *Comput Cardiol* 1990;687–690.
31. Holman ER, Buller VGM, de Roos A, et al. Detection and quantification of dysfunctional myocardium by magnetic resonance imaging: a new three-dimensional method for quantitative wall-thickening analysis. *Circulation* 1997;95:924–931.
32. Buller VGM, van der Geest RJ, Kool MD, et al. Assessment of regional left ventricular wall parameters from short-axis MR imaging using a 3D extension to the improved centerline method. *Invest Radiol* 1997;32(9):529–539.
33. Guttman MA, Prince JL, McVeigh ER. Tag and contour detection in tagged MR images of the left ventricle. *IEEE Trans Med Imaging* 1993;13(1):74–88.
34. Moore CC, McVeigh ER, Zerhouni EA. Quantitative tagged magnetic resonance imaging of the normal human left ventricle. *Top Magn Reson Imaging* 2000;11(6):359–371.

35. Garot J, Bluemke DA, Osman NF, et al. Fast determination of regional myocardial strain fields from tagged cardiac images using harmonic phase MRI. *Circulation* 2000;101(9):981–988.

36. Osman NF, McVeigh ER, Prince JL. Imaging heart motion using harmonic phase MRI. *IEEE Trans Med Imaging* 2000; 19(3):186–202.

37. Pelc NJ, Drangova M, Pelc LR, et al. Tracking of cyclic motion with phase-contrast cine MR velocity data. *J Magn Reson Imaging* 1995;5:339–345.

38. Hennig J, Schneider B, Peschl S, et al. Analysis of myocardial motion based on velocity measurements with a black blood prepared segmented gradient-echo sequence: methodology and applications to normal volunteers and patients. *J Magn Reson Imaging* 1998;8(4):868–877.

39. McInerney T, Terzopoulos D. A dynamic finite element surface model for segmentation and tracking in multidimensional medical images with application to cardiac 4D image analysis. *Comput Med Imaging Graph* 1995;19:69–83.

40. Matsumura K, Nakase E, Haiyama T, et al. Automatic left ventricular volume measurements on contrast-enhanced ultrafast cine magnetic resonance imaging. *Eur J Radiol* 1995; 20(2):126–132.

41. Goshtasby A, Turner DA. Segmentation of cardiac cine MR images for right and left ventricular chambers. *IEEE Trans Med Imaging* 1995;14:56–64.

42. Baldy C, Doueck P, Croisille P, et al. Automated myocardial edge detection from breath-hold cine-MR images: evaluation of left ventricular volumes and mass. *Magn Reson Imaging* 1994;12:589–598.

43. van der Geest RJ, Buller VGM, Jansen E, et al. Comparison between manual and automated analysis of left ventricular volume parameters from short axis MR images. *J Comput Assist Tomogr* 1997;21(5):756–765.

44. Butler SP, McKay E, Paszkowski AL, et al. Reproducibility study of left ventricular measurements with breath-hold cine MRI using a semiautomated volumetric image analysis program. *J Magn Reson Imaging* 1998;8(2):467–472.

45. Kaushikkar SV, Li D, Haacke EM, et al. Adaptive blood pool segmentation in three-dimensions: application to MR cardiac evaluation. *J Magn Reson Imaging* 1996;6:690–697.

46. Singleton HR, Pohost GM. Automatic cardiac MR image segmentation using edge detection by tissue classification in pixel neighborhoods. *Magn Reson Med* 1997;37:418–424.

47. Furber A, Balzer P, Cavaro-Menárd C, et al. Experimental validation of an automated edge-detection method for a simultaneous determination of the endocardial and epicardial borders in short-axis cardiac MR images: application in normal volunteers. *J Magn Reson Imaging* 1998;8: 1006–1014.

48. Nachtomy E, Cooperstein R, Vaturi M, et al. Automatic assessment of cardiac function from short-axis MRI: procedure and clinical evaluation. *Magn Reson Imaging* 1998;16(4): 365–376.

49. Lalande A, Legrand L, Walker PM, et al. Automatic detection of left ventricular contours from cardiac cine magnetic resonance imaging using fuzzy logic. *Invest Radiol* 1999;34(3): 211–217.

50. Amini AA, Weymouth TE, Jain RC. Using dynamic programming for solving variational problems in vision. *IEE Trans PAMI* 1990;12(9):855–867.

51. van Assen HC, Danilouchkine MG, Behloul F, et al. Cardiac LV segmentation using a 3D active shape model driven by fuzzy inference. *LNCS* 2003;2878:533–540.

52. Angelié A, de Koning PJH, Danilouchkine M, et al. Optimizing the automated segmentation of the left ventricle in magnetic resonance images. *Med Phys* 2005;32(2):1–7.

53. Pattynama PMT, Lamb HJ, van der Velde EA, et al. Left ventricular measurements with cine and spin-echo MR imaging: a study of reproducibility with variance component analysis. *Radiology* 1993;187:261–268.

54. Lamb HJ, Doornbos J, van der Velde EA, et al. Echo-planar MRI of the heart on a standard system: validation of measurement ofleft ventricular function and mass. *J Comput Assist Tomogr* 1996;20(6):942–949.

55. Cootes TF, Beeston C, Edwards GJ, et al. A unified framework for atlas matching using active appearance models. *LNCS* 1999;1613:322–333.

56. Mitchell SC, Lelieveldt BPF, van der Geest RJ, et al. Multistage hybrid active appearance model matching: segmentation of left and right ventricles in cardiac MR images. *IEEE Trans Med Imaging* 2001;20(5):415–423.

57. Mitchell SC, Lelieveldt BPF, van der Geest RJ, et al. Segmentation of cardiac MR images: an active appearance model approach. *Proc. SPIE Medical Imaging* 2000;3979:224–234.

58. van der Geest RJ, Lelieveldt BPF, Angelié A, et al. Evaluation of a new method for automated detection of left ventricular boundaries in time series of magnetic resonance images using an active appearance motion model. *J Cardiovasc Magn Reson* 2004;6(3):609–617.

59. Karwatowski SP, Brecker SJD, Yang GZ, et al. Mitral valve flow measured with cine MR velocity mapping in patients with ischemic heart disease: comparison with Doppler echocardiography. *J Magn Reson Imaging* 1995;5:89–92.

60. Beerbaum P, Körperich P, Barth P, et al. Noninvasive quantification of left-to-right shunt in pediatric patients. Phase-contrast cine magnetic resonance imaging compared with invasive oximetry. *Circulation* 103, 2476–2482. 2001.

61. Kondo C, Caputo GR, Semelka R, et al. Right and left ventricular stroke volume measurements with velocity-encoded cine MR imaging: in vitro and in vivo validation. *AJR Am J Roentgenol* 1991;157:9–16.

62. de Roos A, Helbing WA, Niezen RA, et al. Magnetic resonance imaging in adult congenital heart disease. In: Higgins CB, Inwall JS, Pohost GM, eds. *Current and future applications of magnetic resonance in cardiovascular disease.* Armonk, NY: Futura Publishing Company, Inc., 1988:163–172.

63. Powel AJ, Geva T. Blood flow measurement by magnetic resonance imaging in congenital heart disease. *Pediatr Cardiol* 2000;21:47–58.

64. van der Geest RJ, Niezen RA, van der Wall EE, et al. Automated measurement of volume flow in the ascending aorta using MR velocity maps: evaluation of inter- and interobserver variability in healthy volunteers. *J Comput Assist Tomogr* 1998;22(6):904–911.

65. Kim RJ, Fieno DS, Parrish TH, et al. Relationship of MRI delayed contrast enhancement to irreversible injury, infarct age, and contractile function. *Circulation* 1999;100(19): 1992–2002.

66. Kim RJ, Wu E, Rafael A, et al. The use of contrast-enhanced magnetic resonance imaging to identify reversible myocardial dysfunction. *New Engl J Med* 2000;343:1445–1453.

67. Oshinski JN, Yang ZQ, Jones JR, et al. Imaging time after Gd-DTPA injection is critical in using delayed enhancement to determine infarct size accurately with magnetic resonance imaging. *Circulation* 2001;104(23):2838–2842.

68. Schuijf JD, Kaandorp TA, Lamb HJ, et al. Quantification of myocardial infarct size and transmurality by contrast-enhanced magnetic resonance imaging in men. *Am J Cardiol* 2005;94(3): 284–288.

69. Amado LC, Gerber BL, Gupta VK, et al. Accurate and objective infarct sizing by contrast-enhanced magnetic resonance imaging in a canine myocardial infarction model. *J Am Coll Cardiol* 2004;44(12):2383–2389.

7

Magnetic Resonance Contrast Media

Maythem Saeed and Charles B. Higgins

OVERVIEW

Magnetic resonance (MR) contrast media, paramagnetic and super-paramagnetic metal complexes, are made from metals containing unpaired electrons. These agents are used to enhance the capability of magnetic resonance imaging (MRI) and MR angiography (MRA). The inherent contrast of the blood and myocardium on MR depends largely on proton concentration and longitudinal (T1) and transverse (T2) relaxation times. MR contrast media and pulse sequences can manipulate tissue contrast. The effects of MR contrast agents on signal intensity (SI) are described in terms of T1 and T2 relaxivities (R1 and R2). For any contrast medium, the R2/R1 ratio can be used in determining whether the agent is causing predominantly T2 shortening (decrease in SI) or T1 shortening (increase in SI).

Classification of MR contrast media is based on (a) distribution in tissues, (b) changes in tissue contrast, and (c) specificity for special cells or tissues. MR contrast media have three distribution compartments, namely, blood pool, extracellular space, and intracellular compartment. The difference between extracellular and blood-pool MR contrast media is based on residence times in the blood pool and presence in the extracellular compartment. Extracellular gadolinium-based MR contrast media constitute the largest group and are considered very safe. After intravenous administration they distribute within the blood pool (arterial and venous) and then diffuse rapidly into the interstitial space in a similar fashion as water-soluble iodinated contrast agents. Images acquired during the first pass are useful for demonstrating vascular anatomy, extent of myocardial area at risk, and relative myocardial perfusion. On the other hand, images obtained during the equilibrium phase are useful for detecting microvascular obstruction (MO), and images at 10 to 15 minutes after contrast injection are useful for assessing myocardial viability. The development of blood-pool contrast media may be crucial for coronary MRA and for the assessment of microvascular permeability and obstruction. These agents can be used in guiding endovascular guidewires and catheters during interventional procedures. Intracellular MR contrast media are localized inside the myocytes. Labeled cells can be used for monitoring cell trafficking and therapies that are based on the use of stem cells and progenitors. Porphyrin derivatives labeled with gadolinium have the affinity to bind specific tissues. This class of cellular or tissue-specific MR contrast media has been used for mapping necrotic myocardium and detecting vulnerable plaque. The design objectives for the next generation of MR contrast media will likely focus on prolonging intravascular retention (blood-pool contrast media) and improving tissue targeting (tissue-specific contrast media and probes) and molecular imaging. This chapter focuses on the current status of different classes of MR contrast media and summarizes its applications in the cardiovascular system.

MAGNETIC PROPERTIES

MRI measures the characteristics of hydrogen nuclei of water and nuclei with similar chemical shifts, modified by chemical environment across the image. It gives spatial distribution of the intensity of the proton signals in the tissue. The inherent signal on MRI can be manipulated by using different MR pulse sequences, contrast media, and magnetic field strengths (B0) (1,2). The magnitude of signal arises from tissue depends on the amount of water and on longitudinal (T1) and transverse (T2) relaxation times.

T1 is defined as the time constant, which characterizes the rate at which spins align with an external field. The longitudinal relaxivity of T1-enhancing agent describes the amount of T1 relaxation rate (R1 = 1/T1) enhancement produced per quantity of the agent ($s^{-1}mM^{-1}$). R1 is often used in describing the effect of contrast media on tissue relaxation. The T1 process occurs when spins experience B0 fluctuations with frequency components that are close to precessional (Larmor) frequency (3).

T2 is defined as the time constant, which characterizes loss of phase coherence of spin population. The T2 process occurs from the T1 process and by slower B0 fluctuation, including time invariant field differences through space (B0 inhomogeneity). On T2* images, however, the signal loss stems from dephasing of the transverse magnetization as a result of spin moving through a magnetic field disturbance. Tissue SI tends to increase with increasing R1 and decrease with increasing R2. MR pulse sequences that address changes in R1 and R2 are referred to as T1- and T2-weighted images, respectively (4).

MAGNETIC RESONANCE CONTRAST MEDIA

MR contrast media are used to better visualize regions of interest by introducing them into or around these regions. Metals and molecules containing unpaired electrons demonstrate a paramagnetic behavior when placed in an external magnetic field. MR contrast media can be simple substances (such as O_2 and CO_2), stable radical substances (such as nitroxide radical) or metals (such as gadolinium (III), manganese (II), high-spin iron (III), or dysprosium (III)). These metals exert a strong stimulation of either T1 relaxation or T2 relaxation (5–11). They have a different number of unpaired electrons (e.g., seven in gadolinium, five in iron, and five in manganese) and at least one site for water coordination. The efficacy of these metals to affect the proton relaxation times in tissue and blood is related to the magnetic moment of the unpaired electron, electron spin relaxation rate of the metal, and number of coordination sites available for water ligation. Perhaps the most important parameter that influences relaxivity is the rate of rotational diffusion. As rotational diffusion is slowed, the

metal complex fluctuates at a frequency closer to the proton Larmor frequency and the relaxation efficiency can be improved markedly. A particularly useful way to slow rotational rates is to incorporate a targeting functionality capable of binding the complex to a macromolecule. One example of this is MS-325, a derivative of Gd-DTPA, where DTPA ligand was modified to bind noncovalently to plasma albumin (12). Other factors that alter the potency of the paramagnetic agents are molecular tumbling rate, size of the chelate, solvent viscosity, magnetic field strength, and magnetic moment of the paramagnet (5,8,13–15).

Unlike x-ray contrast agents, MR agents are not directly measurable on imaging, but their effects on adjacent proton nuclei are measurable. The longitudinal (r1) and transverse (r2) relaxivity ($L/mmol^{-1}/sec^{-1}$) refer to the amount of increase in 1/T1 and 1/T2 per mmolar of the contrast medium, respectively. The observed longitudinal relaxation rate of protons in aqueous solution containing a paramagnetic complex is the sum of the following factors: (a) a diamagnetic factor that corresponds to the relaxation rate, (b) a paramagnetic factor that arises from the exchange of water molecules from the inner coordination sphere of the metal ion with the bulk water, and (c) a paramagnetic factor that derives from the diffusion of water in the outer coordination sphere of the paramagnetic center (6–10,16–18). Whereas shortening of T1 increases SI, shortening of T2 decreases SI of the blood and tissues (19,20).

CLASSIFICATION

MR contrast media have been classified according to their distribution in the body, alteration of tissue SI, or affinity for specific cells or tissues. Table 7.1 shows the different types of MR contrast media and their stages of development.

DISTRIBUTION IN THE BODY

MR contrast media can be classified on the basis of the distribution in the tissues, namely, extracellular, intracellular, and blood-pool contrast media. This classification is the most widely used and based on the capability of the contrast media to pass across the vascular endothelium and cell membrane. In general, microvessels have small gaps between endothelial cells, allowing diffusion of low molecular weight compounds, such as extracellular and intracellular MR contrast media. Extracellular agents have low molecular weights; thus they diffuse rapidly into the extracellular space (Fig. 7.1) and have a short plasma half-life (<20 minutes).

Blood-pool MR contrast media can be defined as agents having higher molecular weights (>50 kDa) than extracellular media (<2 kDa), therefore slowing their exit from the vascular system (13–15). Large molecules, such as Gd-DTPA-albumin, are not eliminated easily by the kidneys and called "slow-clearance blood-pool media" (21). The most commonly used backbones in blood-pool gadolinium-based MR contrast media are dextran, polylysine, and dendrimer (13–15). Superparamagnetic iron oxide particles are also used as blood-pool agents. Reticuloendothelial phagocytosis plays an important role in clearing superparamagnetic iron oxide particles from the blood (plasma half-life <10 minutes) (7). The superparamagnetic blood-pool iron oxide particles have a larger diameter (4–50 times) than Gd-DTPA-albumin (6 nm). Ultrasmall superparamagnetic iron oxide particles are

TABLE 7-1	Cardiovascular Magnetic Resonance Contrast Media and Their Development Stage

T1-enhancing (relaxivity) contrast media

Gadopentate dimeglumine (Gd-DTPA), Magnevist™, Schering, for sale
Gadodiamide (Gd-DTPA-BMA), Omniscan™, Nycomed, for sale
Gadoterate meglumine (Gd-DOTA), Dotarem™, Guerbet, for sale
Gadoversetamide, Gd-DTPA-BMEA, Optimark™, Mallinckrodt, phase III
Gadoteridol (Gd-HP-DO3A), ProHance™, Bracco, for sale
Gadobutrol (Gd-BT-DO3A), Gadovist™, Schering, phase III
Gadobenate dimeglumine (Gd-BOPTA), MultiHance™, Bracco, for sale
Gadoxetic acid (Gd-EOB-DTPA), III Eovist™, Schering, phase III

Susceptibility (T2*) contrast media

Dysprosium diethylenetriamine pentaacetic acid-bismethylamide (Dy-DTPA-BMA), sprodiamide Nycomed, preclinical phase
Dy-DTPA, preclinical phase
Dy-tetraphenyl-porphyrin sulfonate, Dy-TPPS or Ho-TPPS, preclinical phase

Blood-Pool Agents

(A) Gadolinium chelates
Angiomark (MS-325), Epix, phase II
Gadopentetate-dimeglumine-polylysine, Schering, preclinical phase
Gadomer 17 (Gadomer™), Schering, phase I
Gd-DTPA-dextran, Nycomed, preclinical phase
P792 (macromolecular Gd-DOTA derivate, Vistarem™), clinical trials phase II
(B) Dysprosium-chelates
Albumin(Dy-DTPA)x, preclinical phase
(C) Superparamagnetic iron oxides
Ferrixan, SHU 555a (Resovist), Schering, phase III
AMI-277 (Sinirem, Guerbet™) and (Combidrex™), Advanced Magnetics, phase III
AMI-25 (Endorem™), Guerbet, (Feridex IV™), Berlex, for sale
OMP (Abdoscan), Nycomed
AMI-121 (Lumirem), Guerbet, (Gastromark), Advanced Magnetics, for sale
PION, polycrystalline iron oxide nanoparticles (larger particles = DDM 128, PION-ASF), preclinical phase
MION, monocrystalline iron oxide nanoparticles, preclinical phase
Fe O-BPA USPIO, preclinical phase

Intracellular Agents

Mangafodipir trisodium, (Teslascan™), Nycomed, for sale in Europe

Cellular and Tissue-Specific Contrast Media

Gadophrin II and III, Schering AG, preclinical phase
Gadofluorine-8, Schering, preclinical phase
Iron oxide particles with MION-antimyosin, preclinical phase
Iron particles, for vascular plaque

the small version of these particles. They have relatively long plasma half-lives (>1 hour) and provide strong enhancement of the vascular system and information on microvascular leakage in ischemic myocardium. Blood-pool MR contrast media have a greater T1 relaxivity (r1) than extracellular media because they have (a) multiple paramagnetic ions attached to each polymeric molecule and (b) slower molecular rotational correlation times of each paramagnetic subunit.

The shape of MR contrast media plays an important role in tissue distribution and renal excretion (22–24). For exam-

ple, physiologic studies have shown that the capillaries in myocardium are not permeable to Gadomer (18 kDa) and Vistarem (6.47 kDa and molecular size = 10 nm). The kidneys can easily eliminate Gadomer and Vistarem; thus they are called rapid-clearance blood-pool MR contrast media. Vistarem is an analog of the extracellular contrast medium Dotarem (Gd-DPTA), which has a molecular weight of 0.56 kDa and a diameter of 10.0 Å. Vistarem has a diameter of 50.5 Å. Gadomer has an actual molecular weight of 18 kDa, but because of the globular shape of the molecule, the appar-

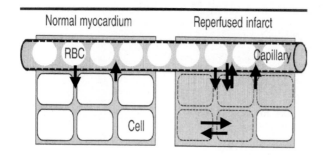

Figure 7.1. Ischemic model illustrates the distribution of extracellular MR contrast media in normal and infarcted myocardium. Extracellular MR contrast media distribute exclusively in the extracellular space in normal myocardium (10%–18% of the tissue volume, *left*). For infarction the fractional distribution volume of the contrast agent increases because of the formation of interstitial edema and loss of membrane integrity of the necrotic cells.

ent molecular mass is 30 to 35 kDa. The quantity of blood-pool agent, which diffuses into the interstitium, is inversely related to the molecular weight, shape, and volume. Blood-pool MR contrast media enhance myocardium to a lesser degree than extracellular agents, because they have a smaller distribution volume (5%–10% vs. 15%–20%) (25).

The third group of agents is the intracellular MR contrast media. Contrast media in this group, represented by Mn^{+2}, have a smaller molecular weight than extracellular and blood-pool contrast media. Manganese passes passively through vascular endothelium and actively through the cell membrane to reach the intracellular space. The transport of Mn^{+2} is through voltage-dependent calcium channels at the cell membrane. Mn^{+2} is rapidly taken up by normal myocardium, with less or no uptake and retention by ischemic and infarcted myocardium (26–29). The uptake pattern of manganese is analogous to that of thallium-201. Skjold et al (30) assessed the magnitude and duration of changes in R1 in human hearts after the administration of 0.05 mmol/kg Mn^{+2}-releasing contrast medium Mn-DPDP. They found that this agent increased myocardial R1 by 34% to 46% for at least 2 hours, but that the increased R1 was not linear with higher doses (30).

MR contrast media have been widely applied in cardiovascular imaging (Table 7.2). The effects of extracellular (Gd-DTPA-BMA), blood-pool (Gd-DTPA-albumin) and in-tracellular ($MnCl_2$) MR contrast media on the relaxation rate (R1) of normal and reperfused infarcted myocardium have been compared in rat hearts (25). The data indicate the following: (a) Gd-based contrast medium increased R1 of infarcted myocardium significantly more compared with normal myocardium at 5 minutes, followed by a gradual, but parallel, decline in R1 of both regions; (b) Gd-DTPA-albumin produced a small increase in R1 of normal and infarcted myocardium at an early phase, followed by a sharp increase in R1 of infarcted, but not normal, myocardium; (c) Mn^{+2}-based contrast medium caused an identical increase in R1 of both regions in the first 5 minutes because of the nonspecific distribution of the contrast medium, followed by a rapid decrease in R1 of infarcted, but not normal, myocardium. Overall, Mn^{+2}-based contrast medium provided the largest R1 difference between normal and infarcted myocardium at a later time than Gd-based media.

CHANGES IN TISSUE CONTRAST

Gadolinium-based MR contrast media act predominantly on T1 relaxation, which results in signal enhancement and "positive" contrast, and to a lesser extent on T2 relaxation, which results in signal reduction and "negative" contrast (31). The T1 and T2 values are changed by changing the number of fluctuating magnetic fields near a nucleus. Positive contrast media are compounds containing either Gd or Mn^{+2}. All clinically approved Gd-based contrast media cause positive enhancement at the recommended doses (0.1–0.3 mmol/kg). It should be noted that the effect of MR contrast media on SI of the blood or tissue is not pure T1 or T2. The T1- and T2-sensitive MR pulse sequences can enhance both effects of MR contrast media. Adding an inversion pulse enhances the T1 capability of echo planar and gradient-echo sequences. The inversion time plays an important role in enhancing regions with different T1 values (Fig. 7.2).

The relaxivities of clinically approved gadolinium chelates are 4 mM/s for r1 and 6 mM/s for r2 at 1.5 T. Negative contrast media are compounds containing either dysprosium or iron (32,33). These agents produce predominantly spin–spin relaxation effects, but ultrasmall iron oxide particles (<300 nm) also produce substantial T1 relaxation. Experimental cardiac studies have shown that the contrast between healthy and diseased tissue can be manipulated using a single MR contrast agent but different MR pulse sequences,

TABLE 7-2	Applications of Magnetic Resonance Contrast Media in Cardiac Imaging

Assessing myocardial perfusion and perfusion reserve
Assessing myocardial viability
Measuring the spatial extent of myocardial stunning, acute and chronic (scar) infarctions
Discriminating acute infarctions from scar tissue
Demonstrating reperfusion at microvascular level and microvascular obstruction
Labeling of stem and progenitor cells
Enhancing plaque and vascular wall imaging
Guiding endovascular catheters during intervention
Anatomy of the coronary arteries

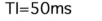

TI=50ms   TI=190ms

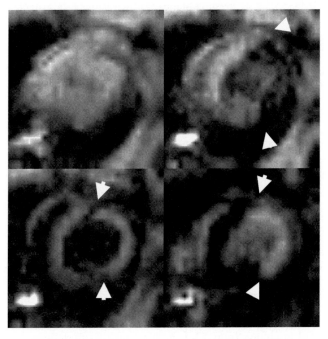

TI=280ms   TI=400ms

Figure 7.2. Inversion recovery echo planar images showing the effect of increasing inversion time (TI) on signal intensity (SI) of normal and acute infarcted myocardium after administration of Gd-based magnetic resonance (MR) contrast medium. The magnitude image (*top left*) with extremely short TI shows no differential enhancement. Increasing TI allows the region with the shortest T1 to pass through null point first and appears as a dark zone. In this case, infarcted myocardium (*arrows*) passed first (*top right*), then left ventricle blood (*bottom left*) and finally the normal remote myocardium (*bottom right*).

which are sensitive to the different contrast mechanisms (29,34–36). Bolus injection of positive MR contrast media proved to be superior to negative contrast media in cardiac imaging (34) because they resolve the saturation by restoring a good part of the longitudinal magnetization between pulses. The R2/R1 ratios of agents can be used to determine whether the agent is causing predominantly T2 or T1 shortening. The R2/R1 ratios are more than 5 for T2-enhancing agents and less than 2 for T1-enhancing agents.

AFFINITY FOR SPECIFIC CELLS AND TISSUES

Cellular and tissue-specific MR contrast media are synthesized to target certain cells or tissues (9,37–39). Their effect is independent of blood volume (37) or distribution volume (Table 7.1) (9,37–39). These agents diffuse or convect to ischemic regions even in the presence of coronary occlusion. They act as T1-enhancing agents (gadophrin II and III) (40,41) or T2*-enhancing agents (iron antimyosin antibody) (42). The necrosis-specific properties of gadophrin II and III have been used to map necrotic myocardium and to demonstrate the high sensitivity of hypertrophied hearts to ischemia (Fig. 7.3).

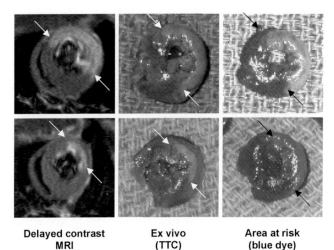

| Delayed contrast MRI | Ex vivo (TTC) | Area at risk (blue dye) |

Figure 7.3. Delayed contrast-enhanced MR images of hypertrophied (*top*) and control (*bottom*) hearts subjected to the same duration of ischemia (25 minutes) followed by reperfusion in a rat model. Note the close relation between the extent of contrast-enhanced medium on magnetic resonance imaging (MRI) and the gold standard triphenyltetrazolium chloride (TTC, *center slices*). The necrosis-specific MR contrast medium, gadophrin II (0.05 mmol/kg), accurately delineated infarcted myocardium in hypertrophied and control hearts. The extent of infarction in hypertrophied heart is substantially larger (almost identical to the area at risk defined by infusion of blue dye in situ, *right slices*) than control heart, suggesting the high sensitivity of hypertrophied hearts to ischemia.

Other vascular specific MR contrast media such as perfluorocarbon nanoparticles and gadofluorine have been used for detecting vulnerable vascular plaques and atherosclerosis-associated inflammatory process in the vascular wall (43–46). Flacke et al (43) proposed the use of ligand-directed, lipid-encapsulated liquid perfluorocarbon nanoparticles (Gd-DTPA-BOA at the outer lipid monolayer) to specifically detect vulnerable plaques. Technical advances in MRI will further increase the efficacy of specific MR contrast media.

CLEARANCE, TOLERANCE, AND SAFETY

Paramagnetic metals are chelated to a ligand to reduce the inherent toxicity and modify their distribution in tissues. The chelation approach has culminated in the development of several Food and Drug Administration-approved gadolinium chelates (Table 7.1). Drawbacks of the chelation are that (a) it decreases the T1 rate constant (47) and that (b) it alters the pharmacokinetic properties of the paramagnetic ions. For example, the rate of renal excretion of gadolinium chelates increased by 550-fold compared with pre-chelation values (47–49).

Transmetallation is another factor contributing to the toxicity of gadolinium. Investigators found that there are some differences in the physicochemical properties of MR contrast media, which arise from the use of linear versus macrocyclic structures for the organic ligands (48), but the difference seems to have little consequence in diagnostic efficacies and safety profiles.

Dissociation of the paramagnetic metal from the chelate is a major factor contributing to the potential toxicity of gadolinium. The integrity of the paramagnetic metal and chelate complex must be maintained in vivo to create a safe and efficacious MR contrast medium. Dissociation of the paramagnetic metal from the chelate is undesirable because both free metal and chelate are highly toxic. The dissociated compounds have a tendency to precipitate in liver, lymph nodes, and bones and obstruct calcium-ion passage into cardiac cells, muscle cells, and nerve tissue cells, potentially causing the arrest of neuromuscular transmission (7,8).

The overall incidence of adverse reactions to extracellular MR contrast media ranges from 0.9% to 2.4%. This rate is relatively low compared with iodinated contrast agents (3% for nonionic and 12.6% for ionic). Runge (50) addressed the issue of safety of the clinically available MR contrast media. He found that these agents produce minor adverse reactions, including nausea (1%–2%) and hives (<1%), and concluded that they are safe and well tolerated in adult and pediatric patients. Mn-DPDP and ferumoxides have a higher percentage of adverse reactions (7%–17% and 15%, respectively).

CARDIAC APPLICATIONS OF MAGNETIC RESONANCE CONTRAST MEDIA

CHARACTERIZATION OF AREA AT RISK

Accurate sizing of the area at risk using noninvasive method provides valuable information for guiding therapeutic interventions aimed at enhancing collateral blood flow (angiogenesis), preserving peri-infarction zones, and preventing LV remodeling. It has been shown that T1- and T2-weighted sequences provide no differential contrast between the normal myocardium and the area at risk (23,51–56). First-pass MR perfusion demonstrates the wash-in of the contrast medium in normal and ischemic myocardium. In coronary artery occlusion (22,52) and stenosis models (23,53–56) remote myocardium appears bright in seconds, and at this time the area at risk appears relatively dark because of delayed arrival of the contrast agent. Recent animal studies indicated that some of the blood-pool contrast media (Gadomer, Gd-DTPA-24-cascade-polymer, and MS-325) provide longer delineation of area at risk than extracellular media (22,23,57). Another study used first-pass perfusion MRI to detect and quantify the spatial extent of the area at risk during brief coronary artery occlusion and reperfusion relative to the "true" size of the area at risk as defined in ex vivo using histochemical stain (23). Investigators found that there is a linear relationship between the regional contrast enhancement of the area at risk and the blood flow during postocclusive hyperemia, but that the size of the area at risk was significantly smaller than at postmortem. This difference in size may reflect an influence of coronary collateral circulation.

Functional and first-pass perfusion MRI were also used in a canine model of coronary artery stenosis for the quantification of functional and perfusion deficits in the area at risk before and after dipyridamole administration (53). It was found that the extent of functional defect was smaller than the perfusion defect during vasodilation. Other studies have

shown that the region demarcated by extracellular MR contrast media underestimates the size of area at risk by at least 10% (53,55,58) because of the rapid diffusion of these agents into the territory through collateral vessels (55). The spatial extent of the area at risk has been recently measured using intracellular manganese-based MR contrast media (28). The size of area at risk on MRI was identical to that measured at postmortem. The definition of the area at risk on MRI was based on the reduce uptake of Mn^{+2} and weak T1 changes compared with normal myocardium. Table 7.2 shows the applications of MR contrast media in the heart.

CHARACTERIZATION OF OCCLUSIVE INFARCTION

A number of clinical studies have indicated that the site of acute infarction can be visualized as a bright region on T2-weighted spin echo and T2-weighted triple inversion recovery sequence (59–63). Although T2-weighted images can detect the presence of myocardial damage, a portion of the area that exhibits increased SI is probably related to the presence of myocardial edema, rather than the myocardial infarction. Especially in the acute phase the demarcated region likely encompasses both viable and nonviable tissue. Furthermore, the difficulty in measuring the extent of myocardial infarction from T2-weighted images is in defining the boundaries of infarction (63) and the lack of differential enhancement in chronic infarction (59–62).

Investigators found that the detection of acute and chronic myocardial infarction can be made with a great deal of certainty after contrast injection (64–68) and application of a segmented inversion-recovery fast low-angle shot (IR-FLASH) pulse sequence (64). It has been shown that preparation of the magnetization before image acquisition, using an inversion pulse, significantly increases the magnitude of T1 enhancement. In a group of patients with chronic ischemic heart disease, Kim et al (67) reported that SI in regions of interest within the hyperenhanced infarcted area was always more than 6 standard deviations above that of nonenhanced remote regions. Thus, this pulse sequence has been widely used in clinical cardiac studies to delineate acute and chronic infarctions (64,66,67–71). The mechanism by which extracellular MR contrast media concentrate in infarcted myocardium is most likely related to the increase in fractional distribution volume because of the loss of cell membrane integrity in acute infarctions and increase in extracellular matrix structure in chronic (dense collagenous scar tissue) infarctions. Despite the marked structural difference between acute and chronic infarctions, hyperenhancement is observed for both with the use of extracellular agents. A recent study (72) showed that blood-pool contrast media can discriminate acute from chronic infarction. The study showed that the blood-pool agent Vistarem enhances acute myocardial infarction, but not chronic (scar) infarction. The lack of enhancement of scar tissue can be attributed to poor vascularization and intact residual vessels.

CHARACTERIZATION OF REPERFUSED INFARCTION

MR contrast media and inversion-recovery fast low-angle shot (IR-FLASH) sequences have proven to be a very useful tool to identify reperfused myocardial infarctions (69), predict functional recovery after coronary revascularization (67), and discriminate transmural from nontransmural myocardial infarction (73). The IR-FLASH technique provides high spatial resolution ($1.5 \times 2.0 \times 6$ mm) compared with SPECT's spatial resolution ($10 \times 10 \times 10$ mm), which underestimates the extent of infarction (Fig. 7.4) (68,69). Reperfused infarction appears bright on delayed contrast-enhanced MRI. The spatial extent of hyperenhancement has been shown to predict functional improvement of stunned myocardium in dogs and in patients (73,74).

The significance of the enhanced region on contrast-enhanced MRI, however, is still debatable. Some observers have suggested that the enhanced region represents only necrotic myocardium (bright is dead) (66,67). Fienno et al (66) and Kim et al (67) reported that the hyperenhanced region on MRI reflects true infarction measured by histochemical stain. They also found that 10 to 20 minutes is the optimum time for measuring the extent of infarction after administration of 0.1 to 0.2 mmol/kg Gd-DTPA and that this time frame is suitable to assess acute (1 day old, $r = 0.99$), subacute (3 days old, $r = 0.99$), and chronic infarctions (8 weeks old, $r = 0.97$).

A second view is that the enhanced region encompasses viable and nonviable myocardium, and that the 10- to 20-minute time frame cannot be applied in acute, subacute, and chronic infarctions. Oshiniski et al (75) demonstrated that the size of the enhanced region varies with the time imaging is performed after Gd-DTPA injection in a model of reperfused acute myocardial infarction. It has been shown that the enhanced region overestimates the true infarct size by 20% to 40% depending on the time after injection. The time for the enhanced zone to correspond closely to the true infarct size was 21 ± 4 minutes. Furthermore, several investigators also demonstrated in acute infarction that extracellular MR contrast media enhance both infarcted and peri-infarcted viable myocardium (76,77). This observation has been supported by histologic evidence in animal models. In a recent study (72) it was shown that the kinetics of the blood-pool agent Vistarem differs in acute and chronic infarction. This agent enhances acute, but not chronic, infarctions (Fig. 7.5).

van Rossum et al (78) were able to discriminate occlusive from reperfused infarctions at early contrast-enhanced MRI (8–10 minutes). SI ratio between infarct and remote myocardium was significantly higher in reperfused than occlusive infarction. A more recent contrast-enhanced MR study by Dendale et al (65) confirmed these results. Patients with open and occluded infarct-related coronary artery occlusion revealed a different temporal pattern of enhancement after Gd-DTPA-BMA. Investigators found that occlusive infarctions enhance more slowly compared with reperfused infarctions; they attributed the difference to the speed of wash-in of the contrast medium into the infarction.

Both T1- and T2-enhancing agents have also been used in sizing reperfused infarction. The size of infarction was smaller by 8% on dysprosium-enhanced MRI compared with the true infarction size on histochemical staining (79). In contrast, the size of reperfused infarction was larger by 10% to 14% on Gadolinium-enhanced MRI compared with histochemical staining. The overestimated enhanced zone likely represents the peri-infarction zone (76,77). In a recent canine study of reperfused infarction, Amado et al (80) found that Gd-DTPA consistently overestimates infarction by 20% when compared with ex vivo measurement using histochemical stain.

CHARACTERIZATION OF MYOCARDIAL VIABILITY AND SALVAGE

Five contrast-enhanced MRI approaches have been proposed to achieve a differential contrast between viable and nonviable myocardium (81). These potential methods used (a) extracellular MR contrast media for quantification of fractional distribution volume, (b) extracellular MR contrast media for delayed contrast enhancement, (c) necrotic tissue-specific contrast media represented by gadophrin and gadofluorine, (d) susceptibility (T2*) contrast media, represented by dysprosium-DTPA-BMA, and (e) ion transport contrast media, represented by $MnCl_2$ and the Mn^{+2}-releasing agent Mn-DPDP.

Extracellular contrast media have been used as markers of viability by measuring the fractional distribution volume (partition coefficient) in normal, ischemic, and infarcted myocardium. An increase in partition coefficient of the tissue means that there is edema and/or loss of cellular membrane integrity. Figure 7.1 shows a schematic model of the distribution of extracellular MR contrast media in the blood and remote normal and ischemically injured myocardium. The partition coefficient has been validated to grade the severity of myocardial injury in animal models (25,82) and used in humans (83). Figure 7.6 shows the effect of various duration of ischemia-reperfusion on the partition coefficient of Gd-DTPA-BMA. Several groups have shown that regions of acute reperfused infarctions appear hyperenhanced on T1-weighted images acquired between 5 and 20 minutes after administration of extracellular and blood-pool MR contrast media (25,64,68,82,83). Another approach for assessing myocardial viability is to use necrotic tissue-specific MR contrast media. For example, gadophrin II and III bind specifically necrotic cells. Because of this unique feature of gadophrin we used the combination of the extracellular Gd-DTPA and gadophrin MR contrast media to compare the extents of enhanced reperfused regions. The major hypothe-

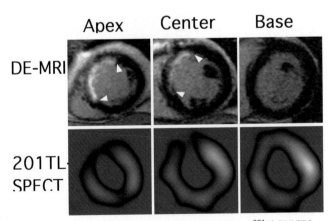

Apex   Center   Base

DE-MRI

201Tl-SPECT

Figure 7.4. Delayed Gd-DTPA-enhanced MR and ^{201}Tl-SPECT images showing acute myocardial infarction in a patient after revascularization. Note that the location of the contrast-enhanced region on MRI (*arrows*) corresponds to the uptake defect on ^{201}Tl-SPECT, but that the extent of the infarction is underestimated on ^{201}Tl-SPECT (courtesy of Gunnar Lund, MD, Hamburg, Germany).

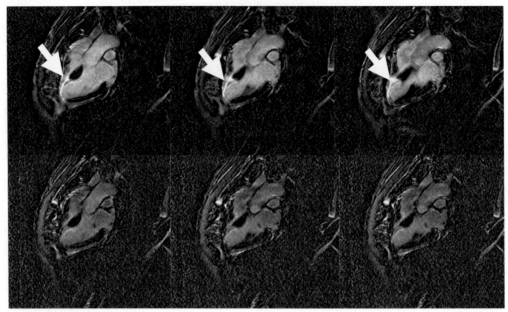

Figure 7.5. Infrared gradient-echo MR images of acute (*top*) and chronic infarction (*bottom*) after administration of 0.026 mmol/kg of the blood-pool agent Vistarem in swine model of reperfused infarction. Note the differential enhancement of acute myocardial infarction, but not chronic (scar) infarction.

sis of the study was that the difference in the hyperenhanced regions demarcated by the two agents is the salvageable border zone. It was found that the Gd-DTPA–enhanced region overestimated the extent of infarction size, and that the gadophrin-enhanced area matched the true infarct size. It was confirmed that the difference in the hyperenhanced regions on contrast-enhanced T1- and T2-weighted sequences encompasses both viable and nonviable myocardium

(63,76,77,84–86). Different methods have been used to confirm the presence of the peri-infarction zone in acute infarctions. Investigators found that the observed contractile dysfunction extends beyond the borders of the infarcted area and includes the peri-infarction viable myocardium (Fig. 7.7) (71,77). Oshiniski et al (75) and Choi et al (86) found viable

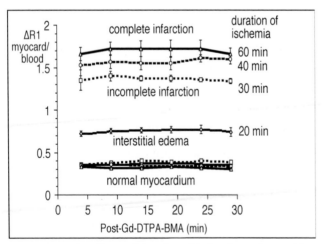

Figure 7.6. The effects of duration of ischemia on the partition coefficients (λ) of extracellular MR contrast media in myocardium. During repetitive measurements the ΔR1 ratios for myocardium/blood remain constant during the initial 29 minutes after injection of 0.2 mmol/kg Gd-DTPA-BMA, suggesting a near equilibrium state. This means that ΔR1 ratios represent partition coefficients (λ), which allows calculation of fractional distribution volume. Note the increase in ΔR1 ratio in hearts subjected to 20, 30, 40, and 60 minutes of coronary occlusion followed by 1 hour of reperfusion.

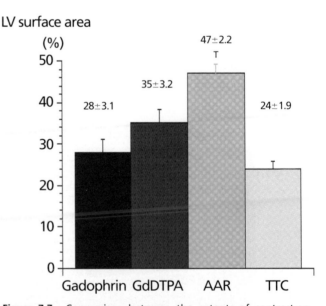

Figure 7.7. Comparison between the extents of contrast-enhanced MR regions (using necrosis-specific gadophrin II and extracellular Gd-DTPA contrast media) and postmortem true infarction size [using triphenyltetrazolium chloride (TTC)] and area at risk (AAR) using phthalocyanine blue dye. The difference in the extent of gadophrin and Gd-DTPA–enhanced regions represents the peri-infarction zone. *$p < 0.01$ compared with gadophrin and TTC and $^{T}p < 0.01$ compared with Gd-DTPA.

myocardium and interstitial edema in the contrast-enhanced peri-infarction zone on electron microscopy. Krombach et al (87,88) confirmed the hyperpermeability of microvessels in the peri-infarction zone after administration of ultrasmall iron oxide particles. Kellman et al (89) used phase-sensitive inversion recovery sequence to demonstrate that the periphery of the infarction has a high transient T1 value and corresponds to reversibly injured myocardium. Another approach in assessing myocardial viability is to use Mn^{+2}-based MR contrast media. The principle of this Mn^{+2}-based approach resembles the thallium approach in SPECT, in which viable cells retain the tracers and necrotic cells release it quickly (26,27,29,82).

MR contrast media can be used in conditions accentuating ischemic injury in hypertrophied hearts (Fig. 7.3) (90,91). The contrast-enhanced technique accurately depicts the higher incidence of myocardial infarction in hypertrophied hearts after reperfusion (90,91) and illustrates the reduction in infarction size after treatment with verapamil, a calcium channel blocker, and nicorandil, a potassium channel opener, in hypertrophied hearts (92,93).

CHARACTERIZATION OF MICROVASCULAR INTEGRITY

The MO zone (no-reflow zone) has been observed as the hypoenhanced zone on contrast-enhanced MRI in acute myocardial infarctions in animal models and patients (53,74,80–83,94–96). This phenomenon has been observed in large reperfused large infarctions. The hypoenhanced zone occupies the core of the infarction after administration of MR contrast media. The no-reflow zone is characterized by persistent hypoperfusion. The presence of hypoenhancement in the core of the enhanced region is the result of microvascular damage and/or obstruction that impedes the delivery of the contrast medium. Extracellular MR contrast media accumulate relatively rapidly in the no-reflow zone compared with blood-pool agents.

The extents of MO zones vary because it is unlikely that the degree of microvascular damage is identical throughout the entire infarction. Small no-reflow zones enhance rapidly because of diffusion of extracellular contrast medium from surrounding regions with intact microvessels (95). Others

areas may have extensive microvascular damage, resulting in prolonged hypoenhancement even on late contrast-enhanced images (68).

The evolution of MO in the first 48 hours after reperfusion has been monitored in experimental animals (97). Contrast-enhanced MRI performed at 2, 6, and 48 hours after reperfusion to define MO zones was correlated to blood flow and MO defined on fluorescent stain. They found that the extent of MO zone on MRI increased threefold during 48 hours after reperfusion. In another study, Wu et al (98) compared the extent of MO on days 2 and 9 in a reperfused infarction canine model using contrast-enhanced echocardiography and contrast-enhanced MRI. No change was found in the extent of MO zone between 2 and 9 days. Gerber et al (99) used the extent of MO on contrast-enhanced MRI to monitor the alterations in the mechanical properties of LV. A strong inverse relationship was found between the magnitude of first principal strain ($r = -0.80$, $p < 0.001$) and the relative extent of MO. In another study in 20 patients, Gerber et al found that early hypoenhancement in reperfused myocardium is highly specific for necrosis and dysfunction, but that its absence is not sensitive to prediction of functional improvement because its extent greatly underestimates the size of infarction (100). Numerous clinical and experimental studies have shown that MO, delineated on contrast-enhanced MRI, is associated with worse prognosis (99,100).

It has been recently suggested that blood-pool contrast media are more suitable than extracellular media for providing prolonged delineation of MO (Fig. 7.8) and defining small (few pixels) MO zones (94). Blood-pool contrast media can demonstrate the progression in the extent of MO zone in mild, moderate, and severe reperfused myocardial injury (95) and the effect of duration of reperfusion on the extent of the MO zone (96).

QUANTIFICATION OF MYOCARDIAL PERFUSION

Extracellular and blood-pool MR contrast media have been used to measure myocardial perfusion (mL/min/g) (101–105). The MR measurement of perfusion is based on Kety's two compartmental-model (101) and validated using a gold standard method, namely, microspheres. Close corre-

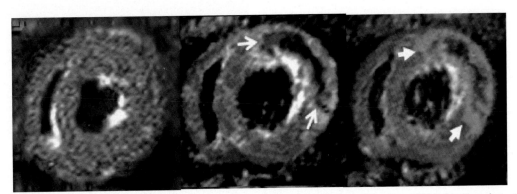

Figure 7.8. Short-axis view spin-echo MR images of a rat heart subjected to reperfused myocardial infarction show the no-reflow zone (microvascular obstruction [MO]). The images were acquired before (*left*) and 9 minutes (*center*) and 15 minutes (*right*) after administration of 0.05 mmol/kg Gadomer. Note the prolonged delineation of the no-reflow zone (*dark core*) and the slow convection of the blood-pool contrast medium Gadomer into infarcted myocardium (*arrows*).

lation was found between the two methods (101,103). A relatively low dose (0.02–0.03 mmol/kg) of MR contrast media was used for measurement of myocardial perfusion. The low dose ensures that the measured changes in regional SI (blood and myocardium) are proportional to the changes in contrast concentration (17,101,103). At a high dose, saturation effects occur and the relationship no longer exists. The saturation effect starts first in the left ventricle chamber blood after the high bolus dose, leading to miscalculation of perfusion.

The use of blood-pool MR media simplifies the modeling of myocardial perfusion because one does not need to model contrast diffusion, but such media are not available at the present time for routine clinical use. The following points need to be considered when using MR contrast agent for myocardial perfusion: (a) the selection of dose must take into account the distance between the injection site and the heart, (b) the bolus of contrast agent dilutes as it passes through the veins and lungs, and (c) it is important to time the delivery of the contrast bolus to the central portion of k-space to achieve maximum effect.

First-pass methods have been implemented in clinical practice to estimate myocardial perfusion, such as maximum enhancement, transit time, and upslope of enhancement. Al-Saadi et al (105) evaluated the diagnostic accuracy of MR first-pass perfusion measurements for the detection of significant coronary artery stenosis in 15 patients with single-vessel coronary artery disease and in five patients without significant coronary artery disease. The SI time curves of the first pass of a Gd-DTPA bolus were evaluated before and after dipyridamole infusion. The diagnostic accuracy was then examined prospectively in 34 patients with coronary artery disease and was compared with coronary angiography. A significant difference in myocardial perfusion reserve between ischemic and normal myocardial segments was found that resulted in a cutoff value of 1.5. The sensitivity, specificity, and diagnostic accuracy for the detection of coronary artery stenosis of 75% or greater were 90%, 83%, and 87%, respectively. Others used contrast-enhanced MRI in detecting and sizing of hypoperfused myocardium and compared this technique with positron emission tomography and quantitative coronary angiography (106). The positron emission tomography data had a sensitivity and specificity of 91% and 94%, respectively. The sensitivity and specificity for contrast-enhanced MRI were slightly lower, 87% and 85%, respectively. Wilke et al (103) addressed the issue of the sensitivity and specificity of contrast-enhanced perfusion MRI in a recent literature review of 22 studies in 559 patients. They observed that the sensitivity and specificity of MR perfusion imaging are $82\% \pm 9\%$ and $88\% \pm 9.6\%$, respectively.

FUTURE PERSPECTIVE

Interventional MRI is a rapidly growing field that aims to reduce radiation exposure during interventional procedures. Contrast media can be used in interventional MRI for tracking the endovascular catheter, enhancing the blood pool during intervention, enhancing the target, and monitoring the

distribution of drugs mixed with contrast media or labeled cells. The contrast-enhanced MRI approach combines tracking and road mapping into a single acquisition and potentially avoids the need of subtraction and overlay images (107–110). In a recent study, the blood-pool MR contrast medium (Gd-DTPA-albumin) was administered to brighten the signal of the blood pool and to track the endovascular catheter on real-time, steady-state free precession imaging. Administration of Gd-DTPA-albumin improved visibility of the dysprosium markers on the shaft of the catheter (109). Dion et al (108) used the intravascular agent MS-325 to visualize the vascular tree during the deployment of femoral artery stents.

Contrast-enhanced MRI may play an important role in local delivery of drugs or progenitor cells (111,112). Figure 7.9 shows the intramyocardial delivery of MR contrast media into myocardium under MR guidance. Mixing angiogenic growth factors or labeling progenitor cells with MR contrast media can be used to monitor the distribution of injected growth factors and cells in situ. Labeling of progenitor and stem cells has been pursued using iron oxide particles and manganese-based MR contrast media (113–115). Superparamagnetic iron oxide particles can be detected at micromolar concentrations of iron and offer sufficient sensitivity for T2*-weighted imaging. Hill et al (116) and Dick et al (117) found that cardiovascular stem and progenitor cells can accumulate iron oxide-based magnetic intracellular contrast media with preservation of viability and with relaxivity characteristics that permit MRI detection. Although not yet fully

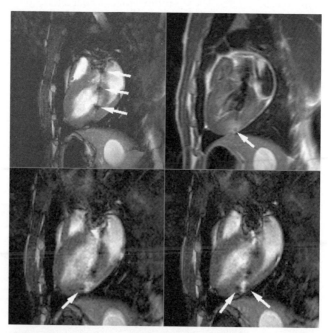

Figure 7.9. Steady-state free precession **(A,C,D)** and dual inversion T1-weighted turbo spin-echo **(B)** MR images showing the catheter in the left ventricle (*arrows* in **A**), transendocardial delivery of low-concentration Gd-DTPA-BMA **(B)**, and after hitting the target from both sides with high-concentration Gd-DTPA-BMA (*arrows* in **C, D**). The gadolinium-oxide markers on the catheter's shaft are clearly visualized as dark spots inside the left ventricle chamber **(A)**.

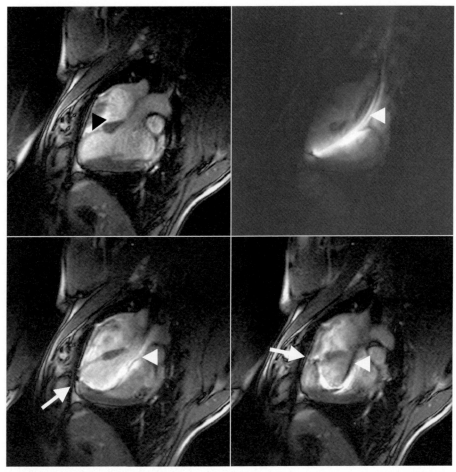

Figure 7.10. Inversion recovery gradient-echo image shows the delayed Dotarem-enhanced scar tissue (*black arrowhead, top left*). Real-time balanced fast field echo images showing the shaft of the endovascular catheter in the left ventricle (*white arrowhead, top right*) and the site of Dys-DTPA-BMA injections (*arrows, bottom left and right*). These images demonstrate the dark sites of the two injections of dysprosium-chelate.

addressed, there might be toxicologic problems associated with the metabolic fate of iron oxide particles. In a typical experiment the amount of cell-internalized iron may be as high as 10 times the amount of endogenous iron. Moreover, it has been shown that the distribution and morphology of endosomes filled with iron oxide particles are highly sensitive to the effects of the external static magnetic field (118).

Because positive enhancement by clinically approved MR contrast media is used to delineate infarcted myocardium, we recently used the extracellular T2*-enhancing contrast medium dysprosium-DTPA-BMA for monitoring the distribution of therapeutic solutions. This nonionic contrast medium can be mixed with potential drugs, genes, or cells during delivery to define the site of injection. More important, extracellular agents clear quickly from the tissue, thus eliminating the potential effects of intracellular agents (e.g., iron particles or manganese) on cell viability or immune system. Figure 7.10 shows the effect of intravenous injection of Gd-DOTA on the scar tissue and intramyocardial delivery of dysprosium-DTPA-BMA on the rim of the scar tissue. The former produces hyperenhancement, whereas the latter causes hypoenhancement. Crich et al (119) described a simple labeling procedure of stem/progenitor cells based on the use of Gd-HPDO3A and Eu-HPDO3A, respectively, where

Gd-chelate acts as the T1 agent for MRI visualization, and Eu-chelate acts as the reporter in fluorescence microscopy. Labeling of progenitor and stem cells with MR contrast media may open the door for studying stem-cell migration, retention, and differentiation in the heart and blood vessels.

REFERENCES

1. Wehrli FW, MacFall JR, Glover GH, et al. The dependence of nuclear magnetic resonance (NMR) imaging contrast on intrinsic and pulse sequence timing parameters. *Magn Reson Imaging* 1984;2:3–16.
2. Moran PR. A general approach to T1, T2 and spin-density discrimination sensitivities in MR imaging sequences. *Magn Reson Imaging* 1984;2:17–22.
3. Fullerton GD. Physiologic basis of magnetic relaxation. In: Stark DD, Bradley WG, eds. *Magnetic resonance imaging.* St. Louis, MO: Mosby-Year Book, Inc.; 1992:88–108.
4. Buxton RB, Edelmann RR, Rosen BR, et al. Contrast in rapid MRI: T1- and T2-weighted imaging. *J Comput Assist Tomogr* 1987;11:7–16.
5. Lauffer RB. Magnetic resonance contrast media: principles and progress. *Magn Reson Q* 1990;6:65–84.

6. Wood ML, Hardy PA. Proton-relaxation enhancement. *J Magn Reson Imaging* 1993;3:149–156.

7. Rocklage SM, Watson AD. Chelates of gadolinium and dysprosium as contrast agents for MR imaging. *J Magn Reson Imaging* 1993;3:167–178.

8. Caravan P, Ellison JJ, McMurry TJ, et al. Gadolinium (III) chelates as MRI contrast agents: structure, dynamics and applications. *Chem Rev* 1999;99;2293–2352.

9. Aime S, Botta M, Fasano M, et al. Lanthanide(III) chelates for NMR biomedical applications. *Chem Soc Rev* 1998; 27,19–29.

10. Aime S, Cabella C, Colombatto S, et al. Insights into the use of paramagnetic Gd(III) complexes in MR-molecular imaging investigations. *J Magn Reson Imaging* 2002;16:394–406.

11. Zhang S, Merritt M, Woessner DE, et al. PARACEST Agents: modulating MRI contrast via water proton exchange. *Chem Res* 2003;36:783–790.

12. Lauffer RB, Parmelle DJ, Dunham SU, et al. MS-325: albumin-targeted contrast agent for MR angiography. *Radiology* 1998;207:529–538.

13. Vexler VS, Clement O, Schmitt-Willich H, et al. Effect of varying the molecular weight of the MR contrast agent GdDTPA-polylysine on blood pharmacokinetic and enhancement patterns. *J Magn Reson Imaging* 1994;4:381–388.

14. Wang SC, Wikstrom MG, White DL, et al. Evaluation of Gd-DTPA-labeled dextran as an intravascular MR contrast agent: imaging characteristics in normal rat tissues. *Radiology* 1990; 175:483–488.

15. Wiener EC, Brechbiel MW, Brothers H, et al. Dendrimer-based metal chelates: a new class of magnetic resonance imaging contrast agents. *Magn Reson Med* 1994;31:1–8.

16. Koenig SH, Brown RD. Field-cycling relaxometry of protein solutions and tissue: implications for MRI. *Prog NMR Spectrosc* 1990;22:487–567.

17. Wedeking P, Sotak CH, Telser J, et al. Quantitative dependence of MR signal intensity on tissue concentration of Gd(HP-DO3A) in the nephrectomized rat. *Magn Reson Imaging* 1992;10:97–108.

18. Tweedle MF, Wedeking P, Telser J, et al. Dependence of MR signal intensity on Gd tissue concentration over a broad dose range. *Magn Reson Med* 1991;22:191–194.

19. Rink PA, Muller RN. Field strength and dose dependence of contrast enhancement by gadolinium-based MR contrast agent. *Eur Radiol* 1999;9:998–1004.

20. Saeed M, Wendland MF, Sakuma H, et al. Inversion recovery and driven equilibrium prepared fast gradient echo imaging of first passage of T1- and T2*-enhancing contrast media in dogs subjected to acute myocardial ischemia. *J Magn Reson Imaging* 1995;5:515–524.

21. Bourasset F, Dencausse A, Bourrinet P, et al. Comparison of plasma and peritoneal concentrations of various categories of MRI blood pool agents in a murine experimental pharmacokinetic model. *MAGMA* 2001;12:82–87.

22. Roberts HC, Saeed M, Roberts TPL, et al. MRI of acute myocardial ischemia: comparing a new contrast agent, Gd-DTPA-24-cascade-polymer, with Gd-DTPA. *J Magn Reson Imaging* 1999;9:204–209.

23. Gerber BL, Blumeke DA, Chin BB, et al. Single-vessel coronary artery stenosis: myocardial perfusion imaging with Gadomer-17 first-pass MR imaging in a swine model of comparison with gadopentate dimeglumine. *Radiology* 2002;225: 104–112.

24. Port M, Corot C, Raynal I, et al. Physicochemical and biological evaluation of P792, a rapid-clearance blood-pool agent for magnetic resonance imaging. *Invest Radiol* 2001;36: 445–454.

25. Saeed M, Higgins CB, Geschwind JF, et al. T1-relaxation kinetics of extracellular, intracellular and intravascular MR contrast agents in normal and acutely reperfused infarcted myocardium using echo planar MR imaging. *Eur Radiol* 2000;10:310–318.

26. Bremerich J, Saeed M, Arheden H, et al. Normal and infarcted myocardium: differentiation with cellular uptake of manganese at MR imaging in a rat model. *Radiology* 2000;216: 524–530.

27. Wendland MF, Saeed M, Bremerich J, et al. Thallium-like test for myocardial viability with Mn-DPDP-enhanced MRI. *Acad Radiol* 2002;9(suppl 1):82–83.

28. Krombach GA, Saeed M, Higgins CB, et al. Contrast enhanced MRI of stunned myocardium using Mn-based MRI contrast media. *Radiology* 2004;230:183–190.

29. Flacke S, Allen JS, Chia JM, et al. Characterization of viable and nonviable myocardium at MR imaging: comparison of gadolinium-based extracellular and blood pool contrast materials versus manganese-based contrast materials in a rat myocardial infarction model. *Radiology* 2003;223:731–738.

30. Skjold A, Vangberg TR, Kristofferson A, et al. Relaxation enhancing properties of Mn DPDP in human myocardium. *J Magn Reson Imaging* 2004;20:948–952.

31. Chu SC, Xu Y, Balschi JA, et al. Bulk magnetic susceptibility shifts in NMR studies of compartmentalized samples: use of paramagnetic reagents. *Magn Reson Med* 1990;13:239–262.

32. Rosen BR, Belliveau JW, Vevea JM, et al. Perfusion imaging with NMR contrast agents. *Magn Reson Med* 1990;14: 249–265.

33. Rozenman Y, Zou X, Kantor H. Cardiovascular MR imaging with iron oxide particles: utility of a superparamagnetic contrast agent and the role of diffusion in signal loss. *Radiology* 1990;175:655–659.

34. Sakuma H, O'Sullivan M, Lucas J, et al. Effect of magnetic susceptibility contrast medium on myocardial signal intensity with fast gradient-recalled echo and spin-echo MR imaging: initial experience in humans. *Radiology* 1994;190:161–166.

35. Saeed M, Wendland MF, Yu KK, et al. Dual effects of gadodiamide injection in depiction of the region of myocardial ischemia. *J Magn Reson Imaging* 1993;3:21–29.

36. Wendland MF, Saeed M, Masui T, et al. Echo-planar MR imaging of normal and ischemic myocardium with gadodiamide injection. *Radiology* 1993;186:535–542.

37. Marchal G, Ni Y, Herijgers P, et al. Paramagnetic metalloporphyrins: infarct avid contrast agents for diagnosis of acute myocardial infarction by MRI. *Eur Radiol* 1996;6:2–8.

38. Li WH, Fraser SE, Meade TJ, et al. A calcium-sensitive magnetic resonance imaging contrast agent. *J Am Chem Soc* 1999; 121:1413–1421.

39. Louie AY, Huber MM, Ahrens ET, et al. In vivo visualization of gene expression using magnetic resonance imaging. *Nat Biotechnol* 2000;18:321–325.

40. Choi SII, Choi SH, Kim ST, et al. Irreversibly damaged myocardium at MR imaging with a necrosis tissue-specific contrast agent in a cat model. *Radiology* 2000;215:863–868.

41. Pislaru SV, Ni Y, Pislaru C et al. Noninvasive measurements of infarct size after thrombolysis with a necrosis-avid MRI contrast agent. *Circulation* 1999;99:690–696.

42. Weissleder R, Lee A, Khaw B, et al. Detection of myocardial infarction with MION-antimyosin. *Radiology* 1992;182: 381–385.

43. Flacke S, Fischer S, Scott MJ, et al. Novel MRI contrast agent for molecular imaging of fibrin: implications for detecting vulnerable plaques. *Circulation* 2001;104:1280–1285.

44. Ruehm SG, Corot C, Vogt P, et al. Magnetic resonance imaging of atherosclerotic plaque with ultrasmall superparamagnetic particles of iron oxide in hyperlipidemic rabbits. *Circulation* 2001;103:415–422.

45. Sirol M, Itskovich VV, Mani V, et al. Lipid-rich atherosclerotic plaques detected by gadofluorine-enhanced in vivo magnetic resonance imaging. *Circulation* 2004;109:2890–2896.

46. Barkhausen J, Ebert W, Heyer C, et al. Detection of atherosclerotic plaque with Gadofluorine-enhanced magnetic resonance imaging. *Circulation* 2003;108:605–609.

47. Cacheris W, Quay S, Rocklaye S. The relationship between thermodynamics and the toxicity of gadolinium complexes. *Magn Reson Imaging* 1980;8:467–481.

48. Tweedle MF, Wedeking P, Krishan K. Biodistribution of radiolabeled, formulated gadopentetate, gadoteridol, gadoterate, and gadodiamide in mice and rats. *Invest Radiol* 1995; 30:372–380.

49. Chang C. Magnetic resonance imaging contrast agents. Designs and physiochemical properties of gadodiamide. *Invest Radiol* 1993;28(Suppl 1):521–527.

50. Runge VM. Safety of approved MR contrast media for intravenous injection. *J Magn Reson Imaging* 2000;12:205–213.

51. Sakuma H, Wendland MF, Saeed M, et al. Multislice measurement of first pass transit of Gd-BOPTA/Dimeg in normal and ischemic myocardium in dogs. *Acad Radiol* 1995;2:864.

52. Saeed M, Wendland MF, Lauerma K, et al. Detection of myocardial ischemia using first pass contrast-enhanced inversion recovery and driven equilibrium fast GRE imaging. *J Magn Reson Imaging* 1995;5:61–70.

53. Schwitter J, Saeed M, Wendland MF, et al. Assessment of myocardial function and perfusion in a canine model of nonocclusive coronary artery stenosis using fast magnetic resonance imaging. *J Magn Reson Imaging* 1999;9:101–110.

54. Kraitchman DL, Wilke N, Hexeberg, et al. Myocardial perfusion and function in dogs with moderate coronary stenosis. *Magn Reson Med* 1996;35:771–780.

55. Saeed M, Wendland MF, Szolar D, et al. Quantification of the extent of area at risk with fast contrast-enhanced magnetic resonance imaging in experimental coronary artery stenosis. *Am Heart J* 1996;132:921–932.

56. Szolar DH, Saeed M, Wendland M, et al. Quantification of area at risk during coronary occlusion and reperfusion by means of MR perfusion imaging. *Acta Radiol* 1997;38:479–488.

57. Kraitchman DL, Chin BB, Heldman AW, et al. MRI detection of myocardial perfusion defects due to coronary artery stenosis with MS-325. *J Magn Reson Imaging* 2002;15:149–58.

58. Szolar DH, Saeed M, Wendland MF, et al. MR imaging characterization of postischemic myocardial dysfunction ("stunned myocardium"): relationship between functional and perfusion abnormalities. *J Magn Reson Imaging* 1996;6:615–624.

59. Been M, Smith MA, Ridgway P. Serial changes in the T1 magnetic relaxation parameter after myocardial infarction in man. *Br Heart J* 1988;59:178–194.

60. McNamara MT, Higgins CB. Magnetic resonance imaging of chronic myocardial infarcts in man. *Am J Roentgenol* 1984; 143:1135–1141.

61. Thompson RC, Liu P, Brady TJ, et al. Serial magnetic resonance imaging in patients following acute myocardial infarction. *Magn Reson Imaging* 1991;9:155–158.

62. Abdel-Aty H, Zagrosek A, Schultz-Menger J, et al. Delayed enhancement and T2-weighted cardiovascular magnetic resonance imaging differentiate acute from chronic myocardial infarction. *Circulation* 2004;109:2411–2416.

63. Dymarkowski S, Ni Y, Miao Y, et al. Value of T2-weighted magnetic resonance imaging early after myocardial infarction in dogs. *Invest Radiol* 2002;37:77–85.

64. Simonetti OP, Kim RJ, Fieno DS, et al. An improved MR imaging technique for the visualization of myocardial infarction. *Radiology* 2001;218:215–223.

65. Dendale P, Franken PR, Block P, et al. Contrast-enhanced and functional magnetic resonance imaging for the detection of viable myocardium after infarction. *Am Heart J* 1998;135:875–880.

66. Fienno DS, Kim RJ, Chen EL, et al. Contrast-enhanced MRI of myocardium at risk: distinction between reversible injury throughout infarct healing. *J Am Coll Cardiol* 2000;36:1985–1991.

67. Kim RJ, Wu E, Rafael A, et al. The use of contrast-enhanced magnetic resonance imaging to identify reversible myocardial dysfunction. *N Engl J Med* 2000;343;1445–1453.

68. Lund G, Stork A, Saeed M, et al. Characterization of patients with acute myocardial infarction by first-pass perfusion and delayed enhancement magnetic resonance imaging validated by 201Tl-SPECT. *Radiology* 2004;232:49–57.

69. Wagner A, Mahrhold H, Elliott MD, et al. Contrast-enhanced MRI and routine single photon emission computed tomography (SPECT) perfusion imaging for detection of subendocardial myocardial infarcts: an imaging study. *Lancet* 2003;361:374–379.

70. Sandestede JJW, Lipke C, Baer M, et al. Analysis of first-pass and delayed contrast-enhancement patterns of dysfunctional myocardium on MR imaging: use in the prediction of myocardial viability. *Am J Roentgenol* 2000;174;1737–1740.

71. Rogers WJ, Kramer CM, Geskin G, et al. Early contrast-enhanced MRI predicts late functional recovery after reperfused myocardial infarction. *Circulation* 1999;99:744–750.

72. Saeed M, Weber O, Lee R, et al. Discrimination of myocardial acute and chronic (scar) infarctions using a blood pool MR contrast media. In press, 2005.

73. Choi KM, Kim RJ, Gubernikoff G, et al. Transmural extent of acute myocardial infarction predicts long-term improvement in contractile function. *Circulation* 2001;104:1101–1107.

74. Gerber J, Garot DA, Bluemke KC, et al. Accuracy of contrast-enhanced magnetic resonance imaging in predicting improvement of regional myocardial function in patients after acute myocardial infarction. *Circulation* 2002;106:1083–1089.

75. Oshiniski JN, Yang Z, Jones JR, et al. Imaging time after Gd-DTPA injection is critical in using delayed enhancement to determine infarct size accurately with magnetic resonance imaging. *Circulation* 2001;104:2838–2842.

76. Lim T-H, Choi SH. MRI of myocardial infarction. *J Magn Reson Imaging* 1999;10:686–693.

77. Saeed M, Bremerich J, Wendland MF, et al. Reperfused myocardial infarction as seen with use of necrosis-specific versus standard extracellular MR contrast media in rats. *Radiology* 1999;213:247–257.

78. van Rossum AC, Visser FC, Van Eenige MJ, et al. Value of gadolinium-diethylene-triamine pentaacetic acid dynamics in magnetic resonance imaging of acute myocardial infarction with occluded and reperfused coronary arteries after thrombolysis. *Am J Cardiol* 1990;65:845–851.

79. Saeed M, Wendland MF, Masui T, et al. Myocardial infarctions on T1- and susceptibility-enhanced MRI: evidence for loss of compartmentalization of contrast media. *Magn Reson Med* 1994;31:31–39.

80. Amado LC, Kraitchman DL, Gerber BL, et al. Reduction of "no-reflow" phenomenon by intra-aortic balloon counterpulsation in a randomized magnetic resonance imaging experimental study. *J Am Coll Cardiol* 2004;43:1291–1298.

81. Saeed M, Wendland MF, Watzinger N, et al. MR contrast media for myocardial viability, microvascular integrity and perfusion. *Eur J Radiol* 2000;34:179–195.

82. Arheden H, Saeed M, Higgins CB, et al. Reperfused rat myocardium subjected to various durations of ischemia: estimation of the distribution volume of contrast material with echoplanar MRI. *Radiology* 2000;215:520–528.

83. Flacke SJ, Fischer SE, Lorenz CH. Measurement of the gadopentate dimeglumine partition coefficient in human myocardium in vivo: normal distribution and elevation in acute and chronic infarction. *Radiology* 2001;218:703–710.

84. Ni Y, Pislaru C, Bosmans H, et al. Intracoronary delivery of Gd-DTPA and Gadophrin-2 for determination of myocardial viability with MR imaging. *Eur Radiol* 2001;11:876–883.

85. Jeong AK, Choi SI, Kim DH, et al. Evaluation by contrast-enhanced MR imaging of the lateral border zone in reperfused myocardial infarction in a cat model. *Korean J Radiol* 2001; 2:21–27.

86. Choi SII, Choi SH, Kim ST, et al. Irreversibly damaged myocardium at MR imaging with a necrosis tissue-specific contrast agent in a cat model. *Radiology* 2000;215:863–868.

87. Krombach GA, Higgins CH, Chujo M, et al. Blood pool enhanced MRI detects suppression of microvascular permeability in early post-infarction reperfusion after nicorandil therapy. *Magn Reson Med* 2002;47:896–902.

88. Krombach GA, Wendland MF, Higgins CH, et al. MR imaging of spatial extent of microvascular injury in reperfused ischemically injured rat myocardium: value of blood pool ultrasmall superparamagnetic particles of iron oxide. *Radiology* 2002;225:479–486.

89. Kellman P, Arial AE, McVeigh ER, et al. Phase-sensitive inversion recovery for detecting myocardial infarction using gadolinium-delayed hyperenhancement. *Magn Reson Med* 2002;47:372–383.

90. Lauerma K, Saeed M, Wendland MF, et al. The use of contrast-enhanced magnetic resonance imaging to define ischemic injury after reperfusion: comparison in normal and hypertrophied hearts. *Invest Radiol* 1994;29:527–535.

91. Schalla S, Wendland MF, Higgins CB, et al. Accentuation of high susceptibility of hypertrophied myocardium to ischemia: gadophrin-enhanced and cardiac function assessment using magnetic resonance imaging. *Magn Reson Med* 2004;51: 552–558.

92. Lauerma K, Saeed M, Wendland MF, et al. Verapamil reduces the size of reperfused ischemically injured myocardium in hypertrophied rat hearts as assessed by magnetic resonance imaging. *Am Heart J* 1996;131:14–23.

93. Schalla S, Higgins CB, Chujo M, et al. Effect of potassium-channel opener therapy on reperfused infarction in hypertrophied hearts: demonstration of preconditioning using functional and contrast-enhanced magnetic resonance imaging. *J Cardiovasc Pharmacol Ther* 2004;9:193–202.

94. Krombach GA, Higgins CB, Chujo M, et al. Gadomer-enhanced MRI for detection of microvascular obstruction: alleviation by nicorandil therapy. *Radiology,* 2004. In press.

95. Schwitter J, Saeed M, Wendland MF, et al. Influence of severity of myocardial injury on the distribution of macromolecules: extravascular versus intravascular gadolinium-based MR contrast media. *J Am Coll Cardiol* 1997;30:1086–1094.

96. Bremerich J, Wendland MF, Higgins CB, et al. Microvascular injury in reperfused infarcted myocardium: non-invasive assessment with contrast enhanced echoplanar MR imaging. *J Am Coll Cardiol* 1998;32:787–793.

97. Rochitte CE, Lima JA, Bluemke DA, et al. Magnitude and time course of microvascular obstruction and tissue injury after acute myocardial infarction. *Circulation* 1998;98: 1006–1014.

98. Wu E, Judd RM, Vargas JD, et al. Visualization of presence, location, and transmural extent of healed Q-wave and non-Q-wave myocardial infarction. *Lancet* 2001;357:21–28.

99. Gerber BL, Rochitte CE, Melin JA, et al. Microvascular obstruction and left ventricular remodeling early after acute myocardial infarction. *Circulation* 2000;101:2734–2741.

100. Wu KC, Zerhouni EA, Judd RM, et al. Prognostic significance of microvascular obstruction by magnetic resonance imaging in patients with acute myocardial infarction. *Circulation* 1998;97:765–772.

101. Wilke N, Kroll K, Merkle H, et al. Regional myocardial blood volume estimated with MR first pass imaging and polylysine-GdDTPA in the dog. *J Magn Reson Imaging* 1995;5;227–237.

102. Cullen JHS, Horsefield MA, Reek CR, et al. A myocardial perfusion reserve index in humans using first-pass contrast-enhanced magnetic resonance imaging. *J Am Coll Cardiol* 1999;33:1386–1394.

103. Wilke N, Jerosch-Herold M, Zenovich A, et al. Magnetic resonance first-pass myocardial perfusion: clinical validation and future applications. *J Magn Reson Imaging* 1999;10: 676–685.

104. Panting JR, Gatehouse PD, Yang GZ, et al. Abnormal subendocardial perfusion in cardiac syndrome X detected by cardiovascular magnetic resonance imaging. *N Engl J Med* 2002; 346:1948–1953.

105. Al-Saadi N, Nagel E, Gross M, et al. Noninvasive detection of myocardial ischemia from perfusion reserve based on cardiovascular magnetic resonance. *Circulation* 2000;101: 1379–1383.

106. Schwitter J, Nanz D, Kneifel S, et al. Assessment of myocardial perfusion in coronary artery disease by magnetic resonance: a comparison with positron emission tomography and coronary artery angiography. *Circulation* 2001;103: 2230–2235.

107. Bakker CJ, Bos G, Weinmann HJ. Passive tracking of catheters and guidewires by contrast-enhanced MR fluoroscopy. *Magn Reson Med* 2001;45:17–23.

108. Dion YM, Ben El Kadi H, Boudoux C, et al. Endovascular procedures under near real-time magnetic resonance imaging guidance: an experimental feasibility study. *J Vasc Surg* 2000,32:1006–1014.

109. Martin AJ, Roberts TPL, Saeed M, et al. Steady state imaging for visualization of endovascular interventions. *Magn Reson Med* 2003;50:434–438.

110. Schalla S, Saeed M, Higgins CB, et al. Transcatheter atrial septal defect closure in an animal model: magnetic resonance imaging assessment and validation. *J Magn Reson Imaging,* 2004. In press.

111. Wang JS, Shum-Tim D, Galipeau J, et al. Marrow stromal cells for cellular cardiomyoplasty: feasibility and potential clinical advantages. *J Thorac Cardiovasc Surg* 2000;120: 999–1005.

112. Orlic D, Kajstura J, Chimenti S, et al. Bone marrow cells regenerate infarcted myocardium *Nature* 2001;410:701–705.

113. Bulte JW, Zhang S, van Gelderen P, et al. Neurotransplantation of magnetically labeled oligodendrocyte progenitors: MR tracking of cell migration and myelination. *Proc Natl Acad Sci U S A* 1999;96:15256–15261.

114. Lewin M, Carlesso N, Tung CH, et al. Tat peptide-derivatized magnetic nanoparticles allow in vivo tracking and recovery of progenitor cells. *Nat Biotechnol* 2000;18:410–414.

115. Frank JA, Miller BR, Arbab AS, et al. Clinically applicable labeling of mammalian and stem cells by combining superparamagnetic iron oxides and transfection agents. *Radiology* 2003;228:480–487.

116. Hill JM, Dick AJ, Raman VK, et al. Serial cardiac magnetic resonance imaging (MRI) of injected mesenchymal stem cells. *Circulation* 2003;108:1009–1014.

117. Dick AJ, Guttman MA, Raman VK, et al. Magnetic resonance fluoroscopy allows targeted delivery of mesenchymal stem cells to infarct borders in swine. *Circulation* 2003;108: 2899–2904.

118. Wilhelm C, Cebers A, Bacri JC, et al. Deformation of intracellular endosomes under a magnetic field. *Eur Biophys J* 2003; 32:655–660.

119. Crich SG, Biancone L, Cantaluppi V, et al. Improved route for the visualization of stem cells labeled with a Gd-/Eu-chelate as dual (MRI and fluorescence) agent. *Magn Reson Med* 2004;51:938–944.

8

Magnetic Resonance of Cardiomyopathies and Myocarditis

Matthias G. Friedrich and Ralf Wassmuth

Cardiomyopathies are chronic, progressive myocardial diseases with distinct morphologic, functional, and electrophysiologic characteristics. On clinical, morphologic, and histologic grounds they have been classified into four categories: dilated cardiomyopathy (DCM), hypertrophic cardiomyopathy (HCM), restrictive cardiomyopathy (RCM), and arrhythmogenic right ventricular cardiomyopathy (ARVC) (1).

Although originally understood as "primary" or "idiopathic," several etiologic factors leading to the phenotype have been identified for each of the cardiomyopathies. A genetic predisposition with a possible additional effect of inflammatory or toxic injuries of the myocardium may contribute to the development of DCM (2) and ARVC (3). Genetic defects are made responsible for HCM (4). RCM may be idiopathic, but it may also be the result of infiltrative systemic diseases such as amyloidosis, which is also often inherited.

The diagnosis of cardiomyopathies must be established by exclusion of other cardiovascular causes, and the specific type of cardiomyopathy must be confirmed, because it has great impact for therapy and prognosis. However, a specific cause cannot be identified in many of them (5). Therapy is guided by the individual stage and hemodynamic relevance of the disease, which is frequently a long-term management problem. Thus, imaging techniques are of paramount importance for both diagnosis and therapy. The modalities frequently used in these diseases are echocardiography, conventional angiography, radionuclide ventriculography, and magnetic resonance imaging (MRI).

THE ROLE OF OTHER DIAGNOSTIC MODALITIES IN CARDIOMYOPATHIES: GENERAL ASPECTS

ECHOCARDIOGRAPHY

In routine clinical care, transthoracic echocardiography serves as the standard technique to assess left ventricular parameters, including M mode, two-dimensional (2D), and Doppler methods. The technique is widely available, noninvasive, fast, and easily performed in most patients. Ejection fraction is estimated with end-diastolic and end-systolic diameters obtained in the parasternal view with the Teichholz formula or, especially in case of regional wall motion abnormalities, with ventricular area/length measurements from apical views using Simpson's rule.

Although there are a variety of applications of echocardiography in cardiomyopathies (6), results feature substantial interstudy and interobserver variability, which is a limiting factor in their use (7–9). Thus, the reliability of phenotyping a patient with a cardiomyopathy may be limited and follow-up data may be inconsistent, especially when different observers are involved (10,11). Because of the poor ultrasound transmission of adjacent tissues such as pulmonary air and sternal or costal bones, the echocardiographic fields of view may be restricted to a small number of transducer positions. Consequently, M mode and 2D echocardiography are highly susceptible to angular errors of the ultrasonic plane and diameters. The shortening fraction can easily be overestimated. Control for plane localization is oftentimes not adequate. Another source of M mode and 2D echo inconsistencies is a parallel shift of the ultrasonic plane out of the targeted center of the ventricle. This shift may result in an underestimation of (especially systolic) intraventricular dimensions and subsequent overestimation of the ejection fraction (12). The use of transesophageal echocardiography (TEE) or techniques such as acoustic quantification (13), automated border detection (14), application of contrast (15), and three-dimensional (3D) postprocessing (12) may improve this state of affairs to some degree. Doppler echocardiography allows for quantification of left ventricular outflow tract (LVOT) obstruction (16) and for the assessment of intracavital flow including abnormalities of valve function. Mitral inflow characteristics, for example, show distinct patterns in different stages of progressive diastolic dysfunction. However, the waveforms go through phases of "pseudonormalization" and thus may have a lack of sensitivity. Tissue Doppler imaging might resolve some of the difficulties (17–20).

The endocardial border often is very difficult to detect, especially in the apex, and comparative data underscore this (21). Recently, different efforts have been made to overcome this problem. The intravenous administration of various air or fluorocarbon-filled microbubbles as contrast materials improves edge detection in patients with impaired image quality and increases the consistency by more than 20%, compared with MRI findings (22,23). However, the use of these contrast agents is limited by their expense and the fact that microbubbles are destroyed by conventional ultrasound frequencies (24,25). The agents have a short half-life of a few minutes. Harmonic imaging includes the signal from the second ultrasound echo into the analysis and was found to reduce both the proportion of unacceptable images by up to 46% (26) and reproducibility (27).

Comparative studies indicate that 3D postprocessed echocardiography may be as accurate as cardiovascular magnetic resonance (CMR) (27,28). Still, the reliability of volumetric results relies on the quality of the raw image data set, which depending on the disease may be nondiagnostic in approximately 15% of patients. TEE may overcome some of the limitations in the transthoracic approach. However, TEE (29) is semi-invasive, uncomfortable, and not free of risks for patients with cardiovascular disease (30).

One of the most important limitations of echocardiographic (as well as other "ray" modalities) is the lack of techniques to analyze tissue pathology itself. Despite the initial hope to identify specific pathology-related changes of echogenicity (31), results to date have generally been disappointing.

LEFT VENTRICULAR CINEANGIOGRAPHY

Left ventricular angiography after intraventricular injection of contrast media reveals an accurate projection of the contracting left ventricle (LV). Biplane data acquisition is possible with high temporal and in-plane spatial resolution (32). Intraventricular thrombi or tumors may be easily detected, albeit the exact localization is not identifiable by projection images. The investigation of coronary vessels in the same session is important to exclude coronary artery disease.

As a strong limitation of the method, invasive angiography poses substantial risks to the patient, including vessel injury, plaque disruption, volume overload, and arrhythmia, leading to an overall mortality of 0.14% (33). During the procedure, both the patient and the physician are exposed to radiation. The luminographic character of the procedure precludes a complete visualization of myocardial anatomy. Furthermore, the setting of such a study affects the results by adrenergic stimulation of the patient's cardiovascular system (34).

In patients with DCM, the main task of left ventricular angiography is the exclusion of significant coronary artery disease. In the setting of HCM it is applied to measure or exclude a pressure gradient within the LV or the outflow tract. A right ventricular angiography visualizes regional or global disturbances of systolic RV function in ARVC. Therefore, left ventricular angiography should be restricted to those indications in which it can really add information beyond echo or CMR.

RADIONUCLIDE LEFT VENTRICULAR ANGIOGRAPHY

Left ventricular angiography using 99-m Technetium derivatives is an acceptable method to assess ventricular function. It has been applied for years and is still widely used to assess anthracycline cardiotoxicity (35). However, the reproducibility of radionuclide angiography does not exceed that of 3D echo or CMR (36–38) and was found to be lower than that of CMR in patients with regional wall motion abnormalities (39). Because this technique is burdened by the use of radioactive substances, its future relevance in cardiology will presumably be limited.

COMPUTED TOMOGRAPHY

Computed tomography and electron beam computed tomography (EBCT) have been applied to assess LV function and mass (40–42); clinical applications are reported in congestive heart failure (43), HCM (44–46), and ARVC (47–49). EBCT has been shown to noninvasively visualize coronary anatomy and thus may be useful for the exclusion of an ischemic cause in a patient with a cardiomyopathy. Another very important and unique contribution of EBCT may be the visualization of fibrosis (50). However, these techniques are limited by radiation and application of contrast media.

CARDIOVASCULAR MAGNETIC RESONANCE IN CARDIOMYOPATHIES: GENERAL ASPECTS

CMR noninvasively visualizes left and right ventricular morphology and function with a very high degree of accuracy and reproducibility (51,52). CMR is superior to 2D echocardiography in determination of ventricular mass (7,53) and volumes (54). In the last few years, the upsurge of cardiac CMR as the in vivo gold standard for identifying the phenotype of cardiomyopathies in the diagnosis and follow-up of these patients is increasingly apparent.

The power of CMR to obtain visual information on the pathologic processes of the myocardium and perform tissue analysis in cardiomyopathies has not yet been fully exploited. The MRI technique will most likely overcome the limitations of density projections, such as radiography or analysis of reflected ultrasound. Because proton relaxivity depends on the chemical environment, pathologic processes with a more or less distinct local chemistry may allow a specific identification of diseased tissue. This principle was recognized rather early on and will be more and more applied for imaging (55,56).

CARDIOVASCULAR MAGNETIC RESONANCE APPROACH TO THE PATIENT WITH CARDIOMYOPATHY

MORPHOLOGY AND FUNCTION

Cardiomyopathies are characterized by specific alterations of ventricular and myocardial geometry, and/or function. To assess volumes and mass, generally white-blood steady state free precession (SSFP) gradient-echo sequences are applied during a breath hold with approximately 30 phases per heartbeat. A stack of short-axis slices covering the entire LV

from the mitral plane to the apex can be considered the gold standard to assess left ventricular volumes and mass (38,57). Recent developments in parallel imaging allow complete left ventricular coverage in one breath hold but are not yet considered routine (58–60). Under routine clinical circumstances, a biplanar approach (long- and short-axis views) may be sufficient (61,62) to estimate mass and systolic function. To cover the whole diastolic phase, techniques have been developed with continuous data acquisition and retrospective gating. The inclusion of the end-diastolic phase is important for the analysis of time-volume curves with respect to late diastole (63). Reliable angulation of the images by a series of angulated scouts obtained during breath hold is crucial because the anatomic axis of the heart is not perpendicular to any of the orthogonal planes of the magnetic field. The slice thickness should be 8 to 10 mm; in case of circumscribed or subtle global changes, it should be reduced adequately. It is important to notice that there is a substantial shortening of the ventricular long axis (64) leading to a smaller number of slices covering the heart in systole compared with diastole. Commercially available software for automated edge detection may facilitate the evaluation process in clinical routine (65,66) but is so far not capable of including papillary muscles and may therefore not be sufficient for precise measurements.

A frequent finding in patients with cardiomyopathies is mild-to-moderate mitral regurgitation. Promoting factors are dilatation of the mitral valve ring (DCM, infiltrative cardiomyopathies) and papillary muscle dysfunction caused by infiltration (sarcoidosis, amyloidosis, hemochromatosis, or tumor). If quantification of mitral regurgitation is required for therapeutic decision-making, an established technique using flow analysis should be performed (67). "Eyeball" quantification of the regurgitant jet, as used in ventriculography or echocardiography (68), may be misleading and should be used with great caution, in particular because the application of SSFP sequences results in a greater homogeneity of the blood pool and might therefore induce underestimation of valvular turbulences.

TISSUE

For delineation of cardiac anatomy, "black-blood" T1-weighted spin-echo techniques are preferable because there is an excellent contrast between the myocardium and adjacent structures such as epicardial fat and intracavital blood. Slice orientation depends on the question being posed to the MR study; however, the orientation should include views orthogonal to the anatomic axis of the heart. Gadolinium (Gd) administration followed by a repeat T1 study may be helpful in infiltrative and inflammatory myocardial disease. T2-weighted image quality has markedly improved with short T1 inversion recovery techniques, and fluid accumulation such as edema and effusion in inflammatory or malignant diseases may be sensitively visualized. Visualization of intramyocardial fibrosis is certainly desirable for the workup of cardiomyopathies. Preliminary studies with contrast-enhanced CMR suggest that the increase of interstitial space in fibrotic tissue may be reflected by Gd accumulation (69). The finding of delayed hyperenhancement in nonischemic cardiomyopathies further support this concept (70). However, comprehensive data including histologic confirmation of patchy fibrosis in areas of delayed enhancement are not yet available.

Beyond imaging focal lesions, the quantification of absolute T1 or T2 is a reliable marker to detect diffuse myocardial changes (56,71–73). However, this approach requires several time-consuming measurements with various echo or inversion times prone to motion artifacts.

METABOLISM

Magnetic resonance spectroscopy (MRS) has generally relied on 1H and 31P and has been applied in several studies of cardiomyopathy. Changes of high-energy phosphates as studied by 31P-MRS in cardiomyopathy were reported for DCM (74,75) and HCM (76). However, MRS remains an experimental approach for several reasons: 1H MRS is limited by a strong signal from water-bound protons and difficulties in spectral interpretation, and 31P MRS is limited by the weakness of the phosphorus signal. Thus, voxels must be sufficiently large to cover circumscribed myocardial regions, and spectra are often altered by blood or adjacent tissue (e.g., skeletal muscle). Newer techniques feature irregularly shaped voxels and a significantly lower degree of spectral contamination (77). This approach may allow reproducible acquisition of reliable and highly informative myocardial spectra and even identify local pathology. Buchthal et al (78) demonstrated changes in the ratio of myocardial phosphocreatine to adenosine triphosphate in women with chest pain but normal angiograms. However, MRS techniques require extensive experience and are prone to motion artifacts (79). Thus, the number of centers with access to this promising tool is currently limited.

DILATED CARDIOMYOPATHY

DCM is characterized by a progressive dilatation of the heart with loss of contractile function. Its cause is not clarified in approximately half of the cases (80). However, the typical pattern may be the final result of a disease process with multiple possible triggers, such as infectious organisms, toxic agents like anthracyclines, autoantibodies, or genetic disorders. The histologic hallmark of DCM is a progressive interstitial fibrosis with a numeric decrease of contractile myocytes. In advanced stages, DCM is also associated with at least relative wall thinning. Endomyocardial biopsy may be of prognostic value and is part of the diagnostic approach. However, sensitivity and specificity of classic criteria were disappointing (81), and such data on more recent techniques such as immunohistochemistry are scarce.

Echocardiography is a standard tool and provides information on LV size and function, although the variability of 2D results may limit its value. Transesophageal (82) and 3D echo techniques may improve the accuracy. Several authors have described the use of dobutamine echo for DCM to gain prognostic information (83,84), but the results were mixed with only moderate predictive power (85).

CARDIOVASCULAR MAGNETIC RESONANCE

Main targets of CMR studies in DCM are LV morphology and function using SSFP gradient-echo sequences (Fig. 8.1). CMR has been proven to have low interobserver and intraobserver variabilities of left ventricular mass and volume measurements (51,54,86) with a good correlation to results obtained with positron emission tomography (87). It is likely to be more accurate than standard echocardiography (53,88) and radionuclide ventriculography (89). CMR was also used to analyze wall thickening in DCM (90), visualize impaired fiber shortening (91), and calculate end-systolic wall stress, which may be a very sensitive parameter for changes of LV function (92). The right ventricle (RV) is also frequently affected in DCM, and its morphology and function are accurately and reproducibly assessed by CMR (93,94).

In patients with DCM, enlargement and reduction of the atrial ejection fraction were found (95). CMR may be the method of choice for a longitudinal follow-up in patients with DCM under pharmacologic interventions (96), and its reproducibility allows for a substantial reduction of the required sample size of clinical trials in DCM (54,97). Thus, costs could be reduced markedly and time could be saved in clinical research.

Recently, CMR was shown to successfully detect fibrotic patterns, which allow for differentiating dilated from ischemic cardiomyopathy (98). A specific pattern involving intramural and especially subepicardial areas is often found in patients with myocarditis (Fig. 8.2). CMR seems to be the tool of choice to visualize the underlying pathology in heart failure.

The high accuracy enables the physician to adequately adjust the therapy, thereby increasing benefits for the pa-

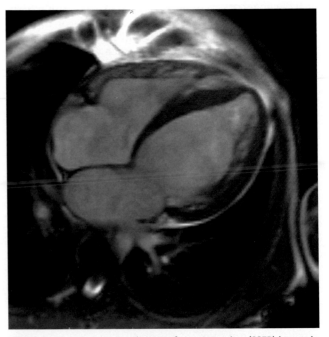

Figure 8.1. Diastolic steady-state free precession (SSFP) image in a patient with severe left ventricular dilatation and dysfunction in dilated cardiomyopathy.

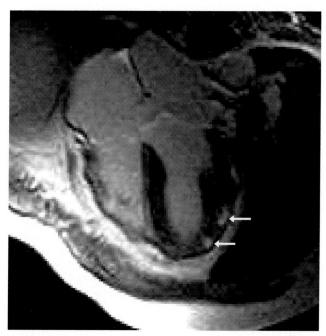

Figure 8.2. Inversion-recovery prepared gradient-echo image ("delayed enhancement") in a patient with recent myocarditis showing focal necrosis of typical subepicardial localization (*arrows*).

tient's quality of life and prognosis. Both improvements in therapy and reduction in hospital admissions for repeat studies are likely to overcome the additional costs of a CMR study. However, an analysis of cost effectiveness has not been prospectively conducted.

Spectroscopic studies have shown that high-energy phosphate metabolism is altered in DCM (99), and a low ratio of phosphocreatine to adenosine triphosphate as assessed by MRS was shown to be of prognostic value in DCM (75). Recent data indicate a role in the early detection of metabolic changes of the myocardium (100). Future studies will shed more light on this exciting field of research, and further clinical studies are warranted.

MYOCARDITIS

Investigating the early onset of DCM is an important clinical issue. The incidence of inflammation-induced forms of DCM is unclear (2); however, a substantial proportion of patients with DCM may in fact have viral myocarditis (101). In a series of endomyocardial biopsies in patients with clinically suspected hypertrophic and DCM the proportion of inflammatory changes as detected in biopsy material was as high as 25% (102). Thus, inflammation may serve as a trigger to initiate myocardial tissue transformation. Autoimmunologic mechanisms as well as the persistence of active viruses are currently under investigation. In these cases, an ongoing inflammatory process is likely to be present. The clinical course of the disease is highly variable and requires a close follow-up. Although clinicopathologic criteria for myocarditis have been further refined, endomyocardial bi-

opsy is limited in general by sample error and variability in pathologic evaluation (81,103), resulting in poor concordance between clinical and pathologic diagnosis (104,105). It is further questionable whether a potentially risky procedure should be undertaken as long as therapeutic consequences are limited. As a valuable tool for noninvasive monitoring, contrast-media enhanced T1-weighted CMR images visualize reversible myocardial signal changes in acute myocarditis (106–112). The signal changes are presumably caused by a combination of increased inflow (inflammatory hyperemia), slow interstitial wash-in/wash-out kinetics (capillary leakage and edema), and diffusion into cells (necrosis). Myocardial Gd-DTPA accumulation is significantly higher in patients with myocarditis than in healthy volunteers. Long-term follow-up may reveal persisting changes in patients with clinical and functional evidence for ongoing inflammation (113). Signal enhancement is also found to be increased in patients with Chagas myocarditis (114,115). Associated edema during acute inflammation may be detected by conventional and breath-hold T2-weighted CMR (Fig. 8.3) (116).

Recently, the sensitivity of contrast-enhanced CMR using an inversion recovery sequence to detect myocarditis was confirmed and validated by myocardial biopsy (111).

Abdel-Aty et al (116) showed that an approach combining contrast enhanced T1- and T2-weighted techniques may be preferable for clinical routine.

Progressive fibrotic replacement of the myocardium characterizes advanced stages of the disease. In a pilot study, the attempt was made to visualize myocardial fibrosis by contrast-enhanced CMR (69), and preliminary experience in humans has been obtained, but histologic validation has to be awaited. The observed lesions showed a patchy distribution, not consistent with a subendocardial, coronary pattern. Detection of fibrosis may be clinically relevant because it may represent an arrhythmogenic substrate (117).

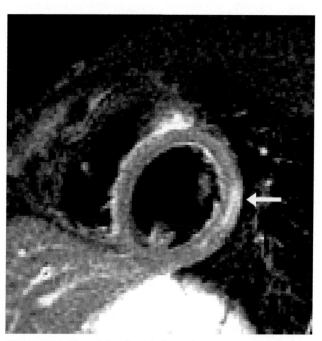

Figure 8.3. T2-weighted triple inversion recovery (STIR) spin-echo image of myocardial edema in myocarditis (*arrow*).

HYPERTROPHIC CARDIOMYOPATHY

HCM features inappropriate myocardial hypertrophy with loss of diastolic function. In addition, a subgroup of patients with hypertrophic obstructive cardiomyopathy features a narrowing of the LVOT. The condition is an important cause of sudden death in young people (118). Histologically, areas of hypertrophy reveal a pattern of myofibrillar disarray and patchy areas of necrotic tissue caused by relative coronary insufficiency.

Endomyocardial biopsy is mainly performed for investigative reasons such as analysis of gene expression. However, for clinical decision-making the sensitivity and specificity in terms of exclusion of restrictive cardiomyopathy and pressure-induced hypertrophy are not satisfying for an invasive procedure with inherent risks.

Echocardiographic findings include wall thickening and accelerated flow in the LVOT in obstructive HCM. For the clinical follow-up, the pressure gradient is estimated from measurements of velocity and according to a modified Bernoulli formula. In a small series of patients, the correlation with direct catheter measurements was satisfactory (119). However, there is an unacceptably high intraindividual variation of results, probably because of the susceptibility of flow velocities to the hemodynamic status (120). Moreover, the pressure gradient may be easily overestimated (121). Tissue Doppler imaging has been used to visualize regional heterogeneity in ventricular motion that might have great impact on functional capacity (122). Thus, although frequently used, echocardiography has substantial limitations in defining the morphology and hemodynamics in individual HCM cases.

CMR studies have been applied to mass, function, morphology, tissue characterization, and hemodynamic relevance of obstruction. Because of its high sensitivity for detecting regional morphologic changes and its noninvasive character, CMR may be of special importance in screening families of index patients.

CMR is more reliable than standard 2D echo to quantify mass (123,124) or determine regional hypertrophy patterns (125,126). Postsurgical changes after myectomy can be reliably monitored and quantified (127).

SSFP gradient-echo sequences are suitable for functional studies, visualization of turbulent flow in LVOT obstruction, and mass quantification. In severe forms, the contracting ventricular walls may oppose each other and the end-systolic volume may remain less than 10 mL. Thus, a very careful contour definition and a contiguous set of short-axis slices are necessary to prevent underestimation of end-systolic volume, which is likely to occur when only long-axis views are used.

Mitral valve regurgitation, probably caused by a pathologic change of leaflet geometry, occurs frequently and should be included in a CMR workup.

Blood flow analysis in the coronary sinus using MR is feasible, and a preliminary study suggested alterations of coronary flow reserve in patients with HCM (128).

Diastolic function (or dysfunction) is a powerful clinical and prognostic factor in hypertrophy but does not yet belong to the routine measurements of CMR. Preliminary clinical results suggest that tagging analysis of the early untwisting motion of the apical myocardium may be a helpful tool to assess diastolic dysfunction in hypertrophic heart diseases (129,130). Other functional changes detected by the use of myocardial tagging are reduced posterior rotation, reduced radial displacement of the inferior septal myocardium (131), heterogeneities of regional function (132), and reduced three-dimensional myocardial shortening (133,134). These findings may be more sensitive in the detection and quantification of functional impairment than conventional parameters such as mitral valve inflow patterns in echocardiography.

Beyond quantification of left ventricular mass and function, CMR is capable in characterizing hypertrophic tissue. Delayed hyperenhancement reveals myocardial heterogeneity in HCM (Fig. 8.4) (135). On the basis of similar lesions in myocardial infarctions, these areas most likely represent zones of focal fibrosis, although no direct histologic comparison has been published. The detection of fibrotic lesions in HCM might have a huge clinical impact because they might represent a risk factor for sudden death (117). Recently, abnormal perfusion patterns have been reported as a feature of HCM (136).

MR techniques have been established to investigate phosphate metabolism in HCM. Myocardial phosphocreatine/adenosine triphosphate ratio and the signal of phosphomonoesters were found to be changed in patients with HCM (76) regardless of the presence of hypertrophy (137). Spindler et al (138) were able to correlate diastolic dysfunction to a decrease of myocardial energy reserve related to high-energy phophate metabolism. Phosphorus metabolism was also found to be altered in skeletal muscles of patients with HCM (139).

The turbulent jet during systolic LVOT obstruction is easily detected when suitable echo times (~4 ms for typical

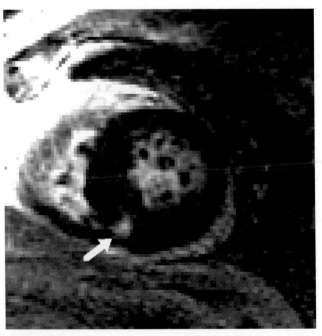

Figure 8.4. Inversion-recovery prepared gradient-echo image ("delayed enhancement") in a patient with hypertrophic cardiomyopathy (HCM) showing focal fibrosis (*arrow*).

72. Marie PY, Angioi M, Carteaux JP, et al. Detection and prediction of acute heart transplant rejection with the myocardial T2 determination provided by a black-blood magnetic resonance imaging sequence. *J Am Coll Cardiol* 2001;37(3):825–831.

73. Anderson LJ, Holden S, Davis B, et al. Cardiovascular T2-star (T2*) magnetic resonance for the early diagnosis of myocardial iron overload. *Eur Heart J* 2001;22(23):2171–2179.

74. Neubauer S, Krahe T, Schindler R, et al. 31P magnetic resonance spectroscopy in dilated cardiomyopathy and coronary artery disease. Altered cardiac high-energy phosphate metabolism in heart failure. *Circulation* 1992;86(6):1810–1818.

75. Neubauer S, Horn M, Cramer M, et al. Myocardial phosphocreatine-to-ATP ratio is a predictor of mortality in patients with dilated cardiomyopathy. *Circulation* 1997;96(7):2190–2196.

76. Jung WI, Sieverding L, Breuer J, et al. 31P NMR spectroscopy detects metabolic abnormalities in asymptomatic patients with hypertrophic cardiomyopathy. *Circulation* 1998;97(25):2536–2542.

77. Loffler R, Sauter R, Kolem H, et al. Localized spectroscopy from anatomically matched compartments: improved sensitivity and localization for cardiac 31P MRS in humans. *J Magn Reson* 1998;134(2):287–299.

78. Buchthal SD, den Hollander JA, Merz CN, et al. Abnormal myocardial phosphorus-31 nuclear magnetic resonance spectroscopy in women with chest pain but normal coronary angiograms. *N Engl J Med* 2000;342(12):829–835.

79. Cannon RO 3rd, Balaban RS. Chest pain in women with normal coronary angiograms. *N Engl J Med* 2000;342(12):885–887.

80. Kasper EK, Agema WR, Hutchins GM, et al. The causes of dilated cardiomyopathy: a clinicopathologic review of 673 consecutive patients [see comments]. *J Am Coll Cardiol* 1994;23(3):586–590.

81. Hrobon P, Kuntz KM, Hare JM. Should endomyocardial biopsy be performed for detection of myocarditis? A decision analytic approach. *J Heart Lung Transplant* 1998;17(5):479–486.

82. Jedlinski I, Michalski M, Dankowski R, et al. Transoesophageal Doppler echocardiography provided important parameters in patients with dilated cardiomyopathy during bisoprolol therapy. *Acta Cardiol* 2002;57(1):38–40.

83. Pratali L, Picano E, Otasevic P, et al. Prognostic significance of the dobutamine echocardiography test in idiopathic dilated cardiomyopathy. *Am J Cardiol* 2001;88(12):1374–1378.

84. Dagdeviren B, Akdemir O, Bolca O, et al. Myocardial texture analysis in idiopathic dilated cardiomyopathy: prediction of contractile reserve on dobutamine echocardiography. *J Am Soc Echocardiogr* 2002;15(1):36–42.

85. Pinamonti B, Perkan A, Di Lenarda A, et al. Dobutamine echocardiography in idiopathic dilated cardiomyopathy: clinical and prognostic implications. *Eur J Heart Fail* 2002;4(1):49–61.

86. Semelka RC, Tomei E, Wagner S, et al. Interstudy reproducibility of dimensional and functional measurements between cine magnetic resonance studies in the morphologically abnormal left ventricle. *Am Heart J* 1990;119(6):1367–1373.

87. Schaefer WM, Lipke CS, Nowak B, et al. Validation of an evaluation routine for left ventricular volumes, ejection fraction and wall motion from gated cardiac FDG PET: a comparison with cardiac magnetic resonance imaging. *Eur J Nucl Med Mol Imaging* 2003;30(4):545–553.

88. Friedrich MG, Strohm O, Osterziel KJ, et al. Growth hormone therapy in dilated cardiomyopathy monitored with MRI. *MAGMA* 1998;6:152–154.

89. Kondo C, Fukushima K, Kusakabe K. Measurement of left ventricular volumes and ejection fraction by quantitative gated SPET, contrast ventriculography and magnetic resonance imaging: a meta-analysis. *Eur J Nucl Med Mol Imaging* 2003;30(6):851–858.

90. Buser PT, Auffermann W, Holt WW, et al. Noninvasive evaluation of global left ventricular function with use of cine nuclear magnetic resonance. *J Am Coll Cardiol* 1989;13(6):1294–1300.

91. MacGowan GA, Shapiro EP, Azhari H, et al. Noninvasive measurement of shortening in the fiber and cross-fiber directions in the normal human left ventricle and in idiopathic dilated cardiomyopathy. *Circulation* 1997;96(2):535–541.

92. Fujita N, Duerinekx AJ, Higgins CB. Variation in left ventricular regional wall stress with cine magnetic resonance imaging: normal subjects versus dilated cardiomyopathy. *Am Heart J* 1993;125(5 Pt 1):1337–1345.

93. Lytrivi ID, Ko HH, Srivastava S, et al. Regional differences in right ventricular systolic function as determined by cine magnetic resonance imaging after infundibulotomy. *Am J Cardiol* 2004;94(7):970–973.

94. Grothues F, Moon JC, Bellenger NG, et al. Interstudy reproducibility of right ventricular volumes, function, and mass with cardiovascular magnetic resonance. *Am Heart J* 2004;147(2):218–223.

95. Jarvinen VM, Kupari MM, Poutanen VP, et al. Right and left atrial phasic volumetric function in mildly symptomatic dilated and hypertrophic cardiomyopathy: cine MR imaging assessment. *Radiology* 1996;198(2):487–495.

96. Osterziel KJ, Strohm O, Schuler J, et al. Randomised, double-blind, placebo-controlled trial of human recombinant growth hormone in patients with chronic heart failure due to dilated cardiomyopathy. *Lancet* 1998;351(9111):1233–1237.

97. Bellenger N, Davies L, Francis J, et al. Reduction in sample size for studies of remodeling in heart failure by the use of cardiovascular magnetic resonance. *J Cardiovasc Magn Res* 2000;2(4):271–278.

98. McCrohon JA, Moon JC, Prasad SK, et al. Differentiation of heart failure related to dilated cardiomyopathy and coronary artery disease using gadolinium-enhanced cardiovascular magnetic resonance. *Circulation* 2003;108(1):54–59.

99. Hardy CJ, Weiss RG, Bottomley PA, et al. Altered myocardial high-energy phosphate metabolites in patients with dilated cardiomyopathy. *Am Heart J* 1991;122(3 Pt 1):795–801.

100. Scheuermann-Freestone M, Madsen PL, Manners D, et al. Abnormal cardiac and skeletal muscle energy metabolism in patients with type 2 diabetes. *Circulation* 2003;107(24):3040–3046.

101. Pankuweit S, Ruppert V, Maisch B. Inflammation in dilated cardiomyopathy. *Herz* 2004;29(8):788–793.

102. Leatherbury L, Chandra RS, Shapiro SR, et al. Value of endomyocardial biopsy in infants, children and adolescents with dilated or hypertrophic cardiomyopathy and myocarditis. *J Am Coll Cardiol* 1988;12(6):1547–1554.

103. Shanes JG, Ghali J, Billingham ME, et al. Interobserver variability in the pathologic interpretation of endomyocardial biopsy results. *Circulation* 1987;75(2):401–405.

104. McKenna WJ, Davies MJ. Immunosuppression for myocarditis. *N Engl J Med* 1995;333(5):312–313.

105. Feldman AM, McNamara D. Myocarditis. *N Engl J Med* 2000;343(19):1388–1398.

106. Friedrich MG, Strohm O, Schulz Menger J, et al. Contrast media-enhanced magnetic resonance imaging visualizes myocardial changes in the course of viral myocarditis. *Circulation* 1998;97(18):1802–1809.

107. Roditi GH, Hartnell GG, Cohen MC. MRI changes in myocarditis—evaluation with spin echo, cine MR angiography and contrast enhanced spin echo imaging. *Clin Radiol* 2000;55(10):752–758.

108. Laissy JP, Messin B, Varenne O, et al. MRI of acute myocarditis: a comprehensive approach based on various imaging sequences. *Chest* 2002;122(5):1638–1648.

109. Geluk CA, Otterspoor IC, de Boeck B, et al. Magnetic resonance imaging in acute myocarditis: a case report and a review of literature. *Neth J Med* 2002;60(5):223–227.

110. Ohata S, Shimada T, Shimizu H, et al. Myocarditis associated with polymyositis diagnosed by gadolinium-DTPA enhanced magnetic resonance imaging. *J Rheumatol* 2002;29(4):861–862.

111. Mahrholdt H, Goedecke C, Wagner A, et al. Cardiovascular magnetic resonance assessment of human myocarditis: a comparison to histology and molecular pathology. *Circulation* 2004;109(10):1250–1258.

112. Chun W, Grist TM, Kamp TJ, et al. Images in cardiovascular medicine. Infiltrative eosinophilic myocarditis diagnosed and localized by cardiac magnetic resonance imaging. *Circulation* 2004;110(3):e19.

113. Wagner A, Schulz-Menger J, Dietz R, et al. Long-term follow-up of patients paragraph sign with acute myocarditis by magnetic paragraph sign resonance imaging. *MAGMA* 2003; 16(1):17–20.

114. Kalil R, Bocchi EA, Ferreira BM, et al. [Magnetic resonance imaging in chronic Chagas cardiopathy. Correlation with endomyocardial biopsy findings]. *Arq Bras Cardiol* 1995;65(5): 413–416.

115. Bellotti G, Bocchi EA, de Moraes AV, et al. In vivo detection of Trypanosoma cruzi antigens in hearts of patients with chronic Chagas' heart disease. *Am Heart J* 1996;131(2): 301–307.

116. Abdel-Aty H, Boye P, Zagrosek A, et al. Diagnostic performance of cardiovascular magnetic resonance in patients with suspected acute myocarditis: comparison of different approaches. *J Am Coll Cardiol* 2005;45:1815–1822.

117. Moon JC, McKenna WJ, McCrohon JA, et al. Toward clinical risk assessment in hypertrophic cardiomyopathy with gadolinium cardiovascular magnetic resonance. *J Am Coll Cardiol* 2003;41(9):1561–1567.

118. Eckart RE, Scoville SL, Campbell CL, et al. Sudden death in young adults: a 25-year review of autopsies in military recruits. *Ann Intern Med* 2004;141(11):829–834.

119. Sasson Z, Yock PG, Hatle LK, et al. Doppler echocardiographic determination of the pressure gradient in hypertrophic cardiomyopathy. *J Am Coll Cardiol* 1988;11(4):752–756.

120. Kizilbash AM, Heinle SK, Grayburn PA. Spontaneous variability of left ventricular outflow tract gradient in hypertrophic obstructive cardiomyopathy. *Circulation* 1998;97(5): 461–466.

121. Levine RA, Jimoh A, Cape EG, et al. Pressure recovery distal to a stenosis: potential cause of gradient "overestimation" by Doppler echocardiography. *J Am Coll Cardiol* 1989;13(3): 706–715.

122. Nagueh SF, Bachinski LL, Meyer D, et al. Tissue Doppler imaging consistently detects myocardial abnormalities in patients with hypertrophic cardiomyopathy and provides a novel means for an early diagnosis before and independently of hypertrophy. *Circulation* 2001;104(2):128–130.

123. Missouris CG, Forbat SM, Singer DR, et al. Echocardiography overestimates left ventricular mass: a comparative study with magnetic resonance imaging in patients with hypertension. *J Hypertens* 1996;14(8):1005–1010.

124. Alfakih K, Bloomer T, Bainbridge S, et al. A comparison of left ventricular mass between two-dimensional echocardiography, using fundamental and tissue harmonic imaging, and cardiac MRI in patients with hypertension. *Eur J Radiol* 2004; 52(2):103–109.

125. Posma JL, Blanksma PK, van der Wall EE, et al. Assessment of quantitative hypertrophy scores in hypertrophic cardiomyopathy: magnetic resonance imaging versus echocardiography. *Am Heart J* 1996;132(5):1020–1027.

126. Pons Llado G, Carreras F, Borras X, et al. Comparison of morphologic assessment of hypertrophic cardiomyopathy by magnetic resonance versus echocardiographic imaging. *Am J Cardiol* 1997;79(12):1651–1656.

127. Franke A, Schondube FA, Kuhl HP, et al. Quantitative assessment of the operative results after extended myectomy and surgical reconstruction of the subvalvular mitral apparatus in hypertrophic obstructive cardiomyopathy using dynamic three-dimensional transesophageal echocardiography. *J Am Coll Cardiol* 1998;31(7):1641–1649.

128. Kawada N, Sakuma H, Yamakado T, et al. Hypertrophic cardiomyopathy: MR measurement of coronary blood flow and vasodilator flow reserve in patients and healthy subjects. *Radiology* 1999;211(1):129–135.

129. Stuber M, Scheidegger M, Fischer S, et al. Alterations in the local myocardial motion pattern in patients suffering from pressure overload due to aortic stenosis. *Circulation* 1999 27; 100(4):361–368.

130. Nagel E, Stuber M, Burkhard B, et al. Cardiac rotation and relaxation in patients with aortic valve stenosis. *Eur Heart J* 2000;21(7):582–589.

131. Maier SE, Fischer SE, McKinnon GC, et al. Evaluation of left ventricular segmental wall motion in hypertrophic cardiomyopathy with myocardial tagging. *Circulation* 1992;86(6): 1919–1928.

132. Kramer CM, Reichek N, Ferrari VA, et al. Regional heterogeneity of function in hypertrophic cardiomyopathy. *Circulation* 1994;90(1):186–194.

133. Dong SJ, MacGregor JH, Crawley AP, et al. Left ventricular wall thickness and regional systolic function in patients with hypertrophic cardiomyopathy. A three-dimensional tagged magnetic resonance imaging study. *Circulation* 1994;90(3): 1200–1209.

134. Young AA, Kramer CM, Ferrari VA, et al. Three-dimensional left ventricular deformation in hypertrophic cardiomyopathy. *Circulation* 1994;90(2):854–867.

135. Choudhury L, Mahrholdt H, Wagner A, et al. Myocardial scarring in asymptomatic or mildly symptomatic patients with hypertrophic cardiomyopathy. *J Am Coll Cardiol* 2002; 40(12):2156–2164.

136. Sipola P, Lauerma K, Husso-Saastamoinen M, et al. First-pass MR imaging in the assessment of perfusion impairment in patients with hypertrophic cardiomyopathy and the Asp175Asn mutation of the alpha-tropomyosin gene. *Radiology* 2003;226(1):129–137.

137. Crilley JG, Boehm EA, Blair E, et al. Hypertrophic cardiomyopathy due to sarcomeric gene mutations is characterized by impaired energy metabolism irrespective of the degree of hypertrophy. *J Am Coll Cardiol* 2003;41(10):1776–1782.

138. Spindler M, Saupe KW, Christe ME, et al. Diastolic dysfunction and altered energetics in the alphaMHC403/+ mouse model of familial hypertrophic cardiomyopathy. *J Clin Invest* 1998;101(8):1775–1783.

139. Jung WI, Sieverding L, Breuer J, et al. Detection of phosphomonoester signals in proton-decoupled 31P NMR spectra of the myocardium of patients with myocardial hypertrophy. *J Magn Reson* 1998;133(1):232–235.

140. White RD, Obuchowski NA, Gunawardena S, et al. Left ventricular outflow tract obstruction in hypertrophic cardiomyopathy: presurgical and postsurgical evaluation by computed tomography magnetic resonance imaging. *Am J Card Imaging* 1996;10(1):1–13.

141. Schulz-Menger J, Strohm O, Waigand J, et al. The value of magnetic resonance imaging of the left ventricular outflow tract in patients with hypertrophic obstructive cardiomy-

opathy after septal artery embolization. *Circulation* 2000; 101(15):1764–1766.

142. Suzuki J, Shimamoto R, Nishikawa J, et al. Morphological onset and early diagnosis in apical hypertrophic cardiomyopathy: a long term analysis with nuclear magnetic resonance imaging. *J Am Coll Cardiol* 1999;33(1):146–151.

143. Amano Y, Takayama M, Amano M, et al. MRI of cardiac morphology and function after percutaneous transluminal septal myocardial ablation for hypertrophic obstructive cardiomyopathy. *AJR Am J Roentgenol* 2004;182(2):523–527.

144. McKenna WJ, Thiene G, Nava A, et al. Diagnosis of arrhythmogenic right ventricular dysplasia/cardiomyopathy. Task Force of the Working Group Myocardial and Pericardial Disease of the European Society of Cardiology and of the Scientific Council on Cardiomyopathies of the International Society and Federation of Cardiology. *Br Heart J* 1994;71(3): 215–218.

145. Fontaine G, Fontaliran F, Frank R. Arrhythmogenic right ventricular cardiomyopathies: clinical forms and main differential diagnoses [editorial; comment]. *Circulation* 1998;97(16): 1532–1535.

146. Basso C, Wichter T, Danieli GA, et al. Arrhythmogenic right ventricular cardiomyopathy: clinical registry and database, evaluation of therapies, pathology registry, DNA banking. *Eur Heart J* 2004;25(6):531–534.

147. Basso C, Thiene G, Corrado D, et al. Arrhythmogenic right ventricular cardiomyopathy. Dysplasia, dystrophy, or myocarditis? *Circulation* 1996;94(5):983–991.

148. Corrado D, Basso C, Thiene G, et al. Spectrum of clinicopathologic manifestations of arrhythmogenic right ventricular cardiomyopathy/dysplasia: a multicenter study. *J Am Coll Cardiol* 1997;30(6):1512–1520.

149. Committees UI-US. Survivors of out-of-hospital cardiac arrest with apparently normal heart. Need for definition and standardized clinical evaluation. Consensus Statement of the Joint Steering Committees of the Unexplained Cardiac Arrest Registry of Europe and of the Idiopathic Ventricular Fibrillation Registry of the United States. *Circulation* 1997;95(1): 265–272.

150. Fontaliran F, Arkwright S, Vilde F, et al. [Arrhythmogenic right ventricular dysplasia and cardiomyopathy. Clinical and anatomic-pathologic aspects, nosologic approach]. *Arch Anat Cytol Pathol* 1998;46(3):171–177.

151. Blomstrom Lundqvist C, Beckman Suurkula M, Wallentin I, et al. Ventricular dimensions and wall motion assessed by echocardiography in patients with arrhythmogenic right ventricular dysplasia. *Eur Heart J* 1988;9(12):1291–1302.

152. Kisslo J. Two-dimensional echocardiography in arrhythmogenic right ventricular dysplasia. *Eur Heart J* 1989;10:22–26.

153. Schick F, Miller S, Hahn U, et al. Fat- and water-selective MR cine imaging of the human heart: assessment of right ventricular dysplasia. *Invest Radiol* 2000;35(5):311–318.

154. Ricci C, Longo R, Pagnan L, et al. Magnetic resonance imaging in right ventricular dysplasia. *Am J Cardiol* 1992;70(20): 1589–1595.

155. Blake LM, Scheinman MM, Higgins CB. MR features of arrhythmogenic right ventricular dysplasia. *AJR Am J Roentgenol* 1994;162(4):809–812.

156. Auffermann W, Wichter T, Breithardt G, et al. Arrhythmogenic right ventricular disease: MR imaging vs angiography. *AJR Am J Roentgenol* 1993;161(3):549–555.

157. Midiri M, Finazzo M. MR imaging of arrhythmogenic right ventricular dysplasia. *Int J Cardiovasc Imaging* 2001;17(4): 297–304.

158. Castillo E, Tandri H, Rodriguez ER, et al. Arrhythmogenic right ventricular dysplasia: ex vivo and in vivo fat detection with black-blood MR imaging. *Radiology* 2004;232(1): 38–48.

159. Bluemke DA, Krupinski EA, Ovitt T, et al. MR Imaging of arrhythmogenic right ventricular cardiomyopathy: morphologic findings and interobserver reliability. *Cardiology* 2003; 99(3):153–162.

160. Globits S, Kreiner G, Frank H, et al. Significance of morphological abnormalities detected by MRI in patients undergoing successful ablation of right ventricular outflow tract tachycardia. *Circulation* 1997;96(8):2633–2640.

161. Proclemer A, Basadonna PT, Slavich GA, et al. Cardiac magnetic resonance imaging findings in patients with right ventricular outflow tract premature contractions [see comments]. *Eur Heart J* 1997;18(12):2002–2010.

162. White RD, Trohman RG, Flamm SD, et al. Right ventricular arrhythmia in the absence of arrhythmogenic dysplasia: MR imaging of myocardial abnormalities. *Radiology* 1998; 207(3):743–751.

163. Sievers B, Addo M, Franken U, et al. Right ventricular wall motion abnormalities found in healthy subjects by cardiovascular magnetic resonance imaging and characterized with a new segmental model. *J Cardiovasc Magn Reson* 2004;6(3): 601–608.

164. Tandri H, Bluemke DA, Ferrari VA, et al. Findings on magnetic resonance imaging of idiopathic right ventricular outflow tachycardia. *Am J Cardiol* 2004;94(11):1441–1445.

165. Tandri H, Friedrich MG, Calkins H, et al. MRI of arrhythmogenic right ventricular cardiomyopathy/dysplasia. *J Cardiovasc Magn Reson* 2004;6(2):557–563.

166. Kushwaha SS, Fallon JT, Fuster V. Restrictive cardiomyopathy. *N Engl J Med* 1997;336(4):267–276.

167. Talreja DR, Edwards WD, Danielson GK, et al. Constrictive pericarditis in 26 patients with histologically normal pericardial thickness. *Circulation* 2003;108(15):1852–1857.

168. Jarvinen VM, Kupari MM, Poutanen VP, et al. A simplified method for the determination of left atrial size and function using cine magnetic resonance imaging. *Magn Reson Imaging* 1996;14(3):215–226.

169. Barkhausen J, Hunold P, Eggebrecht H, et al. Detection and characterization of intracardiac thrombi on MR imaging. *AJR Am J Roentgenol* 2002;179(6):1539–1544.

170. Flora GS, Sharma OP. Myocardial sarcoidosis: a review. *Sarcoidosis* 1989;6(2):97–106.

171. Meyer A, Schafer H, Doring V, et al. [Heart transplantation in myocardial sarcoidosis. Studies on the explanted heart]. *Dtsch Med Wochenschr* 1999;124(39):1131–1134.

172. Syed J, Myers R. Sarcoid heart disease. *Can J Cardiol* 2004; 20(1):89–93.

173. Sugie T, Hashimoto N, Iwai K. [Clinical and autopsy studies on prognosis of sarcoidosis]. *Nippon-Rinsho* 1994;52(6): 1567–1570.

174. Perry A, Vuitch F. Causes of death in patients with sarcoidosis. A morphologic study of 38 autopsies with clinicopathologic correlations. *Arch Pathol Lab Med* 1995;119(2): 167–172.

175. Ratner SJ, Fenoglio JJ Jr., Ursell PC. Utility of endomyocardial biopsy in the diagnosis of cardiac sarcoidosis. *Chest* 1986;90(4):528–533.

176. Uemura A, Morimoto S, Hiramitsu S, et al. Histologic diagnostic rate of cardiac sarcoidosis: evaluation of endomyocardial biopsies. *Am Heart J* 1999;138(2 Pt 1):299–302.

177. Kurashima K, Shimizu H, Ogawa H, et al. MR and CT in the evaluation of sarcoid myopathy. *J Comput Assist Tomogr* 1991;15(6):1004–1007.

178. Otake S, Banno T, Ohba S, et al. Muscular sarcoidosis: findings at MR imaging. *Radiology* 1990;176(1):145–148.

179. Riedy K, Fisher MR, Belic N, et al. MR imaging of myocardial sarcoidosis. *AJR Am J Roentgenol* 1988;151(5):915–916.

180. Smedema JP, van Kroonenburgh MJ, Snoep G, et al. Images in cardiovascular medicine. Cardiac sarcoidosis in a patient

with hypertrophic cardiomyopathy demonstrated by magnetic resonance imaging and single photon emission computed tomography dual-isotope scintigraphy. *Circulation* 2004; 110(24):e529–531.

181. Schulz-Menger J, Strohm O, Dietz R, et al. Visualization of cardiac involvement in patients with systemic sarcoidosis applying contrast-enhanced magnetic resonance imaging. *MAGMA* 2000;11(1–2):82–83.

182. Doherty MJ, Kumar SK, Nicholson AA, et al. Cardiac sarcoidosis: the value of magnetic resonance imaging in diagnosis and assessment of response to treatment. *Respir Med* 1998; 92(4):697–699.

183. Shimada T, Shimada K, Sakane T, et al. Diagnosis of cardiac sarcoidosis and evaluation of the effects of steroid therapy by gadolinium-DTPA-enhanced magnetic resonance imaging. *Am J Med* 2001;110(7):520–527.

184. Vignaux O, Dhote R, Duboc D, et al. Clinical significance of myocardial magnetic resonance abnormalities in patients with sarcoidosis: a 1-year follow-up study. *Chest* 2002; 122(6):1895–1901.

185. Dupuis JM, Victor J, Furber A, et al. [Value of magnetic resonance imaging in cardiac sarcoidosis. Apropos of a case]. *Arch Mal Coeur Vaiss* 1994;87(1):105–110.

186. Gertz MA, Kyle RA, Thibodeau SN. Familial amyloidosis: a study of 52 North American-born patients examined during a 30-year period. *Mayo Clin Proc* 1992;67(5):428–440.

187. Plehn JF, Southworth J, Cornwell GG. Brief report: atrial systolic failure in primary amyloidosis [see comments]. *N Engl J Med* 1992;327(22):1570–1573.

188. Kyle RA, Spittell PC, Gertz MA, et al. The premortem recognition of systemic senile amyloidosis with cardiac involvement. *Am J Med* 1996;101(4):395–400.

189. Koyama J, Ray-Sequin PA, Falk RH. Prognostic significance of ultrasound myocardial tissue characterization in patients with cardiac amyloidosis. *Circulation* 2002;106(5):556–561.

190. Benson L, Hemmingsson A, Ericsson A, et al. Magnetic resonance imaging in primary amyloidosis. *Acta Radiol* 1987; 28(1):13–15.

191. Simons M, Isner JM. Assessment of relative sensitivities of noninvasive tests for cardiac amyloidosis in documented cardiac amyloidosis. *Am J Cardiol* 1992;69(4):425–427.

192. Matsuoka H, Hamada M, Honda T, et al. Precise assessment of myocardial damage associated with secondary cardiomyopathies by use of Gd-DTPA-enhanced magnetic resonance imaging. *Angiology* 1993;44(12):945–950.

193. Fattori R, Rocchi G, Celletti F, et al. Contribution of magnetic resonance imaging in the differential diagnosis of cardiac amyloidosis and symmetric hypertrophic cardiomyopathy. *Am Heart J* 1998;136(5):824–830.

194. Celletti F, Fattori R, Napoli G, et al. Assessment of restrictive cardiomyopathy of amyloid or idiopathic etiology by magnetic resonance imaging. *Am J Cardiol* 1999;83(5):798–801, a710.

195. Maceira AM, Joshi J, Prasad SK, et al. Cardiovascular magnetic resonance in cardiac amyloidosis. *Circulation* 2005; 111(2):186–193.

196. Billingham ME, Cary NR, Hammond ME, et al. A working formulation for the standardization of nomenclature in the diagnosis of heart and lung rejection: Heart Rejection Study Group. The International Society for Heart Transplantation. *J Heart Transplant* 1990;9(6):587–593.

197. Nishimura T, Sada M, Sasaki H, et al. Identification of cardiac rejection with magnetic resonance imaging in heterotopic heart transplantation model. *Heart Vessels* 1987;3(3): 135–140.

198. Almenar L, Igual B, Martinez-Dolz L, et al. Utility of cardiac magnetic resonance imaging for the diagnosis of heart transplant rejection. *Transplant Proc* 2003;35(5):1962–1964.

199. Kober F, Caus T, Riberi A, et al. Objective and noninvasive metabolic characterization of donor hearts by phosphorous-31 magnetic resonance spectroscopy. *Transplantation* 2002; 74(12):1752–1756.

200. Muehling OM, Wilke NM, Panse P, et al. Reduced myocardial perfusion reserve and transmural perfusion gradient in heart transplant arteriopathy assessed by magnetic resonance imaging. *J Am Coll Cardiol* 2003;42(6):1054–1060.

201. Olson LJ, Edwards WD, McCall JT, et al. Cardiac iron deposition in idiopathic hemochromatosis: histologic and analytic assessment of 14 hearts from autopsy. *J Am Coll Cardiol* 1987;10(6):1239–1243.

202. Mavrogeni SI, Gotsis ED, Markussis V, et al. T2 relaxation time study of iron overload in b-thalassemia. *MAGMA* 1998; 6(1):7–12.

203. Ooi GC, Chen FE, Chan KN, et al. Qualitative and quantitative magnetic resonance imaging in haemoglobin H disease: screening for iron overload. *Clin Radiol* 1999;54(2):98–102.

204. Papanikolaou N, Ghiatas A, Kattamis A, et al. Non-invasive myocardial iron assessment in thalassaemic patients. T2 relaxometry and magnetization transfer ratio measurements. *Acta Radiol* 2000;41(4):348–351.

205. Jensen PD, Jensen FT, Christensen T, et al. Evaluation of myocardial iron by magnetic resonance imaging during iron chelation therapy with deferrioxamine: indication of close relation between myocardial iron content and chelatable iron pool. *Blood* 2003;101(11):4632–4639.

206. Anderson LJ, Wonke B, Prescott E, et al. Comparison of effects of oral deferiprone and subcutaneous desferrioxamine on myocardial iron concentrations and ventricular function in beta-thalassaemia. *Lancet* 2002;360(9332):516–520.

207. D'Silva SA, Kohli A, Dalvi BV, et al. MRI in right ventricular endomyocardial fibrosis. *Am Heart J* 1992;123(5): 1390–1392.

208. Huong DL, Wechsler B, Papo T, et al. Endomyocardial fibrosis in Behcet's disease. *Ann Rheum Dis* 1997;56(3):205–208.

209. Oechslin EN, Attenhofer Jost CH, Rojas JR, et al. Long-term follow-up of 34 adults with isolated left ventricular non-compaction: a distinct cardiomyopathy with poor prognosis. *J Am Coll Cardiol* 2000;36(2):493–500.

210. Ritter M, Oechslin E, Sutsch G, et al. Isolated non-compaction of the myocardium in adults. *Mayo Clin Proc* 1997;72(1): 26–31.

211. Jenni R, Hany TF, Debatin JF. MR appearance of isolated non-compaction of the left ventricle. *J Magn Reson Imaging* 1997;7(2):437–438.

212. Junga G, Kneifel S, Von Smekal A, et al. Myocardial ischaemia in children with isolated ventricular non-compaction. *Eur Heart J* 1999;20(12):910–916.

213. Borreguero LJ, Corti R, de Soria RF, et al. Images in cardiovascular medicine. Diagnosis of isolated non-compaction of the myocardium by magnetic resonance imaging. *Circulation* 2002;105(21):E177–178.

214. Baumhakel M, Janzen I, Kindermann M, et al. Images in cardiovascular medicine. Cardiac imaging in isolated non-compaction of ventricular myocardium. *Circulation* 2002; 106(5):e16–17.

215. McCrohon JA, John AS, Lorenz CH, et al. Images in cardiovascular medicine. Left ventricular involvement in arrhythmogenic right ventricular cardiomyopathy. *Circulation* 2002;105(11):1394.

216. Petersen S, Selvanayagam J, Wiesmann F, et al. Left ventricular non-compaction: insights from cardiovascular magnetic resonance imaging. *J Am Coll Cardiol* (in press).

9

Pericardial Diseases

Karen G. Ordovás and Charles B. Higgins

IMAGING OF PERICARDIUM

The imaging modality of choice for initial evaluation of patients with suspected pericardial effusion is transthoracic echocardiography. This widely available and relatively low-cost method has a high accuracy for detection of pericardial effusion and signs of tamponade. It is also a good method for guiding diagnostic or therapeutic pericardiocenteses (1).

The main limitation of echocardiography for this purpose is its inability to assess the entire pericardial extension. It is also not very accurate for depiction of pericardial thickening associated with pericarditis, because echogenicity of the pericardium is similar to adjacent tissues (1).

Major indications for further investigation with cross-sectional imaging are the visualization of loculated pericardial effusion, evaluation of complicated pericardial effusion (hemorrhagic versus nonhemorrhagic), measurement of pericardial thickness, and assessment of enhancement of the pericardium (2–4).

Computed tomography (CT) and magnetic resonance imaging (MRI) provide excellent delineation of the mediastinal anatomy, with high soft-tissue contrast and spatial resolution. The visualization of the entire chest can also give important information for differential diagnosis and extent of pericardial diseases. Both methods provide some information on tissue characterization, which is useful for the diagnosis of pericardial masses (5,6).

CT is the best method for depiction of pericardial calcification, a finding suggestive of constrictive pericarditis in the appropriate clinical setting (7,8). CT-guided pericardiocenteses is a well-established technique for management of loculated pericardial effusions. Electrocardiogram-gated CT can eliminate the artifacts related to cardiac motion and is superior to nongated studies for the evaluation of pericardial abnormalities (4).

MRI has the advantage of avoiding iodinated contrast media and ionizing radiation as well as providing imaging in multiple planes (9–12). The major indication for MRI is the measurement of pericardial thickness, which is useful for diagnosis of constrictive pericarditis in patients with constrictive/restrictive physiology (13,14). Cine MRI can usually differentiate a small pericardial effusion from pericardial thickening, which can be misinterpreted by CT (4).

TECHNIQUES

Multidetector CT imaging with retrospective cardiac gating is used to assess pericardial anatomy and cardiac function with adequate temporal and high spatial resolution. The use of β-blockers to reduce heart rate during image acquisition may be useful to reduce pulsation artifacts and increased signal-to-noise ratio (15).

Electrocardiogram-gated MRI studies with morphologic and functional sequences allow a complete evaluation of the pericardium with high soft-tissue contrast and spatial resolution. Images of the entire heart can be acquired with a few breath holds or during free-breathing. New techniques with a spatial-arrayed coil can image the heart with a high temporal resolution (16).

Turbo spin-echo (SE) T1-weighted images are usually acquired at least in the axial and coronal planes for morphologic assessment of the pericardium. SE or inversion recovery gradient-echo (GRE) images after administration of gadolinium chelates may be used to detect enhancement of inflammatory processes of the pericardium. Cine MR images using GRE or steady-state free precession sequences are acquired to evaluate ventricular function, ventricular sliding motion over the pericardium, and diastolic ventricular septal motion.

NORMAL PERICARDIUM AND NORMAL VARIANTS

The pericardium is a compliant sac that envelops the heart and the origin of the great vessels. It is attached to the sternum anteriorly and to the diaphragm inferiorly. The left atrium is only partially covered by the pericardium. Parietal pericardium consists of fibrous tissue with an inner layer of mesothelial cells that reflect in the regions of pericardial attachment and cover the surface of the heart, forming the visceral pericardium (17). On MRI and CT studies, the normal pericardium is usually less than 2 mm thick (Fig. 9.1). A thickness greater than 4 mm is considered abnormal (9,18). CT can overestimate pericardial thickness in the presence of isodense effusion (2,4). Visualization of the pericardium on both CT and MRI is possible because of its position between two fat planes (epicardial and pericardial). Although the pericardium is visible over the right cardiac chambers in most studies, it may not be visible over the lateral and posterior walls of the left ventricle (9).

The pericardial cavity normally contains up to 50 mL of serous fluid that distributes diffusely around the heart surface and inside the pericardial recesses (17). The complex con-

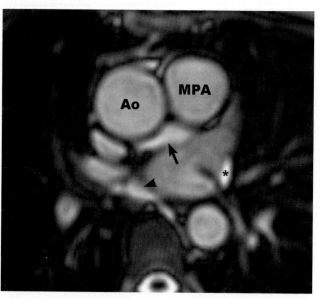

Figure 9.2. Transverse sinus of the pericardium. Axial cine magnetic resonance (MR) image at the level of the main pulmonary artery (MPA) and ascending aorta (Ao) shows the transverse sinus of the pericardium (*arrow*). Note that the pericardial fluid inside the sinus has the same signal intensity of the flowing blood. Also shown are the oblique sinus (*arrowhead*) and left pulmonic vein recess (*asterisk*).

figuration of the pericardial cavity can be understood as two connected complex spaces surrounding the heart and great vessels (19). The first region surrounds the proximal two thirds of the ascending aorta and pulmonary artery out to its bifurcation, and is known as transverse sinus (19,20). The second region surrounds the attachment of inferior vena cava, superior vena cava, and pulmonary veins, delineating a cul-de-sac behind the left atrium called oblique sinus (Figs. 9.2 and 9.3). The pericardial cavity has several recesses that can be recognized on CT and MR images: These are the superior and inferior aortic recesses, left and right pulmonic

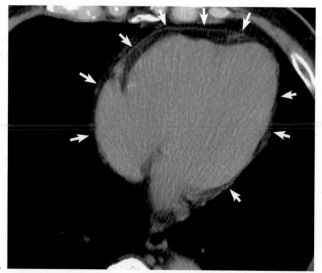

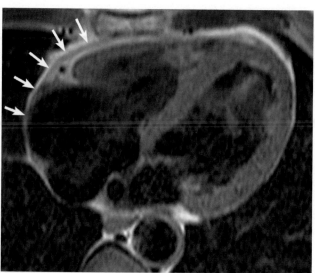

Figure 9.1. Normal pericardium. Computed tomography (CT) **(A)** and axial spin-echo (SE) images **(B)** show the normal appearance of the pericardium (*arrows*).

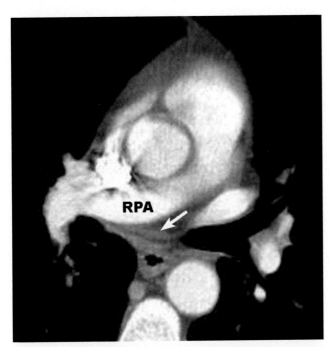

Figure 9.3. Oblique sinus of the pericardium. Contrast-enhanced CT image at the level of the right pulmonary artery (RPA) shows fluid inside the oblique sinus of the pericardium (*arrow*). Note that a fat plane separates this pericardial sinus from the anterior esophageal wall.

recesses, posterior pericardial recess, left and right pulmonary vein recesses, and postcaval recess (Figs. 9.2 and 9.4) (19,21,22).

Knowledge of the cross-sectional anatomy of the pericardial recesses is essential for its differentiation from lymph nodes or abnormalities of adjacent mediastinal structures (23–26). In the setting of malignancy, a misinterpretation of a normal recess as lymphadenomegaly could lead to inappropriate staging and mismanagement of patients (27). On electron-beam CT of normal pericardium, the superior and inferior aortic recesses, left pulmonary recess, and posterior pericardial recess are the most frequently identified (80%–95%) (26). Occasionally, one of the recesses can be much more prominent than the others, increasing the chances of misinterpretation (Fig. 9.5) (28).

PERICARDIAL EFFUSION

Collections of fluid within the pericardial cavity can represent transudate or exudate. The latter include serous, fibrinous, purulent, and hemorrhagic or (rarely) chylous pericardial effusion (29).

Simple pericardial effusion (transudate) has a density close to water on CT (Fig. 9.6) (8). The typical presentation on MRI is absent or hypointense signal in T1-weighted SE as well as a high signal intensity in T2-weighted SE, cine-GRE, and steady state free precession sequences (Fig. 9.7) (11,13,14,30).

Differentiation of transudate from exudate is usually not possible based on imaging appearance alone. However, in-

creased fluid density and heterogeneity on CT suggest the presence of exudate (30). On MRI, intermediate signal intensity on T1-weighted SE images also suggest exudate (Fig. 9.8) (3,4,14).

The appearance of pericardial hematoma depends on the age of the pericardial blood. Acute hemopericardium has a high density on CT, whereas subacute hematomas present with a heterogeneous density (Fig. 9.9) (8). MRI of acute pericardial hematoma shows a high signal intensity on SE T1-weighted sequences and a low signal intensity on cine-GRE images (31,32). Subacute and chronic hematomas are usually heterogeneous with both high- and low-signal intensity regions on T1-weighted images (Fig. 9.10) (33,34).

Chylous effusion is extremely rare. It has been described as a low-density pericardial collection on CT studies (8).

Small amounts of pericardial fluid can be misinterpreted on CT imaging because of similar appearance to pericardial thickening (4,30). MRI is an excellent method for depiction of small pericardial effusions based on the typical signal intensities (13). Typically, even a small volume of fluid appears as a high signal space between the epicardial layers. Pericardial fluid motion during the cardiac cycle on cine-GRE sequences may help in differentiating pericardial fluid and pericardial thickening, as well as excluding the presence of adherences in the regions where fluid motion is visualized between parietal and visceral pericardium (30). Pericardial effusion shows no increase in signal on T1-weighted images after administration of gadolinium chelate. This feature aids in distinguishing between pericardial fluid and pericardial or myocardial tumor on T1-weighted SE images.

ACUTE PERICARDITIS

The causes of acute pericarditis can be separated into infectious and noninfectious. The most common infectious agents are viruses (coxsackie, influenza). Among the noninfectious causes are vasculitis and connective-tissue diseases, diseases of adjacent mediastinal structures, metabolic disorders (uremia, myxoedema), neoplasm, radiation, and trauma (35). Thickening of the pericardium can be related to an acute pericarditis as well as a chronic or postinflammatory process. The abnormality may be diffuse or localized, and pericardial effusion can be associated (35,36).

With an appropriate clinical presentation, acute pericarditis can be recognized on CT and MRI because of an early contrast enhancement of the thickened pericardial layers, which are more frequently smooth in contour (Fig. 9.11). However, pericardial enhancement is nonspecific and can be related to various causes such as inflammation, infection, and tumor. Variable amounts of pericardial effusion are usually present (4,30).

Chronic pericarditis may be suggested by the presence of an irregular contour of the thickened enhancing pericardium in a patient with an insidious clinical course (36,37). However, imaging findings usually cannot predict chronicity of the disease; this determination is dependent on clinical features.

text continues on page 143

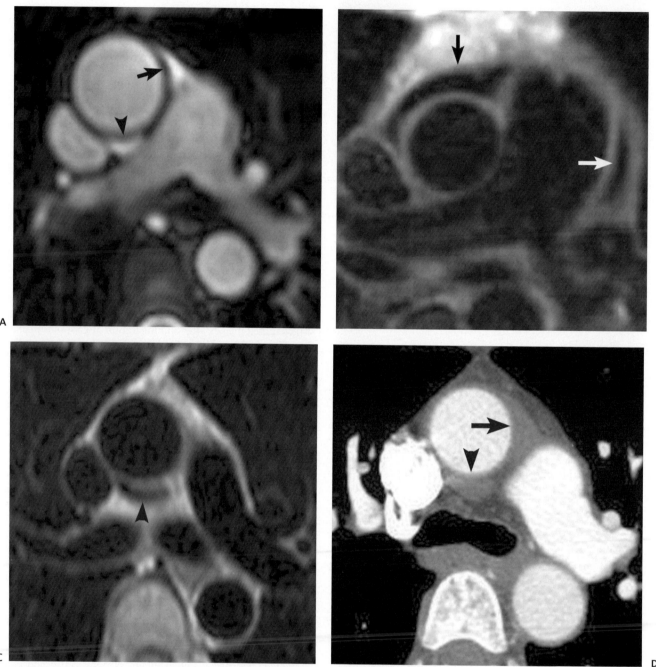

Figure 9.4. Pericardial recesses. Axial cine MR **(A)** and axial SE **(B)** images at the level of the pulmonary artery bifurcation show the anterior (*black arrow*) and posterior (*arrowhead*) portions of the superior aortic recess and the left pulmonic recess (*white arrow*). Axial SE image **(C)** and contrast-enhanced CT **(D)** at the level of the left pulmonary artery also show the anterior (*arrow*) and posterior (*arrowhead*) portions of the superior aortic recess.

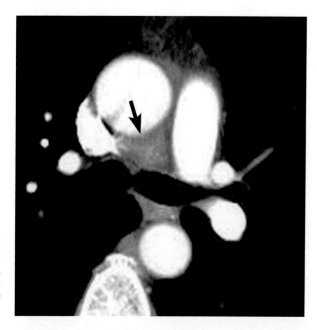

Figure 9.5. Prominent superior aortic recess. Contrast-enhanced CT at the level of the carina shows more than usual volume of pericardial fluid inside the posterior portion of the superior aortic recess (*arrow*).

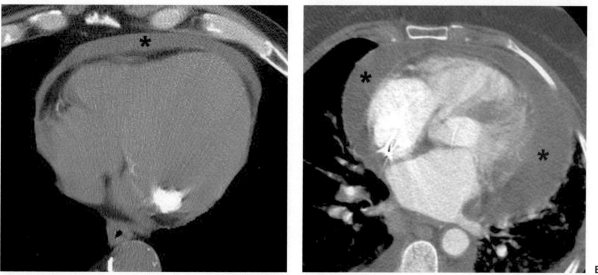

A   B

Figure 9.6. Pericardial effusion on CT. CT image **(A)** demonstrates homogeneous small pericardial effusion with water density (*asterisk*). Contrast-enhanced CT **(B)** shows a large pericardial effusion (*asterisk*).

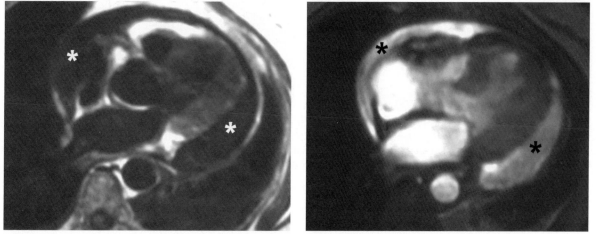

A   B

Figure 9.7. Pericardial effusion on magnetic resonance imaging (MRI). Axial T1-weighted SE image **(A)** shows the low signal intensity of a pericardial effusion (*asterisk*). High signal intensity of the effusion (*asterisk*) is observed on axial cine MR image **(B)**.

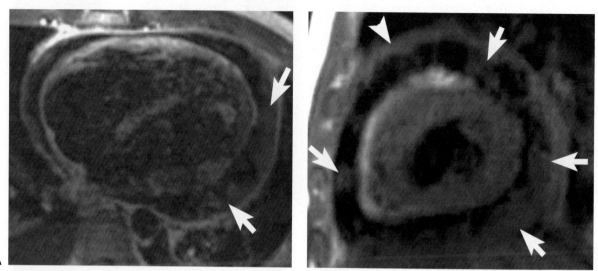

Figure 9.8. Pericardial exudate. SE MR images in the axial **(A)** and sagittal **(B)** planes show an heterogeneous pericardial effusion with areas of intermediate signal in the fluid (*arrows*). A thickened pericardium is also visible (*arrowhead*), consistent with an inflammatory process.

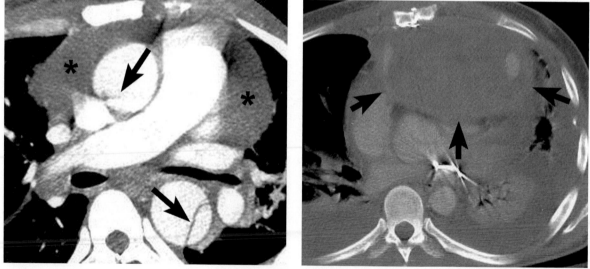

Figure 9.9. Pericardial hematoma on CT. Contrast-enhanced CT at the level of the right pulmonary artery **(A)** shows a type A aortic dissection (*arrows*) associated with a high-density pericardial effusion (*asterisk*) consistent with acute hemopericardium. CT image at the level of the base of the heart **(B)** in another patient after cardiac surgery shows a large heterogeneous collection on the anterior aspect of the pericardium (*arrows*). Note the compression of the right ventricle by the hematoma.

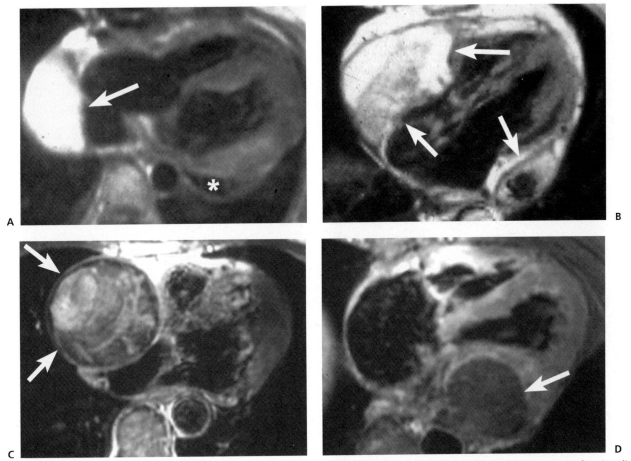

Figure 9.10. MR appearance of pericardial hematoma. Axial SE MR images at the midventricular level show different ages of pericardial blood. The homogeneous high-intensity collection adjacent to the right atrium (*arrow*) is an acute hematoma **(A)**. Note the low intensity of simple pericardial effusion at the left side of the cavity (*asterisk*). Subacute pericardial hemorrhage with areas of low and high signal intensity is shown in loculated **(B,C)** pericardial hematomas (*arrows*). The homogeneous low-intensity collection compressing the left ventricle **(D)** is a typical presentation of an old chronic hematoma (*arrow*).

CONSTRICTIVE PERICARDITIS

Constrictive pericarditis presents clinically as diastolic ventricular dysfunction, with dyspnea, orthopnea, peripheral edema, and occasionally liver enlargement and ascites. Currently, the most common causes of constrictive pericarditis are thoracic radiation therapy and cardiac surgery. In developing countries, tuberculosis is still the leading cause of pericardial constriction (29,35,38,39). The most frequent causes are listed in Table 9.1.

As a result of inflammatory processes, fibrosis of the pericardium and/or pericardial adhesions may occur, sometimes with concomitant calcifications. The less compliant pericardium impedes ventricular and/or atrial filling, depending on the extent of the disease. Another consequence of the rigid pericardium is an increased ventricular interdependence. Because the free walls of ventricular chambers have restricted expansion during diastole, the volumetric capacity of one ventricle is strictly related to the filling of the opposite-sided ventricle. Therefore, minimal differences in ventricular pressures result in diastolic ventricular septal motion toward the ventricle with instantaneously lower diastolic pressure (29,39).

There are four different presentations of constrictive pericarditis: acute inflammatory, effusive constrictive, adhesive, and chronic fibrous. The classic picture is classified as chronic fibrous constrictive pericarditis and consists of fibrotic changes with or without associated calcifications consequent to a previous chronic inflammatory process (Fig. 9.12). Adhesive constrictive pericarditis is characterized by the presence of fibrous bridges between the parietal and visceral pericardium and is usually related to previous suppurative or caseous pericarditis (Fig. 9.13). Acute inflammatory constrictive pericarditis presents as an acute pericarditis with marked thickening of the pericardium associated with constrictive physiology (Fig. 9.14). The inflammatory process can resolve completely or become a chronic constriction. Effusive-constrictive pericarditis is basically chronic constrictive pericarditis mainly involving the visceral pericardium and associated with a chronic pericardial effusion (Fig. 9.15). It is usually recognized when constrictive physiology remains after drainage of the pericardial effusion (35,36).

Various patterns of distribution have been described including global, right-sided, left-sided, and focal (Fig. 9.16) (36). The focal type usually involves the atrioventricular

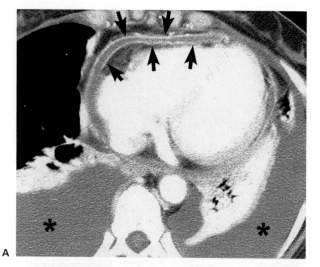

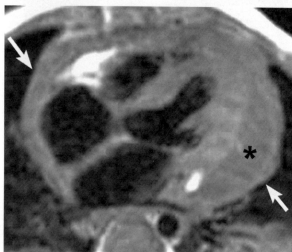

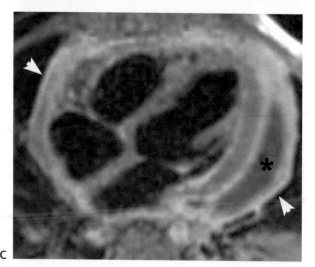

Figure 9.11. Acute pericarditis. Contrast-enhanced CT image **(A)** shows enhancement of the pericardial layers (*arrows*) and a small pericardial effusion. Note the large pleural effusions (*asterisk*). Axial T1-weighted SE images before **(B)** and after **(C)** administration of gadolinium chelate show thickening of the pericardium (*arrows*) and pericardial effusion (*asterisk*). After administration of contrast material, the pericardium enhances (*arrowheads*). Note the intermediate signal intensity of the effusion, consistent with an exudate.

TABLE 9-1	Causes of Constrictive Pericarditis

Injury

Acute myocardial infarction
Postmyocardial infarction syndrome
Pericardiotomy
Irradiation

Infection

Virus
Bacterium
Tuberculosis
Fungus
Parasite

Connective-Tissue Disease

Rheumatoid arthritis
Lupus erythematosus

Metabolic Disorder

Uremia

Neoplasm

Breast and lung carcinoma
Sarcoma
Lymphoma and leukemia
Mesothelioma

Idiopathic

groove and thereby may impede right atrial, and less frequently, left atrial emptying (Fig. 9.17).

The distinction between constrictive pericarditis and restrictive cardiomyopathy is difficult clinically because both diseases present with symptoms of diastolic heart insufficiency and frequently have similar findings of increased and equalized atrial and ventricular pressures on both sides of the heart on cardiac catheterization. This differentiation is crucial for the patient's management because constrictive pericarditis is treated surgically and has a good prognosis, whereas restrictive cardiomyopathy is treated medically and has a poor outcome (40–42).

CT and MRI are the methods of choice for measuring pericardial thickness. MRI has a reported accuracy of 93% for the diagnosis of constrictive pericarditis based on the presence of pericardial thickness (≥ 4 mm) in the appropriate clinical setting (42). It is important to emphasize that rarely constrictive pericarditis can occur with normal pericardial thickness. An additional advantage of CT is its high sensitivity for detection of pericardial calcification, a finding highly suggestive of constrictive pericarditis (7).

Other morphologic characteristics that can be visualized in constrictive pericarditis are the presence of adhesions between visceral and parietal pericardium, a tube-like configuration of one or both ventricles, the enlargement of one or both atrium, and the enlargement of superior and inferior vena cavae (43).

text continues on page 148

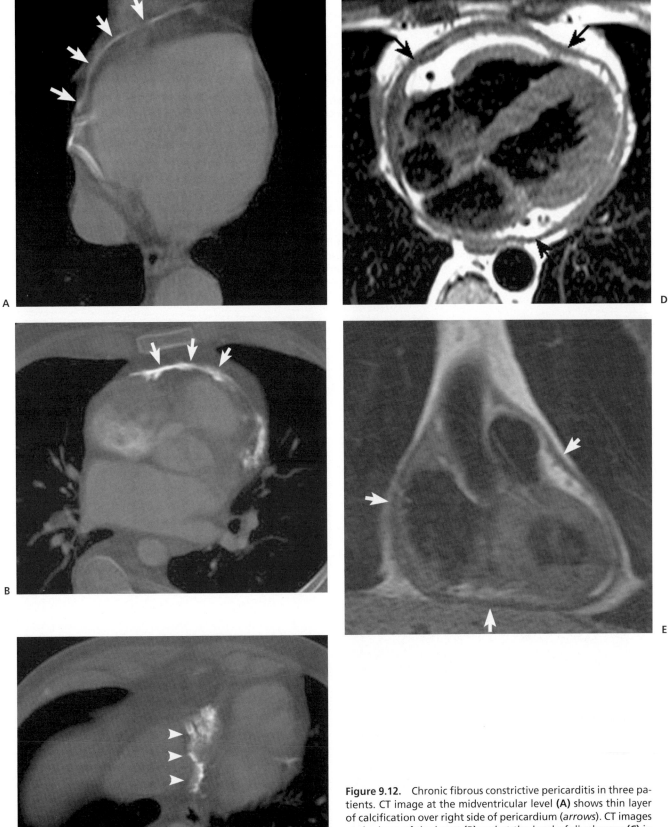

Figure 9.12. Chronic fibrous constrictive pericarditis in three patients. CT image at the midventricular level **(A)** shows thin layer of calcification over right side of pericardium (*arrows*). CT images at the base of the heart **(B)** and at the level of diaphragm **(C)** in another patient demonstrate thick and irregular calcifications in the anterior pericardial region (*arrows*) and the atrioventricular groove (*arrowheads*). Axial **(D)** and coronal **(E)** SE MR images in a third patient show diffuse thickening of the pericardium (*arrows*).

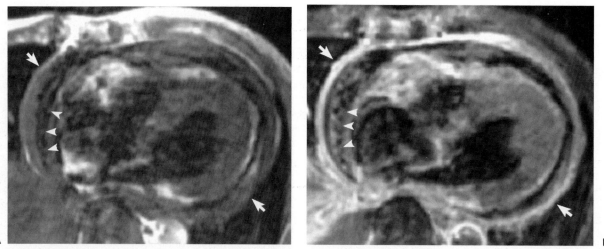

Figure 9.13. Adhesive constrictive pericarditis. Axial SE images at the midventricular level before **(A)** and after **(B)** administration of contrast media show a diffusely thick and irregular pericardium (*arrows*) and pericardial effusion with heterogeneous signal intensity. Note the presence of adhesions between the pericardial layers (*arrowheads*). After the administration of gadolinium chelate, there is enhancement of the pericardium and the adhesions in this patient with chronic pericardial tuberculosis.

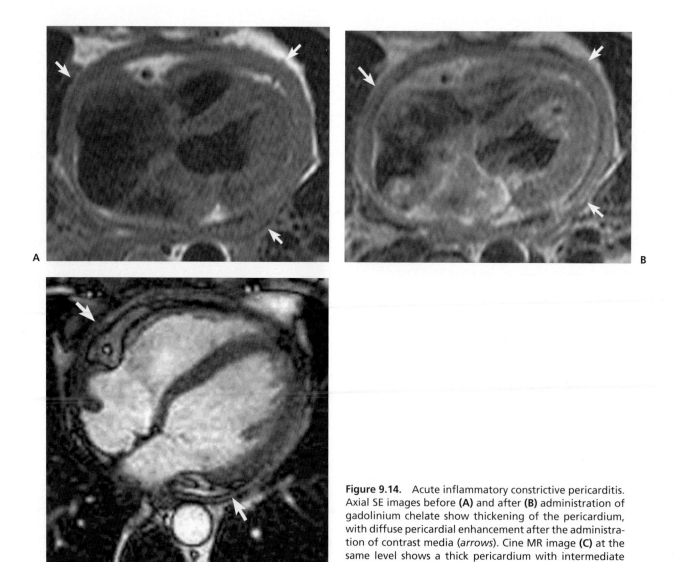

Figure 9.14. Acute inflammatory constrictive pericarditis. Axial SE images before **(A)** and after **(B)** administration of gadolinium chelate show thickening of the pericardium, with diffuse pericardial enhancement after the administration of contrast media (*arrows*). Cine MR image **(C)** at the same level shows a thick pericardium with intermediate signal intensity (*arrows*).

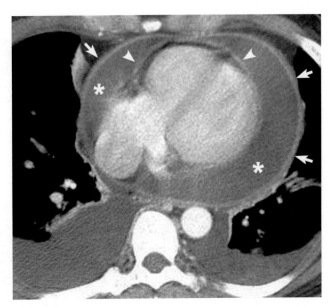

Figure 9.15. Effusive-constrictive pericarditis. Contrast-enhanced CT at the midventricular level shows thickening and enhancement of both the visceral (*arrowheads*) and parietal (*arrows*) pericardium associated with a large pericardial effusion (*asterisk*).

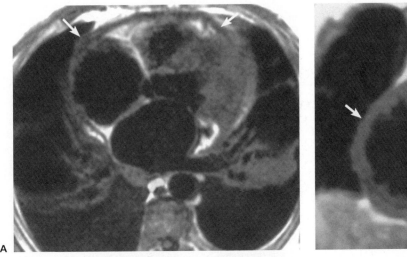

A

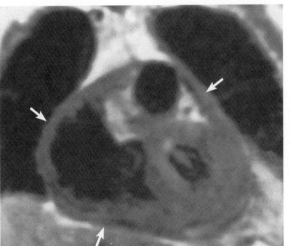

B

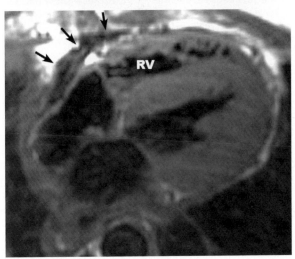

C

Figure 9.16. Different distributions of constrictive pericarditis. SE MR images in the axial **(A)** and coronal **(B)** planes demonstrate the global distribution of the pericardial thickening (*arrows*). Axial SE MR image at the midventricular level **(C)** shows thickening of the pericardium over the right atrium and right ventricle (*arrows*) (right-sided distribution). Note the tubular configuration of the right ventricle (RV).

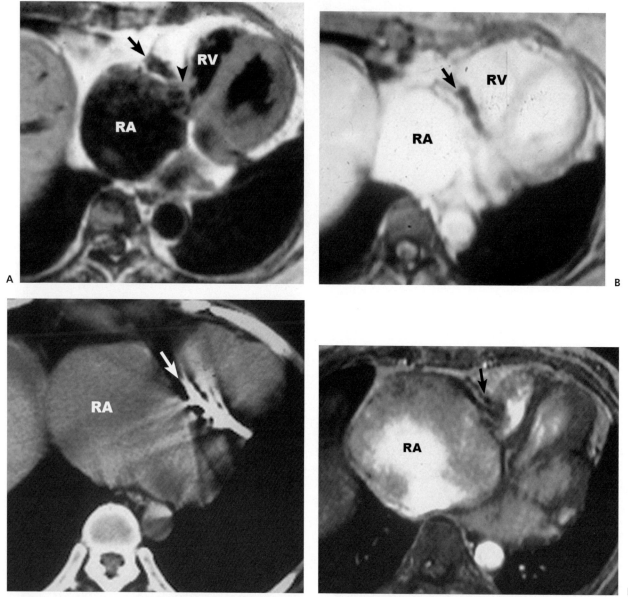

Figure 9.17. Focal constrictive pericarditis. Axial SE **(A)** and axial cine MR **(B)** images at the midventricular level show thickening of the pericardium at the atrioventricular groove (*arrow*). Note that the focal pericardial constriction compresses the tricuspid annulus (*arrowhead*). The right atrium (RA) is enlarged, whereas the right ventricle (RV) is small and has a tubular shape. Axial CT image **(C)** and axial cine MR image **(D)** of another patient demonstrate calcification localized at the atrioventricular groove (*arrow*) with narrowing of the tricuspid annulus and a very large right atrium (RA).

Cine MRI with high temporal resolution can depict abnormal ventricular septal motion toward the left ventricle in early diastole (Fig. 9.18) (44,45). Previously described on echocardiography, this finding is related to the characteristic increased ventricular interdependence present in constrictive pericarditis (46). This finding also has high sensitivity and specificity for the diagnosis of constrictive pericarditis when clinically interrogated (45).

ABSENCE OF PERICARDIUM

Pericardial defects are rare and usually asymptomatic congenital abnormalities. The defect is more commonly partial and on the left side, but can rarely present at the right side, at the diaphragmatic surface, or even be complete. CT and MRI can depict herniation of cardiac structure through the defect. Discontinuation of the pericardial line can occasionally be detected in the partial form. The most reliable signs of complete absence of the left pericardium is interposition of lung between the aorta and main pulmonary artery, in the aortopulmonary window, and a rotation of the cardiac axis to the left side (Fig. 9.19) (47,48). The usual presentation is in an asymptomatic person with an abnormal chest radiograph with a configuration of the chest suggestive of complete or partial absence of pericardium. A possible complication is bulging of the left atrial appendage and base of the heart through the defect (4). The edges of the defect can compress the left coronary artery when the base of the left

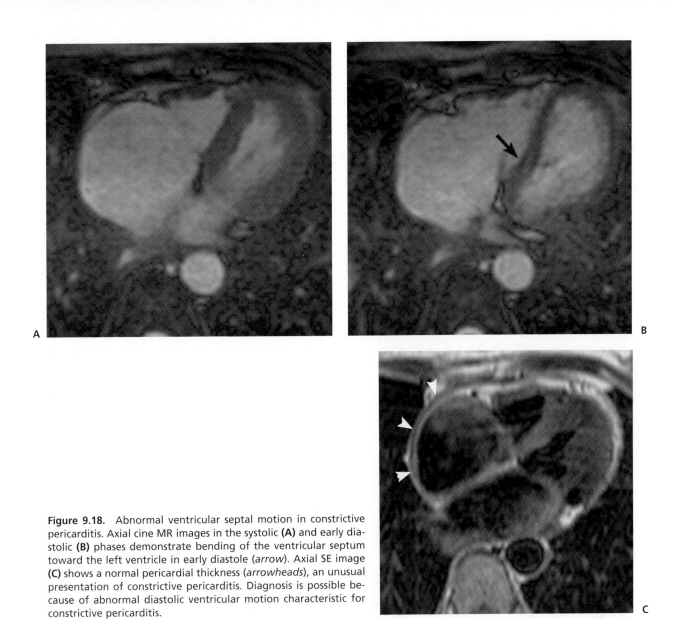

Figure 9.18. Abnormal ventricular septal motion in constrictive pericarditis. Axial cine MR images in the systolic **(A)** and early diastolic **(B)** phases demonstrate bending of the ventricular septum toward the left ventricle in early diastole (*arrow*). Axial SE image **(C)** shows a normal pericardial thickness (*arrowheads*), an unusual presentation of constrictive pericarditis. Diagnosis is possible because of abnormal diastolic ventricular motion characteristic for constrictive pericarditis.

Figure 9.19. Absence of pericardium. Axial SE images at the level of the great vessels **(A)** and ventricles **(B)**. There is interposition of the lung between the aortic knob and the main pulmonary artery (*arrow*) associated with a leftward shift of the heart. Ao, aorta; PA, pulmonary artery; RV, right ventricle; LV, left ventricle.

ventricle herniates through the partial defect causing chest pain, ventricular arrhythmias, or sudden death.

PERICARDIAL MASSES

PERICARDIAL CYST AND DIVERTICULUM

Congenital pericardial cysts are usually located at the right cardiophrenic angle and have smooth walls without internal septations. Typically, they do not communicate with the pericardial cavity. On CT imaging, they usually have the attenuation value of water. A high signal intensity on T2-weighted sequences and an intermediate to low intensity on T1-weighted sequences is the characteristic appearance on SE MRI (Fig. 9.20). However, occasionally a highly proteinaceous content causes a moderate to high signal intensity on T1-weighted images. A lack of contrast enhancement is seen in these lesions (Fig. 9.21) (49,50).

Pericardial diverticula are rare and consist of an outpouching of the pericardial sac. Distinction from a cyst, when possible, is based in the presence of a communication with the pericardial space, identified by changes in size related to body positioning (50,51).

PERICARDIAL TUMORS

Primary pericardial tumors are rare, with mesothelioma being the most frequent. Sarcoma, lipoma, hemangioma, dermoid, and teratoma can also occur in the pericardium (52).

Secondary tumors of the pericardium are far more common. These involve local invasion of lung and mediastinal malignancies and distal metastases. Lymphomas, melanomas, lung, and breast carcinomas are the most common primary tumors that involve the pericardium (Fig. 9.22) (25,40,53–55).

Most neoplasms have medium signal intensity on T1-weighted SE images and high signal intensity on T2-weighted SE images (4,56,57). Melanoma is an exception with characteristic high intensity on T1-weighted images (58,59).

Pericardial hemorrhagic effusion caused by a malignant primary or secondary tumor of the heart or pericardium can

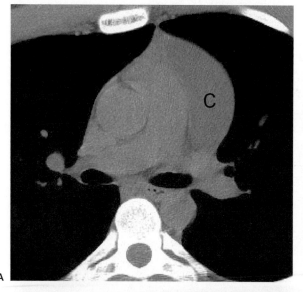

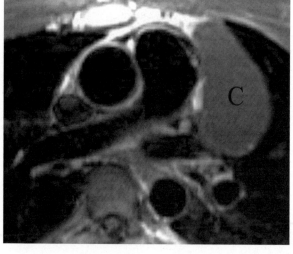

Figure 9.20. Pericardial cyst. CT image **(A)**, axial T1-weighted **(B)** and T2-weighted **(C)** SE images. Cystic mass *(C)* conforms to the contour of the heart and main pulmonary artery. The cyst has water density on CT, homogeneous low to intermediate signal intensity on the T1-weighted images, and homogeneous high signal intensity on the T2-weighted images.

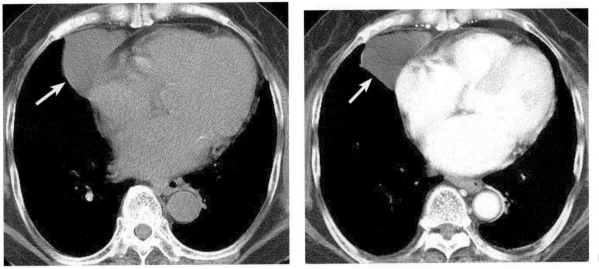

Figure 9.21. Pericardial cyst. CT images before **(A)** and after **(B)** the administration of contrast media show a homogeneous mass at the right cardiophrenic angle with water attenuation (*arrow*). No enhancement is observed in the postcontrast image.

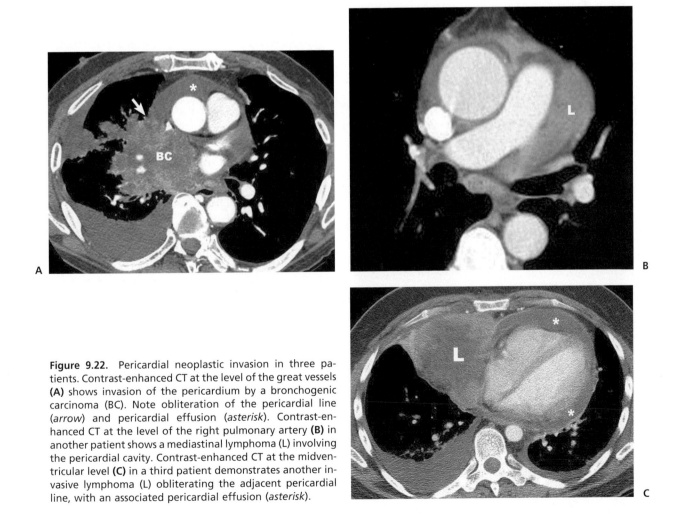

Figure 9.22. Pericardial neoplastic invasion in three patients. Contrast-enhanced CT at the level of the great vessels **(A)** shows invasion of the pericardium by a bronchogenic carcinoma (BC). Note obliteration of the pericardial line (*arrow*) and pericardial effusion (*asterisk*). Contrast-enhanced CT at the level of the right pulmonary artery **(B)** in another patient shows a mediastinal lymphoma (L) involving the pericardial cavity. Contrast-enhanced CT at the midventricular level **(C)** in a third patient demonstrates another invasive lymphoma (L) obliterating the adjacent pericardial line, with an associated pericardial effusion (*asterisk*).

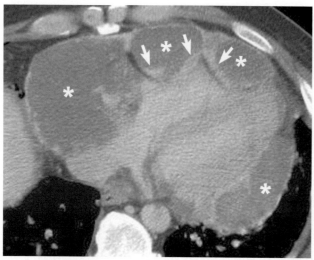 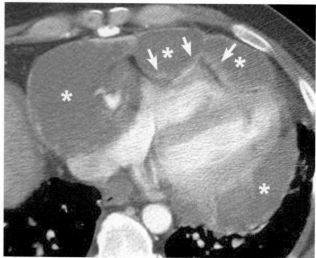

Figure 9.23. Pericardial metastases. CT images before **(A)** and after **(B)** administration of contrast media show a loculated pericardial effusion (*asterisks*). There are enhancing pericardial nodules on the visceral pericardium (*arrows*).

be recognized by MRI and CT. A hemorrhagic effusion should raise suspicion for tumor involvement of the pericardium. Pericardial metastases can also be recognized as enhancing nodules or masses on the visceral or parietal pericardium after administration of contrast media (Fig. 9.23) (4).

The characteristic signal intensity of masses such as cyst, lipoma, hemangioma, and melanoma metastases allows a high probability of a correct histologic diagnosis based on MRI. However, detection, evaluation of the tumor extension, and differentiation between benign and malignant appearance are the most important roles of cross-sectional imaging in this setting. Nevertheless, definitive differentiation between benign and malignant tumors is frequently not possible (60).

REFERENCES

1. Engel PJ. Echocardiographic findings in pericardial disease. In: Fowler NO, ed. *The pericardium in health and disease.* Armonk, NY: Futura; 1985:99.
2. Yousem D, Traill TT, Wheeler PS, et al. Illustrative cases in pericardial effusion misdetection: correlation of echocardiography and CT. *Cardiovasc Intervent Radiol* 1987;10:162.
3. Mulvagh SL, Rokey R, Vick GWD, et al. Usefulness of nuclear magnetic resonance imaging for evaluation of pericardial effusions, and comparison with two-dimensional echocardiography. *Am J Cardiol* 1989;64:1002.
4. Wang ZF, Reddy GP, Gotway MB, et al. CT and MR imaging of pericardial disease. *Radiographics* 2003;23:S167.
5. Silverman PM, Harell GS. Computed tomography of the normal pericardium. *Invest Radiol* 1983;18:141.
6. White CS. MR evaluation of the pericardium. *Top Magn Reson Imaging* 1995;7:258.
7. Isner JM, Carter BL, Bankoff MS, et al. Computed tomography in the diagnosis of pericardial heart disease. *Ann Intern Med* 1982;97:473.
8. Tomoda H, Hoshiai M, Furuya H, et al. Evaluation of pericardial effusion with computed tomography. *Am Heart J* 1980; 99:701.
9. Sechtem U, Tscholakoff D, Higgins CB. MRI of the normal pericardium. *AJR Am J Roentgenol* 1986;147:239.
10. Pope CF, Gore JC, Sostman D, et al. The apparent pericardium on cardiac NMR images. *Circulation* 1985;72(Suppl III):124.
11. Smith WHT, Beacock DJ, Goddard AJP, et al. Magnetic resonance evaluation of the pericardium. *Br J Radiol* 2001;74:384.
12. Frank H, Globits S. Magnetic resonance imaging evaluation of myocardial and pericardial disease. *J Mag Reson Imaging* 1999;10:617.
13. Sechtem U, Tscholakoff D, Higgins CB. MRI of the abnormal pericardium. *AJR Am J Roentgenol* 1986;147:245.
14. Stark DD, Higgins CB, Lanzer P, et al. Magnetic resonance imaging of the pericardium: normal and pathologic findings. *Radiology* 1984;150:469.
15. Breen JF. Imaging of the pericardium. *J Thorac Imaging* 2001; 16:47.
16. Weiger M, Pruessmann KP, Boesinger P. Cardiac real-time imaging using SENSE. *Magn Reson Med* 2000;43:177.
17. Edwards ED. Applied anatomy of the heart. In: Giuliani ER, Fuster V, eds. *Cardiology: fundamentals and practice.* 2nd ed. St Louis Mo: Mosby-Year Books; 1991:47.
18. Bull RK, Edwards PD, Dixon AK. CT dimensions of the normal pericardium. *Br J Radiol* 1998;71:923.
19. Vesely TM, Cahill DR. Cross-sectional anatomy of the pericardial sinuses, recesses, and adjacent structures. *Surg Radiol Anat* 1986;8:221.
20. Im JG, Rosen A, Webb WR, et al. MR imaging of the transverse sinus of the pericardium. *AJR Am J Roentgenol* 1988; 150:79.
21. McMurdo KK, Webb WR, von Schulthess GK, et al. Magnetic resonance imaging of the superior pericardial recesses. *AJR Am J Roentgenol* 1985;145:985.
22. Black CM, Hedges LK, Javitt MC. The superior pericardial sinus: normal appearance on gradient-echo MR images. *AJR Am J Roentgenol* 1993;160:749.
23. Solomon SL, Brown JJ, Glazer HS, et al. Thoracic aortic dissection: pitfalls and artifacts in MR imaging. *Radiology* 1990; 177:223.
24. Batra P, Bigoni B, Manning J, et al. Pitfalls in the diagnosis of thoracic aortic dissection at CT angiography. *RadioGraphics* 2000;20:309.
25. Chiles C, Baker ME, Silverman PM. Superior pericardial recess simulating aortic dissection on computed tomography. *J Comput Assist Tomogr* 1986;10:421.

26. Groell R, Schaffler GJ, Rienmueller R. Pericardial sinuses and recesses: findings at electrocardiographically triggered electron-beam CT. *Radiology* 1999;212:69.

27. Truong MT, Erasmus JJ, Gladish GW, et al. Anatomy of pericardial recesses on multidetector CT: implications for oncologic imaging. *AJR Am J Roentgenol* 2003;181:1109.

28. Shin MS, Jolles PR, Ho KJ. CT evaluation of distended pericardial recess presenting as a mediastinal mass. *J Comput Assist Tomogr* 1986;10:860.

29. Spodick DH. Pericardial diseases. In: Braunwald E, Zipes DP, Libby P, eds. *Heart disease: a textbook of cardiovascular medicine.* 6th ed. Philadelphia: WB Saunders; 2001:1823.

30. Axel L. Assessment of pericardial disease by magnetic resonance and computed tomography. *J Magn Reson Imaging* 2004;19:816.

31. Seelos KC, Funari M, Chang JM, et al. Magnetic resonance imaging in acute and subacute mediastinal bleeding. *Am Heart J* 1992;123:1269.

32. Vilacosta I, Gomez J, Dominguez J, et al. Massive pericardiac hematoma with severe constrictive pathophysiologic complications after insertion of an epicardial pacemaker. *Am Heart J* 1995;130:1298.

33. Brown DL, Ivey TD. Giant organized pericardial hematoma producing constrictive pericarditis: a case report and review of the literature. *J Trauma* 1996;41:558.

34. Ferguson ER, Blackwell GG, Murrah CP, et al. Evaluation of complex mediastinal masses by magnetic resonance imaging. *J Cardiovasc Surg* (Torino) 1998;39:117.

35. Troughton RW, Asher CR, Klein AL. Pericarditis. *Lancet* 2004;363:717.

36. Rienmuller R, Groll R, Lipton MJ. CT and MRI imaging of pericardial disease. *Radiol Clin N Am* 2004;42:587.

37. Kovanlikaya A, Burke LP, Nelson MD, Wood J. Characterizing chronic pericarditis using steady-state free-precession cine MR imaging. *AJR Am J Roentgenol* 2002;179:475.

38. Fowler NO. Constrictive pericarditis: its history and current status. *Clin Cardiol* 1995;18:341.

39. Myers RBH, Spodick DH. Constrictive pericarditis: clinical and pathophysiologic characteristics. *Am Heart J* 1999;138:219.

40. Hancock EW. Differential diagnosis of restrictive cardiomyopathy and constrictive pericarditis. *Heart* 2001;86:343.

41. Nishimura RA. Constrictive pericarditis in the modern era: a diagnostic dilemma. *Heart* 2001;86:619.

42. Masui T, Finck S, Higgins CB. Constrictive pericarditis and restrictive cardiomyopathy: evaluation with MR imaging. *Radiology* 1992;182:369.

43. Higgins CB. Acquired heart disease. In: Higgins CB, Hricak H, Helms CA, ed. *Magnetic resonance imaging of the body.* Philadelphia, PA: Lippincott-Raven; 1997:409.

44. Giorgi B, Mollet NRA, Dymarkowski S, et al. Clinically suspected constrictive pericarditis: MR imaging assessment of ventricular septal motion and configuration in patients and healthy subjects. *Radiology* 2003;228:417.

45. Ordovás KG, Reddy GP, Sharp MJ, et al. MRI evaluation of ventricular septal motion abnormality (septal bounce): differentiation of constrictive pericarditis from restrictive cardiomyopathy. *Radiology* 2004;233(P): 668.

46. Himelman RB, Lee E, Schiller NB. Septal bounce, vena cava plethora, and pericardial adhesion: informative two-dimensional echocardiographic signs in the diagnosis of pericardial constriction. *J Am Soc Echo* 1988;1:333.

47. Letanche G, Gayer C, Souquet PJ, et al. Agenesis of the pericardium: clinical echocardiographic and MRI aspects. *Rev Pneumol Clin* 1988;44:105.

48. Gutierrez FR, Shackelford GD, McKnight RC, et al. Diagnosis of congenital absence of left pericardium by MR imaging. *J Comput Assist Tomogr* 1985;9:551.

49. Vinée P, Strover B, Sigmund G, et al. MRI of the paracardial cyst. *J Magn Reson Imaging* 1992;2:593.

50. Higgins CB. Pericardial cysts and diverticula. In: Higgins CB, ed. *CT of the heart and the great vessels.* Mount Kisco, New York: Futura Publishing; 1983:296.

51. Jeung MY, Gasser B, Gangi A, et al. Imaging of cystic masses of the mediastinum. *Radiographics* 2002;22:S79.

52. Grebenc ML, Rosado de Christenson ML, Burke AP, et al. Primary cardiac and pericardial neoplasms: radiologic-pathologic correlation. *Radiographics* 2000;20:1073.

53. Abraham KP, Reddy V, Gattuso P. Neoplasms metastatic to the heart: review of 3314 consecutive autopsies. *Am J Cardiovasc Pathol* 1990;3:195.

54. Klatt EC, Heitz DR. Cardiac metastases. *Cancer* 1990;65: 1456.

55. Schoen FJ, Berger BM, Guerina NG. Cardiac effects of noncardiac neoplasms. *Cardiol Clin* 1984;2:657.

56. Hanock EW. Pericardial disease in patients with neoplasm. In: Reddy PS, Leon DF, Shaver JA, eds. *Pericardial disease.* New York: Raven Press; 1982:325.

57. Hoffmann U, Globits S, Frank H. Cardiac and paracardiac masses: current opinion on diagnostic evaluation by magnetic resonance imaging. *Eur Heart J* 1998;19:553.

58. Enochs WS, Petherick P, Bogdanova A, et al. Paramagnetic metal scavenging by melanin: MR imaging. *Radiology* 1997; 204:417.

59. Mousseaux E, Meunier P, Azancott S, et al. Cardiac metastatic melanoma investigated by magnetic resonance imaging. *Magn Reson Imaging* 1998;16:91.

60. Higgins CB, Krombach G. Cardiac and paracardiac masses. In: Webb WR, Higgins CB, eds. *Thoracic imaging.* Philadelphia, PA: Lippincott-Raven; 2004:735.

10

Arrhythmogenic Right Ventricular Cardiomyopathy

Peter T. Buser, Dagmar I. Keller, and Jens Bremerich

CLINICAL BACKGROUND

Arrhythmogenic right ventricular cardiomyopathy (ARVC) is an inheritable disease characterized by fibrofatty infiltration of the right ventricular myocardium with ventricular arrhythmias and sudden death (1,2). It has been reported to account for 3% to 10% of unexplained sudden cardiac death in patients less than 65 years old (3,4). Patients with ARVC are therefore candidates for an active therapeutic management, including antiarrhythmic medication, invasive electrophysiologic procedures, and implantation of a cardioverter-defibrillator (5).

It is a rare disorder, but it is the most common cause of sudden cardiac death in younger populations. The major pathologic findings are replacement of the myocardium by fatty and fibrous tissue and numerous structural abnormalities of the right ventricle including areas of wall thinning with single or multiple aneurysms or formation of diverticula. Current opinion indicates that this replacement process is caused by one of three mechanisms: apoptosis, inflammatory myocardial disease, or genetically determined myocardial dystrophy. Four stages of the disease have been proposed: (a) a concealed phase, in which anatomic changes are subtle and arrhythmias may be minor, but in which sudden cardiac death may be the first indication of the disease; (b) an overt electrical disorder presenting with ventricular tachycardias or sudden cardiac death, in which structural and functional abnormalities of the right ventricle are more apparent; (c) progressive right ventricular failure with preserved left ventricular function; and (d) biventricular dysfunction (6).

ARVC is a progressive disease and may be familial in 30% to 50% of cases with both autosomal dominant and recessive patterns. ARVC presents with a wide spectrum of clinical manifestations ranging from symptomatic patients with ventricular tachycardias, syncope, sudden cardiac death, or heart failure to asymptomatic relatives of patients with ARVC. A wide range of prognoses has been suggested including long-term favorable outcome and adverse events such as sudden cardiac death or severe heart failure. It is therefore mandatory to correctly diagnose this disease to indicate the necessary treatment and to make decisions for familial screening examinations.

The diagnosis of ARVC is based on the identification of structural abnormalities, fatty replacement of right ventricular myocardium, electrocardiographic changes, arrhythmias of right ventricular origin, and history of familial disease. Because the diagnosis of ARVC is difficult to make with certainty and in view of the fact that the only accepted gold standard for this diagnosis is autopsy proof of specific morphologic and histologic alterations of the right ventricular myocardium, a Task Force has proposed diagnostic criteria (7). Individual criteria were listed as major or minor, and combinations of these were judged to indicate the presence of the disease. Among the major criteria, severe or marked structural abnormalities of the right ventricle and fibrofatty replacement of the myocardium on endomyocardial biopsy were included. Therefore, identification of structural and functional abnormalities of the right ventricular myocardium and replacement of right ventricular myocardium by fatty and fibrous tissue remain a cornerstone for the diagnosis of ARVC, which preferably should be made by noninvasive means. Cardiac magnetic resonance (CMR) has the unique advantage to be an absolutely noninvasive technique, providing information on dimensions, geometry, shape, volumes, and function of all cardiac chambers, tissue characterization such as differentiation of fat from myocardium, and identification of fibrous formations such as myocardial scar. CMR, therefore, has been increasingly used for the evaluation of right ventricular disease and has evolved as the noninvasive imaging modality of choice in ARVC.

CARDIAC MAGNETIC RESONANCE TECHNIQUES

There is no widely accepted standard imaging protocol for the investigation of patients with suspected ARVC using CMR. The CMR imaging protocol is aimed at recognizing three major aspects of ARVC: (a) global and regional morphology of the right ventricle; (b) global and regional function of the right and left ventricle; and (c) infiltration of the myocardium with fibrous and fatty tissue. The right ventricle has a complex geometry, is asymmetric, and is highly trabeculated. The mean right ventricular free wall thickness in healthy individuals is only 2.7 ± 0.4 mm and only 1.9 ± 1.1 mm at the right ventricular apex (7). Epicardial fat is usually present, especially in association with the right coronary artery within the right atrioventricular groove and with the left anterior descending coronary artery in the apical region. Tongues of epicardial fat may extend into the myocardium in healthy individuals (8,9). The identification of small morphologic alterations of the thin right ventricular free wall, the analysis of regional wall-motion abnormalities of a complex geometric structure, and the identification of intramural or transmural fatty infiltrates of the right ventricular myocardium require high-resolution images without significant arti-

facts. Retrospective analysis of static magnetic resonance (MR) images of 39 patients from a ARVC registry revealed an excellent image quality in less than 10% of cases (10). Thus, basic requirements for equipment, software, imaging protocol, readout, and documentation should be fulfilled for the CMR investigation of patients with suspected ARVC. A cardiac phased array coil is preferred, and gradient coil strength should minimally be 20 mT/m. Cardiac gating and breath-hold imaging are required (11). Black-blood imaging is used to depict morphologic abnormalities of the right ventricle and intramyocardial fatty infiltration. Additional application of fat saturation sequences can improve identification of fatty tissue and therefore interobserver variability for bright T1 signals within the myocardium of the free right ventricular wall (12). Bright-blood cine imaging is used for visualizing global and regional ventricular function and to measure end-diastolic and end-systolic volumes for calculation of stroke volume and ejection fraction. In addition, significant valvular disease can be demonstrated or excluded. Diastolic dysfunction of the right ventricle can be assessed by measurement of blood-flow velocities across the tricuspid valve during the whole cardiac cycle by application of MR velocity mapping (13).

BLACK-BLOOD IMAGING

For black-blood techniques, breath-hold imaging with double-inversion recovery fast spin-echo (DIR-FSE) techniques is preferred to traditional spin-echo (SE) imaging. These techniques substantially shorten imaging time and virtually eliminate respiratory motion artifacts. Black-blood inversion prepared, half Fourier single-shot turbo spin-echo (HASTE) imaging currently is not recommended because of blurring of subtle anatomic details. Frequent ventricular ectopy can substantially deteriorate image quality. In patients with suspected ARVC and frequent ventricular ectopy, a low dose of oral beta-blocker (e.g., 50 mg metoprolol) can be given 1 hour before the CMR examination to reduce ventricular ectopy. However, contraindications for beta-blockade must be considered.

Right ventricular morphology is best shown in axial and sagittal imaging planes. Axial imaging planes should encompass the whole heart starting from the pulmonary artery to the diaphragm. Axial imaging planes provide the best view of the right ventricular anterior wall up to the proximal parts of the right ventricular outflow tract. Because the anatomic course of the right ventricular outflow tract toward the pulmonary valve and the common pulmonary artery progresses from ventral to dorsal, axial planes will not be optimal for the assessment of dimensions and morphology of the subpulmonary part of the right ventricular outflow tract. Sagittal planes through the right ventricular outflow tract will depict this portion optimally. This is especially important when high signal intensity areas can be detected within the myocardium, which are suspicious for fatty infiltrates. It has been shown that intramyocardial fat detection is superior with application of fast SE imaging alone and combined with fat suppression than with gated SE imaging (14).

BRIGHT-BLOOD IMAGING

For bright-blood imaging, steady state free precession imaging (FIESTA, true FISP, balanced fast field echo) is the preferred technique because it allows better endocardial definition when compared with fast gradient-echo imaging. Alternatively, segmental k-space cine gradient-echo images (FLASH, FAST-CARD) can be used. Cine imaging in the axial plane is optimal to assess right ventricular global and regional function. Again, the whole heart is covered from the pulmonary artery to the diaphragm. Contraction abnormalities of the right ventricular outflow tract, areas of wall thinning and reduced contraction, aneurysm formation, regions of focal hypokinesia, and akinesia or dyskinesia of the right ventricular free wall can be best depicted in axial imaging planes. However, at least one additional imaging plane should be used to assess function of the diaphragmatic right ventricular wall segments, function of the right ventricular outflow tract, and left ventricular volumes and function. In sagittal imaging planes, the right ventricular outflow tract is usually well depicted along its long axis as well as diaphragmatic segments of the right ventricular wall. To assess, in addition, left ventricular regional and global function accurately and to measure right ventricular and left ventricular volumes, proper left ventricular short-axis planes encompassing the whole left ventricle from above the atrioventricular plane to the apex should be used. Quantification of ventricular volumes is performed by contouring the end-diastolic and end-systolic frames of the entire right ventricle and left ventricle, using a summation of disks method (Simpson's rule) with integration over the image slices. For further evaluation of left ventricular abnormalities, especially in the anterior and apical segments, two-chamber and/or four-chamber long-axis imaging planes should be added.

INTERPRETATION OF CARDIAC MAGNETIC RESONANCE FINDINGS

INTRAMYOCARDIAL FAT

On black-blood images normal myocardium shows an intermediate signal similar to that of skeletal muscle. Fat appears as a bright signal. In healthy individuals, epicardial fat is usually seen in the atrioventricular groove and around the right ventricular apex. However, distribution of epicardial fat varies considerably in healthy individuals and may cover the whole aspect of the right ventricular free wall as a thick bright tissue layer. There is often a clear demarcation line between the myocardium and the epicardial fat. Disruption of this demarcation line and extension of the bright signals into the myocardium are frequently seen (Fig. 10.1). This is not a specific sign of ARVC, and it can also be observed in healthy individuals (9,15). It is important to realize that findings of increased intramyocardial fat signals on CMR are not part of the Task Force criteria for the diagnosis of ARVC and that experts in the field do not recommend equating intramyocardial fat signal on CMR with fatty infiltration found on endomyocardial biopsy. On the other hand, there

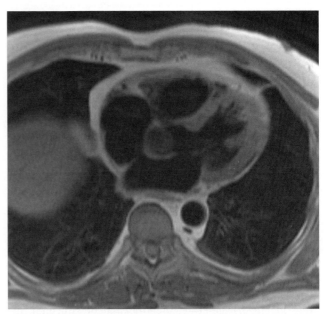

Figure 10.1. T1-weighted turbo spin-echo (SE) image in an axial plane of a patient without clinical suspicion of arrhythmogenic right ventricular cardiomyopathy (ARVC). Thick layer of epicardial fat that partially infiltrates into the myocardium in the right ventricular (RV) apical region.

is currently no gold standard that can be used to definitely diagnose or exclude ARVC, and the Task Force criteria have so far not been validated.

Hyperintense intramyocardial signals on T1-weighted images have been described in 20% to 100% of patients with ARVC (10,11,16–20). Auffermann et al (17) investigated 36 patients with biopsy-proven ARVC and found intramyocardial hyperintense signals on T1-weighted SE images in 22%. In this study, fatty infiltration on CMR, but not on endomyocardial biopsy, predicted the inducibility of ventricular tachycardias on electrophysiologic testing. In 8 of 15 patients with the clinical diagnosis of ARVC, Ricci et al (16) found myocardial areas with hyperintense signals in anatomic sites of the right ventricle usually affected by the disease. In addition, in seven of these eight patients these areas showed an overlap with a-dyskinetic areas assessed with gradient-echo cine MR or echocardiography. In the explanted heart of one patient undergoing heart transplantation, an excellent correlation between the localizations of the fatty infiltrates described in CMR and histologic examination was found. Molinari et al (18) investigated 124 patients with ventricular arrhythmias and left bundle branch block (LBBB) morphology and 38 control subjects with one of three different MR scanners. In one system, fat-suppression techniques were applied for identification of intramyocardial fat. In this retrospective study with three different MR systems and patients with a wide range of LBBB ventricular tachycardias, an increased rate of myocardial replacement by adipose tissue was found with increasing complexity of arrhythmias. Intramyocardial hyperintense signals were also described in the left ventricular myocardium in 5% of the subjects with sustained ventricular tachycardias and polymorphic premature beats. Menghetti et al (19) described findings with SE imaging in 15 patients with ARVC accord-

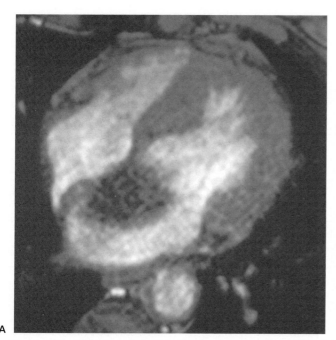

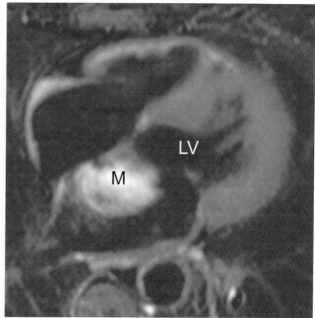

A   B

Figure 11.3. Myxoma of the LA. Cine magnetic resonance (MR) image **(A)** and T1-weighted SE image after the administration of contrast medium. Myxoma (M) is attached by a narrow pedicle to the atrial septum. LV, left ventricle.

must raise the suspicion of such a process. The extent of attachment may be difficult to assess for large tumors, which nearly fill the entire cavity, so that they are compressed against the septum. As a result, the tumor appears to have broad contact with the atrial septum on static MR images. Myxomas can grow through a patent foramen ovale and extend into both atria, a condition that has been described as a "dumbbell" appearance (19). Cine MRI permits an evaluation of tumor motion and may help to identify the site and length of attachment of the tumor to the wall(s) of cardiac chamber(s) (20). With this technique, myxomas have been demonstrated to prolapse into the corresponding ventricle during diastole (21).

Usually, myxomas display an intermediate signal intensity (isointense to the myocardium) on T1-weighted SE images (22–24). On T2-weighted SE images, myxomas usually have a higher signal intensity than myocardium. However, myxomas with lower signal intensity have also been observed (25). This variable appearance is the consequence of a variable content of water-rich myxomatous stroma in comparison with the components that have a short T2 relaxation time. Fibrous stroma, calcification, and deposition of paramagnetic iron after interstitial hemorrhage can reduce the signal intensity of the tumor on T2-weighted SE images (26,27). Rarely, myxomas have been reported to be invisible on SE images because of a lack of contrast with the dark blood pool (25). Such tumors can be delineated with cine MRI, on which they appear with high contrast against the surrounding bright blood (Fig. 11.4). Most myxomas show increased signal intensity after administration of Gd-DTPA on T1-weighted images, which is most probably secondary to an increased interstitial space and therefore larger distribution volume of the contrast agent within the tumor than in normal tissue.

LIPOMA AND LIPOMATOUS HYPERTROPHY OF THE ATRIAL SEPTUM

Lipomas are reported to be the second most common benign cardiac tumor in adults but may actually be the most common. They may occur at any age but are encountered most frequently in middle-aged and elderly adults. Lipomas consist of encapsulated mature adipose cells and fetal fat cells. The tumor consistence is soft, and lipomas may grow to a large size without causing symptoms. Large atrial lipomas or intramural lipomas have been reported to cause atrial or ventricular arrhythmia (28). Lipomas are typically located in the RA (Figs. 11.5 and 11.6) or atrial septum (29). They arise from the endocardial surface and have a broad base of attachment. Lipomas have the same signal intensity as subcutaneous and epicardial fat on all MRI sequences. Because fat has a short T1 relaxation time, lipomas have high signal intensity on T1-weighted images, which can be suppressed with fat-saturating pulse sequences (Fig. 11.7). Usually, they appear with homogeneous signal intensity but may have a few thin septations. They do not enhance after the administration of contrast material (30). On T2-weighted images, lipomas have intermediate signal intensity. On cine images, acquired with a balanced steady state free precession sequence, and lipomas have margins with low signal intensity. It has been proposed that this appearance results from intravoxel phase cancellation effects from blood and fat (31).

Lipomas are considered to be distinct from lipomatous hypertrophy of the atrial septum. Lipomatous hypertrophy of the atrial septum is more common and may have clinical significance, because this lesion can be a cause of supraventricular arrhythmias. It is usually associated with older age, but not with obesity. Lipomatous hypertrophy is defined as a deposition of fat, in the atrial septum around the fossa

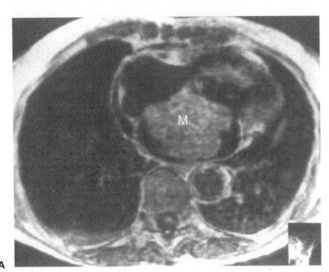

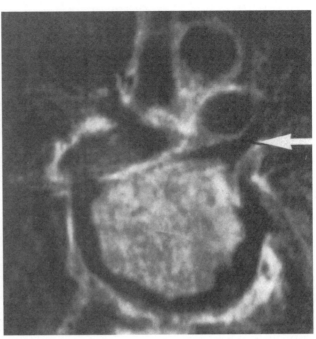

A   B

Figure 11.4. Left atrial myxoma. Transaxial **(A)** and coronal **(B)** T1-weighted SE images demonstrate the large mass (M) arising from the atrial septum. Tumor shows a broad base of attachment to the atrial septum. Nearly the entire LA is filled by the tumor. Pericardial effusion is present. Pulmonary vein (*arrow*). (Courtesy of A. Lomonoco, M.D., Tucson, Arizona.)

ovalis, that exceeds 2 cm in transverse diameter (32). It spares the fossa ovalis, a characteristic feature that is clearly delineated with T1-weighted SE images. Lipomatous hypertrophy has the same cellular composition as lipoma but is not encapsulated and infiltrates into the tissue of the atrial septum. It is not a true neoplasm. Fatty tissue may extend from the septum into both atria to a considerable degree. Signal intensity on MRI is similar to that of lipomas (33,34). MRI is used for tissue characterization, delineation of extent of the fat, and evaluation of possible caval obstruction (35).

PAPILLARY FIBROELASTOMA

Papillary fibroelastoma constitutes approximately 10% of benign primary cardiac tumors (36), but up to 70% of primary cardiac valve tumors (37). Fibroelastomas usually present in the seventh decade of life. These tumors consist of avascular fronds of connective tissue lined by endothelium. Papillary fibroelastomas are attached to the valves by a short pedicle in approximately 90% of cases (Fig. 11.8). They usually do not exceed 1 cm in diameter. Papillary fibroelastomas have been

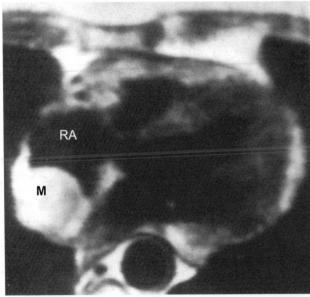

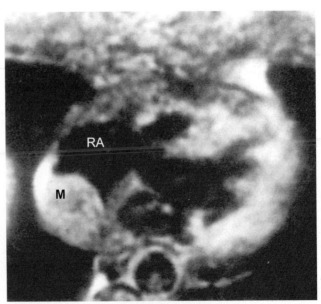

A   B

Figure 11.5. Lipoma. T1-weighted SE images without **(A)** and with **(B)** fat saturation show a mass (M) in the right atrium (RA). Tumor has a sharp border to the myocardium. There is decrease of signal intensity after application of fat saturation.

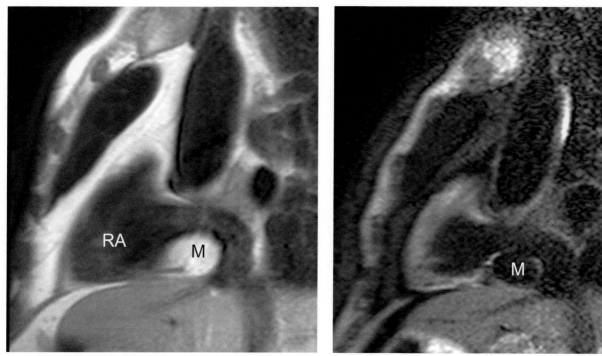

Figure 11.6. Lipoma. T1-weighted SE images without **(A)** and with **(B)** fat saturation show a mass (M) in the RA. Fat saturation nearly completely diminished the signal of the tumor. RA, right atrium.

found to occur on the aortic (29%), mitral (25%), pulmonary (13%), and tricuspid valves (17%) (38). Right-sided tumors usually remain asymptomatic. Symptoms associated with fibroelastoma typically relate to the embolization from thrombi, which accumulate on the tumor. Because of their high content of fibrous tissue, they have low signal intensity on T2-weighted images (39). The diagnosis of these valvular tumors is challenging because of their small size, low contrast relative to the blood pool on SE images, and location on the rapidly moving valves. However, with recent advances in fast MR sequences and improved homogeneity of the bright-blood pool signal, the visualization of valve motion during the cardiac cycle has become possible (40). Small masses at-

tached to valves have been accurately depicted with MRI (41). In many cases, such lesions can be assessed only with cine MRI. In these cases, signal intensity characteristics after the administration of Gd-DTPA cannot be evaluated, and the differential diagnosis between thrombus and tumor may not be feasible (42). Cine MRI can be used to assess the effect of valvular tumors on valve function; it demonstrates jet flow caused by either obstruction or regurgitation (42).

RHABDOMYOMA

In children, rhabdomyomas are the most common cardiac tumor, comprising 40% of all cardiac tumors in this age

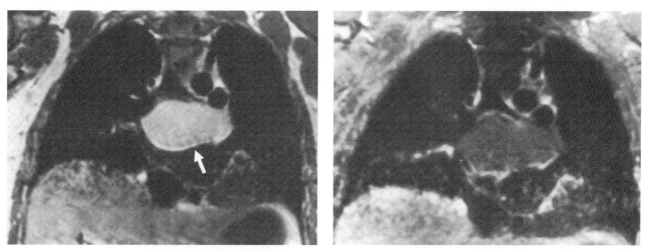

Figure 11.7. Paracardiac lipoma. Coronal T1-weighted SE images, without **(A)** and with **(B)** fat saturation. Mass is located above the LA and demonstrates sharp borders (*arrow*). The bright signal of the tumor is depleted by fat saturation.

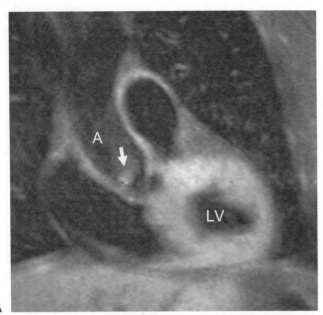
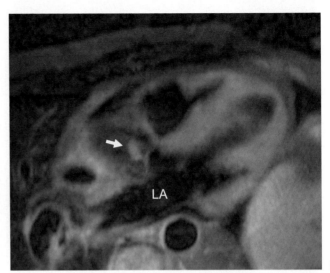

Figure 11.8. Fibroelastoma. Coronal **(A)** and parasagittal **(B,** three-chamber-view) T1-weighted SE images show a small mass (*arrows*) attached to the aortic valve. A, Aorta; LA, left atrium; LV, left ventricle. (Courtesy of Arno Bucker, M.D., Aachen, Germany.)

group. One third to one half of rhabdomyomas are found in patients with tuberous sclerosis. Rhabdomyomas may vary in size and are frequently multiple (Fig. 11.6). They are characterized by an intramural location and involve equally the left ventricle (LV) and right ventricle (RV). Small, entirely intramural tumors may be difficult to identify (43). Larger tumors distort the shape of the myocardial wall or may bulge into the cavity. Larger tumors can also distort the epicardial contour of the heart. Rhabdomyomas may have a signal intensity similar to that of normal myocardium on SE images, cine MRI, and contrast-enhanced T1-weighted SE images (20). They also have been reported to have a high signal intensity on T1-weighted SE images and may display hyperenhancement after the administration of contrast medium (44).

FIBROMA

Fibroma is the second most common benign cardiac tumor in children. It is a connective tissue tumor that is composed of fibroblasts interspersed among collagen fibers. It arises within the myocardial walls. Unlike most other primary cardiac tumors, fibromas usually do not display cystic changes, hemorrhage, or focal necrosis, but dystrophic calcification is common. Fibromas may cause arrhythmias and have been reported to be associated with sudden death (45). Approximately 30% of these tumors remain asymptomatic and may be discovered incidentally because of heart murmurs, electrocardiogram changes, or abnormalities on chest x-ray film. Fibromas occur most often within the septum or the anterior wall of the RV and can reach a large diameter. On T2-weighted MR images, they are characteristically hypointense to the surrounding myocardium, which is compatible with the short T2 relaxation time of fibrous tissue. On T1-weighted images, fibromas may appear isointense to the myocardium. Usually, fibromas show little or no contrast

enhancement after the administration of Gd-DTPA (46). However, Gd-DTPA has been effectively used to demarcate these intramural tumors more clearly from normal myocardium (Figs. 11.9 and 11.10) (9). Enhancement of normal myocardium has been shown to be as high as 42% ± 17% (19). Hyperenhancement of compressed myocardium at the margin of the tumor facilitates delineation of the borders of the nonenhancing tumor (19). On delayed inversion-recovery GE images at 10 to 15 min after Gd-DTPA, fibromas show hyperenhancement.

The differential diagnosis for intramural masses in children is rhabdomyoma. If the tumor is solitary and has low signal intensity on T2-weighted images, fibroma is more likely. If multiple tumors are present, especially in cases of tuberous sclerosis, rhabdomyoma can confidently be diagnosed (47,48).

PHEOCHROMOCYTOMAS

Pheochromocytomas arise from neuroendocrine cells clustered in the visceral paraganglia in the posterior wall of the LA, roof of the RA, atrial septum, and along the coronary arteries. Pheochromocytomas can be found at each of these locations but are predominantly encountered in and around the LA (Fig. 11.11). Most are paracardiac in location. They usually have a broad interface with the heart. Hypertension, the most common symptom, is related to catecholamine overproduction by the mass. The average age of the patient at diagnosis is 30 to 50 years (6). Although cases of metastatic spread of cardiac pheochromocytomas have rarely been reported, these tumors are usually benign (49). Pheochromocytomas are generally highly vascularized. The average size ranges from 3 to 8 cm at the time of diagnosis. Pheochromocytomas are hyperintense to the myocardium on T2-weighted images and isointense on T1-weighted images. After the administration of Gd-DTPA, they show strong sig-

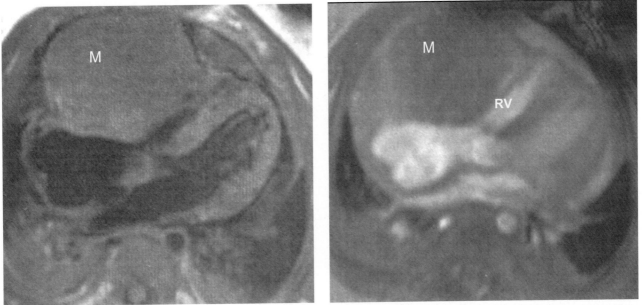

Figure 11.9. Fibroma of the right ventricle (RV). Axial T1-weighted SE **(A)** and cine MR **(B)** images show a large mass (M) centered in the right ventricular free wall, which narrows the RV. Mass demonstrates homogeneously intermediate signal intensity on the SE image and low signal intensity on the cine MR image.

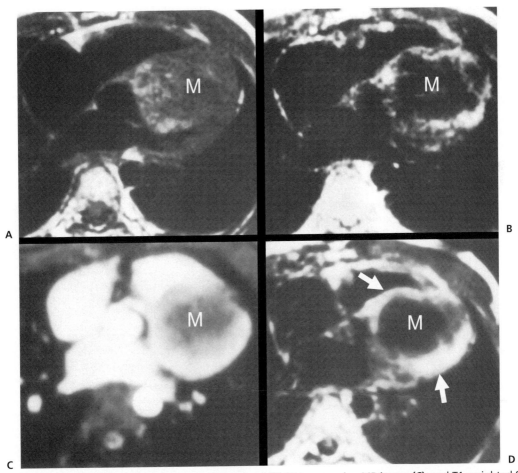

Figure 11.10. Fibroma of the LV. T1-weighted **(A)** and T2-weighted **(B)** SE images, cine MR image **(C)**, and T1-weighted SE image **(D)** after the administration of Gd-DTPA. SE images demonstrate the mass (M), arising from the ventricular septum. The mass has low signal intensity on the T2-weighted image. The mass projects into the bright-blood pool on the cine MR image. Contrast enhancement of the myocardium surrounding the mass is seen after the administration of Gd-DTPA (*arrows*). The mass does not show enhancement within the first few minutes after contrast administration.

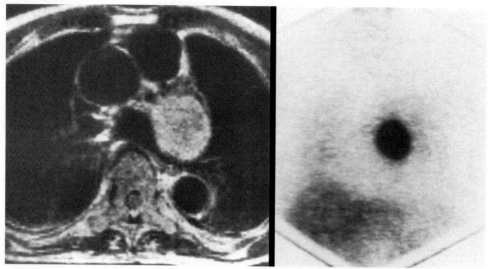

Figure 11.11. Pheochromocytoma. T1-weighted SE image **(A)** and metaiodobenzylguanidine scan **(B)**. A mass adjacent to the LA shows uptake of this radionuclide.

nal enhancement because of their high vascularity (50,51). Enhancement may be heterogeneous, with central non-enhancing areas related to tumor necrosis (52). The combination of imaging findings, clinical symptoms, and biochemical evidence of catecholamine overproduction usually permits a confident diagnosis.

HEMANGIOMA

Cardiac hemangiomas are composed of endothelial cells that line interconnecting vascular channels. These vascular cavities are separated by connective tissue. According to the size of the vascular channels, hemangiomas are divided into capillary, cavernous, or venous types. Calcification is often present in these tumors (53). Hemangiomas may involve the endocardium, myocardium, or epicardium. They have been found in all chambers and the pericardium (53). On T2-weighted images, hemangiomas are hyperintense. On T1-weighted images, they vary from hyperintense to intermediate signal intensity. Because of interspersed calcifications and possible flow voids at areas of blood flow in the channels of hemangiomas, they may have inhomogeneous signal intensity (54,55). They usually show intense enhancement after the administration of gadolinium contrast medium because of their rich vascularity (56).

MALIGNANT PRIMARY CARDIAC TUMORS

One fourth of primary cardiac tumors are malignant; sarcomas comprise the largest number, followed by mesotheliomas and lymphomas. The features of malignant cardiac tumors are the following: involvement of more than one cardiac chamber, extension into pulmonary veins or pulmonary arteries, wide point of attachment to the heart, necrosis

within the tumor, extension outside the heart, and hemorrhagic pericardial effusion. A combined intramural and intracavitary location is another feature of malignant tumors (Fig. 11.12). MRI is effective for demonstrating invasion of the pericardium and extension into the pericardial fat (Figs. 11.13 and 11.14). Pericardial infiltration is displayed on MRI as a disruption, thickening, or nodularity of the pericardium, often combined with pericardial effusion. Cardiac tamponade as a consequence of hemorrhagic pericardial effusion may be demonstrated (42).

Extension into the mediastinum and metastasis is also a clear sign of malignancy. The organs most frequently in-

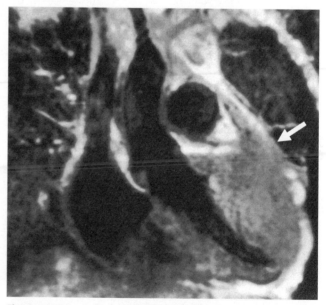

Figure 11.12. Left ventricular lymphosarcoma. Coronal T1-weighted SE image at the level of the LV show the mass arising from the left ventricular free wall. Mass invades the pericardium (*arrow*).

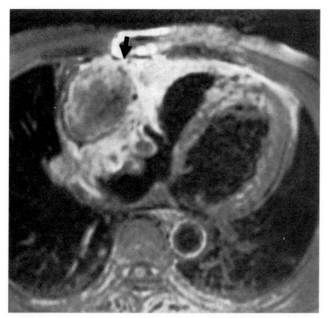

Figure 11.13. Right atrial angiosarcoma. Transaxial T1-weighted SE image after the administration of contrast medium demonstrates a mass that fills the RA and extends into the pericardium. Disruption of the pericardial fat (*arrow*).

volved are lungs, pleura, mediastinal lymph nodes, and liver. The inherent contrast between pericardium, which is delineated with a low signal intensity, and mediastinal fat, which has a high signal intensity, permits a clear delineation of mediastinal invasion (43).

The rapid growth of malignant cardiac tumors may cause focal necrosis in the central part of the tumor. Necrotic areas are delineated as regions of lower signal intensity, within a hyperenhancing mass after the administration of Gd-DTPA (Fig. 11.15).

ANGIOSARCOMA

Angiosarcomas are the most common malignant cardiac tumor in adults and constitute one third of malignant cardiac tumors. They occur predominately in men between 20 and 50 years of age. This entity has been divided into two clinicopathologic forms (57). Most frequently, angiosarcomas are found in the RA and usually arise from the atrial septum. In this form, no evidence of Kaposi sarcoma is found. Another form is characterized by evolvement of the epicardium and/or pericardium in the presence of Kaposi sarcoma. These lesions are usually small, localized, and asymptomatic. This form is associated with acquired immunodeficiency syndrome (58).

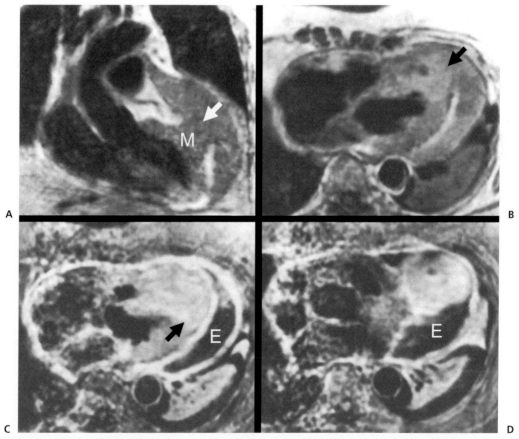

Figure 11.14. Angiosarcoma of the LV. T1-weighted SE images in the coronal **(A)** and transaxial planes **(B)** and transaxial images with fat saturation after administration of contrast medium at the base of the heart **(C)** and near the apex **(D)**. Before the administration of contrast material, the tumor (M) cannot readily be distinguished from the pericardial effusion, especially in regions where pericardial fat is absent (*arrows* in **A** and **B**). After the administration of Gd-DTPA, the tumor and pericardium demonstrate hyperenhancement. Effective differentiation from the surrounding normal myocardium (*arrows* in **C**) and from the pericardial effusion **(E)** is possible.

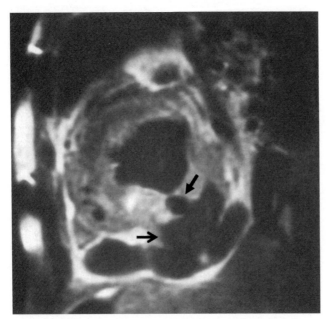

Figure 11.15.   Left ventricular rhabdomyosarcoma. Sagittal T1-weighted SE image after the administration of contrast medium demonstrates a mass with central necrosis (*arrow*). There is loculated pericardial effusion adjacent to the necrotic area (*arrow*).

Angiosarcomas usually grow within the myocardial wall. The myocardial infiltration by the tumor may trigger arrhythmia or cause conducting disorders (59). However, symptoms usually occur late, which impairs the therapeutic options (60). The tumor tissue is friable and characterized by a tendency of bleeding. Thus, they are often associated with pericardial effusion and cardiac tamponade. Myocardial rupture caused by tumor infiltration and necrosis of the wall has been observed in several cases (61). Prognosis of cardiac angiosarcoma is poor, and mean life expectancy after diagnosis is only several months (62).

Angiosarcomas consist of ill-defined anastomotic vascular spaces that are lined by endothelial cells and avascular

clusters of moderately pleomorphic spindle cells surrounded by collagen stroma. T1-weighted SE imaging usually demonstrates heterogeneous signal intensity of the tumor with focal areas of high signal intensity, which presumably represent hemorrhage (63). However, angiosarcomas can also have homogeneous signal intensity (Fig. 11.16). After the administration of contrast medium, angiosarcomas show hyperenhancement (Fig. 11.17). Some of the tumors show regions of low signal intensity on both T1- and T2-weighted images. These central regions have a high signal intensity on cine GE images and represent vascular channels. This finding is often described as a "cauliflower appearance" (64). Cases with diffuse pericardial infiltration have been found to show linear hyperenhancement along vascular spaces (65).

RHABDOMYOSARCOMA

Rhabdomyosarcomas are the most common malignant cardiac tumors in children. They can arise anywhere in the myocardium. Rhabdomyosarcomas are often multiple. Their signal intensity on MRI is variable. Rhabdomyosarcomas may be isointense to the myocardium on T1- and T2-weighted images, but areas of necrosis can exhibit heterogeneous signal intensity and patchy hyperenhancement after the administration of Gd-DTPA (Fig. 11.15) (43,66). Extracardiac extension into the pulmonary arteries and descending aorta has been clearly delineated with MRI (67).

OTHER SARCOMAS (FIBROSARCOMA, OSTEOSARCOMA, LEIOMYOSARCOMA, LIPOSARCOMA)

Other possible primary sarcomas are fibrosarcoma, osteosarcoma, leiomyosarcoma, and liposarcoma. These all are rare tumors, comprising approximately 4% of primary cardiac masses (12). Radical resection of cardiac sarcomas has been shown to increase median survival from approximately 12 to 16 months to approximately 38 months (68). Detailed

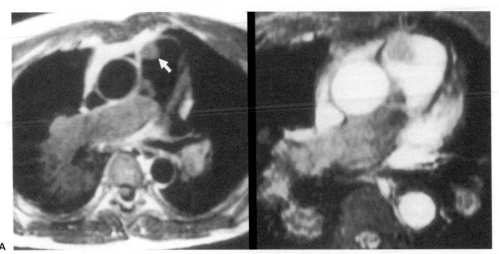

Figure 11.16.   Angiosarcoma of the pulmonary artery. T1-weighted SE **(A)** and cine MR **(B)** images at the level of the main and right pulmonary arteries. A mass fills the right pulmonary artery. A tumor nodule is attached to the wall of the main pulmonary artery (*arrow*). Mass shows intermediate signal intensity on the cine MR image, which indicates tumor rather than subacute or chronic clot.

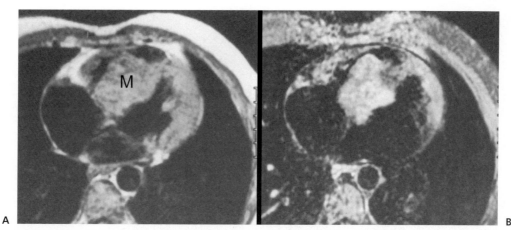

Figure 11.17. Angiosarcoma arising from the ventricular septum. T1-weighted SE images before **(A)** and after **(B)** the administration of Gd-DTPA and fat saturation. Mass (M) shows hyperenhancement after administration of contrast material. Hyperenhancement facilitates demarcation from normal myocardium.

assessment of infiltration of anatomic structures is required for evaluation of feasibility of resection and can be reliably performed by MRI (69).

The signal intensity characteristics of these entities are nonspecific (70). On T1-weighted images, signal intensity is isointense to normal myocardium (Fig. 11.18), whereas it is hyperintense on T2-weighted images. Most of these tumors show increased signal intensity on T1-weighted images after the administration of Gd-DTPA (43,71), so that the lesions are more conspicuous and the delineation of the tumor margins is increased. As mentioned previously, findings on MRI that suggest malignancy are involvement of more than one chamber or great vessel, extension to the pericardium or beyond, and necrosis of the tumor (72).

LYMPHOMA

Primary cardiac lymphoma is less common than secondary lymphoma, involving the heart, which usually represents the spread of non-Hodgkin lymphoma (73). Primary cardiac lymphoma is defined as an extranodal non-Hodgkin lymphoma, which is exclusively located in the heart or pericardium. Almost all primary cardiac lymphomas are B-cell lymphomas (73,74). Primary lymphoma of the heart most often occurs in immunocompromised patients, in whom it is highly aggressive. Although primary cardiac lymphoma is rare, it is mandatory to suspect this entity in the diagnosis because early chemotherapy seems to be effective (75). The tumor arises most often on the right side of the heart, especially in the RA (Fig. 19), but has also been found in the other chambers. A large pericardial effusion is frequently present and might even be the only sign of primary cardiac lymphoma (76). Variable morphology of the masses has been described; both circumscribed polypoid and ill-defined infiltrative lesions have been reported. Lymphomas may appear hypointense to the myocardium on T1-weighted and hyperintense on T2-weighted images (77,78). After the administration of Gd-DTPA, homogeneous or heterogeneous enhancement of the tumor, depending on the presence of

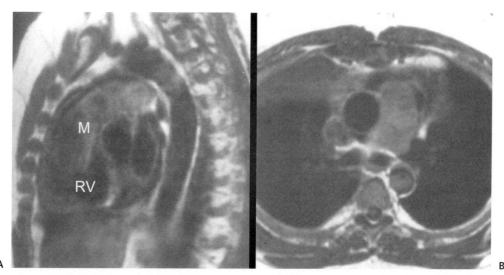

Figure 11.18. Liposarcoma. Sagittal **(A)** and transaxial **(B)** T1-weighted SE images demonstrate the tumor (M) in the RV, which extends into the right ventricular outflow tract and pulmonary artery.

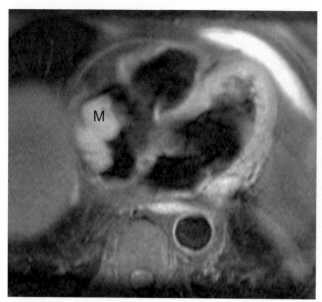

Figure 11.19. Lymphoma. T1-weighted SE image after the administration of contrast medium shows a mass (M) in the RA. Mass shows homogenous enhancement.

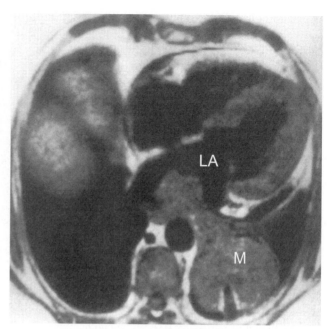

Figure 11.20. Lung cancer extending into the LA. T1-weighted SE image demonstrates the mass (M) extending into the left atrium (LA). Pericardial effusion is present.

necrosis, may be seen (Fig. 11.19) (79). Recent reports showed that delayed-enhancement MR images show hyperintensity of the lymphoma and clearly delineated the extension of the lymphoma (80).

SECONDARY CARDIAC TUMORS

Secondary tumors of the heart are 30- to 40-fold more frequent than primary tumors. In patients with malignancies, the reported frequency ranges from 3% to 18% (81). In general, three different patterns of involvement of the heart can be distinguished: (a) direct extension from intrathoracic tumors (mediastinum or lung), (b) spread from the abdomen through the inferior vena cava into the RA, and (c) metastasis.

DIRECT EXTENSION FROM ADJACENT TUMORS

Tumors of the lung and mediastinum can infiltrate the pericardium and heart directly (Fig. 11.20). It is important to recognize invasion of the heart because such a tumor is usually nonresectable. In mediastinal lymphoma, possible invasion of the pericardium can change the staging of the tumor. MRI is especially suited for delineating of paracardiac tumors and possible extension into the heart because of its wide field of view. MRI clearly shows extension of these tumors to the cardiac structures and possible evidence of hemorrhagic or nonhemorrhagic pericardial effusion. In

studies comparing the accuracy of computed tomography with that of MRI for staging advanced lung cancer invading the cardiac cambers, MRI was more effective in demonstrating invasion of the pericardium and myocardium (82).

METASTASIS

Melanomas, leukemias, and lymphomas (Figs. 11.21, 11.22, and 11.23) most frequently metastasize to the heart, but cardiac metastasis can arise from almost any malignant tumor in the body. Melanomas have the highest frequency of seeding into the heart and have been found in 64% of patients with this entity at autopsy (83). The mechanism of metastatic spread to the heart is direct seeding at the endocardium, passage of tumor emboli through the coronary arteries, or retrograde lymphatic flow through bronchomediastinal lymphatic channels (7). MRI is highly effective for delineating the extent of secondary cardiac tumors (Figs. 11.24, 11.25, and 11.26) and assessing potential resectability (8).

TRANSVENOUS EXTENSION INTO THE HEART

The third pathway for the entry of secondary tumors into the heart is tumor infiltration of vessels connecting with cardiac cambers. Tumor thrombus arising from carcinoma of the kidney, liver, or adrenal gland can extend through the inferior vena cava into the RA (Fig. 11.27), and primary carcinoma of the thymus can extend through the superior vena cava into the RA. Carcinoma of the lung can invade pulmonary veins and grow into the LA or invade the superior vena cava (Fig. 11.28). The evaluation of the possible attachment

text continues on page 178

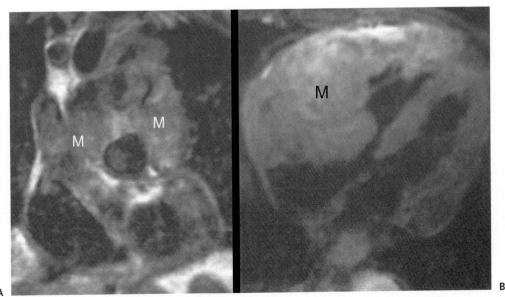

Figure 11.21. Lymphoma. Coronal T1-weighted SE image before the administration of contrast material **(A)** and transaxial T1-weighted SE image with fat saturation after the administration of Gd-DTPA **(B)**. Large mediastinal mass (M) encases the main mediastinal vessels. Mass invades the wall of the RV and extends into the right ventricular chamber. After the administration of Gd-DTPA the mass enhances.

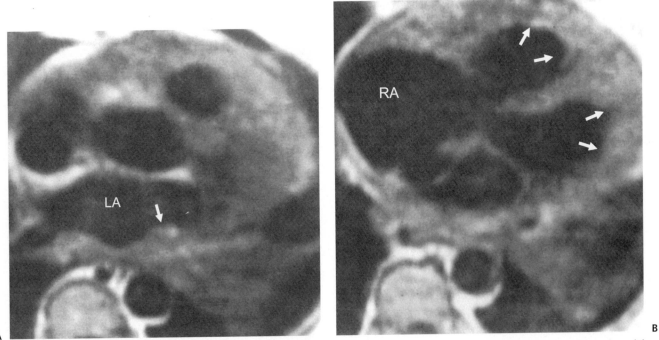

Figure 11.22. Mediastinal lymphoma extending into the LA and LV. Transaxial SE images at the level of the LA **(A)** and LV **(B)** demonstrate the mass infiltrating the pericardium and the posterior wall (*arrow* in **A**) of the LA. Mass invades the posterior left ventricular wall (*arrowhead*). There is thickening of the ventricular walls (*arrows* in **B**), which was confirmed at autopsy to be caused by spread of lymphoma (RA, right atrium).

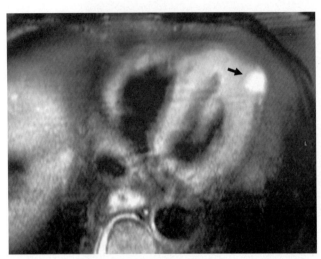

Figure 11.23. Intramural metastasis in the LV. Transaxial T1-weighted SE image after the administration of contrast medium shows an enhancing mass (*arrow*) in the free wall of the LV. Mass extends into the pericardium. (Courtesy of Elmar Spuentrup, M.D., Aachen, Germany.)

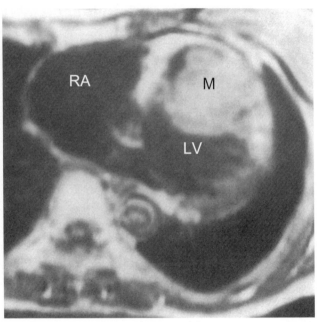

Figure 11.25. Metastatic tumor of the RV. SE image demonstrates the tumor (M) in the RV. LV, left ventricle; RA, right atrium; RV, right ventricle.

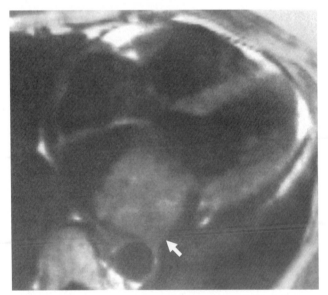

Figure 11.24. Metastatic tumor in the LA. SE image demonstrates a mass in the left atrial cavity. Tumor has a narrow point of attachment to the left atrial wall (*arrow*).

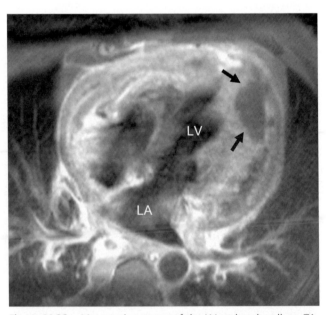

Figure 11.26. Metastatic tumour of the LV and pericardium. T1-weighted transaxial SE image after the administration of contrast medium shows a mass (*arrows*) in the wall of the LV and thickening of the pericardium. LA, left atrium; LV, left ventricle.

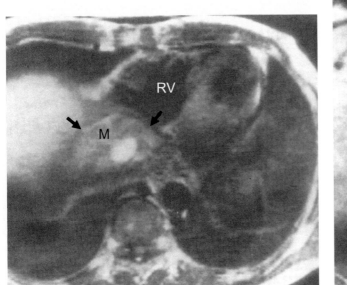

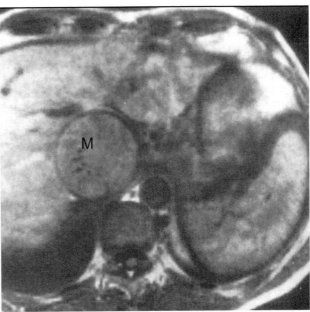

A

B

Figure 11.27.   Adrenal tumor with extension through the inferior vena cava into the RA. T1-weighted SE images at the level of the RA **(A)** and liver **(B)** demonstrate the mass (M) extending through the inferior vena cava into the RA (*arrows*). High signal intensity within the tumor is to the result of hemorrhage. RV, right ventricle.

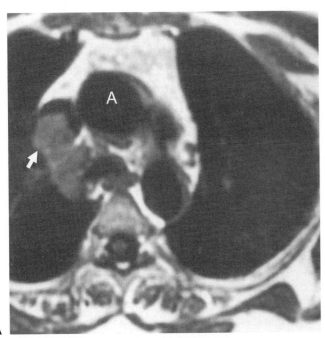

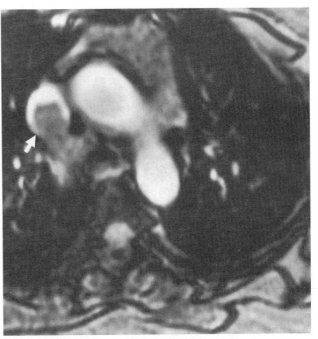

A

B

Figure 11.28.   Lung cancer invading the superior vena cava. Transaxial T1-weighted SE **(A)** and cine MR **(B)** images show a mass adjacent to the superior vena cava. Mass has invaded the vessel and fills it partially (*arrow*). A, aorta.

of such tumors to the atrial wall is mandatory for surgical planning. If the atrial walls are not infiltrated, complete resection of the tumor may still be possible.

INTRACARDIAC THROMBUS

Thrombus is the most common intracardiac mass, involving most frequently the LV or LA. Atrial thrombus is most often seen in patients with mitral valve disease or atrial fibrillation. Mural thrombus is associated with akinetic or dyskinetic regions of the ventricle. It is most often located in the LV after myocardial infarction or in dilated cardiomyopathy (Fig. 11.29). However, any region of the ventricular cavity with stasis of blood is prone to thrombus formation (Fig. 11.30). MRI is especially advantageous for detecting thrombus in the left atrial appendage, which may be difficult to assess by means of transthoracic echocardiography. The risk of embolism from cardiac thrombi depends on morphologic features, which can easily be assessed on MRI. Mobile or protruding emboli carry a risk of approximately 50% for embolic events, whereas flat or nonmobile thrombi carry a risk of 10% for causing emboli (84). However, embolism is more likely to occur with subacute thrombi than with organized thrombi.

On SE images, the signal intensity of thrombus can vary from low to high depending on age-related changes in the composition of the thrombus (85). Thrombus can with time acquire paramagnetic hemoglobin breakdown products, such as intracellular methemoglobin and hemosiderin, or superparamagnetic substances, such as ferritin. Fresh thrombus

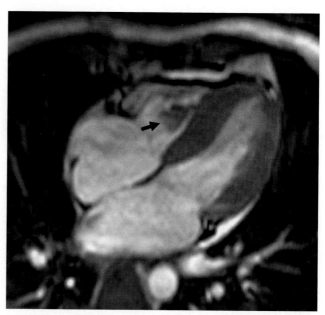

Figure 11.30. Right ventricular thrombus. Transaxial cine MR image. Signal intensity of the thrombus (*arrow*) is low.

usually shows high signal intensity on T1- and T2-weighted SE images, whereas older thrombus may have low signal intensity on T1- and T2-weighted images (86,87). An intracavitary high signal on SE images caused by slowly flowing blood may be difficult to distinguish from thrombus (88,89). However, this problem can be overcome either by using the SE sequences after inversion recovery pulses to null intracavitary signal or by using cine MRI (90,91). The inversion recovery, turbo FLASH sequence, which has been developed for late enhancement imaging of myocardial infarction (92), is well suited for delineation of intracavitary thrombi (Fig. 11.31) (93).

DIFFERENTIATION BETWEEN TUMOR AND BLOOD CLOT

The distinction between blood clot and tumor is more reliably attained with GE sequences. The GE technique is more sensitive to susceptibility and T2* effects than is the SE technique. As the various blood degeneration products pass through the different stages of magnetic susceptibility, they continue to cause shortening of T2* relaxivity; the result is low signal intensity of the thrombus on GE images (Fig. 11.26). An exception to this generalization is fresh thrombus, which can have high signal intensity (86). Tumor tissue usually is hyperintense in comparison with myocardium and skeletal muscle on T2-weighted SE images. However, some myxomas can produce low signal and so mimic thrombus. Another method for differentiating between tumor and clot is to use Gd-DTPA–enhanced T1-weighted images. Thrombus does not enhance after the administration of Gd-DTPA, whereas tumors show enhancement (9). Tumor can usually be differentiated from thrombus by combining GE images and T1-weighted SE images after the administration of

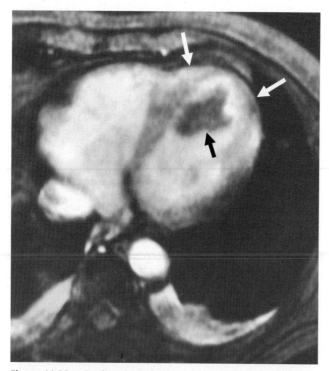

Figure 11.29. Cardiac thrombus associated with apical left ventricular aneurysm. Transaxial cine MR image. Thrombus demonstrates with low signal intensity (*black arrow*). Apical left ventricular aneurysm (*white arrows*).

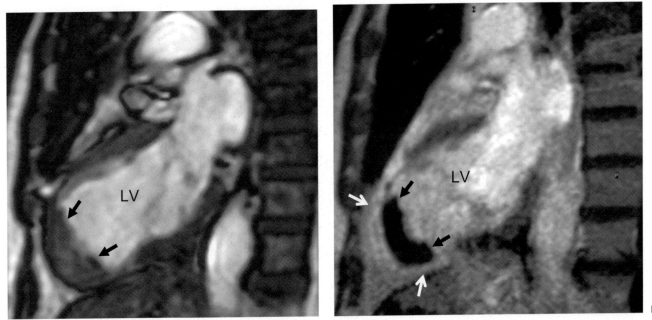

A

B

Figure 11.31.   Left ventricular thrombus associated with apical left ventricular aneurysm. Thrombus (*arrows*) is isointense to the myocardium on the parasagittal cine MR image (A). After the administration of contrast medium, the hypointense thrombus (*black arrows*) can be distinguished from the enhancing infracted myocardium (*white open arrows*). LV, left ventricle. (Courtesy of Marcus Katoh, M.D., Aachen, Germany.)

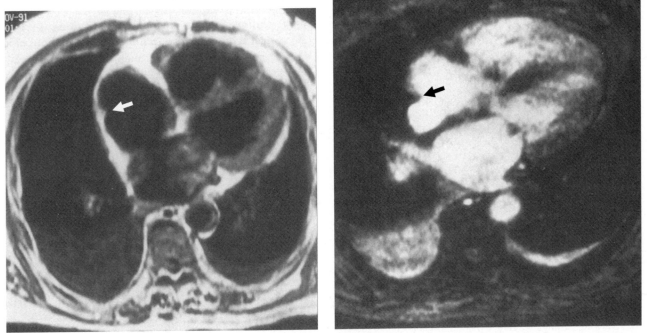

A

B

Figure 11.32.   Axial SE **(A)** and cine MR **(B)** image demonstrate prominence of crista terminalis projecting into the RA (*arrow*). (From Meier RA, Martnell G.G. MRI of right atrial pseudomass: is it really a diagnostic problem? *J Comput Assist Tomogr* 1994;18:398, with permission.)

Gd-DTPA. However, organized thrombus may have areas that enhance (93,94).

PITFALLS: DIFFERENTIATION OF CARDIAC MASSES FROM NORMAL ANATOMIC VARIATIONS

Diagnostic difficulties may arise from the misdiagnosis of normal anatomic variants, such as a prominent crista terminalis, Eustachian valve, or Chiari network (95). The crista terminalis is a fibromuscular band extending between the ostia of the superior and inferior venae cavae on the posterior right atrial wall and represents a residuum of the septum spurium, where the sinus venosus was embryonically incorporated into the right atrial wall (Fig. 11.32) (96). The Chiari network is a reticulum situated in the RA. It is attached to the region of the crista terminalis and extends to the valves of the inferior vena cava and coronary sinus, or sometimes to the floor of the RA near the ostium of the coronary sinus. The Chiari network is derived from the valvulae venosa (96). These structures regress to variable degrees, and nodule-like forms in the RA may be visible on MRI in some patients (Fig. 11.27). Awareness of these variations can prevent misinterpretation as mass lesions.

REFERENCES

1. Lam KY, Dickens P, Chan AC. Tumors of the heart. A 20-year experience with a review of 12,485 consecutive autopsies. *Arch Pathol Lab Med* 1993;117:1027.
2. Blondeau P. Primary cardiac tumors—French studies of 533 cases. *Thorac Cardiovasc Surg* 1990;38(Suppl 2):192–195.
3. Link KM, Lesko NM. MR evaluation of cardiac/juxtacardiac masses. *Top Magn Reson Imaging* 1995;7:232.
4. Kaminaga T, Takeshita T, Kimura I. Role of magnetic resonance imaging for evaluation of tumors in the cardiac region. *Eur Radiol* 2003;13(Suppl 4):L1.
5. Brown JJ, Barakos JA, Higgins CB. Magnetic resonance imaging of cardiac and paracardiac masses. J *Thorac Imaging* 1989;4:58
6. Hoffmann U, Globits S, Schima W, et al. Usefulness of magnetic resonance imaging of cardiac and paracardiac masses. *Am J Cardiol* 2003;92:890.
7. Fujita N, Caputo GR, Higgins CB. Diagnosis and characterization of intracardiac masses by magnetic resonance imaging. *Am J Card Imaging* 1994;8:69.
8. Barakos JA, Brown JJ, Higgins CB. MR imaging of secondary cardiac and paracardiac lesions. *AJR Am J Roentgenol* 1989;153:47.
9. Funari M, Fujita N, Peck WW, et al. Cardiac tumors: assessment with Gd-DTPA enhanced MR imaging. *J Comput Assist Tomogr* 1991;15:953.
10. Niwa K, Tashima K, Terai M, et al. Contrast-enhanced magnetic resonance imaging of cardiac tumors in children. *Am Heart J* 1989;118:424.
11. Araoz PA, Mulvagh SL, Tazelaar HD, et al. CT and MR imaging of benign primary cardiac neoplasms with echocardiographic correlation. *Radiographics* 2000;20:1303.
12. Araoz PA, Eklund HE, Welch TJ, et al. CT and MR imaging of primary cardiac malignancies. *Radiographics* 1999;19:1421.
13. MacGowan SW, Sidhu P, Aherne T, et al. Atrial myxoma: national incidence, diagnosis and surgical management. *Ir J Med Sci* 1993;162:223.
14. Carney JA. Carney complex: the complex of myxomas, spotty pigmentation, endocrine overactivity, and schwannomas. *Semin Dermatol* 1995;14:90.
15. Acebo E, Val-Bernal JF, Gomez-Roman JJ, et al. Clinicopathologic study and DNA analysis of 37 cardiac myxomas: a 28-year experience. *Chest* 2003;123:1379.
16. Dubois CL, Herijgers P. Imaging of a huge atrial myxoma. *Heart* 2003;89:99.
17. Sakamoto H, Sakamaki T, Sumino H, et al. Production of endothelin-1 and big endothelin-1 by human cardiac myxoma cells. *Circ J* 2004;68:1230.
18. Grebenc ML, Rosado-de-Christenson ML, Green CE, et al. Cardiac myxoma: imaging features in 83 patients. *Radiographics* 2002;22:673.
19. Semelka RC, Shoenut JP, Wilson ME, et al. Cardiac masses: signal intensity features on spin-echo, gradient-echo, gadolinium-enhanced spin-echo, and TurboFLASH images. *J Magn Reson Imaging* 1992;2:415.
20. Go RT, O'Donnell JK, Underwood DA, et al. Comparison of gated cardiac MRI and 2D echocardiography of intracardiac neoplasms. *AJR Am J Roentgenol* 1985;145:21.
21. Spuentrup E, Mahnken AH, Kuhl HP, et al. Fast interactive real-time magnetic resonance imaging of cardiac masses using spiral gradient echo and radial steady-state free precession sequences. *Invest Radiol* 2003;38:288.
22. Sievers B, Fritzsche D, Bias-Franken R, et al. Magnetic resonance imaging in the detection of a large left atrial myxoma. *Am J Med* 2003;115:155.
23. Roberts-Thomson KC, Teo KS, Stuklis R, et al. Left atrial myxoma: magnet or echo? *Intern Med J* 2004;34:210.
24. Conces DJ Jr., Vix VA, Klatte EC. Gated MR imaging of left atrial myxomas. *Radiology* 1985;156:445.
25. Pflugfelder PW, Wisenberg G, Boughner DR. Detection of atrial myxoma by magnetic resonance imaging. *Am J Cardiol* 1985;55:242.
26. Masui T, Takahashi M, Miura K, et al. Cardiac myxoma: identification of intratumoral hemorrhage and calcification on MR images. *AJR Am J Roentgenol* 1995;164:850.
27. Matsuoka H, Hamada M, Honda T, et al. Morphologic and histologic characterization of cardiac myxomas by magnetic resonance imaging. *Angiology* 1996;47:693.
28. Oyama N, Oyama N, Komatsu H, et al. Images in cardiovascular medicine. Left ventricular asynchrony caused by an intramuscular lipoma: computed tomographic and magnetic resonance detection. *Circulation* 2003;107:e200.
29. Mousseaux E, Idy-Peretti I, Bittoun J, et al. MR tissue characterization of a right atrial mass: diagnosis of a lipoma. *J Comput Assist Tomogr* 1992;16:148.
30. Comeau CR, Berke AD, Wolff SD. Ventricular lipoma detection by magnetic resonance imaging. *Circulation* 2001;103:1485.
31. Salanitri JC, Pereles FS. Cardiac lipoma and lipomatous hypertrophy of the interatrial septum: cardiac magnetic resonance imaging findings. *J Comput Assist Tomogr* 2004;28:852.
32. Kaplan KR, Rifkin MD. MR diagnosis of lipomatous infiltration of the interatrial septum. *AJR Am J Roentgenol* 1989;153:495.
33. Heyer CM, Kagel T, Lemburg SP, et al. Lipomatous hypertrophy of the interatrial septum: a prospective study of incidence, imaging findings, and clinical symptoms. *Chest* 2003;124:2068.
34. Gaerte SC, Meyer CA, Winer-Muram HT, et al. Fat-containing lesions of the chest. *Radiographics* 2002;22(Spec No):S61–S78.

35. Aziz YF, Julsrud PR. Can cardiac magnetic resonance imaging reliably differentiate between benign and neoplastic fat? *Int J Cardiovasc Imaging* 2002;18:227.

36. Gowda RM, Khan IA, Nair CK, et al. Cardiac papillary fibroelastoma: a comprehensive analysis of 725 cases. *Am Heart J* 2003;146:404

37. Edwards FH, Hale D, Cohen A, et al. Primary cardiac valve tumors. *Ann Thorac Surg* 1991;52:1127.

38. Grinda JM, Couetil JP, Chauvaud S, et al. Cardiac valve papillary fibroelastoma: surgical excision for revealed or potential embolization. *J Thorac Cardiovasc Surg* 1999;117:106.

39. al Mohammad A, Pambakian H, Young C. Fibroelastoma: case report and review of the literature. *Heart* 1998;79:301.

40. Atkinson DJ, Edelman RR. Cineangiography of the heart in a single breath hold with a segmented turboFLASH sequence. *Radiology* 1991;178:357.

41. Shiraishi J, Tagawa M, Yamada T, et al. Papillary fibroelastoma of the aortic valve: evaluation with transesophageal echocardiography and magnetic resonance imaging. *Jpn Heart J* 2003;44:799.

42. Wintersperger BJ, Becker CR, Gulbins H, et al. Tumors of the cardiac valves: imaging findings in magnetic resonance imaging, electron beam computed tomography, and echocardiography. *Eur Radiol* 2000;10:443.

43. Rienmuller R, Lloret JL, Tiling R, et al. MR imaging of pediatric cardiac tumors previously diagnosed by echocardiography. *J Comput Assist Tomogr* 1989;13:621.

44. Winkler M, Higgins CB. Suspected intracardiac masses: evaluation with MR imaging. *Radiology* 1987;165:117.

45. Cina SJ, Smialek JE, Burke AP, et al. Primary cardiac tumors causing sudden death: a review of the literature. *Am J Forensic Med Pathol* 1996;17:271.

46. Brechtel K, Reddy GP, Higgins CB. Cardiac fibroma in an infant: magnetic resonance imaging characteristics. *J Cardiovasc Magn Reson* 1999;1:159.

47. Beghetti M, Gow RM, Haney I, et al. Pediatric primary benign cardiac tumors: a 15-year review. *Am Heart J* 1997;134:1107.

48. Kiaffas MG, Powell AJ, Geva T. Magnetic resonance imaging evaluation of cardiac tumor characteristics in infants and children. *Am J Cardiol* 2002;89:1229.

49. Arai A, Naruse M, Naruse K, et al. Cardiac malignant pheochromocytoma with bone metastases. *Intern Med* 1998;37:940.

50. Hamilton BH, Francis IR, Gross BH, et al. Intrapericardial paragangliomas (pheochromocytomas): imaging features. *AJR Am J Roentgenol* 1997;168:109.

51. Sahdev A, Sohaib A, Monson JP, et al. CT and MR imaging of unusual locations of extra-adrenal paragangliomas (pheochromocytomas). *Eur Radiol* 2005;15:85–92. Epub 2004 Jul 28.

52. Orr LA, Pettigrew RI, Churchwell AL, et al. Gadolinium utilization in the MR evaluation of cardiac paraganglioma. *Clin Imaging* 1997;21:404.

53. Brodwater B, Erasmus J, McAdams HP, et al. Case report. Pericardial hemangioma. *J Comput Assist Tomogr* 1996;20:954.

54. Oshima H, Hara M, Kono T, et al. Cardiac hemangioma of the left atrial appendage: CT and MR findings. *J Thorac Imaging* 2003;18:204.

55. Seline TH, Gross BH, Francis IR. CT and MR imaging of mediastinal hemangiomas. *J Comput Assist Tomogr* 1990;14:766.

56. Kemp JL, Kessler RM, Raizada V, et al. Case report. MR and CT appearance of cardiac hemangioma. *J Comput Assist Tomogr* 1996;20:482.

57. Janigan DT, Husain A, Robinson NA. Cardiac angiosarcomas. A review and a case report. *Cancer* 1986;57:852.

58. Silver MA, Macher AM, Reichert CM, et al. Cardiac involvement by Kaposi's sarcoma in acquired immune deficiency syndrome (AIDS). *Am J Cardiol* 1984;53:983.

59. Corso RB, Kraychete N, Nardeli S, et al. Spontaneous rupture of a right atrial angiosarcoma and cardiac tamponade. *Arq Bras Cardiol* 2003;81:611.

60. Vogt FM, Hunold P, Ruehm SG. Images in vascular medicine. Angiosarcoma of superior vena cava with extension into right atrium assessed by MD-CT and MRI. *Vasc Med* 2003;8:283.

61. Mukohara N, Tobe S, Azami T. Angiosarcoma causing cardiac rupture. *Jpn J Thorac Cardiovasc Surg* 2001;49:516.

62. Rettmar K, Stierle U, Sheikhzadeh A, et al. Primary angiosarcoma of the heart. Report of a case and review of the literature. *Jpn Heart J* 1993;34:667.

63. Bruna J, Lockwood M. Primary heart angiosarcoma detected by computed tomography and magnetic resonance imaging. *Eur Radiol* 1998;8:66.

64. Kim EE, Wallace S, Abello R, et al. Malignant cardiac fibrous histiocytomas and angiosarcomas: MR features. *J Comput Assist Tomogr* 1989;13:627.

65. Yahata S, Endo T, Honma H, et al. Sunray appearance on enhanced magnetic resonance image of cardiac angiosarcoma with pericardial obliteration. *Am Heart J* 1994;127:468.

66. Villacampa VM, Villarreal M, Ros LH, et al. Cardiac rhabdomyosarcoma: diagnosis by MR imaging. *Eur Radiol* 1999;9:634.

67. Szucs RA, Rehr RB, Yanovich S, et al. Magnetic resonance imaging of cardiac rhabdomyosarcoma. Quantifying the response to chemotherapy. *Cancer* 1991;67:2066.

68. Hoffmeier A, Deiters S, Schmidt C, et al. Radical resection of cardiac sarcoma. *Thorac Cardiovasc Surg* 2004;52:77.

69. Clarke NR, Mohiaddin RH, Westaby S, et al. Multifocal cardiac leiomyosarcoma. Diagnosis and surveillance by transoesophageal echocardiography and contrast enhanced cardiovascular magnetic resonance. *Postgrad Med J* 2002;78:492.

70. Watanabe AT, Teitelbaum GP, Henderson RW, et al. Magnetic resonance imaging of cardiac sarcomas. *J Thorac Imaging* 1989;4:90.

71. Schvartzman PR, White RD. Imaging of cardiac and paracardiac masses. *J Thorac Imaging* 2000;15:265.

72. Siripornpitak S, Higgins CB. MRI of primary malignant cardiovascular tumors. *J Comput Assist Tomogr* 1997;21:462.

73. Roberts WC, Glancy DL, DeVita VT Jr. Heart in malignant lymphoma (Hodgkin's disease, lymphosarcoma, reticulum cell sarcoma and mycosis fungoides). A study of 196 autopsy cases. *Am J Cardiol* 1968;22:85.

74. Ceresoli GL, Ferreri AJ, Bucci E, et al. Primary cardiac lymphoma in immunocompetent patients: diagnostic and therapeutic management. *Cancer* 1997;80:1497.

75. Anghel G, Zoli V, Petti N, et al. Primary cardiac lymphoma: report of two cases occurring in immunocompetent subjects. *Leuk Lymphoma* 2004;45:781.

76. Nakakuki T, Masuoka H, Ishikura K, et al. A case of primary cardiac lymphoma located in the pericardial effusion. *Heart Vessels* 2004;19:199.

77. Tada H, Asazuma K, Ohya E, et al. Images in cardiovascular medicine. Primary cardiac B-cell lymphoma. *Circulation* 1998;20;97:220.

78. Dorsay TA, Ho VB, Rovira MJ, et al. Primary cardiac lymphoma: CT and MR findings. *J Comput Assist Tomogr* 1993;17:978.

79. Hoffmann U, Globits S, Frank H. Cardiac and paracardiac masses. Current opinion on diagnostic evaluation by magnetic resonance imaging. *Eur Heart J* 1998;19:553.

80. Kubo S, Tadamura E, Yamamuro M, et al. Primary cardiac lymphoma demonstrated by delayed contrast-enhanced magnetic resonance imaging. *J Comput Assist Tomogr* 2004;28:849.

81. Hanfling SM. Metastatic cancer to the heart. Review of the literature and report of 127 cases. *Circulation* 1960;22:474–483.

82. Mader MT, Poulton TB, White RD. Malignant tumors of the heart and great vessels: MR imaging appearance. *Radiographics* 1997;17:145.

83. Glancy DL, Roberts WC. The heart in malignant melanoma. A study of 70 autopsy cases. *Am J Cardiol* 1968;21:555.

84. van Dantzig JM, Delemarre BJ, Bot H, et al. Left ventricular thrombus in acute myocardial infarction. *Eur Heart J* 1996; 17:1640.

85. Seelos KC, Caputo GR, Carrol CL, et al. Cine gradient refocused echo (GRE) imaging of intravascular masses: differentiation between tumor and nontumor thrombus. *J Comput Assist Tomogr* 1992;16:169.

86. Dooms GC, Higgins CB. MR imaging of cardiac thrombi. *J Comput Assist Tomogr* 1986;10:415.

87. Gomes AS, Lois JF, Child JS, et al. Cardiac tumors and thrombus: evaluation with MR imaging. *AJR Am J Roentgenol* 1987; 149:895.

88. Yousem DM, Balakrishnan J, Debrun GM, et al. Hyperintense thrombus on GRASS MR images: potential pitfall in flow evaluation. *AJNR Am J Neuroradiol* 1990;11:51.

89. von Schulthess GK, Fisher M, Crooks LE, et al. Gated MR imaging of the heart: intracardiac signals in patients and healthy subjects. *Radiology* 1985;156:125.

90. von Schulthess GK, Augustiny N. Calculation of T2 values versus phase imaging for the distinction between flow and thrombus in MR imaging. *Radiology* 1987;164:549.

91. Jungehulsing M, Sechtem U, Theissen P, et al. Left ventricular thrombi: evaluation with spin-echo and gradient-echo MR imaging. *Radiology* 1992;182:225.

92. Simonetti OP, Kim RJ, Fieno DS, et al. An improved MR imaging technique for the visualization of myocardial infarction. Radiology 2001;218:215–223.

93. Barkhausen J, Hunold P, Eggebrecht H, et al. Detection and characterization of intracardiac thrombi on MR imaging. *AJR Am J Roentgenol* 2002;179:1539.

94. Paydarfar D, Krieger D, Dib N, et al. In vivo magnetic resonance imaging and surgical histopathology of intracardiac masses: distinct features of subacute thrombi. *Cardiology* 2001;95:40.

95. Mirowitz SA, Gutierrez FR. Fibromuscular elements of the right atrium: pseudomass at MR imaging. *Radiology* 1992;182: 231.

96. Meier RA, Hartnell GG. MRI of right atrial pseudomass: is it really a diagnostic problem? *J Comput Assist Tomogr* 1994;18:398.

12

Valvular Heart Disease

Jan Bogaert, Steven Dymarkowski, Marie-Christine Herregods, and Andrew M. Taylor

Although the incidence of valvular heart disease (VHD) in developed countries is relatively low compared with the incidence of ischemic heart disease, it continues to cause considerable morbidity and mortality, and in many patients surgical valve repair or replacement will be indicated (1). The diagnosis of VHD is usually based on the patients' symptoms (e.g., dyspnea on exertion, exertional syncope, angina, shortness of breath, palpitations, fatigue, and heart failure) and abnormal cardiac auscultation (e.g., diastolic or systolic murmur). The role of additional imaging procedures, usually echocardiography with Doppler flow measurements and less frequently cardiac catheterization, is to assess the severity of VHD and evaluate the impact on cardiac function. Cardiac imaging is also indicated to monitor the disease progress and help in determining the optimal timing for surgical intervention. In contrast with other cardiac diseases, such as assessment of myocardial infarction and viability, in which magnetic resonance imaging (MRI) can be considered as the reference technique, the role of MRI in assessing patients with VHD is currently not well established. This is in part because of the availability of a good and well-accepted noninvasive first-line imaging modality, i.e., echocardiography. Moreover, clinicians are still unaware of the potential clinical applications of MRI for assessing cardiac diseases (2). This chapter focuses on the different approaches to study VHD with MRI in the clinical setting.

MAGNETIC RESONANCE IMAGING STRATEGIES TO EVALUATE VALVULAR HEART DISEASE

Cardiac valves are essential structures for normal cardiac function. In normal conditions, they guarantee unidirectional blood flow through the heart. When opened, valves do not hamper the blood flow, and when closed, they prevent return of blood, although a small amount of "physiologic" regurgitation is not uncommonly found in the normal population (usually the tricuspid and pulmonary valve, less frequently the mitral valve). In the diseased state, the valve orifice may become narrowed, leading to an obstruction of the blood flow (*valvular stenosis*), and/or the valve leaflets may not completely coapt, leading to a pathologic regurgitation of blood into the proximal chamber (*valvular regurgitation*). As a consequence, this leads to changes in preload and/or afterload conditions of the involved cardiac chamber. The role of imaging in patients suspected of VHD is to obtain information on the following issues: (a) definition of valvular anatomy, i.e., number of valve leaflets, leaflet thickness, and presence of infective endocarditis; (b) assessment of valvular function, i.e., degree of valvular stenosis or regurgitation; (c) definition of the consequences of the valvular dysfunction on ventricular/atrial size, function and mass, and pulmonary artery pressure; (d) assessment of associated morphologic abnormalities, e.g., great vessel anatomy or thrombus formation; and (e) exclusion of non–VHD-related cardiac pathology, such as coronary artery disease and prior myocardial infarction. Much of this required information can be obtained with cardiovascular MRI: a single investigation that is safe, noninvasive, and without irradiation exposure.

VALVULAR MORPHOLOGY

Although fast spin-echo MRI techniques with dark-blood prepulses, obtained during mid-diastole, provide high-quality morphologic images of the heart, they are seldom of diagnostic quality to evaluate the valvular anatomy (3). This is mainly related to the lack of contrast between the low-proton density of valve leaflets and the surrounding dark blood (Fig. 12.1). With bright-blood MRI, using either the spoiled gradient-echo (GE) or balanced steady state free precession (b-SSFP) techniques, valve leaflets are visible as low signal intensity structures surrounded by the bright blood (Fig. 12.1). More-

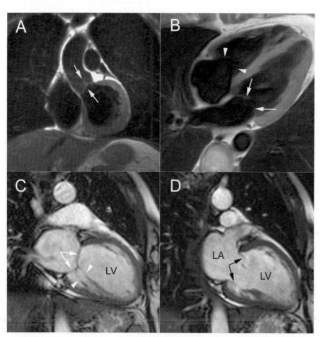

Figure 12.1. Valvular morphology on dark-blood **(A,B)** and bright-blood magnetic resonance imaging (MRI) **(C,D)**. **(A)** Coronal fast spin-echo MRI of the aortic valve (*arrows*). **(B)** Fast spin-echo MRI of the mitral (*arrows*) and tricuspid valve (*arrowheads*) in the horizontal long-axis plane. The valve leaflets appear as low signal intensity structures surrounded by the dark blood. Vertical long-axis bright-blood MRI using the balanced steady-state free precession (b-SSFP) technique at end-systole **(C)** and during early ventricular filling **(D)**. The leaflets of the mitral valve (*arrows*) and the tendinous chords (*arrowheads*) are well visible. The mobility of the leaflets (*black arrows*) can be well appreciated. LA, left atrium; LV, left ventricle.

over, their depiction is greatly enhanced by using the cine-viewing mode, allowing for better visualization of the number of valve leaflets, leaflet morphology, and integrity, as well as leaflet mobility and motion. On the new b-SSFP techniques combining a good spatial with an excellent contrast resolution, the subvalvular apparatus (e.g., tendinous chords) of the atrioventricular valves is also clearly seen (Fig. 12.1). Although echocardiography remains the investigation of choice for imaging valve leaflet anatomy, MRI can be helpful for unraveling valvular anatomy in patients with poor subjects for echocardiography, for example, because of a heavily calcified mitral valve ring or aortic valvular calcifications. The best imaging planes are a combination of longitudinal and perpendicular views through the diseased valve(s). It should be emphasized that in patients with endocarditis, echocardiography is superior to MRI in detecting valvular vegetations because of its real-time imaging features, whereas for endocarditis-related complications, such as abscess or pseudoaneurysm formation, MRI is often complementary to echocardiography (Fig. 12.2).

VALVULAR REGURGITATION

Accurate definition of the degree of valvular regurgitation with MRI is appealing because none of the conventional imaging techniques (i.e., cardiac ultrasound and cardiac catheterization) are well suited to perform this task (4). Cardiovascular MRI can image the regurgitant jet in any plane, and thus provide a three-dimensional (3D) appreciation of the regurgitant jet. In addition, MRI can quantify blood flow and thus provide accurate information on the regurgitant volume, either as an absolute value or as a regurgitant fraction. This information in combination with global ventricular function is of particular clinical relevance for the timing of valve replacement. The following techniques can be applied to evaluate the severity of valvular regurgitation:

- Qualitative assessment of signal loss on cine MRI.
- Quantitative assessment by velocity-encoded cine MRI.
- Quantitative assessment of ventricular volumes, function, and mass.

Qualitative Assessment of Signal Loss with Cine Magnetic Resonance Imaging

The bright-blood phenomenon on spoiled GE cine MRI techniques is based on the laminar inflow of fully magnetized spins. Intravoxel dephasing of the proton spins because of flow disturbance (turbulence, acceleration) leads to loss in signal. This principle can be applied to assess valvular regurgitation. Imaging over multiple frames throughout the cardiac cycle enables visual assessment of flow disturbance caused by the regurgitation. Depending on the severity, a dark signal is visible extending from the diseased valve into the receiving chamber, either pencil-beam–like or fan-like, during a variable time period of the cardiac cycle (Fig. 12.3). With a combination of contiguous cine MRI slices, the direction of the regurgitant jet can be well visualized. Because of the continuous-changing loading conditions, the jet direction is often variable (Fig. 12.4). Similar to cardiac catheterization and cardiac ultrasound, the extent of signal loss in

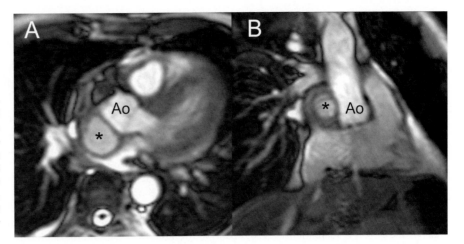

Figure 12.2. Pseudoaneurysm formation in a 56-year-old patient with renal transplant and history of endocarditis. b-SSFP cine MRI in axial plane **(A)** and vertical long-axis through aortic root **(B)**. The infectious pseudoaneurysm is visible as a well-defined hyperintense structure (*asterisk*) behind the aortic root (Ao). MRI is indicated to detect and follow up the formation of these pseudoaneurysms in patients with endocarditis.

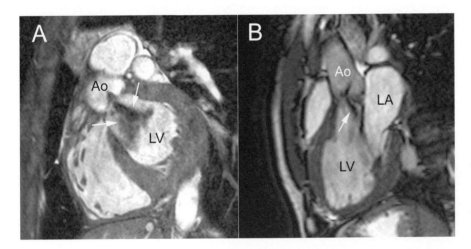

Figure 12.3. Typical appearance of aortic regurgitation on bright-blood b-SSFP MRI. The regurgitant jet is typically visible as a black fan-like **(A)** or pencil-like jet **(B)** extending from the aortic valve (*arrows*) into the left ventricle (LV). Ao, aorta; LA, left atrium.

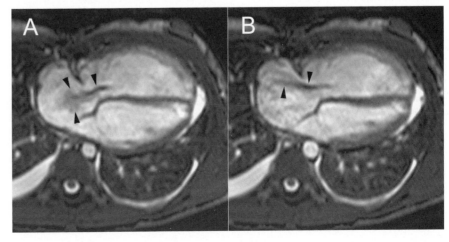

Figure 12.4. Severe tricuspid regurgitation in a 25-year-old patient with transposition of the great arteries treated with the Mustard procedure. Secondary to the right ventricular dilation, there is a severe tricuspid regurgitation visible as a black jet into the right atrium. Note the change in direction of the holosystolic jet (*arrowsheads*) on an early **(A)** and later **(B)** systolic time frame. Note the bilateral pleural effusion.

the receiving chamber can be used to grade the severity of regurgitation. This semiquantitative approach, however, has similar shortcomings as the approach used by the other conventional imaging techniques. The signal loss is highly dependent on the imaging parameters (e.g., echo time), and several studies have shown poor reproducibility of the technique between centers (5–7). The severity is underestimated when the jet impinges on the cardiac chamber wall, and this method is unable to separate turbulent volumes when dual valve disease exists. Nevertheless, cine MRI remains an interesting approach to rapidly evaluate the presence or absence of valvular regurgitation. In case of valve regurgitation, other MRI techniques can be applied to quantify the valvular regurgitation severity. The new standard bright-blood sequence that is now used to study cardiac function; that is, the b-SSFP technique is designed to be relatively flow-insensitive, yielding a better endocardial/blood pool definition than spoiled GE techniques. As a consequence, however, this results in reduced visualization of flow disturbance secondary to valvular regurgitation. In particular, mild regurgitation may not be seen or is less apparent on b-SSFP cine imaging. In a recent study, Krombach et al (8) found a good correlation between b-SSFP cine imaging and color Doppler and cardiac catheterization in patients with known valvular dysfunction. Although the jet phenomenon was slightly more pronounced on spoiled GE cine MRI, the

b-SSFP cine technique resulted in a significantly better image quality.

Quantitative Assessment by Velocity-Encoded Cine Magnetic Resonance Imaging

Noninvasive quantification of blood flow can be achieved with velocity-encoded cine MRI (also called velocity mapping or phase-contrast velocity mapping). For an extensive description of the velocity-encoded cine MRI technique, refer to Chapter 5 on MR blood-flow measurements. In brief, spins moving along a magnetic field gradient are exposed to a different magnetic field than the stationary, nonmoving spins. As a result, these moving spins experience a different degree of dephasing than stationary spins, which is proportional to the distance they move in time (and thus the velocity). This phenomenon can be exploited to measure flow velocities and to extract flow volumes that pass through valves. Velocity-encoded cine MRI can be applied in any direction, although for flow quantification of valvular lesions, through-plane imaging is used. Stationary spins are depicted as middle-gray, whereas increasing velocities in either direction are shown in increasing grades of white or black (Fig. 12.5). Precise determination of the velocity window, as close as possible to the expected peak velocity, is

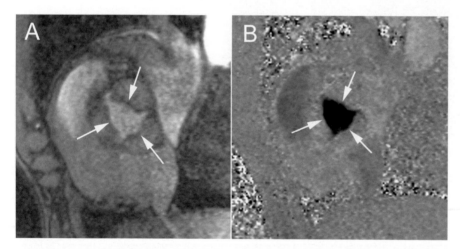

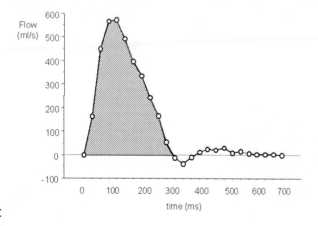

C

Figure 12.5. Quantitative through-plane flow assessment of the aortic valve using the velocity-encoded cine MRI technique. Magnitude image **(A)**, phase image **(B)**, and corresponding phase-contrast velocity map **(C)**. The three leaflets of the aortic valve in opened position are well visible on the magnitude image (*arrows*) **(A)**. Forward flow through the aortic valve is shown as dark signal on the phase image (*arrows*), whereas stationary spins have a middle-gray signal intensity. Delineation of the aortic valve orifice of all images obtained during the entire cardiac cycle yields the phase-contrast velocity map. Forward flow through the aortic valve is shown by positive values, whereas retrograde flow has negative values. The surface under the curve yields the flow volumes and enables calculation of ventricular stroke volumes (*shaded surface*).

important to avoid aliasing while maintaining the highest sensitivity for flow measurements. Measurement of the spatial mean velocity for all pixels in a region of interest enables calculation of the instantaneous flow volume at any point of the cardiac cycle (Fig. 12.5). Calculation of the flow volume per heartbeat can be made by integrating the instantaneous flow volumes for all frames throughout the cardiac cycle. Velocity-encoded cine MRI has been well validated in vitro and in vivo, and can be considered the best available in vivo technique for flow measurements (9–11). In healthy individuals, the output of the left ventricle (LV) and right ventricle (RV) obtained by quantification of the through-plane flow in the proximal ascending aorta and pulmonary trunk has a 1:1 ratio. Differences in ratio can be caused by left-to-right or right-to-left shunt, or by valvular dysfunction.

To obtain reliable measurements of flow velocities and volumes through valves with velocity-encoded cine MRI, several technical issues need to be addressed. To keep phase errors induced by eddy currents and Maxwell terms as low as possible, the area of interest should be as close to the center of the main magnetic field (B_o) as possible. The imaging plane should be perpendicular to the valve. This ensures that the velocity vectors of most voxels are perpendicular to the imaging plane. This can be achieved by a thorough knowledge of cardiac anatomy and cardiac image plane positioning. The best position for flow measurements is not exactly at the level of the valve, but just proximal or distal to the valve annulus. Correction for motion of the valve annulus through the imaging plane during the cardiac cycle can be obtained with the slice-tracking technique (12). However, this promising technique is not yet available for clinical use.

Quantitative Assessment of Ventricular Volumes, Function, and Mass

Cardiac MRI is currently considered the reference technique for in vivo measurement of ventricular volumes and myocardial mass. For this task, breath-hold cine MRI, with the b-SSFP sequence, is used. According to the volumetric approach (Simpson's rule), a set of cardiac short-axis cuts covering the length of the ventricles enables the determination of ventricular volumes and myocardial mass (see Chap. 6). In normal conditions, there is a 1:1 relationship between LV and RV stroke volumes. In the absence of a cardiac shunt, any discrepancy between stroke volumes in a patient with regurgitation will identify the regurgitant volume. Unfortunately, only patients with a single regurgitant valve can be assessed. A combination with velocity-encoded cine MRI, however, allows assessment and quantification of multivalvular disease.

VALVULAR STENOSIS

Exact determination of the stenotic valve area and transvalvular gradient is crucial in assessing patients with valvular stenosis. Although this is usually achieved by echo Doppler and cardiac catheterization, MRI is capable of assessing valvular stenosis. Different strategies are currently available. Valvular stenosis can be identified by signal loss on cine MR images. The orifice area can be measured on perpendicular views through the stenotic valve. Velocity-encoded cine MRI may be used to establish an accurate peak velocity across the valve to quantify the severity of the stenosis, whereas b-SSFP cine MRI enables determination of the impact of valve stenosis on ventricular volumes, function, and mass.

Visual Assessment of Valve Stenosis on Cine Magnetic Resonance Imaging

Use of signal loss extending from a stenotic valve into the distal chamber or vessel is helpful for identification of a stenotic valve (Fig. 12.6). The degree of signal loss, however, is not only dependent on the degree of stenosis but also on the echo time used. For shorter echo times, less spin dephasing occurs. Kilner et al (13) showed that in more severe stenoses, shorter echo times need to be used to prevent signal loss in the images. Similar as for the qualitative assessment of valvular regurgitation, signal loss is less marked on the b-SSFP cine MR images, and therefore it is more difficult to get a feel for the peak velocity with b-SSFP sequences than with conventional spoiled-GE cine imaging.

Valve Orifice Quantification

Valve area or valve orifice can be estimated indirectly using the peak systolic transvalvular gradient (cardiac catheterization) and the continuity equation (echo Doppler), or can be calculated by direct planimetry (transesophageal echocardiography and MRI). MR images perpendicular through the stenotic valve, during maximal opening, allow a planimetric quantification of the valve orifice (14,15). It is currently unclear whether b-SSFP sequences with short echo times are better than the conventional spoiled-GE techniques to obtain reliable estimates of the valve stenosis (16,17). Although spoiled-GE cine MRI, especially when using longer echo times, is sensitive to spin-dephasing artifacts, the b-SSFP technique may have different sources of artifacts, including sensitivity to areas of magnetic field disturbance (e.g., calcifications, tissue interfaces) and sometimes severe artifacts in areas of highly complex flow (16). By using data from velocity-encoded flow curves, the continuity equation (similar as used in echo Doppler) can be used to calculate valve area (17,18) (see "Aortic Valve" section).

Quantitative Evaluation with Velocity-Encoded Cine Magnetic Resonance Imaging

Information from the phase-contrast velocity map, i.e., peak velocity across the valve, can be used to obtain an estimate of the gradient across the valve, using the modified Bernoulli equation:

$$\Delta P = 4\, V^2$$

where P is the pressure decrease across the stenosis (in millimeters of mercury) and V is velocity (in meters per second). The technique is comparable with Doppler echo measurements and has an in vitro accuracy of 4% (19). The main advantage of the technique over cardiac ultrasound is that the velocity jet can be aligned easily in any direction without the limitation of acoustic windows or the interference of (peri-) valvular calcifications.

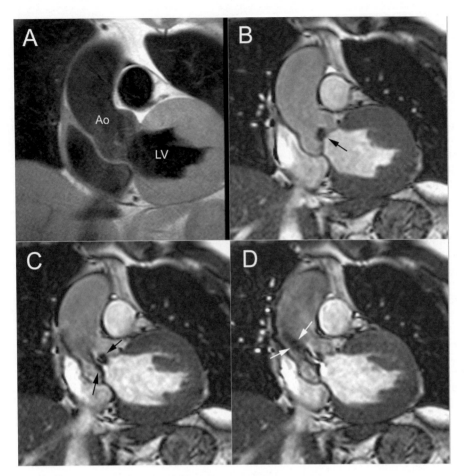

Figure 12.6. Severe aortic stenosis (AS) in a 45-year-old man with bicuspid aortic valve. Coronal T1-weighted fast spin-echo MRI **(A)** and coronal balanced-SSFP cine MRI at end-diastole **(B)** and early **(C)** and mid- **(D)** systole. Hypointense thickening of the tips of the valve leaflets, best visible on balanced-SSFP cine MRI (*black arrows* in **B** and **C**). Severe reduction of the aortic valve opening with black jet in ascending aorta during systole (*arrows* in **D**). Note the dilation of the aortic and ascending aorta secondary to the aortic valve stenosis. Severe concentric hypertrophy of the left ventricle (LV wall mass: 257 g).

The flow through a stenotic valve can be imaged in-plane (velocity jet parallel to the imaging plane) or through-plane (velocity jet perpendicular to the imaging plane). The in-plane method visualizes the entire jet and shows the point within the jet of peak velocity. However, peak velocity may not always be accurately depicted, for instance when the jet is not aligned in a single 2-D plane, or in case of tight narrow jets, there may be partial volume averaging and motion within the imaging slice. For through-plane motion, the jet will always pass through the imaging plane, but because only part of the stenotic jet is sampled, the peak velocity may not be measured. Because both strategies have advantages and disadvantages, it is the best to use a combination of the two strategies with initial definition of the jet in-plane and quantification with through-plane imaging at the site of maximum velocity on the in-plane image.

Use of an appropriate velocity window is essential to maintain sensitivity and accuracy of measurements while avoiding aliasing. An estimate of the peak velocity and ideal velocity window can be obtained with fast, breath-hold, velocity-encoded cine MRI techniques, before progressing to the more time-consuming conventional phase-contrast velocity-mapping sequence.

ASSOCIATED FINDINGS IN VALVULAR HEART DISEASE

It is important to identify the presence of associated findings in patients with VHD. The presence of VHD will have an immediate impact on the loading conditions of the ventricle, eventually leading to a geometric ventricular remodeling with morphologic changes (cavity diameter, wall thickness, and myocardial tissue characteristics) and functional changes (systolic, diastolic [dys-] function). It is commonly accepted that MRI is more accurate than echocardiography in describing this remodeling process (20). A reversed remodeling is found early after valve replacement (20,21). Assessment of the inflow patterns through the atrioventricular valves or flow patterns in the pulmonary and systemic veins with velocity-encoded cine MRI can be used to assess diastolic function, whereas contrast-enhanced inversion-recovery MRI with late or delayed imaging is able to depict abnormal areas of focal (hyper-) enhancement reflecting areas of macroscopic fibrosis or microinfarction in patients with long-standing aortic stenosis (AS). Myocardial tagging can be applied to noninvasively study abnormal myocardial deformation patterns in patients with VHD (22,23).

In the presence of mitral stenosis or VHD with atrial fibrillation, thrombus formation in the atria or atrial appendages needs to be ruled out. A combination of cine MRI sequences (preferably the b-SSFP technique) and contrast-enhanced inversion-recovery MRI is likely the best strategy to depict abnormal intracavity structures (24). The vertical long-axis view is well suited to visualize the left atrial appendage. Abnormalities of the thoracic vessels are not uncommon in pulmonary and/or aortic VHD. Aortic or pulmonary valve stenosis is not infrequently associated with aneurysmal dilatation of the proximal ascending aorta or pulmonary trunk, respectively. Moreover, there is an association between the presence of bicuspid aortic valve and aortic coarctation. MRI offers the possibility of an integrated approach combining valve imaging and great vessel imaging. The arsenal of MRI techniques used to study the thoracic vessels consists of fast spin-echo MRI, b-SSFP cine MRI sequences, and 3D contrast-enhanced MR angiography.

ASSESSMENT OF NONVALVULAR CARDIAC DISEASES

Concomitant non–VHD-related cardiac diseases are not infrequent in patients with VHD. For example, LV dysfunction with low cardiac output in the presence of AS may be related to the AS, but it also may be caused by concomitant coronary artery disease or previous myocardial infarction. To determine the potential benefit of an aortic valve replacement in such patients, other causes of LV dysfunction need to be excluded. As highlighted in other chapters in this book, MRI can be applied to image the proximal and mid-segments of the coronary arteries (Chap. 19) to evaluate the myocardial perfusion in rest and stress conditions (Chap. 13) and to determine the presence and extent of myocardial necrosis and scar tissue (Chap. 16). In this way, MRI is appealing to the clinicians because it offers a comprehensive approach to investigate patients with VHD.

AORTIC VALVE

AORTIC STENOSIS

Severe AS is an important clinical entity because it is the most common valve lesion considered for valve replacement in the United States, especially in older people (1). AS may be congenital (e.g., bicuspid aortic valve) or acquired (i.e., degenerative [fibrocalcific senile AS] and rheumatic heart disease). In addition to stenosis of the aortic valve, subvalvular and supravalvular stenosis may also lead to AS. The hemodynamic consequence of all forms is an increase in LV afterload, leading to concentric LV hypertrophy (Fig. 12.6). It is essential in the diagnosis of AS to obtain information on the gradient across the aortic valve and the absolute aortic

valve area. The gradient as such gives an incomplete assessment of the AS severity. Because the gradient is dependent on the stroke volume, ejection time (both of which are load-dependent and influenced by myocardial contractility), and aortic pressure, it is possible for a mean aortic valve gradient less than 50 mm Hg to be associated with severe, moderate, or even mild AS. Thus, it is important to determine aortic valve area. Severe AS is defined as an aortic valve area ≤ 1.0 cm^2 (≤ 0.60 cm^2/m^2). In patients with severe AS, initially with heart failure (New York Heart Association III/IV), low gradients are not infrequently found. Moreover, because these patients often have comorbid conditions (coronary artery disease, previous myocardial infarction, systemic hypertension, diabetes mellitus, and chronic obstructive pulmonary disease), there is uncertainty about the cause of low LV ejection fraction and the patient outcome after aortic valve replacement.

On longitudinal cine MR images through the aortic valve, the stenotic valve usually presents as a thickened, low-intensity, nearly immobile structure, with a systolic jet (visible as a signal void) through the narrowed valve orifice. There may be concomitant aortic regurgitation, visible as diastolic signal void into the LV. Perpendicular cine views through the aortic valve can clearly show the number of valve leaflets, the mobility of leaflets, and the aortic valve orifice. These images enable direct measurement of the aortic valve area (Fig. 12.7). For this measurement, the area of flow through-plane at the level of the origin of the flow jet is used. The results of this technique to date, however, have been conflicting. Whereas Friedrich et al demonstrated a good agreement between the aortic valve area calculations on MRI and cardiac catheterization ($r = 0.78$), John et al reported a poor agreement between both techniques ($r = 0.44$) (14–16). As an alternative, application of the continuity equation on velocity-encoded cine MRI profiles in the left ventricular outflow tract (LVOT) (velocity measured below the valve) and aorta (above the valve in the aorta) showed a good agreement between MRI and similar data acquired with echocardiography ($r = 0.83$) (17,18). The velocity time integral (VTI) is measured for systolic forward flow in both planes (Fig. 12.8). The aortic valve area A_{Ao} (centimeters squared) is given by:

$$A_{Ao} = A_{LVOT}(VTI_{LVOT}/VTI_{Ao})$$

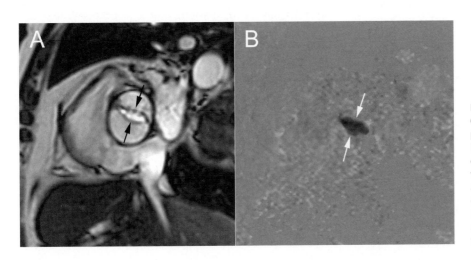

Figure 12.7. Bicuspid aortic valve in a 67-year-old man. Magnitude **(A)** and phase **(B)** images obtained perpendicular through the aortic valve. Note the bicuspid appearance of the aortic valve, as well as the moderate narrowing of the aortic valve orifice (*arrows*), causing a dilatation of the aortic root and ascending aorta (not shown). Planimetry enables direct calculation of the aortic valve orifice.

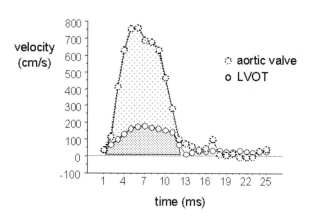

Figure 12.8. Calculation of the functional aortic valve area using the velocity time integral (VTI) continuity equation for AS. The graph shows the velocity-time curves obtained perpendicular through the aortic valve (*dashed line*) and left ventricular outflow tract (LVOT) (*full line*). The peak velocity through the aortic valve is 7.15 m/s and through the LVOT is 1.78 m/s. LVOT area is 4.8 cm². Summation of area under the curve during systole gives the VTI, enabling calculation of the functional aortic valve area.

where A_{LVOT} is LVOT area in square centimeters, VTI_{LVOT} is LVOT VTI, and VTI_{Ao} is AoVTI.

Velocity-encoded cine MRI enables calculation of the gradient through the stenotic aortic valve, using the peak velocity. This approach has shown a good in vivo agreement for a wide range of pressure gradients across the aortic valve between MR velocity mapping and echo Doppler and cardiac catheterization (25). As mentioned, a combination of in-plane and through-plane velocity measurements is the best approach to obtain the highest peak velocities through the stenotic valve. Depending on the severity of AS, velocity windows up to 5 m/s, or in extreme forms up to 10 m/s, need to be chosen.

An important issue when imaging AS is the evaluation of the impact on LV function and mass and on aortic root dimensions. The b-SSFP cine MRI technique can be used to measure the degree of LV hypertrophy and to monitor the reduction in myocardial mass after aortic valve replacement (20,21,26,27). Caliber changes in the proximal thoracic aorta are not infrequent in patients with AS. MRI can be considered the reference technique to measure aortic diameters. In patients with angina and AS, visualization of the coronary arteries is often requested to exclude ischemic heart disease as a contributing factor to the symptoms. To date, the role of coronary MR angiography is unclear, though there may be a role in excluding coronary artery disease in patients with VHD with a low likelihood of coronary artery stenoses.

Several studies, using myocardial tagging, have shown altered myocardial contractility and relaxation patterns in patients with AS. In pressure-overloaded, hypertrophied ventricles, there is an increase in apical rotation with increased LV torsion and a delay and prolongation of diastolic untwisting (21–23). After aortic valve replacement, a normalization of LV torsion is found. A better understanding of cardiac physiology in AS may help in defining the optimal time for operative intervention in AS (21–23).

AORTIC REGURGITATION

Aortic regurgitation is caused by abnormalities of the valve leaflets (e.g., congenital bicuspid aortic valve, rheumatic heart disease, bacterial endocarditis, myxomatous valve associated with cystic medial necrosis, and aortic valve prolapse), or is secondary to dilatation of the aortic root (e.g., Marfan syndrome, syphilitic aortitis, ankylosing spondylitis, Reiter disease, rheumatoid disease, and Ehlers-Danlos syndrome) or to aortic dissection. The impact of aortic regurgitation on cardiac hemodynamics is dependent on the speed of onset of regurgitation. In acute regurgitation, such as in bacterial endocarditis or aortic dissection, the LV has no time for adaptation. LV filling pressures rapidly increase, cardiac output decreases, and left atrial pressures increase. This cascade of events leads to pulmonary edema and ultimately shock. The initial response in chronic aortic regurgitation is LV hypertrophy because compensation for the increased wall stress is secondary to volume overload. This is followed by a progressive LV dilatation and reduction in ventricular function.

Regular follow-up is required to follow-up disease progression and to determine optimal timing of aortic valve replacement. The timing of surgery is important and is a balance between operating too soon (operative risks, insertion of a valve that will not last forever, lifelong anticoagulation), and operating too late (irreversible LV failure). At present, the decision for surgical intervention usually depends on clinical symptoms, chest x-ray film appearance, echocardiographic findings, and longitudinal changes in these parameters (28).

Regurgitant aortic jets are best visualized in the coronal or oblique coronal imaging plane (Fig. 12.3). Although the extent of signal void can be used to obtain a semiquantitative estimate of the aortic regurgitation, the most accurate method for quantifying the regurgitant fraction is velocity-encoded cine MRI. Care should be taken that the majority of flow is measured through-plane (Fig. 12.9). This can be achieved by obtaining two perpendicular images through the ascending aorta and defining an oblique axial plane perpendicular to both. The best position for imaging plane is just above or below the aortic valve. A through-plane velocity window of 1.5 m/s can be recommended in isolated aortic regurgitation. In case of concomitant AS, a dual velocity window, with a high systolic setting of ± 5 m/s, changing to ± 1.5 m/s for the diastolic frames, is necessary to obtain the best sensitivities. Aortic regurgitation is expressed in absolute terms, i.e., millimeters per heartbeat, or liters per minute (milliliters per beat × heart rate) (Fig. 12.9), or as a regurgitant fraction which is given by:

Regurgitant fraction (%) = [aortic retrograde flow (mL/beat)/aortic forward flow (mL/beat)] × 100

The severity of regurgitation can be defined as follows (5):

- Mild: regurgitation fraction 15% to 20%.
- Moderate: regurgitation fraction 20% to 40%.
- Severe: regurgitation fraction >40%.

Because the interstudy reproducibility is high (29), velocity-encoded cine MRI may be an ideal technique in long-term

32. Heidenreich PA, Steffens JC, Fuijta N, et al. The evaluation of mitral stenosis with velocity-encoded cine MRI. *Am J Cardiol* 1992;75:365–369.

33. Mohiaddin RH, Amanuma M, Kilner PJ, et al. MR phase-shift velocity mapping of mitral and pulmonary venous flow. *J Comput Assist Tomogr* 1991;15:227–243.

34. Aurigemma G, Reichek N, Schiebler M, et al. Evaluation of mitral regurgitation by cine MRI. *Am J Cardiol* 1990;66: 621–625.

35. Hundley WG, Li HF, Willard JE, et al. Magnetic resonance imaging assessment of the severity of mitral regurgitation. *Circulation* 1995;92:1151–1158.

36. Fujita N, Chazouillers AF, Hartiala JJ. Quantification of mitral regurgitation by velocity encoded cine nuclear magnetic resonance imaging. *J Am Coll Cardiol* 1994; 23:951–958.

37. Myerson S, Neubauer S. Direct quantification of mitral regurgitation with phase velocity mapping. *J Cardiovasc Magn Reson* 2004;6:49–50.

38. Kivelitz DE, Dohmen PM, Lembcke A, et al. Visualization of the pulmonary valve using cine MR imaging. *Acta Radiologica* 2003;44:172–176.

39. Roest AAW, Helbing WA, Kunz P, et al. Exercise MR imaging in the assessment of pulmonary regurgitation and biventricular function in patients after Tetralogy of Fallot repair. *Radiology* 2002;223:204–211.

40. Tulevski II, Hirsch A, Dodge-Khatami A, et al. Effect of pulmonary valve regurgitation on right ventricular function in patients with chronic right ventricular pressure overload. *Am J Cardiol* 2003; 92:113–116.

41. Therrien J, Siu SC, McLaughin PR, et al. Pulmonary valve replacement in adult late after repair of Tetralogy of Fallot: are we operating too late? *J Am Coll Cardiol* 2000;36:1670–1675.

42. Vliegen HW, Van Straten A, de Roos A, et al. Magnetic resonance imaging to assess the hemodynamic effects of pulmonary valve replacement in adults late after repair of tetralogy of Fallot. *Circulation* 2002;106:1703–1707.

43. Razavi R, Muthurangu V, Taylor AM, et al. Magnetic resonance assessment of percutaneous pulmonary valve-stent implantation (abstract). *J Cardiovasc Magn Reson* 2004;6:429.

44. van Straten A, Vliegen HW, Hazekamp MG, et al. Right ventricular function after pulmonary valve replacement in patients with tetralogy of Fallot. *Radiology* 2004; 223:824–829.

45. Waggoner AD, Quinones MA, Young JB, et al. Pulsed Doppler echocardiography detection of right-sided valve regurgitation. Experimental results and clinical significance. *Am J Cardiol* 1981;47:279–283.

46. Mollet NR, Dymarkowski S, Bogaert J. MRI and CT revealing carcinoid heart disease. *Eur Radiol* 2003;13:L14–L18.

47. Randall PA, Kohman LJ, Scalzetti EM, et al. Magnetic resonance imaging of prosthetic cardiac valves in vitro and in vivo. *Am J Cardiol* 1988;62:973–976.

48. Shellock FG. MR imaging of metallic implants and materials: a compilation of the literature. *Am J Roentgenol* 1988;151: 811–814.

49. Deutsch HJ, Bachmann R, Sechtem U, et al. Regurgitant flow in cardiac valve prosthesis: diagnostic value of gradient echo nuclear magnetic resonance imaging in reference to transesophageal two-dimensional color Doppler echocardiography. *J Am Coll Cardiol* 1992;19:1500–1507.

50. Fontaine AA, Heinrich RS, Walker PG, et al. Comparison of magnetic resonance imaging and laser Doppler anemometry velocity measurements downstream of replacement heart valves: implications for in vivo assessment of prosthetic valve function. *J Heart Valve Dis* 1996;5:66–73.

51. Lepore V, Lamm C, Bugge M, et al. Magnetic resonance imaging in the follow-up of patients after aortic root reconstruction. *Thorac Cardiovasc Surg* 1996;44:188–192.

52. Botnar R, Nagel E, Scheidegger MB, et al. Assessment of prosthetic aortic valve performance by magnetic resonance velocity imaging. *MAGMA* 2000;10:18–26.

53. Kozerke S, Hasenkam JM, Nygaard H, et al. Heart motion-adapted MR velocity mapping of blood velocity distribution downstream aortic valve prostheses: initial experience. *Radiology* 2001;218:548–555.

54. Kozerke S, Hasenkam JM, Pedersen EM, et al. Visualization of flow patterns distal to aortic valve prostheses in humans using a fast approach for cine 3D velocity mapping. *J Magn Reson Imaging* 2001;13:690–698.

13

Myocardial Perfusion in Ischemic Heart Disease

Juerg Schwitter

Coronary artery disease (CAD) is the leading cause of death in the industrialized world. Treatment of CAD has shown much progress in the past few years based on therapeutic strategies aimed at risk factor modifications (e.g., through lipid lowering interventions) and through new options for revascularizations (e.g., the introduction of drug-eluting stents). These improvements, however, are contrasted by a lack of efficient diagnostics. Invasive coronary angiography detects disease reliably but is costly and bears a small risk for complications. Stress echocardiography as a noninvasive technique is safe, but its robustness is suboptimal, resulting in a compromised reproducibility and misdiagnoses depending on reader experience (1). Scintigraphic techniques demonstrate adequate reproducibility, but some limitations in spatial resolution reduce sensitivity, while attenuation artifacts compromise specificity (2,3). Finally, nuclear techniques expose patients to radiation, which becomes important if the test screens patients for the presence of disease and/or monitors progression of disease in patients with known CAD. Similarly, radiation limitations also apply to computed tomographic (CT) coronary angiography.

Magnetic resonance (MR) perfusion imaging is not affected by any of the above limitations. Instead, it shows an unbeatable versatility. Therefore, the pathophysiological events during CAD development will be summarized in order to identify potential imaging targets. These considerations are followed by a technical section that explains pulse sequences, contrast media (CM), and concepts of data analysis. Taking the technical complexity of MR perfusion imaging into account, its performance in multicenter trials is of particular importance, and first positive results are now available (4–6). These and future studies will define the role of MR perfusion imaging in the work-up of cardiac patients.

PATHOPHYSIOLOGY OF CORONARY ARTERY DISEASE

DEVELOPMENT OF CORONARY ARTERY LESIONS

A large number of clinical and experimental studies relate endothelial dysfunction to cardiovascular risk factors, thereby supporting the concept of endothelial dysfunction being a crucial initial step in the development of atherosclerosis (7–9). In dysfunctional endothelium, the production of nitrous oxide (NO) is reduced, which in turn enhances the expression of endothelial adhesion molecules (10). These alterations in endothelial cells of conduit arteries and vasa vasorum promote the recruitment of leucocytes to the vessel intima (10,11). While mononuclear leucocytes typically become foam cells by accumulating lipids and form reversible fatty streaks, accumulation of smooth muscle cells and their production of extracellular matrix may induce the formation of fibrous lesions during this phase of atherogenesis. Inflammatory mediators can impede the ability of smooth muscle cells to maintain the collagen content in atherosclerotic lesions. (12) Activated macrophages are also known to produce matrix-degrading enzymes (13), which can further destabilize the fibrous cap of atheromas, finally resulting in plaque rupture. Repetitive plaque ruptures and subsequent healing, even when clinically silent, may account for an intermittent progression of atherosclerotic lesions (14,15). With progressive disease, ruptures of larger plaques that contain considerable amounts of lipids and tissue factor, a powerful procoagulant, can cause ultimate thrombus formation and acute vessel occlusion (16). In line with this concept, invasive studies demonstrated an increasing risk for rupture of lesions with increasing stenosis severity (15,17–19). Accordingly, vulnerable plaques are characterized by four major criteria (20): (a) thin cap with large lipid core, (b) stenosis >90%, (c) endothelial denudation with superficial platelet aggregation, and (d) fissured plaque. Therefore, a major goal of noninvasive imaging is to identify vulnerable plaques in the various perfusion beds, particularly the heart, the carotids, the renals, and the peripheral arteries of the lower limbs.

Ideally, identification of vulnerable plaques would include determination of location, mass (stenosis severity), and composition of lesions. Direct visualization of plaques in the coronary circulation has been performed in several studies and is discussed in detail in Chapter 4. In this context, it might be useful to consider the following. In a 3-mm coronary vessel imaged with a currently available spatial resolution of 0.5×0.5 mm^2 for coronary magnetic resonance angiography (MRA), signal distribution in as little as 27 pixels would determine the degree of stenosis (criterium two of vulnerable plaque definition). With respect to plaque composition and morphology (criteria 1 and 4), as little as 6 pixels/component would characterize a plaque, causing a 70% luminal reduction (with three components in the plaque—fibrosis, lipid necrotic core, and inflammatory cell-rich components—each occupying one third of the plaque area). Alternatively, the severity of stenosis could be determined by assessing myocardial perfusion disturbances, whereby one would neglect the additional information contained in the plaque composition. In this case, it is assumed that a 3-mm vessel supplies approximately 60 g of muscle tissue (21), which corresponds to approximately 10,500 pixels (considering a spatial resolution for perfusion imaging of 3×3 mm^2 and a cardiac coverage of 50%). Therefore, a change in stenosis severity would be detected more reliably by integrating 10,500 pixels in the myocardium than 27 pixels covering the cross-sectional area of the coronary vessel.

DETECTION OF HEMODYNAMICALLY SIGNIFICANT CORONARY LESIONS

Once the decision is made to assess myocardial perfusion in order to assess the severity of coronary artery stenoses, two major strategies can be used. The first strategy is based on the concept that a hemodynamically significant stenosis limits flow during hyperemia. In order to detect a reduction in hyperemic flow in a given patient, the measured hyperemic flow must be compared with normal values for hyperemic flow. In this approach, hyperemia is typically induced by intravenous (IV) infusion of a pharmacological vasodilator such as adenosine (or dipyridamole). The second strategy uses the determination of the coronary flow reserve (CFR) in order to detect hemodynamically significant stenoses. It "normalizes" hyperemic flow by dividing it through resting flow (flow$_{hyperemic}$ / flow$_{rest}$). Several positron emission tomographic (PET) studies have demonstrated a close correlation of CFR versus percent area stenosis, however, with a tendency toward even better correlations of hyperemic flow versus percent area stenosis (22–24). While the first approach, the stress-only protocol, requires a normal database to provide threshold values for the hyperemic flow state, the CFR approach incorporates measurements of resting flow. Division of hyperemic flow by resting flow can become problematic, taking into account that many factors that influence resting flow (e.g., heart rate, contractility, and loading conditions) cannot be controlled in a clinical setting (25). Furthermore, matching myocardial regions, such as the subendocardial layer, for both rest and hyperemic condition may be difficult (since the geometry of the heart changes with changing heart rate, loading, etc.). Finally, to obtain accurate results for the CFR calculation, the technique must guarantee a linear relationship between MR-derived perfusion parameters and flow over a wide range of flow conditions (resting and hyperemic flow).

TECHNICAL ASPECTS OF MAGNETIC RESONANCE PERFUSION IMAGING

NONCONTRAST MEDIUM-BASED APPROACHES

An elegant approach for perfusion measurements exploits the decrease in T$_2$ relaxation time of deoxygenated and thus paramagnetic hemoglobin (since oxygenated hemoglobin is slightly diamagnetic, causing less of T$_2$ shortening). With this blood oxygen level dependent (BOLD) method, a T$_2$- or T$_2$*-weighted pulse sequence allows for an estimation of an increased content of oxygenated blood, which is expected to occur in the presence of unrestricted hyperemic flow (which is associated with a lower oxygen [O$_2$] extraction). However, this approach is sensitive to magnetic field inhomogeneities, and the robustness of the method is not yet demonstrated (26,27). Also, signal differences in normally perfused regions versus hyperemic regions (with a fourfold increase in flow) were as low as 32% in an experimental setting (28). This low signal difference might be problematic since studies with CM first-pass approaches performed in humans showed differences in signal increase in the range of 80% to 100% to be clinically inadequate, while differences in the range of 250% to 300% were required for reliable detection of ischemic regions in patients (29).

Arterial spin labeling is another technique that does not require the administration of exogenous CM (30–33). This approach is based on T_1 measurements after global and slice-selective spin preparation (using appropriate electrocardiographic [ECG] triggered pulse sequences). Owing to the inflow of unsaturated proton spins, T_1 in tissue is shortened after slice-selective preparation compared with global preparation. Assuming a two-compartment model, absolute tissue perfusion is calculated. However, this concept assumes that direction of flowing blood in intramural vessels can be aligned with the slice orientation, which is not expected to occur for different myocardial layers and is further complicated in in-vivo studies by cardiac contraction. Magnetization transfer techniques are also under investigation to assess myocardial perfusion (34). A schematic of the various pulse sequences for perfusion assessment is given in Figure 13.1.

MAGNETIC RESONANCE PULSE SEQUENCES FOR CONTRAST MEDIA FIRST-PASS STUDIES

Most experience exists with the CM first-pass approach used for the detection of perfusion abnormalities. With this technique, a bolus of CM is injected into a peripheral or central vein, and its effect on myocardial signal during hyperemia (stress-only protocol) and during resting conditions (stress-rest protocol) is monitored with fast MR pulse sequences.

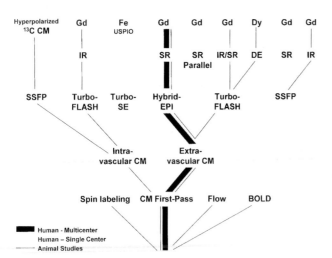

Figure 13.1. Overview of various imaging strategies for perfusion assessment combining various pulse sequences and contrast media (CM). All approaches given in the figure have been reported for cardiac imaging except for hyperpolarized ^{13}C CM, which to date has only been used for cerebral perfusion imaging. BOLD, blood oxygen level dependent (imaging); CM, contrast medium; DE, driven equilibrium (yielding T_2-weighting); Dy, dysprosium-chelate; EPI, echo-planar imaging; Fe, iron-based CM; FLASH, fast low-angle shot (imaging); Gd, gadolinium-chelate; IR, inversion recovery; SE, spin echo; SR, saturation recovery; SSFP, steady state free precession; USPIO, ultra small paramagnetic iron oxide particle.

Requirements for all CM first-pass techniques either under development or in clinical trials include: (a) providing high spatial resolution to permit detection of small subendocardial perfusion deficits, (b) providing adequate cardiac coverage to allow for assessment of the extent of perfusion deficits, and (c) featuring high CM sensitivity to generate optimum contrast between normally and abnormally perfused myocardium during CM first pass. Finally, acquisition of perfusion data should occur every 1 to 2 heartbeats to yield signal intensity time curves of adequate temporal resolution that allow for extraction of various perfusion parameters (to be discussed). To fulfill these requirements, speed of data acquisition and time-efficient magnetization preparation are crucial. Since passage of CM during hyperemic conditions only lasts 5 to 10 seconds, breathing motion is typically minimized by a breath-hold maneuver, and cardiac motion is eliminated by ECG-triggering. In contrast to scintigraphic techniques, control of cardiac and breathing motion preserves the high spatial resolution of the MR perfusion data in the order of 1–3 mm $\times$ 1–3 mm. Most commonly used are the extravascular Gadolinium (Gd-) chelates in combination with heavily T_1-weighted pulse sequences. Signal increase in the myocardium during first pass of these CM is dependent on perfusion of the myocardium and diffusion of CM into the interstitial space. Since these CM are excluded from the intracellular compartment (i.e., of viable cells with intact cell membranes), a perfusion deficit during first pass can reflect either hypoperfused viable myocardium or scar tissue. Conversely, for scintigraphic techniques, the flow tracers are taken up by viable myocytes, causing tracer accumulation and consequently an increase in signal (Fig. 13.2). In order to differentiate by MRI viable hypoperfused myocardium from scar, both demonstrating slow CM wash-in during MR first-pass studies, it is recommended to wait for equilibrium distribution of CM in the various compartments, such as blood and the extracellular-interstitial spaces of viable myocardium and scar. This occurs within 10 to 20 min post-CM injection. Subsequently, late enhancement imaging (with the inversion time set to null normal myocardium) displays hypoperfused but viable myocardium as dark tissue, while scar tissue appears bright owing to the high distribution volume of CM in the enlarged interstitial space of fibrous tissue. For comparison, during equilibrium distribution of scintigraphic tracers (occurring after rest injection or rest reinjection), tracer is not taken up by scar tissue, which consequently appears as a cold spot, while viable tissue appears as a hot spot (Fig. 13.2).

Magnetization Preparation

A high contrast between abnormally and normally perfused myocardium during peak effect of bolus can be achieved by preparing the myocardium by a 180° inversion pulse (inversion recovery [IR]) technique. Maximum contrast is obtained by nulling the signal of precontrast myocardium by applying IR times in the order of 300–400 ms (delay time of preparation recovery [TPR] from preparation to recovery, i.e., readout of central k-space lines) (35–43). However, combining this IR preparation scheme with a turbo fast low-angle shot (FLASH) read out results in a total data acquisition window of 650–750 ms/slice, which precludes the acquisition of multiple slices during 1–2 heartbeats. To circumvent this

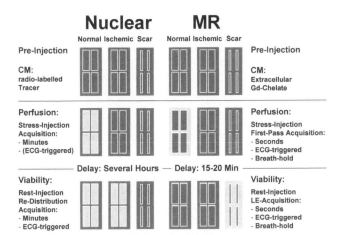

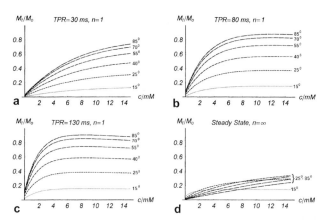

Figure 13.2. Mechanism for MR imaging and scintigraphy for the assessment of myocardial perfusion and viability. Upper row: The three main conditions of myocardium are depicted before administration of contrast media (CM), i.e., normal (nonischemic) myocardium, ischemic myocardium, and chronic scar tissue. Large rectangles represent intact myocytes (within extravascular compartment containing intravascular and extracellular space), and small rectangles represent fibrocytes (within large interstitial compartment). Middle row: Perfusion assessment. Radiolabeled tracer is trapped within viable myocytes (*bright rectangles*); less tracer accumulation occurs in hypoperfused, ischemic tissue (*middle column*), which appears as cold spot (*dark rectangles*). For MR in normally perfused myocardium, MR CM distributes within the extracellular compartment during first pass (intravascular space is not shown for clarity), causing signal increase. In hypoperfused myocardium (*middle column*), first-pass wash-in kinetics are delayed. In hypoperfused scar tissue, negligible accumulation occurs for both radiotracer and MR CM. For viability assessment (*bottom row*), equilibrium distribution is required for both radiotracer and MR CM. In scintigraphy, radiotracer is not accumulated in fibrocytes and scar appears as a cold spot (fixed defect) (*middle row*), while radiotracer accumulates in viable myocytes of ischemic myocardium, yielding a hot spot (reversible defect, as discussed above). For MR, distribution volume of MR CM in scar tissue is large, with consequent high concentration of MR CM. Scar tissue appears bright on late enhancement MR imaging (with inversion time nulling viable myocardium). Of importance, the combined perfusion viability MR study is short since equilibrium distribution is typically achieved within 15–20 min. In addition, data acquisition by MR lasts a few seconds only, allowing the use of breath holding and ECG triggering, which preserves a high spatial resolution of the perfusion and viability data.

Figure 13.3. The simulations show the influence of the delay time between a 90° saturation recovery preparation pulse and readout (time of preparation recovery [TPR]) on the signal response (fast gradient echo-pulse sequence with TR/TE of 5/1 ms) for various contrast medium (CM) concentrations c, with r_1 and r_2 of 4 and 6 mM^{-1}·s^{-1}, respectively (native T_1 and T_2: 1 s and 35 ms, respectively). The signal response curves are shown for the first TR period (n = 1) (**A–C**) and for the steady state (n = ∞) (**D**). The readout flip angles are 15°, 25°, 40°, 55°, 70°, and 85° (with dash lengths increasing with flip angle). The maximum signal and the sensitivity to changes of the CM concentration c at low concentrations increase with TPR (**A–C**). At higher concentrations, however, c cannot be unambiguously inferred from the signal with increasing TPR (clipping of the signal) (**B,C**). The steady state signal no longer depends on details of the magnetization preparation (**D**).

concentration relationship is important, but also the number of excitations required to achieve steady state of magnetization. Further, TPR should result in acquisition windows, which are placed within phases of minimal motion during the cardiac cycle. A TPR of 120 ms in combination with a hybrid echo-planar readout scheme can result in an acquisition window as short as 240 ms/slice (46). This combination avoids data acquisitions during rapid cardiac motion—such as during early systole, early diastole, and late diastole (atrial contraction)—over a wide range of heart rates that may occur during hyperemia. This very fast approach allows for multislice data acquisition while preserving a high sampling rate. To speed up the acquisition, some suggest playing out one single nonslice selective 90° saturation pulse and acquiring all slices in series thereafter (47). With this scheme, however, the delay time varies from slice to slice, and consequently CM sensitivity becomes dependent upon slice position, potentially complicating data analysis. In a modified version of a saturation recovery preparation, the entire myocardium experienced a 90° saturation pulse except for the slice of tissue that was immediately imaged after preparation (48). With this scheme, the time period for read out of slice$_n$ was utilized to prepare slice$_{n+1}$, etc. (i.e., the acquisition window equaled the saturation recovery time). This approach allows acquisition of seven slices every 2 heartbeats at heart rates up to 115 beats/min.

Magnetic Resonance Data Read Out

Conventional turbo-FLASH pulse sequences were often used in the past for perfusion imaging. With this technique,

problem, partial preparation flip angles, such as 45° to 60°, have been suggested, allowing for shorter delay times (TPR) (44,45). However, this limits the dynamic range of signal response (29).

A saturation recovery preparation by a 90° pulse is particularly attractive since it shortens the delay time TPR to 100–150 ms (29) and additionally renders the sequence heart rate independent. Figure 13.3 demonstrates the influence of increasing TPR following a 90° preparation on signal response for a fast gradient echo-pulse sequence (TR/TE 5/1 ms, r_1 and r_2^* of CM is 4 and 6 mmol^{-1}·s^{-1}, respectively). With increasing TPR, the sensitivity of the pulse sequence for low CM concentrations increases; however, at the cost of reduced sensitivity at higher CM concentrations. In order to select the optimum TPR, not only the signal intensity CM

each k-line is preceded by a radiofrequency excitation, which results in a readout duration in the order of 350–450 ms depending on the number of phase-encoding steps and duration of TR (35–42). Since this acquisition window is too long to allow for multislice imaging, faster echo-planar pulse sequences became popular (49–51), particularly when broken up in fewer lines per radiofrequency excitation, known as hybrid echo-planar pulse sequences (29,44–46). This technique reduces TE and consequently renders the sequence more robust with respect to potential susceptibility artifacts. With these accelerated pulse sequences, several k-lines are acquired following one single radiofrequency excitation, reducing the TR per k-line down to <2 ms and consequently substantially reducing total acquisition window/slice. Since fast imaging is inherently conflicting with signal-to-noise ratio, readout strategies during steady state conditions of magnetization appear promising since they preserve magnetization and thus a high signal-to-noise ratio. This technique has been employed successfully in animal models for monitoring CM first pass through the myocardium (52). In a human volunteer study, however, ECG triggering, the presence of artifacts (banding artifact probably due to off-resonance), and a low signal increase (approximately 40% of baseline signal) were problematic (53). A high image quality, reflected by a substantial signal increase in the myocardium during first pass, appears crucial for reliable CAD detection, and even offsets some compromise in cardiac coverage (29). Nevertheless, improving cardiac coverage without the need to reduce spatial and temporal resolution would be beneficial since extent of CAD correlates with outcome. Parallel imaging approaches can increase coverage without a compromise in spatial and temporal resolution. In a recent study in human volunteers, the loss in signal-to-noise ratio given by $g \times \sqrt{R}$ (with g being the so-called geometry factor and R the accelerating factor) was compensated for by a longer TR owing to implementation of TSENSE, a modification of SENSE (54), and increasing the

readout flip angle from 20° to 30°. This accelerated hybrid echo-planar saturation recovery technique yielded twice as many slices as obtained with the nonparallel approach, while signal-to-noise ratio improved by approximately 20% (55). Further studies in patients will certainly define the value of this approach with respect to diagnostic performance.

Imaging Parameters and Myocardial Signal Response

The concept of CM first-pass perfusion imaging is based on the assumption that the CM administered intravenously is delivered to the myocardium in relation to tissue perfusion; consequently, the relationship between signal intensity and CM concentration should be known. With fast gradient echo-pulse sequences, the extravascular Gd-chelates typically show an increase in myocardial signal intensity up to a maximum (T_1-dominated behavior) and signal decreases at higher CM concentrations (T_2-dominated behavior). The pulse sequence applied should show a linear CM concentration signal-intensity relationship. This relationship is dependent on the type of pulse sequence and the imaging parameters such as magnetization preparation, delay time TPR, readout flip angle, k-space trajectories during read out, and others. Figure 13.3 demonstrates that signal response is not only influenced by TPR but also by the readout flip angle. During repetitive radiofrequency excitations, the curves (Fig. 13.3A–C) approach steady state magnetization, which yields the curves shown in Figure 13.3D. Varying signal responses for different TR periods, however, cause signal inhomogeneities in k-space and thus image artifacts. Figure 13.4 shows the course of signal response during successive TR periods in relation to TPR and readout flip angle. At higher flip angles, the steady state is approached earlier for a given TPR, while a shorter TPR of 11.6 ms (at 55° readout flip angle) would achieve steady state already after first TR. These considerations might illustrate that imaging parameters strongly affect

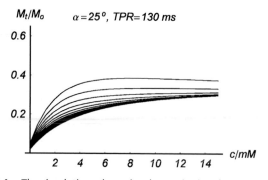
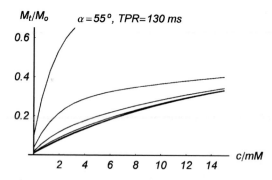

Figure 13.4. The simulations show the change in signal response for different time of recovery (TR) periods, n. Signal response curves for every second of the first 64 TR periods are shown for two different flip angles 25° and 55° in **(A)** and **(B)**, respectively (other assumptions are as for simulations shown in Figure 13.3). Assuming ideal spoiling of transverse magnetization, the steady state is approached in earlier TR periods for higher flip angles. At 55°, all signals acquired after approximately 6 dummy scans well match the steady state signal, which resulted in a homogenous signal response in k-space. This could possibly reduce artifacts along the phase-encoding direction and keep their magnitude at a constant level for all CM concentrations. In contrast, for a flip angle of 25° and a delay TPR of 130 ms, the signal for different TR periods varies considerably. Daniel Nanz, PhD, is acknowledged for performing the simulations, providing the material for Figures 13.3 and 13.4, and for his sound insights in MR physics, which he has shared with the author over the past years.

signal response and should be optimized with respect to dynamic range of signal response, signal intensity CM concentration relationship, homogeneity of signal in k space, and timing of acquisition during the cardiac cycle. A study in phantoms demonstrated that optimization of a hybrid echoplanar pulse sequence (44) with respect to TPR, readout flip angle, and preparation flip angle could improve signal response of Gd-DTPA-doped phantoms from 80% (of no doped phantom) to 250%, which ultimately increased diagnostic performance in patients significantly (29). However, changes in these parameters typically go along with changes in the acquisition window/slice, which can affect cardiac coverage.

Ideally, perfusion data would be evaluated by dedicated algorithms rather than by subjective reading (to be discussed). This approach would allow comparison of signal responses in an individual patient with a normal database, rendering the technique less observer dependent. In this scenario, it should be kept in mind that in case the pulse sequence and/or the imaging parameters are modified (e.g., by a hardware or software upgrade), an adaptation of the normal values in the database is required. These technical considerations illustrate that myocardial signal response is strongly dependent on imaging parameters and that further studies will be needed to generate possible standards for MR perfusion imaging as a prerequisite for a broader application of this technique.

CONTRAST MEDIA

After administration of an exogenous CM into the circulation, such as into a peripheral vein, observed myocardial signal changes reflect changes in the CM concentration and thus are related to perfusion. However, the relation between signal and CM concentration is not only dependent on the type of pulse sequence and the imaging parameters, but also on the type and dose of CM. While conventional T_1-shortening CM, such as extravascular Gd-chelates, induce a signal increase in normally perfused myocardium during first pass, other classes of extravascular CM (e.g., T_2*-shortening CM such as dysprosium chelates) induce a signal loss (Fig. 13.5). Even Gd-chelates at higher concentrations can induce a signal decrease during first pass when combined with a T_2-weighted sequence (56,57). Thus, the signal CM concentration relationship is typically nonlinear and can even be inverse depending on CM type, dose, and pulse sequences applied. This is fundamentally different from ischemia detection based on the assessment of wall motion, where new onset of dysfunction unambiguously indicates the presence of ischemia.

T_1-ENHANCING EXTRAVASCULAR CONTRAST MEDIA

T_1-enhancing extravascular CM are the most frequently used media and represent the conventional extravascular Gd-chelates. Administration of these CM typically induce an

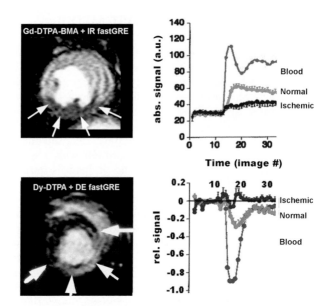

Figure 13.5. Effect of the type of CM and pulse sequence on first-pass signal response in blood and myocardium. Top row: A conventional extravascular Gadolinium-chelate (Gd-DTPA-BMA) is administered in a dog model with critical stenosis of the left circumflex coronary artery during vasodilation (induced by dipyridamole) and combined with an inversion recovery fast gradient echo-pulse sequence (IR-fast GRE). At the peak effect of the bolus (*left*), hypoperfused myocardium appears dark (*arrows*) and normally perfused myocardium appears bright. The gray signal intensity time curve on the right shows normal signal increase, and the black curve shows delayed signal increase of hypoperfused myocardium.

Bottom row: An extravascular Dysprosium-chelate (Dy-DTPA) is applied to the same animal model. In combination with a T_2-weighted (driven-equilibrium) fast gradient echo sequence (DE-fast GRE), the CM induces a signal loss. Consequently, at the peak effect of the CM (*left*), the hypoperfused myocardium appears bright (*arrows*), and normally perfused myocardium appears dark. Accordingly, the signal intensity time curve of normal myocardium shows a signal drop (*gray curve*). (Images courtesy of C.B. Higgins, MD, M. Saeed, PhD, and M. Wendland, PhD, from the University of California, San Francisco.

increase in myocardial signal during first pass, which allows detection of hypoperfused myocardium as territories of lower signal by visual assessment or by a quantitative approach extracting various parameters from the signal intensity time curves (to be discussed). Studies demonstrated a strong impact of maximum achievable myocardial signal increase during first pass on diagnostic performance (29). Therefore, the best test performance is expected for high CM doses (in combination with pulse sequences with strong T_1-weighting). This provides a large dynamic range of signal response in the myocardium, i.e., a large signal difference between normally perfused and hypoperfused territories. However, at higher CM doses, susceptibility artifacts may occur at the subendocardium, where differences in CM concentrations between blood and myocardium are particularly high during first pass. In a multicenter trial, strongly T_1-weighted sequences (saturation recovery preparation and hybrid echo-planar readout) showed absence of a susceptibility induced signal drop in the subendocardial layer up to doses of 0.15 mmol/kg of an extravascular Gd-chelate (4).

INTRAVASCULAR CONTRAST MEDIA

T_1-enhancing intravascular CM such as albumin-targeted MS-325 (45) or polylysine-Gd (58,59) have been applied in animal models. In these studies, differences (for group means) between normally perfused and stenosis-dependent hypoperfused myocardium were reported. However, to the best of our knowledge, these intravascular Gd-based CM have not yet been tested in humans. Intravascular superparamagnetic iron oxide nanoparticles (USPIO) with a starch coating were used for perfusion studies in humans (60). In combination with a T_2-weighted turbo spin-echo sequence, a signal drop in normal myocardium of 59% (in eight patients) was observed; however, this CM is no longer under investigation owing to iron accumulation in the liver. Since susceptibility influences signal drop of T_2*-enhancing CM, not only the concentration of CM in the voxel but also its intravoxel distribution (homogeneous versus inhomogeneous) determines its T_2*-shortening effect, thus rendering such an approach susceptible to vessel architecture (orientation and intervessel distance). This principle was demonstrated with a dysprosium-chelate in an elegant experimental model of reperfusion injury (61). Since T_2* approaches are affected by these geometry factors (which are not known *a priori*), measurements of tissue CM concentrations by T_1 techniques are considered superior.

HYPERPOLARIZED CONTRAST MEDIA

Conventional Gd-chelates act by modulating the signal from surrounding water molecules by accelerating their relaxation rates. The low polarization level of the spin population of the nuclear magnetic resonance active nuclei at the thermal equilibrium at a field strength of 1.5 T is compensated by the vast abundance of water molecules in the human body. One way to increase signal would be to increase the field strength since the polarization level increases with magnetic flux density. Alternatively, however, the polarization level of the spin population of specific nuclei such as liquid ^{13}C in various compounds can be increased by a factor of up to 100,000 (as compared with polarization of water protons at the thermal equilibrium). For this purpose, two techniques—dynamic nuclear polarization (62) and parahydrogen-induced polarization (63)—were recently described. A major advantage of hyperpolarized ^{13}C CM is that the signal is only received from the ^{13}C-nuclei; thus, no signal from background tissue is obtained. This theoretically allows for absolute quantification of perfusion since the signal is directly proportional to the amount of ^{13}C molecules. However, since the spin population of ^{13}C molecules is far from thermal equilibrium, longitudinal magnetization decays with specific time constants (depending on the type of the ^{13}C compound). Thus, CM depolarization must be taken into account similarly to radiotracer modeling that corrects for tracer decay. In addition, depolarization due to repetitive radiofrequency pulsing also has to be considered, which further destroys longitudinal magnetization depending on the pulse sequence type and the imaging parameters. Johansson et al showed that depolarization can be approximated by a monoexponential function with a time constant T_D, and

successfully applied this concept for cerebral perfusion quantification (64).

ANALYSIS OF PERFUSION DATA

A variety of studies have demonstrated that hypoperfused myocardium supplied by stenosed coronary arteries can be detected by visual assessment of first-pass data (4,5,42,43,46,65). A visual approach takes advantage of an experienced observer able to differentiate hypoperfusion that causes reduced myocardial signal from artifacts. Thus, a visual assessment by an experienced reader may yield a high portion of correct diagnoses, but at the cost of some interreader variability (unless reading criteria are strictly defined and easily assessable by different readers). Therefore, a computer-assisted or automatic analysis of perfusion data would be highly desirable and could potentially render MR perfusion analyses fully reproducible. An automatic analysis, of course, not only eliminates observer variability but also saves human resources. Elimination of observer variability is particularly important if individual patient data are compared with a normal database and for repetitive studies performed to monitor disease activity. Since many different analysis procedures were reported, some common definitions for analysis characteristics have been proposed (Fig. 13.6). A quantitative approach is also ideal in order to generate receiver-operator characteristics (ROC) curves, which are the adequate means for assessment of test performance. Once a ROC curve for a specific protocol (including data analysis) is determined, optimum cost-effectiveness of the test can be calculated since cost-effectiveness changes with changing portions of false and true negatives and positives.

Perfusion Data Assessment

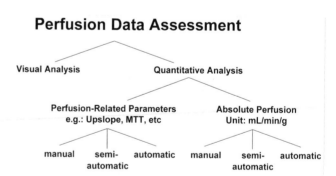

Figure 13.6. Perfusion data can be assessed in many ways and some inconsistency is noted when analysis procedures are reported. A scheme is proposed for better definition of possible analysis strategies. In this scheme, "quantitative" is defined as results that are obtained in numbers, allowing for comparison of studies both in cross section (e.g., patient data vs. normal database) and longitudinally (e.g., monitoring disease activity). Irrespective whether these quantitative analyses yield perfusion-related parameters or absolute perfusion, the results are obtained either (a) manually (and thus are associated with some observer dependence); (b) in a semiautomatic fashion, i.e., some observer interaction with the data set is present (again associated with some minor observer dependence); or (c) such quantitative data are obtained automatically, thus eliminating any observer interaction with the data, which completely eliminates analysis variability. MMT, mean transit time.

VISUAL ASSESSMENT

In order to minimize observer variability, well-defined criteria need to be sensitive to the detection of delayed CM wash in and yet specific in order to differentiate perfusion defects from artifacts. Relatively long persistence of zones with low signal during first pass are suggestive for the presence of hypoperfusion, particularly when located in the subendocardial layer (46,66). It is conceivable that criteria that increase specificity most likely will decrease sensitivity and vice versa. Accordingly, it has been suggested that test performances be based on ROC curves (67,68). These analyses demonstrated that different readers tend to read at different thresholds, resulting in high observer variabilities with kappa values as low as 0.30 (5).

QUANTITATIVE APPROACH: PERFUSION-RELATED PARAMETERS

Since first-pass perfusion studies are typically performed during a breath hold, a first step in any type of a quantitative approach involves registration of the first-pass data over time, (i.e., motion in the data caused by breathing and/or diaphragmatic drift should be eliminated either by a manual procedure or by [semi-] automatic algorithms) (69–71). From the resulting signal intensity (time curves of various transmural or subendocardial segments covering ideally the entire left ventricular myocardium), a variety of parameters can be extracted, such as peak signal intensity (35,36,45,72), signal change over time (slope) (29,39–41,46,72–74), arrival time, time to peak signal, mean transit time (72,73,75,76), area under the signal intensity time curve (52), etc. A candidate parameter for a broader clinical application should demonstrate on one hand a close correlation with tissue perfusion, and on the other hand should prove a low interobserver and intertest variability. For the upslope of the signal intensity time curve, a relatively close correlation with perfusion data is reported in both animal (73,77) and human studies (46), while its robustness was demonstrated in a multicenter trial (4). This upslope parameter is relatively insensitive to CM recirculation since it uses the initial portion of the signal intensity time curve only, and also reduces the sensitivity of this parameter for motion (most patients are able hold their breath for this short time period). Taking into account that cardiac perfusion studies are performed with phased-array coils, analyses of signal intensity time curves have to correct for inhomogeneous coil sensitivities. As a correction, it has been suggested that the precontrast signal be subtracted from the first-pass signal intensities (47). However, signal reception by a phased-array coil does not cause a constant offset of signal over the field-of-view; instead the signal decreases with increasing distance from the coil, which consequently requires a division of first-pass signal by precontrast signal for correction (4,46). Signal response in the myocardium is not only dependent on coil distance but also on the arterial input. To obtain an estimate of the arterial input, myocardial upslope data are often divided by the upslope of signal in the left ventricular blood pool (29,40,41,46,74). This approach is suboptimal for input correction and may fail in situations with substantial variations in hemodynamics. Further, an experimental study demonstrated linearity between the upslope and perfusion measured by microspheres for low perfusion values only (77). At perfusion levels higher than approximately 1.5 mL/min/g, the upslope underestimated true perfusion (77). A similar relationship was described for humans using PET perfusion measurements as the standard of reference (46). This nonlinearity in the high-flow range would be particularly problematic if measurements would involve low- and high-flow states as for CFR calculations. Absolute quantification of perfusion would be helpful for the CFR approach.

QUANTITATIVE APPROACH: ABSOLUTE TISSUE PERFUSION

While several models exist for perfusion measurements, CM first-pass techniques with residue detection will be addressed. It is assumed that CM diluted in blood enters the tissue via the artery, passes through the capillaries, and leaves the tissue through the venous system. The CM concentration in the tissue is then solely determined by the arterial input and venous outflow through the conservation of mass (Fick principle, 1870). The relationship between arterial CM concentration (arterial input function), tissue CM concentration, and tissue perfusion is described by a convolution integral. The model introduced by Kety takes both CM inflow and outflow into account and assumes a freely diffusible CM that is homogeneously mixed within a single tissue compartment (78). It is described by the following formula:

$$\text{Equation 1: } C_T(t) = F \cdot \int_0^t C_A \cdot (\tau) \cdot e^{-F/\lambda\,(t-\tau)}\,d\tau$$
$$= C_A(t) \otimes F \cdot e^{-F/\lambda \cdot t}$$

where C_T is the tissue CM concentration at time t, C_A is the CM concentration in blood, F is tissue perfusion (in mL/min/g), λ is the tissue-blood partition coefficient, and $\otimes$ denotes convolution. This approach does not require assumptions on the shape of the arterial input function, and after measurements of C_T and C_A, F and λ can be determined by a two-parameter fit (by application of a three-parameter fit, blood volume V_B can be incorporated in the model as well). Several deconvolution routines have been used to obtain F (77, 79–82). In the case of nonfreely diffusible CM, the extraction fraction E must also be considered (83–85), where E is related to F by:

$$\text{Equation 2: } K_i = E \times F = F\,(1 - e^{-PS/F})$$

with PS being the permeability-surface-area product (in mL/g/s) and K_i the unidirectional influx constant (in mL/g/s).

For blood pool CM, which are restricted to the intravascular compartment and therefore do not mix homogeneously in the tissue compartment, the so-called bolus tracking approach, based on the central volume principle (Stewart, 1894), is typically applied as follows:

$$\text{Equation 3: } V_B = F \times MTT$$

with MTT being the mean transit time (expected distribution of transit times for the blood through the tissue volume).

Since the extravascular Gd-chelates do not cross the intact blood-brain barrier, this model is the preferred one for cerebral perfusion. However, hyperpolarized ^{13}C CM can act as intravascular tracers (64) and hence, this model could become attractive for cardiac studies using these types of CM.

For all models mentioned, measurement of the arterial CM concentration over time, (i.e., the arterial input function) is crucial. As a prerequisite, an accurate mathematic description of the signal intensity CM concentration relationship over the full range of CM concentrations occurring in the blood pool during first-pass conditions is required (58,80,86,87). As previously mentioned, in order to achieve an appropriate contrast-to-noise level for the signal response in the myocardium, relatively high CM doses would be desirable. However, such high doses are likely to cause a clipping of the signal intensity time curve from which a conversion of signal intensities into CM concentration is not possible. To solve this, Christian et al (77) presented a dual bolus approach, whereby a small CM bolus was injected first for determination of an arterial input function, followed by a larger CM bolus to achieve an adequate signal response in the myocardium. In a canine model, this approach yielded absolute values of tissue perfusion in close agreement with microsphere measurements. Alternatively, Gatehouse et al (88) proposed a dual T_1 sensitivity method that used a single high-dose CM bolus injection, thus providing adequate signal response in the myocardium while preventing clipping of blood signal at peak effect of the bolus. The latter is achieved by applying a short saturation recovery TPR to measure blood signal (low T_1 sensitivity for very short T_1), while TPR is longer for measurement of myocardial signal

(high T_1 sensitivity for longer T_1). Furthermore, to speed up the acquisition for the low T_1-sensitive blood-pool measurements, a low spatial resolution is implemented. With this dual T_1 sensitivity single-bolus approach, perfusion reserve estimates closely matched the dual bolus results in a set of volunteers. Once a reliable arterial input function is obtained, different models for calculation of perfusion may be applied. Since conventional CM exert their effect indirectly through water proton relaxation, diffusion of water molecules between the intravascular and extravascular compartments modifies the MR signal during first pass (89–92). If the effect of an intravascular CM would be confined to the intravascular compartment (e.g., no water exchange), maximum achievable signal during first pass would approximate 10% of fully relaxed magnetization (assuming a blood volume in tissue of 10%), whereas an extravascular CM mixed homogeneously in the extravascular space by diffusion would yield a maximum signal during first pass of 20% of fully relaxed magnetization (assuming an extracellular compartment of 20% and the absence of any water exchange between compartments). As shown in Figure 13.7, intravascular and extravascular CM yielded approximately 50% and 70% of fully relaxed magnetization during first pass, respectively. These results indicate that water exchange across both capillary vessel walls and cell membranes strongly affects the signal generation (89). Generally, water exchange conditions are categorized into fast, intermediate, and slow. For fast water exchange, myocardial signal response in the presence

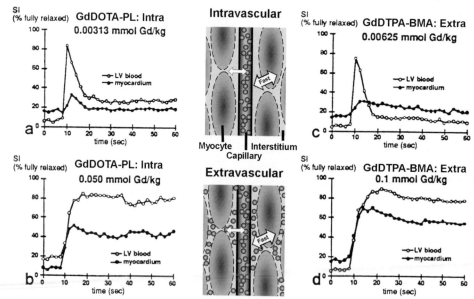

Figure 13.7. **(A,B)** Signal intensity time curves (STC) after administration of an intravascular Gadolinium-chelate (bound to polylysine [PL]). Note the different shape of the STC for blood (*open circles*) with marked clipping of the peak signal for the higher dose **(B)** compared with the lower dose **(A)**. For a series of increasing CM doses (data not shown), myocardial signal for the intravascular CM saturated at approximately 50% of fully relaxed signal **(B)**. This signal behavior is explained by a restricted water exchange between intravascular and extravascular compartment (*small arrow in the corresponding scheme*) and the fast water exchange between extravascular/extracellular and intracellular compartment (*large arrow in the scheme*) (*top*). **(C,D)** STC after administration of an extravascular Gadolinium-chelate (Gd-DTPA-BMA). Again, the STC for blood (*open circles*) is clipped for the higher dose **(D)**. For the extravascular CM, myocardial signal saturates at approximately 70% of fully relaxed signal **(D)**. This signal behavior is explained by perfusion and additional diffusion of CM into the extravascular compartment and the fast water exchange between extravascular/extracellular and intracellular compartment (*large arrow in the scheme*) (*bottom*). (From Wendland MF, Saeed M, Yu KK, et al. Inversion recovery EPI of bolus transit in rat myocardium using intravascular and extravascular gadolinium-based MR contrast media: dose effects on peak signal enhancement. *Magn Reson Med* 1994;32:319–329.)

of a CM would be unaffected be water exchange, i.e., tissue $1/T_1$ ($= r_1$) increases linearly with intravascular r_1 (with the slope of this relationship representing blood volume). Thus, fast water exchange changes in r_1 in tissue reflect changes in r_1 of blood. Fast water exchange exists if the rate of water exchange between compartments is considerably higher than the difference in r_1 between the compartments in the presence of CM. Larsson et al (93) performed simulations on the basis of the tracer kinetic model proposed by Kety (78) to calculate the unidirectional influx constant K_i for diffusion of CM over the capillary membrane (in mL/min/g) using Equations 1 and 2. For low doses of extravascular CM, e.g., 0.1 mmol/kg body weight to limit differences in r_1 between compartments and assuming E greater 0.3, water exchange only minimally affected K_i, while water exchange strongly affected the signal generated by intravascular CM (93). Similar findings were reported by other groups (90–92), demonstrating that intra- and extravascular water exchange is the rate-limiting step for signal generation in tissue (slow exchange regime) (Fig. 13.7). Accordingly, neglecting water exchange for intravascular CM could result in considerable errors in perfusion measurements.

In addition to water exchange in ischemic tissue, leakage of intravascular CM across capillary membranes may occur (94,95). For extravascular CM, Tong et al demonstrated substantial changes of E for different levels of myocardial perfusion similar to radioactive tracers (85). Nevertheless, other investigators assumed no relevant changes in E for resting and hyperemic conditions, allowing them to determine K_i at rest and during hyperemia to calculate a perfusion index or CFR (96,97). Besides precision, the robustness of parameter estimates is another important aspect of different models in combination with extravascular and intravascular CM. Based on simulations, regional blood volume and E were most sensitive for noise when determined by extravascular CM (83), while other studies showed intravascular CM being more reliable for regional blood volume determinations (98,99). Despite a large body of simulations (83,98) and experimental data (58,80), the clinical value of quantitative measures for the detection of CAD in patients still remains unclear.

With hyperpolarized ^{13}C-CM water exchange does not affect the MR signal and consequently, perfusion quantification becomes feasible without assumptions on water exchange. From the signal received from the ^{13}C molecules, their concentration can be readily calculated if the level of polarization is known. Since depolarization of a hyperpolarized CM in an imaged slice is dependent on relaxation times (which are in the order of 30–60 s depending on the specific type of ^{13}C molecules) and the pulse sequence, the time constant T_D of the polarization function can be calculated to enter the appropriate models (e.g., Equation 1 or 3) to take depolarization into account (64).

PERFORMANCE OF MAGNETIC RESONANCE PERFUSION IMAGING

ANIMAL STUDIES

In animal models, the feasibility of MR first-pass perfusion imaging to detect differences in myocardial perfusion has been demonstrated repeatedly (35,36,100,101). In addition, experimental studies offer the possibility of relating estimates of myocardial perfusion derived from MR data sets to microsphere measurements, which are generally accepted as the standard of reference. Table 13.1 lists several contrast-based and noncontrast-based MR techniques and provides the correlations achieved versus microsphere measurements. In a study using BOLD imaging, percent signal enhancement on T_2-weighted images was determined in normally perfused and hyperemic myocardium (28). The ratio for the two myocardial territories correlated closely with the perfusion ratio determined by microspheres. However, the slope of the correlation was far away from unity (Table 13.1). Instead, Δr_2 measurements yielded a slope of 0.94 (102). Despite this excellent correlation, the sensitivity to detect differences in perfusion by this technique appears rather low since a 100% increase in flow yielded a signal increase of only 5% (e.g., change in myocardial r_2 of 0.94/s). Thus, differences in flow of 300% would be required to cause detectable changes in r_2 (102). For another non-CM-based technique, such as arterial spin labeling, an excellent agreement with microsphere measurements was reported; however, these results were obtained in nonbeating rat hearts at 4.7 T (30). While several investigators calculated slope or 1/MTT from γ-variate fits of signal intensity time curves (59,73,76), others demonstrated the possibility of quantifying perfusion in absolute measures of ml/min/g when applying sophisticated kinetic models to the MR data (58,79,80). However, 95% confidence intervals of –57% to +57% to +45% to 82% (58,79) indicate that the sensitivity of these techniques to detect changes in perfusion might be limited. Furthermore, to our knowledge, the utility of these absolute quantitative approaches for the detection of CAD in unselected patient populations has yet to be demonstrated.

HUMAN STUDIES

Single-Center Studies: Visual Assessment

Visual assessment of MR perfusion data is popular since it avoids time-consuming data postprocessing. In addition, artifacts within the data can be "overread" by the observer, at least if he is experienced in interpreting MR perfusion studies. However, this approach also introduces variability depending upon the observer performance, resulting in sensitivities/specificities as high as 83% / 100% in some studies (65), while others showed lower performance of 89% / 44% (43). These studies used quantitative coronary angiography (QCA) as the standard of reference, although the anatomical degree of stenoses did not always match the degree of perfusion abnormalities. In a recent study, MR first-pass perfusion imaging was compared with single photon emission computed tomography (SPECT) in 69 patients (103). At a dose of 0.075 mmol/kg of Gd-DTPA injected into a peripheral vein during vasodilation, visual assessment yielded a sensitivity and specificity of 90% and 85%, respectively, for the detection of stenoses with ≥70% diameter reduction on QCA. In comparison with SPECT, MR performed significantly better with areas under the ROC curves (AUC) of 0.89–0.91 for observer 1 and 2, respectively, versus AUC of 0.71–0.75 for SPECT (103).

TABLE 13-1 Experimental MR Perfusion Imaging: Comparison Versus Microsphere Measurements

Authors	MR approach	CM	Analysis	Corr. r	Slope	Intercept	Animal	No.	Model
BOLD									
Fieno et al (28)	Bold T2-weighted	no	% SI-enhancement ratio	0.80	0.08	0.94	dogs	13	occlusions adeno
Wright et al (102)	Bold 3D T2-weighted	no	ΔR_2 ratio	0.80	0.94	0.02	dogs	9	adeno
Spin-labeling									
Reeder et al (30)	spin-labeling (at 4.7 T)	no	$1/T_{1app}$	0.91 to 0.97	0.62 to 0.67	0.45 to 0.46	rabbits	3	occlusion non-beating heart (Langendorff)
Poncelet et al (31)	spin-labeling	no	$1/T_{1app}$	0.83	0.62	0.64	pigs	6	adeno
Extravascular CM									
Wilke et al (73)	IR turbo-FLASH	extra	γ-variate fit 1/MTT upslope of STC	0.89 0.66	0.02	0.03	dogs	3	occlusions stenosis/dip
Wilke et al (82)	SR turbo-FLASH	extra	fermi function ratio: $R_F(0)$	0.88	0.92	0.10	pigs	8	occlusions adeno
Klocke et al (52)	IR true-Fisp	extra	ratio: AUC	0.93	0.96	0.07	dogs	12	occlusions stenosis/adeno
Christian et al (77)	SR hybrid EPI	extra	dual bolus fermi function upslope of STC	0.95 0.69	0.95	0.10	dogs	16	occlusions adeno
Intravascular CM									
Wilke et al (58)	IR turbo-FLASH	intra	multiple pathway axially distributed model (ml/min/g)	−0.1*	−0.92 to 0.72**	—	dogs	7	stenosis/adeno
Kraitchman et al (59)	IR turbo-FLASH	intra	γ-variate fit ratio: upslope	0.77	—	—	dogs	7	stenosis/dobut
Lombardi et al (76)	IR turbo-FLASH (at 0.5 T)	intra	γ-variate fit 1/MTT	0.70	—	—	pigs	5	stenosis/adeno
Kraitchman et al (45)	Partial presaturation Hybrid echo-planar	intra	% SI-enhancement ratio	0.80	0.58	0.33	pigs	12	stenosis/dip
Jerosch-Herold et al (79)	SR turbo-FLASH	intra	model-indep. decon. blood flow (ml/min/g) perfusion reserve	−0.06* 0.0*	−45% to 45%** −57% to 57%**		pigs	4	occlusions adeno

All studies were performed on 1.5 T systems unless noted otherwise.
Adeno, adenosine; AUC, area under the signal intensity time curve; BOLD, blood oxygen level dependent (imaging); CM, contrast medium; dip, dipyridamole; dobut, dobutamine; EPI, echo-planar imaging; extra, extravascular CM; Fisp, fast imaging with steady-state precession; FLASH, fast low-angle shot acquisition; intra, intravascular CM; IR, inversion recovery; micro, radio-labeled microspheres; mod-indep. decon, model-independent deconvolution; MTT, mean transit time; $R_F(0) = F$, the impulse response amplitude represents relative measure of perfusion; Ratio, ischemic/normal region (for this correlation the same ratio is calculated for microsphere measurements); SI, signal intensity; SR, saturation recovery; STC, signal intensity time curve; T_{1app}, apparent T_1 of myocardium in presence of flow.
* Mean difference in mL/min/g (minus = underestimation by MR).
** Confidence interval of 95%.

Single-Center Studies: Quantitative (Semi-) Automatic Analysis

Calculation of rate of myocardial signal change (upslope) during first-pass conditions is probably the most widely used type of a quantitative (semi-) automatic approach yielding a perfusion-related parameter. On the basis of a single-slice IR acquisition, Al-Saadi et al (41) calculated a CFR index ($slope_{hyperemia}$ / $slope_{rest}$), yielding a sensitivity and specificity of 90% and 83%, respectively, at a CFR threshold of 1.5 for the detection of stenoses with ≥75% area reduction on QCA. In this study, as a rough estimate of the arterial input, the upslope of signal in the left ventricular blood pool was used, and the dose of the extravascular CM Gd-DTPA was kept at 0.025 mmol/kg body weight to minimize clipping of the blood pool signal intensity time curve. Peripheral administration of the same CM dose and acquisition in a multislice mode yielded a similar performance for the CFR index (calculated as previously described), with a sensitivity and specificity of 88% and 90%, respectively (AUC 0.93), for the detection of stenoses with ≥75% area reduction on QCA (47). A stress-only protocol was proposed by our group (46), and a comparable performance of the hyperemic upslope parameter was reported when thresholds were derived from a normal data base, yielding a sensitivity and specificity of 87% and 85%, respectively, for the detection of stenoses of ≥50% diameter reduction on QCA (Fig. 13.8). This stress-only protocol avoids the need for matching myocardial regions for rest and stress condition, and therefore offers easy analysis of the subendocardial layer, where perfusion abnormalities are most severe (46,66). When comparing the MR upslope parameter with PET perfusion imaging, a sensitivity and specificity of 91% and 94%, respectively was reported, with AUC of 0.93 (46).

Multicenter Studies

As previously discussed, MR perfusion imaging provides excellent spatial and temporal resolution for signal monitoring during CM first pass and is potentially the most accurate method currently available for the noninvasive assessment of myocardial perfusion in humans. However, if MR perfusion imaging should become the first line method for clinical work-up of patients with known or suspected CAD, its robustness and reliability has to be demonstrated in multicenter trials. Additionally, the optimum CM dose for CAD detection should be known. In a stress-only protocol, the upslope parameter performed best with relatively high CM doses ranging from 0.10 to 0.15 mmol/kg Gd-DTPA, yielding an AUC of 0.91 ± 0.07 and 0.86 ± 0.08, respectively, with corresponding sensitivity/specificity of 91 / 78 and 94 / 71% for doses of 0.10 and 0.15 mmol/kg, respectively (4). Thus, this multicenter trial confirmed the high diagnostic performance of the stress-only approach in combination with an upslope analysis proposed in an earlier single-center study (46) (Fig. 13.8). However, in this multicenter, single-vendor trial, the high diagnostic performance was achieved only in data with adequate quality (a quality reading was performed first, which eliminated 14% of the studies). An example of a study at the dose of 0.15 mmol/kg is shown in Figure 13.9. At this level of data quality, the upslope approach proved to be sensitive, specific, and robust, with a kappa value of

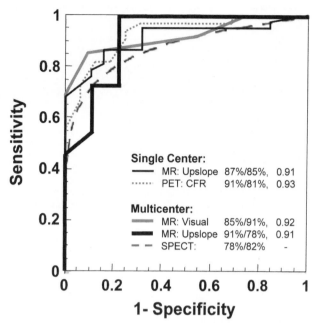

Figure 13.8. Comparison of diagnostic performance of MR perfusion imaging in single center and multicenter trials and with scintigraphic studies. A single-center study (*thin black line*) evaluated a first-pass MR stress-only protocol (saturation recovery hybrid echo-planar pulse sequence) followed by a quantitative semiautomatic analysis yielding upslope as the perfusion-related parameter. A high sensitivity and specificity for the detection of coronary artery stenoses (≥50% diameter reduction in quantitative coronary angiography) was obtained. Numbers represent sensitivity/specificity and the area under the receiver operator characteristics curve, respectively. A similar performance was achieved for positron emission tomography in that study (*dotted gray line*). (From Schwitter J, Nanz D, Kneifel S, et al. Assessment of myocardial perfusion in coronary artery disease by magnetic resonance: a comparison with positron emission tomography and coronary angiography. *Circulation* 2001;103:2230–2235.) These MR results were confirmed in a recent multicenter single-vendor trial that used a visual assessment (best of three blinded core lab readers). This approach (*gray line*), however, is susceptible to interreader variability (Fig. 13.10). Analysis of the upslope parameter (*thick black line*) in a multicenter data set, as performed in the single-center trial, again yielded high sensitivity and specificity, confirming the results of the single-center study. In addition, semiautomatic quantification of a perfusion-related parameter (*upslope*) was associated with fair-to-good interobserver agreement (Fig. 13.10). For comparison, the largest multicenter single photon emission computed tomography study yielded similar diagnostic performance (*dark dotted line*). (With permission from Wolff S, Schwitter J, Coulden R, et al. Myocardial first-pass perfusion magnetic resonance imaging: a multicenter dose-ranging study. *Circulation* 2004;110:732–737; Giang T, Nanz D, Coulden R, et al. Detection of coronary artery disease by Magnetic Resonance myocardial perfusion imaging with various contrast medium doses: first European multicenter experience. *Eur Heart J* 2004; 25:1657–1665; and Hendel RC, Berman DS, Cullom SJ, et al. Multicenter clinical trial to evaluate the efficacy of correction for photon attenuation and scatter in SPECT myocardial perfusion imaging. *Circulation* 1999;99:2742–2749.)

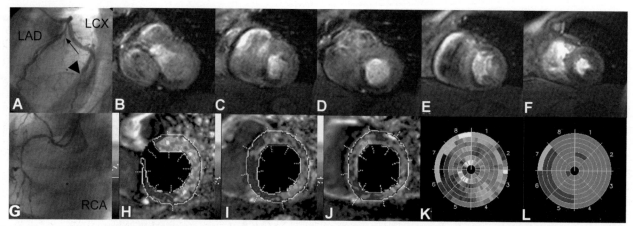

Figure 13.9.   Example of an MR perfusion study for a dose of 0.15 mmol/kg body weight of Gd-DTPA (saturation recovery hybrid echo-planar pulse sequence). **(A)** Distal stenosis in the large left circumflex coronary artery (LCX) is shown (*arrow head*). Another stenosis is present in the small first diagonal branch of the left anterior descending coronary artery (LAD) (*arrow*) on x-ray coronary angiography. Five short-axis MR perfusion images at peak bolus effect **(B–F)** demonstrate low signal areas in the inferior wall and a small hypointense area in the anterior wall **(E,F)**. **(H–J)** Corresponding upslope maps. **(K)** Polar maps for the subendocardial layer are given with thresholds applied pixel-wise and for the entire segments **(L)** with blue/red encoding for upslope values below/above the thresholds, respectively. This study further demonstrates the limitation of using coronary anatomy as a reference for perfusions studies: The perfusion defects in segments 5 and 6 (typically assigned to the right coronary artery) represent a mismatch with the right coronary artery perfusion territory, which is supplied by a large LCX in this patient. (Reproduced with permission from Giang T, Nanz D, Coulden R, et al. Detection of coronary artery disease by Magnetic Resonance myocardial perfusion imaging with various contrast medium doses: first European multicenter experience. *Eur Heart J* 2004;25:1657–1665.)

0.73 for interobserver agreement (4). In comparison, Figure 13.10 shows kappa values for interobserver agreement for a multicenter scintigraphy study (104) as well as for multicenter MR perfusion studies (4–6). Figure 13.10 clearly demonstrates the potential disadvantage of a pure visual assessment of perfusion studies.

Several single-center studies suggested a superiority of MR perfusion imaging over scintigraphic techniques

(46,103). Therefore, a large multicenter, multivendor trial was performed to compare MR perfusion imaging not only with QCA, but also with SPECT imaging (6). Two hundred forty-one patients were studied in 18 centers. This study again confirmed the high diagnostic performance of the MR first-pass perfusion approach and also showed superiority over SPECT imaging (6). As shown in Figure 13.10, the low kappa value for visual reading of these multicenter, mul-

Figure 13.10.   A high reproducibility of perfusion data analysis is crucial for a broader application of a diagnostic technique in both clinical routine and research. Kappa values for interreader agreement are given for three approaches, involving no standardization of visual readings, some standardization for visual reading procedures, and uniform quantitative algorithms (semiautomatic quantitative approach yielding upslope values). In this comparison, visual readings of multicenter, multivendor data with some standardizations performed poorly (*gray bar*), while multicenter, single-vendor data yielded poor-to-fair results (*black bar, middle column*). For a semiautomatic analysis of multicenter single-vendor data (*black bar, right*), however, fair-to-good results were achieved. Similar observations were reported for multicenter, multivendor scintigraphic data (*hashed bars*). (Reproduced with permission from Schwitter J, Bauer W, van Rossum AC, et al. MR perfusion imaging for detection coronary artery disease: a multicenter dose finding study in comparison with x-ray coronary angiography and single photon emission computed tomography. *Circulation* 2004;111:643; Wolff S, Schwitter J, Coulden R, et al. Myocardial first-pass perfusion magnetic resonance imaging: a multicenter dose-ranging study. *Circulation* 2004;110:732–737; Giang T, Nanz D, Coulden R, et al. Detection of coronary artery disease by magnetic resonance myocardial perfusion imaging with various contrast medium doses: first European multicenter experience. *Eur Heart J* 2004;25:1657–1665; and Wackers FJT, Bodenheimer M, Fleiss JL, Brown M, et al. Factors affecting uniformity in interpretation of planar Thallium-201 imaging in a multicenter trial. *J Am Coll Cardiol* 1993;21:1064–1074.)

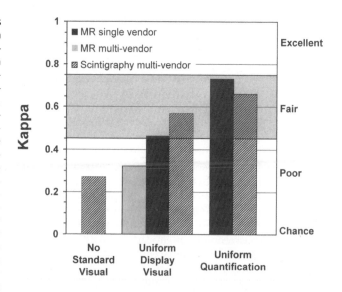

tivendor MR perfusion data underscores the need for standardization of data acquisition and analysis. These goals are aimed at a currently ongoing multicenter, multivendor phase III clinical trial that will include 550 patients world wide.

FUTURE PERSPECTIVE

Several single and multicenter MR perfusion trials could demonstrate a high diagnostic value of this technique, which can perform better than established SPECT techniques if conducted in expert centers. It will be a major challenge for all involved in MR imaging to transfer knowledge of experienced centers into the entire cardiac imaging community. Certainly, large multicenter trials are an invaluable tool for this purpose. In parallel, some improvements in scanner hardware and coil design are expected in the near future. In combination with well-trained personnel, who will perform standardized MR perfusion studies, the data quality will most likely allow for (semi-) automatic analysis. Such a quantitative perfusion assessment, based on a method that can be repeated without affecting patient safety, could well shift the paradigm of "reaction" (testing in case of symptoms) and/or complications to that of "action" (monitoring disease in a preclinical stage before complications occur). This would reduce the number of acute myocardial infarctions, which still show a high mortality despite novel treatment strategies. Monitoring CAD would also allow assessment of the effect of rigorous modifications of risk factors and detect progressive CAD in patients after revascularizations. Finally, standardized MR perfusion performance would be the basis for reliable cost-effectiveness calculations, which are increasingly important. In the near future, a robust MR perfusion approach will be the backbone for the work-up of patients with known or suspected CAD and will be combined with functional and viability tests in patients with advanced CAD.

Further studies will evaluate to what extent perfusion imaging at 3 T would increase test performance. Of particular potential is the novel hyperpolarized CM, which will be studied extensively in the years to come. And finally, revascularizations might be performed in the interventional MR laboratory as the ultimate extension of the "one-stop shop."

REFERENCES

1. Hoffmann R, Marwick TH, Poldermans D, et al. Refinements in stress echocardiographc techniques improve inter-institutional agreement in interpretation of dobutamine stress echocardiograms. *Eur Heart J* 2002;23:821–829.
2. Hendel RC, Berman DS, Cullom SJ, et al. Multicenter clinical trial to evaluate the efficacy of correction for photon attenuation and scatter in SPECT myocardial perfusion imaging. *Circulation* 1999;99:2742–2749.
3. Taillefer R, DeDuey EG, Udelson JE, et al. Comparative diagnostic accuracy of Tl-201 and Tc-99m sestamibi SPECT imaging (perfusion and ECG-gated SPECT) in detecting coronary artery disease in women. *J Am Coll Cardiol* 1997;29:69–77.
4. Giang T, Nanz D, Coulden R, et al. Detection of coronary artery disease by Magnetic Resonance myocardial perfusion imaging with various contrast medium doses: first European multicenter experience. *Eur Heart J* 2004;25:1657–1665.
5. Wolff S, Schwitter J, Coulden R, et al. Myocardial first-pass perfusion magnetic resonance imaging: a multicenter dose-ranging study. *Circulation* 2004;110:732–737.
6. Schwitter J, Bauer W, van Rossum AC, et al. MR perfusion imaging for detection coronary artery disease: a multicenter dose finding study in comparison with X-ray coronary angiography and single photon emission computed tomography. *Circulation* 2004;111:643 (abstract).
7. Celermajer DS, Sorensen KE, Gooch VM, et al. Non-invasive detection of endothelial dysfunction in children and adults at risk of atherosclerosis. *Lancet* 1992;340:1111–1115.
8. Suwaidi JA, Hamasaki S, Higano ST, et al. Long-term follow-up of patients with mild coronary artery disease and endothelial dysfunction. *Circulation* 2000;101:948–954.
9. Clarkson P, Celermajer DS, Donald AE, et al. Impaired vascular reactivity in insulin-dependent diabetes mellitus is related to disease duration and low density lipoprotein cholesterol levels. *J Am Coll Cardiol* 1996;28:573–579.
10. Lefer AM, Ma XL. Decreased basal nitric oxide release in hypercholesterolemia increases neutrophil adherence to rabbit coronary artery endothelium. *Arterioscler Thromb* 1993; 13:771–776.
11. Barker SGE, Beesley JE, Baskerville PA, et al. The influence of the adventitia on the presence of smooth muscle cells and macrophages in the arterial intima. *Eur J Vasc Endovasc Surg* 1995;9:222–227.
12. Libby P. Molecular bases of the acute coronary syndromes. *Circulation* 1995;91:2844–2850.
13. Galis ZS, Sukhova GK, Lark MW, et al. Increased expression of matrix metalloproteinases and matrix degrading activity in vulnerable regions of human atherosclerotic plaques. *J Clin Invest* 1994;94:2493–2503.
14. Davies MJ. A macro and micro view of coronary vascular insult in ischemic heart disease. Circulation 1990;82:II38–46.
15. Bruschke AV, Kramer JR Jr, Bal ET, et al. The dynamics of progression of coronary atherosclerosis studied in 168 medically treated patients who underwent coronary arteriography three times. *Am Heart J* 1989;117:296–305.
16. Wilcox JN, Smith KM, Schwartz SM, et al. Localization of tissue factor in the normal vessel wall and in the atherosclerotic plaque. *Proc Natl Acad Sci USA* 1989;86:2839–2843.
17. Ellis S, Alderman E, Cain K, et al. Prediction of risk of anterior myocardial infarction by lesion severity and measurement method of stenoses in the left anterior descending coronary distribution: a CASS Registry Study. *J Am Coll Cardiol* 1988; 11:908–916.
18. Waters D, Lesperance J, Francetich M, et al. A controlled clinical trial to assess the effect of a calcium channel blocker on the progression of coronary atherosclerosis. *Circulation* 1990;82:1940–1953.
19. Ojio S, Takatsu H, Tanaka T, et al. Considerable time from the onset of plaque rupture and/or thrombi until the onset of acute myocardial infarction in humans: coronary angiographic findings within 1 week before the onset of infarction. *Circulation* 2000;102:2063–2069.
20. Naghavi M, Libby P, Falk E, et al. From vulnerable plaque to vulnerable patient: a call for new definitions and risk assessment strategies: Part I. *Circulation* 2003;108:1664–1672.
21. Seiler C, Kirkeeide RL, Gould KL. Measurement from arteriograms of regional myocardial bed size distal to any point in the coronary vascular tree for assessing anatomic area at risk. *J Am Coll Cardiol* 1993;21:783–797.
22. Uren NG, Melin JA, De Bruyne B, et al. Relation between myocardial blood flow and the severity of coronary artery stenosis. *N Engl J Med* 1994;330:1782–1788.

23. Di Carli M, Czernin J, Hoh CK, et al. Relation among stenosis severity, myocardial blood flow, and flow reserve in patients with coronary artery disease. *Circulation* 1995;91:1944–1951.

24. Sambuceti G, Parodi O, Marcassa C, et al. Alterations in regulation of myocardial blood flow in one-vessel coronary artery disease determined by positron emission tomography. *Am J Cardiol* 1993;72:538–543.

25. Schwitter J, DeMarco T, Kneifel S, et al. Magnetic resonance-based assessment of global coronary flow and flow reserve and its relation to left ventricular functional parameters: a comparison with positron emission tomography. *Circulation* 2000;101:2696–2702.

26. Li D, Dhawale P, Rubin PJ, et al. Myocardial signal response to dipyridamole and dobutamine: demonstration of the BOLD effect using a double-echo gradient-echo sequence. *Magn Reson Med* 1996;36:16–20.

27. Atalay MK, Reeder SB, Zerhouni EA, et al. Blood oxygenation dependence of T1 and T2 in the isolated, perfused rabbit heart at 4.7T. *Magn Reson Med* 1995;34:623–627.

28. Fieno DS, Shea SM, Li Y, et al. Myocardial perfusion imaging based on the blood oxygen level-dependent effect using T2-prepared steady-state free-precession magnetic resonance imaging. *Circulation* 2004;110:1284–1290.

29. Bertschinger KM, Nanz D, Buechi M, et al. Magnetic resonance myocardial first-pass perfusion imaging: parameter optimization for signal response and cardiac coverage. *J Magn Reson Imaging* 2001;14:556–562.

30. Reeder SB, Atalay MK, McVeigh ER, et al. Quantitative cardiac perfusion: a noninvasive spin-labeling method that exploits coronary vessel geometry. *Radiology* 1996;200:177–184.

31. Poncelet BP, Koelling TM, Schmidt CJ, et al. Measurement of human myocardial perfusion by double-gated flow alternating inversion recovery EPI. *Magn Reson Med* 1999;41:510–519.

32. Wendland MF, Saeed M, Lauerma K, et al. Endogenous susceptibility contrast in myocardium during apnea measured using gradient recalled echo planar imaging. *Magn Reson Med* 1993;29:273–276.

33. Belle V, Kahler E, Waller C, et al. In vivo quantitative mapping of cardiac perfusion in rats using a noninvasive MR spin-labeling method. *J Magn Reson Imaging* 1998;8:1240–1245.

34. Prasad PV, Burstein D, Edelman RR. MRI evaluation of myocardial perfusion without a contrast agent using magnetization transfer. *Magn Reson Med* 1993;30:267–270.

35. Saeed M, Wendland MF, Sakuma H, et al. Coronary artery stenosis: detection with contrast-enhanced MR imaging in dogs. *Radiology* 1995;196:79–84.

36. Schwitter J, Saeed M, Wendland MF, et al. Assessment of myocardial function and perfusion in a canine model of non-occlusive coronary artery stenosis using fast magnetic resonance imaging. *JMRI* 1998;9:101–110.

37. Manning WJ, Atkinson DJ, Grossman W, et al. First-pass nuclear magnetic resonance imaging studies using gadolinium-DTPA in patients with coronary artery disease. *J Am Coll Cardiol* 1991;18:959–965.

38. Lauerma K, Virtanen KS, Sipila LM, et al. Multislice MRI in assessment of myocardial perfusion in patients with single-vessel proximal left anterior descending coronary artery disease before and after revascularization. *Circulation* 1997;96:2859–2867.

39. Matheijssen NA, Louwerenburg HW, van Rugge F, et al. Comparison of ultrafast dipyridamole magnetic resonance imaging with dipyridamole SestaMIBI SPECT for detection of perfusion abnormalities in patients with one-vessel coronary artery disease: assessment by quantitative model fitting. *Magn Reson Med* 1996;35:221–228.

40. Eichenberger AC, Schuiki E, Kochli VD, et al. Ischemic heart disease: assessment with gadolinium-enhanced ultrafast MR imaging and dipyridamole stress. *J Magn Reson Imaging* 1994;4:425–431.

41. Al-Saadi N, Nagel E, Gross M, et al. Noninvasive detection of myocardial ischemia from perfusion reserve based on cardiovascular magnetic resonance. *Circulation* 2000;101:1379–1383.

42. Sensky PR, Jivan A, Hudson NM, et al. Coronary artery disease: combined stress MR imaging protocol-one-stop evaluation of myocardial perfusion and function. *Radiology* 2000;215:608–614.

43. Walsh EG, Doyle M, Lawson MA, Blackwell GG, et al. Multislice first-pass myocardial perfusion imaging on a conventional clinical scanner. *Magn Reson Med* 1995;34:39–47.

44. Ding S, Wolff SD, Epstein FH. Improved coverage in dynamic contrast-enhanced cardiac MRI using interleaved gradient-echo EPI. *Magn Reson Med* 1998;39:514–519.

45. Kraitchman DL, Chin BB, Heldman AW, et al. MRI detection of myocardial perfusion defects due to coronary artery stenosis with MS-325. *J Magn Reson Imaging* 2002;15:149–158.

46. Schwitter J, Nanz D, Kneifel S, et al. Assessment of myocardial perfusion in coronary artery disease by magnetic resonance: a comparison with positron emission tomography and coronary angiography. *Circulation* 2001;103:2230–2235.

47. Nagel E, Klein C, Paetsch I, et al. Magnetic resonance perfusion measurements for the noninvasive detection of coronary artery disease. *Circulation* 2003;108:432–437.

48. Slavin GS, Wolff SD, Gupta SN, et al. First-pass myocardial perfusion MR imaging with interleaved notched saturation: feasibility study. *Radiology* 2001;219:258–263.

49. Edelman RR, Li W. Contrast-enhanced echo-planar MR imaging of myocardial perfusion: preliminary study in humans. *Radiology* 1994;190:771–777.

50. Schwitter J, Debatin JF, von Schulthess GK, et al. Normal myocardial perfusion assessed with multishot echo-planar imaging. *Magn Reson Med* 1997;37:140–147.

51. Schwitter J, Sakuma H, Saeed M, et al. Very fast cardiac imaging. *Magn Reson Imaging Clin N Am* 1996;4:419–432.

52. Klocke FJ, Simonetti OP, Judd RM, et al. Limits of detection of regional differences in vasodilated flow in viable myocardium by first-pass magnetic resonance perfusion imaging. *Circulation* 2001;104:2412–2416.

53. Schreiber WG, Schmitt M, Kalden P, et al. Dynamic contrast-enhanced myocardial perfusion imaging using saturation-prepared TrueFISP. *J Magn Reson Imaging* 2002;16:641–652.

54. Pruessmann KP, Weiger M, Scheidegger MB, et al. SENSE: sensitivity encoding for fast MRI. *Magn Reson Med* 1999;42:952–962.

55. Kellman P, Derbyshire JA, Agyeman KO, et al. Extended coverage of first-pass perfusion imaging using slice-interleaved TSENSE. *Magn Reson Med* 2004;51:200–204.

56. Saeed M, Wendland MF, Yu KK, et al. Dual effects of gadodiamide injection in depiction of the region of myocardial ischemia. *J Magn Reson Imaging* 1993;3:21–29.

57. Sakuma H, O'Sullivan M, Lucas J, et al. Effect of magnetic susceptibility contrast medium on myocardial signal intensity with fast gradient-recalled echo and spin-echo MR imaging: initial experience in humans. *Radiology* 1994;190:161–166.

58. Wilke N, Kroll K, Merkle H, et al. Regional myocardial blood volume and flow: first-pass MR imaging with polylysine-Gd-DTPA. *J Magn Reson Imaging* 1995;5:227–237.

59. Kraitchman DL, Wilke N, Hexeberg E, et al. Myocardial perfusion and function in dogs with moderate coronary stenosis. *Magn Reson Med* 1996;35:771–780.

60. Bjerner T, Johansson L, Ericsson A, et al. First-pass myocardial perfusion MR imaging with outer-volume suppression

and the intravascular contrast agent NC100150 injection: preliminary results in eight patients. *Radiology* 2001;221: 822–826.

61. Saeed M, Wendland MF, Masui T, et al. Reperfused myocardial infarctions on T1- and susceptibility-enhanced MRI: evidence for loss of compartmentalization of contrast media. *Magn Reson Med* 1994;31:31–39.

62. Hall DA, Maus DC, Gerfen GJ, et al. Polarization-enhanced NMR spectroscopy of biomolecules in frozen solution. *Science* 1997;276:930–932.

63. Golman K, Axelsson O, Johannesson H, et al. Parahydrogen-induced polarization in imaging: subsecond 13C angiography. *Magn Reson Med* 2001;46:1–5.

64. Johansson E, Mansson S, Wirestam R, et al. Cerebral perfusion assessment by bolus tracking using hyperpolarized 13C. *Magn Reson Med* 2004;51:464–472.

65. Hartnell G, Cerel A, Kamalesh M, et al. Detection of myocardial ischemia: value of combined myocardial perfusion and cineangiographic MR imaging. *AJR Am J Roentgenol* 1994; 163:1061–1067.

66. Keijer JT, van Rossum AC, Wilke N, et al. Magnetic resonance imaging of myocardial perfusion in single-vessel coronary artery disease: implications for transmural assessment of myocardial perfusion. *J Cardiovasc Magn Reson* 2000;2: 189–200.

67. Swets JA. Measuring the accuracy of diagnostic systems. *Science* 1988;240:1285–1288.

68. Metz CE. ROC methodology in radiologic imaging. *Invest Radiol* 1986;21:720–733.

69. Holland AE, Goldfarb JW, Edelman RR. Diaphragmatic and cardiac motion during suspended breathing: preliminary experience and implications for breath-hold MR imaging. *Radiology* 1998;209:483–489.

70. McConnell MV, Khasgiwala VC, Savord BJ, et al. Prospective adaptive navigator correction for breath-hold MR coronary angiography. *Magn Reson Med* 1997;37:148–152.

71. Chuang ML, Chen MH, Khasgiwala VC, et al. Adaptive correction of imaging plane position in segmented k-space cine cardiac MRI. *J Magn Reson Imaging* 1997;7:811–814.

72. Keijer JT, van Rossum AC, van Eenige MJ, et al. Magnetic resonance imaging of regional myocardial perfusion in patients with single-vessel coronary artery disease: quantitative comparison with (201)Thallium-SPECT and coronary angiography. *J Magn Reson Imaging* 2000;11:607–615.

73. Wilke N, Simm C, Zhang J, et al. Contrast-enhanced first pass myocardial perfusion imaging: correlation between myocardial blood flow in dogs at rest and during hyperemia. *Magn Reson Med* 1993;29:485–497.

74. Panting JR, Gatehouse PD, Yang GZ, et al. Abnormal subendocardial perfusion in cardiac syndrome X detected by cardiovascular magnetic resonance imaging. *N Engl J Med* 2002; 346:1948–1953.

75. Keijer JT, van Rossum A, van Eenige M, et al. Semiquantitation of regional myocardial blood flow in normal human subjects by first-pass magnetic resonance imaging. *Am Heart J* 1995;130:893–901.

76. Lombardi M, Jones RA, Westby J, et al. Use of the mean transit time of an intravascular contrast agent as an exchange-insensitive index of myocardial perfusion. *J Magn Reson Imaging* 1999;9:402–408.

77. Christian TF, Rettmann DW, Aletras AH, et al. Absolute myocardial perfusion in canines measured by using dual-bolus first-pass MR imaging. *Radiology* 2004;232:677–684.

78. Kety S. The theory and application of the exchange of inert gas in lung and tissues. *Pharmacol Rev* 1951;3:1–41.

79. Jerosch Herold M, Hu X, Murthy NS, et al. Magnetic resonance imaging of myocardial contrast enhancement with MS-325 and its relation to myocardial blood flow and the perfusion reserve. *J Magn Reson Imaging* 2003;18:544–554.

80. Kroll K, Wilke N, Jerosch Herold M, et al. Modeling regional myocardial flows from residue functions of an intravascular indicator. *Am J Physiol* 1996;271:H1643–1655.

81. Jerosch-Herold M, Swingen C, Seethamraju RV. Myocardial blood flow quantification with MRI by model-independent deconvolution. *Med Phys* 2002;29:886–897.

82. Wilke N, Jerosch HM, Wang Y, et al. Myocardial perfusion reserve: assessment with multisection, quantitative, first-pass MR imaging. *Radiology* 1997;204:373–384.

83. Larsson HB, Fritz Hansen T, Rostrup E, et al. Myocardial perfusion modeling using MRI. *Magn Reson Med* 1996;35: 716–726.

84. Diesbourg L, Prato F, Wisenberg G, et al. Quantification of myocardial blood flow and extracellular volumes using a bolus injection of Gd-DTPA: kinetic modelling in canine ischemic disease. *Mag Reson Med* 1992;23:239–253.

85. Tong CY, Prato FS, Wisenberg G, et al. Measurement of the extraction efficiency and distribution volume for Gd-DTPA in normal and diseased canine myocardium. *Magn Reson Med* 1993;30:337–346.

86. Fritz-Hansen T, Rostrup E, Larsson HB, et al. Measurement of the arterial concentration of Gd-DTPA using MRI: a step toward quantitative perfusion imaging. *Magn Reson Med* 1996;36:225–231.

87. Larsson HB, Stubgaard M, Sondergaard L, et al. In vivo quantification of the unidirectional influx constant for Gd-DTPA diffusion across the myocardial capillaries with MR imaging. *J Magn Reson Imaging* 1994;4:433–440.

88. Gatehouse PD, Elkington AG, Ablitt NA, et al. Accurate assessment of the arterial input function during high-dose myocardial perfusion cardiovascular magnetic resonance. *J Magn Reson Imaging* 2004;20:39–45.

89. Wendland MF, Saeed M, Yu KK, et al. Inversion recovery EPI of bolus transit in rat myocardium using intravascular and extravascular gadolinium-based MR contrast media: dose effects on peak signal enhancement. *Magn Reson Med* 1994; 32:319–329.

90. Judd RM, Atalay MK, Rottman GA, et al. Effects of myocardial water exchange on T1 enhancement during bolus administration of MR contrast agents. *Magn Reson Med* 1995;33: 215–223.

91. Judd RM, Reeder SB, May Newman K. Effects of water exchange on the measurement of myocardial perfusion using paramagnetic contrast agents. *Magn Reson Med* 1999;41: 334–342.

92. Donahue KM, Burstein D, Manning WJ, et al. Studies of Gd-DTPA relaxivity and proton exchange rates in tissue. *Magn Reson Med* 1994;32:66–76.

93. Larsson HB, Rosenbaum S, Fritz Hansen T. Quantification of the effect of water exchange in dynamic contrast MRI perfusion measurements in the brain and heart. *Magn Reson Med* 2001;46:272–281.

94. Dauber IM, VanBenthuysen KM, McMurtry IF, et al. Functional coronary microvascular injury evident as increased permeability due to brief ischemia and reperfusion. *Circ Res* 1990;66:986–998.

95. Svendsen JH, Bjerrum PJ, Haunso S. Myocardial capillary permeability after regional ischemia and reperfusion in the in vivo canine heart. Effect of superoxide dismutase. *Circ Res* 1991;68:174–184.

96. Fritz-Hansen T, Rostrup E, Sondergaard L, et al. Capillary transfer constant of Gd-DTPA in the myocardium at rest and

during vasodilation assessed by MRI. *Magn Reson Med* 1998; 40:922–929.

97. Cullen JH, Horsfield MA, Reek CR, et al. A myocardial perfusion reserve index in humans using first-pass contrast-enhanced magnetic resonance imaging. *J Am Coll Cardiol* 1999; 33:1386–1394.

98. Neyran B, Janier MF, Casali C, et al. Mapping myocardial perfusion with an intravascular MR contrast agent: robustness of deconvolution methods at various blood flows. *Magn Reson Med* 2002;48:166–179.

99. Bjornerud A, Bjerner T, Johansson LO, et al. Assessment of myocardial blood volume and water exchange: theoretical considerations and in vivo results. *Magn Reson Med* 2003; 49:828–837.

100. Wendland MF, Saeed M, Masui T, et al. Echo-planar MR imaging of normal and ischemic myocardium with gadodiamide injection. *Radiology* 1993;186:535–542.

101. Wendland MF, Saeed M, Masui T, et al. First pass of an MR susceptibility contrast agent through normal and ischemic heart: gradient-recalled echo-planar imaging. *J Magn Reson Imaging* 1993;3:755–760.

102. Wright KB, Klocke FJ, Deshpande VS, et al. Assessment of regional differences in myocardial blood flow using T2-weighted 3D BOLD imaging. *Magn Reson Med* 2001;46: 573–578.

103. Ishida N, Sakuma H, Motoyasu M, et al. Noninfarcted myocardium: correlation between dynamic first-pass contrast-enhanced myocardial MR imaging and quantitative coronary angiography. *Radiology* 2003;229:209–216.

104. Wackers FJT, Bodenheimer M, Fleiss JL, et al. Factors affecting uniformity in interpretation of planar Thallium-201 imaging in a multicenter trial. *J Am Coll Cardiol* 1993;21: 1064–1074.

14

Left Ventricular Function in Ischemic Heart Disease

Eike Nagel

I schemic heart disease is one of the most common health problems of the Western world. A variety of tests are available in routine clinical practice for the noninvasive diagnosis of coronary artery disease (CAD), such as exercise electrocardiography (ECG), echocardiography, single photon emission computed tomography (SPECT), positron emission tomography (PET), and cardiovascular magnetic resonance imaging (CMR). The advantages and disadvantages of each technique are summarized in Table 14.1. Many noninvasive diagnostic tools are suboptimal, and both patients and physicians want a reliable diagnosis. Consequently, 40% to 60% of all patients who undergo invasive cardiac catheterization procedures do not require a revascularization procedure such as bypass surgery or angioplasty. Thus, a noninvasive test with a higher rate of diagnostic accuracy might reduce the number of overall cardiac catheterization procedures.

CMR has evolved into a new technique for the noninvasive detection of obstructive CAD. The ability of CMR to visualize global and regional wall motion and systolic thickening of the left ventricle (LV) with a high degree of spatial and temporal resolution makes it possible to detect abnormalities of wall motion. In addition, perfusion defects and reductions in coronary flow reserve can be assessed. Except for high-grade coronary artery stenosis, abnormalities can, for the most part, be identified only under stress conditions. These can be induced by physical exercise or by means of standardized stress protocols with infusions of pharmacologic agents such as dobutamine/atropine, dipyridamole, or adenosine. To date, the most reliable clinical data are based on the analysis of LV wall motion and thickening during pharmacologic stress. In this chapter, the results of recent studies and a detailed description of how to perform stress tests are presented.

PATHOPHYSIOLOGY

Ischemic heart disease can be caused by a variety of pathophysiologic conditions. Stenosis of the coronary arteries (CAD) is the most common of these, but LV hypertrophy, alterations of the microcirculation, and a reduction of energy uptake are other less frequent causes. Patients with CAD usually have sufficient blood flow at rest; however, during stress, which induces a four- to fivefold increase in blood

TABLE 14-1   Different Techniques for the Evaluation of Myocardial Ischemia

	Advantage	Disadvantage
Exercise ECG	Low cost Wide availability	Low diagnostic accuracy Many equivocal results Target heart rate not reached in many patients
Stress Echocardiography	Low cost Wide availability	Nondiagnostic examinations in 10% to 15%
SPECT	Low cost	Radiation Low specificity Attenuation artifacts, especially in women
PET	Quantitative evaluation No attenuation artifacts	Limited availability High cost Radiation
CMR	High diagnostic accuracy Combination of wall motion, perfusion, and anatomy No radiation	Limited availability High cost

CMR, cardiovascular magnetic resonance imaging; ECG, electrocardiography; PET, positron emission tomography; SPECT, single photon emission computed tomography.

flow in healthy persons, the myocardium supplied by the stenotic coronary arteries does not receive enough blood because blood flow is impeded through the narrowed coronary artery lumen. Thus, except in very severe cases in which the patients have ischemia at rest, stress testing is required to induce ischemia.

STRESS TESTING

Stress testing can be performed with either physical or pharmacologic stimulation. In general, to detect ischemic heart disease with a high level of sensitivity and reproducibility, a defined end point (submaximal stress) must be reached. This end point is defined by the heart rate as follows:

$$\text{Target Heart Rate} = 0.85 (220 - \text{Age})$$

ERGOMETRIC STRESS

Ergometric stress is the most physiologic stress test. Patients exercise on a bicycle or treadmill ergometer with incremental workloads. In general, this kind of stress has the disadvantages of relatively low reproducibility and the induction of motion artifacts. Because many patients with CAD also have other vessels that are stenotic (e.g., in their legs), they cannot be adequately stressed and frequently do not reach the required heart rate.

Ergometric stress in combination with CMR has additional limitations. Patients lie on their back within a relatively small-bore magnet so that an optimal setup for ergo-

metric stress is difficult to achieve. As a result, a large number of tests may be nondiagnostic because of an inadequate level of stress. In addition, CMR, which is sensitive to motion artifacts, is not compatible with exercise-induced stress testing. However, new techniques such as real-time imaging may overcome this problem.

PHARMACOLOGIC STRESS

Pharmacologic stress is preferred by many clinicians because the results are highly reproducible and diagnostic in most patients. Careful monitoring is required for patient safety (to be discussed). Two different approaches are used: Oxygen consumption can be increased by increasing the heart rate and contractility (dobutamine/arbutamine), or vasodilation can be induced (dipyridamole/adenosine). The different pharmacologic stress protocols are summarized in Table 14.2.

Dobutamine

Dobutamine is a sympathomimetic drug with β_1-, β_2-, and slight α_1-receptor-stimulating properties. Infusion of the drug increases the cardiac contractility and rate and decreases the systolic vascular resistance. Whereas during low-dose infusion (≤ 10 µg/kg/min) increased contractility is the major effect, at higher doses, the increased consumption of oxygen causes contraction abnormalities in myocardial segments supplied by stenotic coronary arteries.

A low dose of dobutamine is defined as an infusion of up to 10 µg/min/kg of body weight. Such a dose is sufficient to stimulate myocardium that does not contract at rest but

TABLE 14-2 Stress Protocols

Stress Test	Patient Instructions	Protocol	Antidote
Dobutamine for the for assessment of viability		5, 10 µg/kg BW per minute for >3 min	
Dobutamine/atropine for the detection of coronary artery disease (wall motion)	No β-blockers and nitrates 24 hours before the examination	(5), 10, 20, 30, 40 µg/kg BW per minute for 3 min each, up to 1 mg atropine (4 × 0.25 mg) until submaximal heart rate [(220 − age) × 0.85] is reached (half-life 2 min)	β-Blocker (esmolol) 0.5 mg mg/kg as slowly injected bolus, additional bolus of 0.2 mg/kg as needed, sublingual nitroglycerin
Dipyridamole (perfusion)	No caffeine (tea, coffee, Aminophylline 250 mg chocolate, etc.) or medications such as aminophylline or nitrates 24 hours before the examination	0.56 mg/kg BW per minute for 4 min, maximal effect after approximately 3 to 4 min (half-life 30 min)	IV slowly injected with ECG monitoring, sublingual nitroglycerin
Adenosine (perfusion)	Same as for dipyridamole	140 µg/kg BW per minute for 6 min (half-life 4 to 10 s)	Stop infusion (in occasional cases aminophylline 250 mg IV slowly injected with ECG monitoring)

BW, body weight; ECG, electrocardiogram.

may benefit from revascularization (viable or hibernating myocardium); however, this dose is insufficient to induce ischemia.

A high dose of dobutamine is defined as an infusion aimed at inducing ischemia. As previously explained, it is essential that patients reach their target heart rate. To achieve this goal, atropine, which increases the heart rate by an anticholinergic mechanism, is commonly added. The stress protocol most widely used is described in the guidelines of the American Society of Echocardiography. Stress is induced by increasing doses of dobutamine, started at 10 µg/kg of body weight per minute for 3 min and increased in increments of 10 µg/kg of body weight per minute every 3 min, until a maximal dose of 40 µg/kg of body weight per minute is reached. (Some investigators use 50 µg/kg of body weight per minute as a maximum.) If the target heart rate is not reached, up to 1 mg of atropine is added in 0.25 mg fractions. The test must be stopped if certain criteria are fulfilled (Table 14.3).

TABLE 14-3 Dobutamine Termination Criteria

Submaximal heart rate reached [(220 − age) × 0.85]
Systolic pressure decrease >20 mmHg below baseline systolic blood pressure or decrease >40 mm Hg from a previous level
Blood pressure increase >240/120 mm Hg
Intractable symptoms
New or worsening wall-motion abnormalities in at least 2 of 17 adjacent left ventricular segments
Complex cardiac arrhythmias

Dipyridamole (Vasodilation)

Dipyridamole and its metabolic product and active component adenosine are vasodilators. They induce ischemia by a "steal effect" as follows: Coronary arteries with significant stenoses receive local stimuli (e.g., local adenosine produced by the endothelial cells) and are dilated to a maximum at rest. Thus, these vessels are not dilated any further if an external vasodilator is added. In contrast, healthy vessels react with significant vasodilation and increased blood flow after pharmacologic stimulation. This reaction can be measured as flow reserve in perfusion or flow measurements. Because of the increased flow in healthy areas, less blood is delivered to the myocardial areas supplied by diseased coronary arteries (steal effect), so that ischemia develops in these myocardial regions. In clinical practice, a few centers use vasodilators to induce wall-motion abnormalities, usually 140 µg of adenosine per minute for a maximum of 6 min. The sensitivity of wall-motion testing with vasodilators is less than that with dobutamine/atropine, which is more frequently used. However, vasodilators are the preferred stressors for perfusion and flow measurements.

ACCURACY OF STRESS-INDUCED WALL-MOTION ABNORMALITIES IN THE DIAGNOSIS OF ISCHEMIA

The echocardiographic detection of wall-motion abnormalities during high-dose dobutamine or exercise stress has been

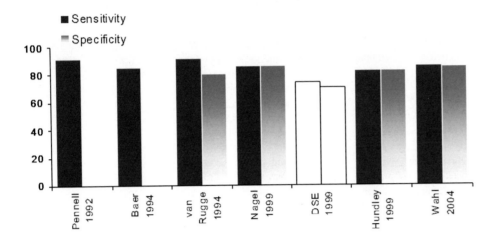

Figure 14.1. Diagnostic performance of dobutamine stress MR from 583 patients in the literature. Note the superiority in comparison to dobutamine stress echocardiography (DSE) and the small variation of results.

shown to be an accurate diagnostic tool for screening patients with suspected CAD. Sensitivities of 54% to 96% and specificities of 60% to 100% have been reported (1), depending on the pretest likelihood of disease and the experience of the stress centers. However, the value of stress echocardiography is limited by a 10% to 15% rate of nondiagnostic results (1) and low specificities for the basal-lateral and basal-inferior segments of the LV (2).

CMR has yielded good results in the detection of wall-motion abnormalities at intermediate doses of dobutamine (maximum of 20 µg/kg of body weight per minute intravenously) (Fig. 14.1) (3–5). However, echocardiographic studies have shown that high-dose dobutamine and additional atropine are required to ensure a high sensitivity. In a prospective study of 208 patients with suspected CAD, stress with high-dose dobutamine/atropine (40 µg of dobutamine per kilogram of body weight per minute plus up to 1 mg of atropine intravenously) was used, and echocardiography and CMR were compared with angiography for the detection of significant CAD (stenosis of >50% the vessel diameter on angiography) (6). This study found significantly better values for the sensitivity (86% vs. 74%), specificity (86% vs. 70%), and diagnostic accuracy (86% vs. 73%) of CMR versus transthoracic echocardiography. These differences were most pronounced in the patients with moderate echocardiographic image quality (Fig. 14.2) (7). In a different study by Hundley et al (8), a similar protocol was used to assess patients with nondiagnostic echocardiographic image quality, and 94% of them could be adequately examined with CMR, for a sensitivity and specificity of 83% in those patients who also underwent coronary angiography. More recently, studies have confirmed the high diagnostic accuracy of dobutamine stress (DS) MR imaging in patients with wall-motion abnormalities at rest or after revascularization (9).

Because high-dose dobutamine stress CMR is highly accurate and can be performed within less than 40 min, it has

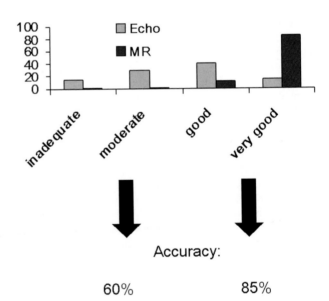

Figure 14.2. Diagnostic accuracy in relation to image quality. Whereas with MR, almost all patients show good or very good image quality, a significant group of patients results in inadequate or moderate echocardiographic image quality. Patients with suboptimal image quality result in a lower diagnostic accuracy, independent of the imaging technique. (With permission from Nagel E, Lehmkuhl HB, Klein C, et al. Influence of image quality on the diagnostic accuracy of dobutamine stress magnetic resonance imaging in comparison with dobutamine stress echocardiography for the noninvasive detection of myocardial ischemia. *Z Kardiol* 1999;88(9):622–630 and Nagel E, Lehmkuhl HB, Bocksch W, et al. Noninvasive diagnosis of ischemia-induced wall motion abnormalities with the use of high-dose dobutamine stress MRI: comparison with dobutamine stress echocardiography. *Circulation* 1999;99(6):763–770.)

replaced dobutamine stress echocardiography for the detection of CAD in patients with nondiagnostic or suboptimal echocardiographic image quality in our institution.

PROGNOSTIC VALUE OF DOBUTAMINE STRESS MAGNETIC RESONANCE IMAGING

Until now, only limited data were available on the prognostic information provided by high-dose DSMR. The presence of inducible wall-motion abnormalities during DSMR identifies those patients at risk of myocardial infarction and cardiac death independent of the presence of traditional risk factors for CAD (10). A low number of cardiac events were found in patients with a negative stress test (2% over 2 years for patients with left ventricular ejection fraction [LVEF] >40%, and 0% over 2 years for patients with LVEF ≥60%).

IMAGE ACQUISITION

For the assessment of wall motion, cine loops of the heart are acquired with steady state free precession (SSFP). In contrast to turbo-gradient echo techniques that have been used in most studies published so far, imaging contrast in SSFP is generated by the difference in magnetization between blood and myocardium rather than inflow of strongly magnetized blood into the imaging slice. This results in a much better delineation of the endocardial border, especially in long-axis views. In our institution we use a SSFP sequence in combination with parallel image acquisition and retrospective ECG gating, resulting in >25 phases/cardiac cycle up to heart rates of 200 beats/min during a breath-hold of 4–6 seconds. The in-plane spatial resolution is in the range of 1.6 mm × 1.6 mm. The heart can be visualized with

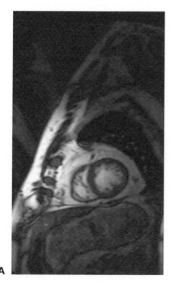

A

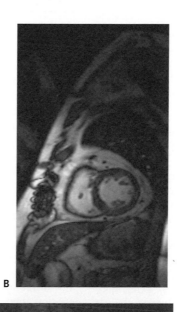

B

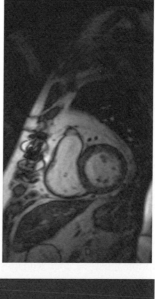

C

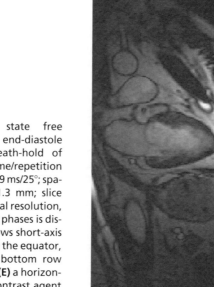

D

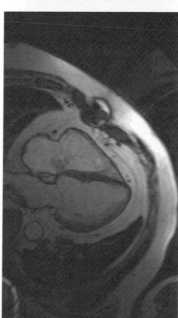

E

Figure 14.3. Steady state free precession images at end-diastole acquired during s breath-hold of 16 heartbeats. Echo time/repetition time/flip angle, 2.1 ms/5.9 ms/25°; spatial resolution, 1.3 × 1.3 mm; slice thickness, 8 mm; temporal resolution, 40 ms. One of 18 cardiac phases is displayed. The top row shows short-axis views at **(A)** the apex, **(B)** the equator, and **(C)** the base; the bottom row shows **(D)** a vertical and **(E)** a horizontal long-axis view. No contrast agent was used.

TABLE 14-4	Contraindications to Magnetic Resonance Stress Tests
MR examination	Incompatible metallic implants (e.g., pacemakers, retro-orbital metal, cerebral artery clips)
	Claustrophobia
Dobutamine	Severe arterial hypertension (≥220/120 mm Hg)
	Unstable angina pectoris
	Significant aortic stenosis (aortic valve gradient >50 mm Hg or aortic valve area >1 cm^2)
	Complex cardiac arrhythmias
	Significant hypertrophic obstructive cardiomyopathy
	Myocarditis, endocarditis, pericarditis
	Other major disease
Dipyridamole/ adenosine	Myocardial infarction <3 days
	Unstable angina pectoris
	Severe arterial hypertension
	Asthma or severe obstructive pulmonary disease
	Atrioventricular block >IIa

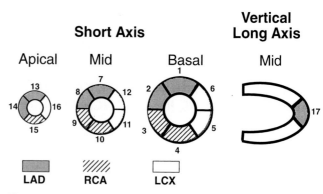

Figure 14.4. Seventeen-segment model suggested by the American Heart Association. The coronary artery territories are shown in the graph.

either contiguous short-axis slices or a combination of several short-axis views (typically three to five) and long-axis (typically 2- and 4-chamber) views (Fig. 14.3).

For high-dose dobutamine stress tests, breath-hold cine imaging with SSFP techniques should be used in preference to conventional non-breath-hold techniques. These fast techniques significantly reduce the scan time, improve image quality, and enable the rapid detection of wall-motion abnormalities. Imaging starts immediately after the dobutamine dose is increased for each stress level. To achieve an adequate number of phases during tachycardia, the temporal resolution must be approximately 25 frames/s (<40 ms). Studies published so far have used a spatial resolution of about 2 × 2 mm or better with a slice thickness of 6 to 10 mm. Images are acquired and reviewed at rest and during each stress level. The stress protocol, details of monitoring, contraindications, and termination criteria are summarized in Tables 14.2 to 14.5.

IMAGE INTERPRETATION

For image interpretation, a multiple cine loop display that allows different stress levels to be assessed at the same time is recommended. The ventricle is typically analyzed at 17 LV segments per stress level according to the standards suggested by the American Society of Echocardiography (11) and the American Heart Association (Fig. 14.4). Each segment is assigned to a specific coronary artery; however, depending on the coronary artery anatomy or degree of collateralization, some segments may be supplied by different arteries. Thus, it is often not possible to define a stenotic coronary artery from a wall-motion study. Image quality is graded as good, acceptable, or bad, and the number of diagnostic segments is reported. Segmental wall motion is classified as normokinetic, hypokinetic, akinetic, or dyskinetic and assigned one to four points (Fig. 14.5). The sum of the points is divided by the number of analyzed segments to yield a wall-motion score. Normal contraction results in a wall-motion score of 1, and a higher score indicates wall-motion abnormality. During stress with increasing doses of dobutamine, either a lack of increase in wall motion or systolic wall thickening or a reduction in wall motion or thickening is regarded as a pathologic finding (Fig. 14.6). Visual interpretation may be facilitated with the use of myocardial tagging (12). Kuijpers et al demonstrated that additional cor-

TABLE 14-5	Monitoring Requirements for Stress Magnetic Resonance Imaging		
Dipyridamole/Atropine		**Dobutamine + Adenosine**	
Heart rate and rhythm (single-lead ECG)	Continuously	Continuously
Blood pressure	Every minute	Every minute
Pulse oximetry*	Continuously	Continuously
Symptoms	Continuously	Continuously
Wall-motion abnormalities	Every dose increment	At peak stress

* Only required for additional rhythm control if no vector ECG is available.
ECG, electrocardiogram.

ages with scintigraphic images is easily accomplished since both techniques are three-dimensional, and identical regions can be matched (34).

To define transmural scar by end-diastolic wall thickness, a cutoff value of 5.5 mm was selected. This value corresponded to the mean end-diastolic wall thickness in normal persons minus 2.5 standard deviations. It also corresponded well with the wall thickness of less than 6 mm found in a histopathologic study of transmural chronic scar (33). Regions that had a mean end-diastolic wall thickness of less than 5.5 mm showed a significantly reduced uptake of FDG in comparison to regions that had an end-diastolic wall thickness of 5.5 mm or more (10). In 29 of 35 patients studied, the determination of viability based on FDG uptake was identical to the determination based on myocardial morphology as assessed by MRI. Importantly, relative FDG uptake did not differ between segments with systolic wall thickening at rest or akinesia at rest as long as wall thickness was preserved. These findings were applied to another group of patients who underwent revascularization and control MRI 3 months after revascularization (11). Of 125 segments with an end-diastolic wall thickness of less than 5.5 mm in 43 patients with chronic infarcts, only 12 segments recovered (corresponding to a negative predictive accuracy of 90% for the finding of end-diastolic wall thinning to predict transmural scar). In contrast, the positive predictive accuracy was only 62% for preserved end-diastolic wall thickness of 5.5 mm or more in predicting the presence of viable myocardium with the potential for recovery. The most likely explanation for this finding is that the amount of viable myocardium cannot be directly visualized on gradient echo MR images. However, it is the amount of viable myocardium present in a particular region of the LV that determines whether the segment will recover function or not. Regions with preserved wall thickness may contain very small rims of epicardially located viable myocardium and yet not exhibit substantial wall thinning. However, such a small rim of viable myocardium may not be sufficient to result in improved wall thickening after revascularization. Reduced end-diastolic wall thickness was also found to be a strong predictor of irreversibly damaged tissue in a study in which resting transthoracic echocardiography was used to assess patients with healed Q wave anterior wall infarcts. This study, which defined myocardial viability as recovery of function after revascularization, found a predictive value of 87% for a pattern of increased acoustic reflectance combined with reduced end-diastolic wall thickness (38).

The relationship between end-diastolic wall thickness and viability has been disputed by other researchers (13) who found FDG uptake on PET images to be largely independent of regional end-diastolic wall thickness. However, this study included recent and chronic infarcts and used a suboptimal conventional spin-echo technique with a short echo time of 20 ms to measure wall thickness. More recently, thallium-201 uptake was correlated with end-diastolic and end-systolic LV wall thickness as measured on cine MR images in patients with acute and healed myocardial infarcts (39). In this study, end-systolic wall thickness correlated better with normalized thallium activity then did end-diastolic wall thickness. Regions with normalized thallium activity of less than 50% showed wall-thickening values of 12.3 ± 30.6%, and wall thickening was only slightly larger in regions with

thallium activities between 50% and 60% (13.8 ± 27.0 %). From a receiver operating curve (ROC), an end-systolic wall thickness value of 9.8 mm had a sensitivity of 90% and a specificity of 94% in identifying regions with a normalized thallium uptake of less than 50%. In our opinion, the study does not really contradict our finding that end-diastolic wall thickness is able to distinguish between scarred and viable myocardium. The patient population of Lawson et al (39) differed in one important aspect from ours: They included patients with hypokinesia in their study, whereas only patients with akinesia were included in ours. Obviously, any degree of wall thickening is related to the presence of contracting and hence viable cells in the region of interest. Nevertheless, it is undoubtedly true that end-systolic wall thickness gives even larger differences between normal and viable myocardium if one includes zones of viability that are still contracting. However, viable zones in our studies did not contract (akinesia or dyskinesia) and systolic wall thickness was therefore not better than end-diastolic wall thickness for distinguishing between viable myocardium and scar.

CONTRACTILE RESERVE DURING LOW-DOSE DOBUTAMINE INFUSION

Although severely reduced end-diastolic wall thickness is very helpful in identifying myocardium that is highly unlikely to recover after revascularization because it is completely scarred (11), the value of a preserved end-diastolic wall thickness for predicting recovery of function following revascularization is disappointingly low. However, MRI offers the possibility to observe and measure wall thickening not only at rest but also during low-dose dobutamine infusion. With the implementation of fast MR sequences, a standard viability study protocol can be completed within 30 min, similar to a dobutamine echocardiography study. Sensitivity of DE-MRI for detection of viable myocardium as defined by a normalized FDG uptake on PET images was reported to be 81% at a specificity of 95% (10). When recovery of wall thickening was considered to be the gold standard, the sensitivity of DE-MRI in predicting recovery of function after revascularization was 89% with a specificity of 94%. The latter analysis was patient-related, which is clinically more meaningful than a segment-by-segment analysis (11). In contrast, Gunning et al (12) studied 30 patients with severe LV dysfunction (mean LV ejection fraction [EF] = 24%) and showed a high specificity of 83% but a low sensitivity of 50% for a visually assessed contractile reserve as a predictor of functional recovery after revascularization. Likewise, Sandstede et al (40) found a low sensitivity (61%) but high specificity (90%) for improved segmental wall motion during dobutamine infusion. The latter two studies are consistent with dobutamine echocardiography findings, which also demonstrated a relatively modest sensitivity but high specificity for prediction of functional improvement (4,7). There are several explanations for these differences in predicting functional outcome, however patient selection is probably the key issue. The higher LVEF (mean LVEF = 41% vs. 24%) in the study by Baer et al (11), with possibly fewer ultrastructural changes and loss of contractile protein in areas of dysfunctional but viable myocardium, may have increased the likelihood of eliciting a dobutamine-stimulated contraction reserve. It is known that evaluation of the contractile reserve has a reduced predictive accuracy if more severe wall-motion abnormality is present at rest. For example, in akinetic or dyskinetic segments at rest, the sensitivity of dobutamine echocardiography for prediction of functional recovery may be as low as 26% (41). Interestingly, a recently published study by Wellnhofer et al (42) reported a sensitivity of 75% and a specificity of 93% for functional recovery of infarct regions as assessed by low-dose dobutamine MRI, resulting in a diagnostic accuracy similar to that reported by Baer et al (11) (Table 15.1). Moreover in this study, low-dose dobutamine MRI was superior to scar quantification by contrast-enhanced MRI in a head-to-head comparison for the prediction of functional recovery (42). This advantage was largest in segments with a delayed enhancement of 1% to 74% transmural extent of MI.

A head-to-head comparison is also available for low-dose dobutamine MRI and dobutamine transesophageal echocardiography (TEE) (29,43) in the assessment of viable myocardium. Normalized FDG uptake on PET images was used as the standard against which both techniques were compared (43). The sensitivity and the specificity of dobutamine TEE and low-dose dobutamine MRI for assessing FDG PET-defined myocardial viability were 77% versus 81% and 94% versus 100%, respectively. In a recently published study, the recovery of regional LV function after revascularization was chosen as the reference standard for the direct comparison of both imaging techniques on a qualitative visual basis (29). The positive and negative predictive accuracy rates of dobutamine TEE and low-dose dobutamine MRI for the prediction of LV functional improvement were 85% versus 92% and 80% versus 85%, respectively. Thus, both imaging techniques provide similar accuracy rates in assessing viability in both quantitative (measurement of wall thickening) (43) and less time-consuming qualitative (evaluation of wall motion) analysis (29). In the choice of an appropriate technique, patient acceptance becomes an important consideration. Al-though claustrophobia and electrocardiogram triggering may be problematic in MRI, only a small number of patients are affected. In contrast, many patients do not like the experience of a TEE examination. On the other hand, TEE offers a clear economic advantage because the cost of an echo probe is only a fraction of that of an MR scanner.

FUTURE DEVELOPMENTS OF LOW-DOSE DOBUTAMINE MAGNETIC RESONANCE IMAGING FOR THE ASSESSMENT OF MYOCARDIAL VIABILITY

Low-dose dobutamine MRI proved to be a valid and clinically robust tool for the detection of viable myocardium and can compete with echocardiography and scintigraphic imaging techniques with respect to the prediction of functional recovery (Fig. 15.5). However, current data originate from a few studies only predominantly enrolling patients with chronic CAD. Therefore, multicenter studies in larger numbers of patients covering the entire spectrum of postischemic dysfunction (acute, subacute, and chronic infarction) are required to fully evaluate this technique. Although a recently published study by Wellnhofer et al (42) pointed out the superiority of low-dose dobutamine MRI in predicting functional recovery compared to the identification of scar tissue by quantification of the transmural extent of DE-MRI, the latter MR technique has some advantages that make it a strong competitor if viability is the question. Both low-dose dobutamine MRI and DE-MRI require intravenous access, but DE-MRI does not require infusion of a pharmacological stressor in the magnet and therefore requires less intensive monitoring, is safer, easier to implement, and faster to complete. On the other hand, low-dose dobutamine MRI can be integrated easily into a diagnostic set up for the combined

| TABLE 15-1 | Stress Echocardiography and Low-Dose Dobutamine Stress MRI for the Prediction of Left Ventricular Functional Recovery after Successful Revascularization |

Method of Viability Assessment	Reference Parameter	Sensitivity (%)	Specificity (%)	No. Patients Included	Study (Ref.)
Dobu-TTE	Wall-motion recovery postrevascularization	82	86	n = 25	Cigarroa et al, 1993 (7)
Dobu-TTE	Wall-motion recovery postrevascularization	86	90	n = 38	Smart et al, 1993 (8)
Dobu-TEE	Wall-motion recovery postrevascularization	92	88	n = 42	Baer et al, 1996 (4)
Dobu-MRI	Wall-motion recovery postrevascularization	50	81	n = 23	Gunning et al, 1998 (11)
Dobu-MRI	Wall-thickening improvement (>2 mm) postrevascularization	89	94	n = 43	Baer et al, 1998 (10)
Dobu-MRI	Wall-motion recovery	75	93	29	Wellnhofer et al, 2004 (42)

Dobu, dobutamine; TEE, transesophageal echocardiography; TTE, transthoracic echocardiography.

Figure 15.5. Diagnostic value of low-dose dobutamine stress MRI in comparison to established imaging techniques for the prediction of left ventricular functional recovery following successful revascularization procedures. LDDE, low-dose dobutamine echocardiography; MRI-DWT, magnetic resonance imaging assessed end-diastolic wall thickness at rest; MRI-SWT, magnetic resonance imaging assessed dobutamine-induced systolic wall thickening; TC-MIBI, technetium-methoxyisobutylisonitril; TI-201re, thallium-201 reinjection scintigraphy (late); TI-201rest, thallium-201 rest scintigraphy. (Adapted from Bax JJ, Wijns W, Cornel JH, et al. Accuracy of currently available techniques for prediction of functional recovery after revascularization in patients with left ventricular dysfunction due to chronic coronary artery disease: comparison of pooled data. *J Am Coll Cardiol* 1997;30:1451–1460.)

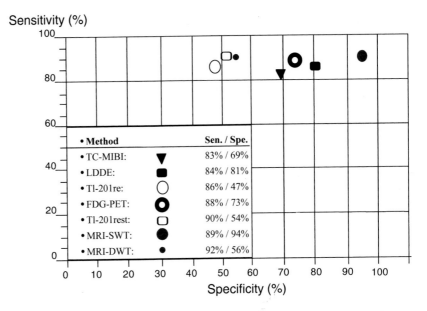

• Method	Sen. / Spe.
• TC-MIBI:	83% / 69%
• LDDE:	84% / 81%
• TI-201re:	86% / 47%
• FDG-PET:	88% / 73%
• TI-201rest:	90% / 54%
• MRI-SWT:	89% / 94%
• MRI-DWT:	92% / 56%

assessment of viability and myocardial ischemia. From a clinical point of view, the question arises whether a substantial amount of viability is sufficient to provide a clinical benefit (improved stress tolerance, reversal of adverse remodeling, prevention of recurrent ischemia, and arrhythmias) without a detectable functional improvement after revascularization, especially in patients with severe myocardial dysfunction. Further studies must show whether the complementary information of low-dose dobutamine MRI (superior predictor of functional recovery) and DE-MRI (localization and quantification of scar tissue) should be used for profound clinical decision-making in patients suspected to have viable myocardium.

REFERENCES

1. Gould KL. Myocardial viability. What does it mean and how to measure it? *Circulation* 1991;83:333–335.
2. Braunwald E, Rutherford J. Reversible ischemic left ventricular dysfunction: evidence of the "hibernating myocardium." *J Am Coll Cardiol* 1986;8:1467–1470.
3. Di Carli MF, Maddahi J, Rokhsar S, et al. Long-term survival of patients with coronary artery disease and left ventricular dysfunction: implications for the role of myocardial viability assessment in management decisions. *J Thoracic Cardiovasc Surg* 1998;116:997–1104.
4. Bax JJ, Wijns W, Cornel JH, et al. Accuracy of currently available techniques for prediction of functional recovery after revascularization in patients with left ventricular dysfunction due to chronic coronary artery disease: comparison of pooled data. *J Am Coll Cardiol* 1997;30:1451–1460.
5. Baer FM, Voth E, Deutsch H, et al. Predictive value of low dose dobutamine transesophageal echocardiography and fluorine-18-fluorodeoxyglucose positron emission tomography for recovery of regional left ventricular function after successful revascularization. *J Am Coll Cardiol* 1996;28:60–69.
6. Lucignani G, Paolini G, Landoni C, et al. Presurgical identification of hibernating myocardium by combined use of technetium-99m hexakis 2-methoxyisobutylisonitrile single photon

emission tomography and fluorine-18 fluoro-2-deoxy-D-glucose positron emission tomography in patients with coronary artery disease. *Eur J Nucl Med* 1992;19:874–881.
7. Bax JJ, Cornel JH, Visser FC, et al. Prediction of recovery of myocardial dysfunction following revascularization: comparison of F18-fluorodeoxyglucose/thallium-201 single photon computed emission tomography, thallium-201 stress-reinjection single photon emission tomography and dobutamine echocardiography. *J Am Coll Cardiol* 1996;28:558–564.
8. Cigarroa CG, deFilippi CR, Brickner ME, et al. Dobutamine stress echocardiography identifies hibernating myocardium and predicts recovery of left ventricular function after coronary revascularization. *Circulation* 1993;88:430–436.
9. Smart SC, Sawada S, Ryan T, et al. Low-dose dobutamine echocardiography detects reversible dysfunction after thrombolytic therapy of acute myocardial infarction. *Circulation* 1993;88:405–415.
10. Baer FM, Voth E, Schneider CA, et al. Dobutamine-gradient echo MRI: a functional and morphologic approach to the detection of residual myocardial viability. *Circulation* 1995;91: 1006–1015.
11. Baer FM, Theissen P, Schneider CA, et al. Dobutamine magnetic resonance imaging predicts contractile recovery of chronically dysfunctional myocardium after successful revascularization. *J Am Coll Cardiol* 1998;31:1040–1048.
12. Gunning MG, Anagnostopoulos C, Knight CJ, et al. Comparison of 201-TL, 99mTc-Tetrofosmin, and dobutamine magnetic resonance imaging for identifying hibernating myocardium. *Circulation* 1998;98:1869–1874.
13. Perrone-Filardi P, Bacharach SL, Dilsizian V, et al. Metabolic evidence of viable myocardium in regions with reduced wall thickness and absent wall thickening in patients with chronic ischemic left ventricular dysfunction. *J Am Coll Cardiol* 1992; 20:161–168.
14. Mallory GK, White PD, Salcedo-Galger J. The speed of healing of myocardial infarction: a study of the pathologic anatomy in 72 cases. *Am Heart J* 1939;18:647–671.
15. Heusch G, Schulz R. Hibernating myocardium: a review. *J Mol Cell Cardiol* 1996;28:2359–2372.
16. Popio KA, Gorlin R, Bechtel D, et al. Postextrasystolic potentiation as a predictor of potential myocardial viability: Preoperative analysis compared with studies after coronary bypass surgery. *Am J Cardiol* 1977;39:944–953.

17. Cigarroa CG, de Filippi CR, Brickner ME, et al. Dobutamine stress echocardiography identifies hibernating myocardium and predicts recovery of left ventricular function after coronary revascularization. *Circulation* 1993;88:430–436.

18. Barkhausen J, Ruehm SG, Goyen M, et al. MR evaluation of ventricular function: true fast imaging with steady-state precession versus fast low-angle shot cine MR imaging: feasibility study. *Radiology* 2001;219:264–269.

19. Cerqueira MD, Weissmann NJ, Dilsizian V, et al. Standardized myocardial segmentation and nomenclature for tomographic imaging of the heart.: a statement for healthcare professionals from the Cardiac Imaging Committee of the Council of Clinical cardiology of the American Heart Association. *Circulation* 2002;105:539–542.

20. van Rugge FP, van der Wall EE, Spanjersberg SJ, et al. Magnetic resonance imaging during dobutamine stress for detection and localization of coronary artery disease. Quantitative wall motion analysis using a modification of the centerline method. *Circulation* 1994;90:127–138.

21. van der Geest RJ, Buller VGM, Jansen E, et al. Comparison between manual and semiautomated analysis of left ventricular volume parameters from short-axis MR images. *J Comp Assist Tomogr* 1997;21:756–765.

22. Kraitchman DL, Sampath S, Castillo E, et al. Quantitative ischemia detection during cardiac magnetic resonance stress testing by use of FastHARP. *Circulation* 2003;107:2025–2030.

23. Mazzadi NA, Janier MF, Brossier B, et al. Tagged MRI and PET in severe CAD: discrepancy between preoperative inotropic reserve and intramyocardial fusnctional outcome after revascularization. *Am J Physiol Heart Circ Physiol* 2004;287: H2226–H2233.

24. Judd R, Lup-Olivieri C, Arai M, et al. Physiological basis of myocardial contrast enhancement in fast magnetic resonance images of 2-day-old reperfused canine infarcts. *Circulation* 1995;92:902–1910.

25. Kim R, Fieno D, Parrish T, et al. Relationship of MRI delayed contrast enhancement to irreversible injury, infarct age and contractile function. *Circulation* 1999;100:1992–2002.

26. Wu KC, Zerhouni EA, Judd RM, et al. Prognostic significance of microvascular obstruction by magnetic resonance imaging in patients with acute myocardial infarction. *Circulation* 1998; 97:765–772.

27. Kim RJ, Chen EL, Lima JA, et al. Myocardial Gd-DTPA kinetics determine MRI contrast enhancement and reflect the extent and severity of myocardial injury after acute reperfused infarction. *Circulation* 1996;94:3318–3326.

28. Rogers WJ, Kramer CM, Geskin G, et al. Early contrast-enhanced MRI predicts late functional recovery after reperfused myocardial infarction. *Circulation* 1999;99:744–750.

29. Baer FM, Theissen P, Crnac J, et al. Head-to-head comparison of dobutamine-transesophageal echocardiography and dobutamine-magnetic resonance imaging for the prediction of left ventricular functional recovery in patients with chronic coronary artery disease. *Eur Heart J* 2000;21:981–991.

30. Pirolo JS, Hutchins GM, Moore GW. Infarct expansion: pathologic analysis of 204 patients with a single myocardial infarct. *J Am Coll Cardiol* 1986;7:349–354.

31. Sayad DE, Willett DL, Bridges WH, et al. Noninvasive quantitation of left ventricular wall thickening using cine magnetic resonance imaging with myocardial tagging. *Am J Cardiol* 1995;76:985–989.

32. Lima JAC, Jeremy R, Guier W, et al. Accurate systolic wall thickening by nuclear magnetic resonance imaging with tissue ragging: Correlation with sonomicrometers in normal and ischemic myocardium. *J Am Coll Cardiol* 1993;21:1741–1751.

33. Dendale P, Franken PR, van der Wall EE, et al. Wall thickening at rest and contractile reserve early after myocardial infarction: correlation with myocardial perfusion and metabolism. *Coron Artery Dis* 1997;8:259–264.

34. Schmidt M, Voth E, Schneider CA, et al. F-18-FDG uptake is a reliable predictor of functional recovery of akinetic but viable infarct regions as defined by magnetic resonance imaging before and after revascularization. *Magn Reson Imaging* 2004; 22:229–236.

35. Dubnow MH, Burchell HB, Titus JL. Postinfarction left ventricular aneurysm. A clinicomorphologic and electrocardiographic study of 80 cases. *Am Heart J* 1965;70:753–760.

36. Braunwald E, Kloner RA. Myocardial reperfusion: a double-edged sword? *J Clin Invest* 1985;76:1713–1719.

37. Baer FM, Smolarz K, Jungehulsing M, et al. Chronic myocardial infarction: assessment of morphology, function, and perfusion by gradient echo magnetic resonance imaging and 99mTc-methoxyisobutyl-isonitrile SPECT. *Am Heart J* 1992;123: 636–645.

38. Faletra F, Crivellaro W, Pirelli S, et al. Value of transthoracic two-dimensional echocardiography in predicting viability in patients with healed Q-wave anterior wall myocardial infarction. *Am J Cardiol* 1995;76:1002–1006.

39. Lawson MA, Johnson LL, Coghlan L, et al. Correlation of thallium uptake with left ventricular wall thickness by cine magnetic resonance imaging in patients with acute and healed myocardial infarcts. *Am J Cardiol* 1997;80:434–441.

40. Sandstede J, Bertsch G, Beer M, et al. Detection of myocardial viability by low-dose dobutamine cine MRI. *Magn Reson Imaging* 1999;17:1437–1443.

41. Bonow RO. Identification of viable myocardium. *Circulation* 1996;94:2674–2680.

42. Wellnhofer E, Olariu A, Klein C, et al. Magnetic resonance low-dose dobutamine test is superior to scar quantification for the prediction of functional recovery. *Circulation* 2004;109: 2172–2174.

43. Baer FM, Voth E, LaRosee K, et al. Comparison of dobutamine transesophageal echocardiography and dobutamine magnetic resonance imaging for detection of residual myocardial viability. *Am J Cardiol* 1996;78:415–419.

16

Assessment of Myocardial Viability by Contrast Enhancement

Raymond J. Kim, Michael D. Elliott, and Robert M. Judd

CLINICAL SIGNIFICANCE OF MYOCARDIAL VIABILITY

In patients with ischemic heart disease, one of the most important determinants of long-term survival is the level of left ventricular (LV) dysfunction (1–3). It is important to recognize, however, that not all dysfunction of the LV is irreversible and represents previous infarction. In the setting of *chronic* coronary artery disease (CAD) and LV dysfunction, it is well established that LV function can improve following revascularization procedures such as percutaneous coronary angioplasty (PTCA) and coronary artery bypass surgery (CABG) (4–9). The mechanism for reversible myocardial dysfunction in this setting is not entirely clear, but terms such as *hibernating myocardium* (4,5) and *repetitive stunning* (10–12) have been used to describe the underlying pathophysiology. Regardless of the actual mechanism, several facts are known about this clinical syndrome. First, the prevalence is not inconsequential. Several studies have demonstrated that in up to one third of patients with chronic CAD and LV dysfunction, LV function improves after revascularization (13–16). Second, it is clear that diagnostic testing before revascularization can be useful in predicting functional improvement after revascularization (Fig. 16.1). Third, more recent studies have shown that patients

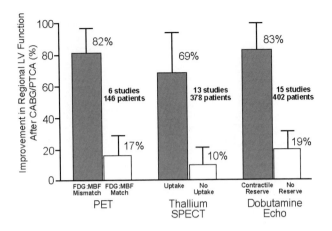

Figure 16.1. Likelihood of improved regional LV function after revascularization based on noninvasive methods to detect viable myocardium. Data are from 34 pooled studies involving over 900 patients. The range of values are reported from the individual studies (*horizontal error lines*). The *shaded bars* represent the positive predictive value and the *open bars* represent the inverse of the negative predictive value. (From Bonow RO. Identification of viable myocardium. *Circulation* 1996;94(11):2674–2680, with permission.)

with reversible dysfunction who undergo revascularization derive benefits beyond improved ventricular function, such as increased survival (17–20). For example, in a meta-analysis of 24 studies representing over 3,000 patients, revascularization of patients with dysfunctional but viable myocardium, as determined by thallium perfusion imaging, F-18 fluorodeoxyglucose (FDG) metabolic imaging, or dobutamine stress echocardiography (DSE), resulted in almost an 80% reduction in annual mortality (21). Furthermore, in patients with viability, there was a direct relationship between the severity of LV dysfunction and the magnitude of benefit with revascularization (21).

In the *acute* setting following an episode of myocardial ischemia and reperfusion, it is recognized that reversible myocardial dysfunction can also occur. In this setting, the underlying process is myocardial "stunning" (10,22,23), and the ventricular dysfunction should improve over time if reperfusion therapy was successful. There are several reasons why it is important to distinguish between stunned and infarcted myocardium. First, the patient prognosis is changed. Several studies have shown that patients with acute ventricular dysfunction primarily resulting from myocardial necrosis have a worse prognosis than patients with ventricular dysfunction that is primarily reversible (24,25). Second, patient management during the acute setting may be changed. Viable but injured myocardium, such as stunned myocardium, is potentially at risk for future infarction if the reperfusion therapy was not complete and significant stenosis remains (25,26). Additionally, a determination of the extent of nonviable and viable myocardium across the ventricular wall in a dysfunctional region may be valuable in selecting patients most likely to benefit from therapy that can modulate ventricular remodeling after acute myocardial infarction (MI), such as angiotensin-converting enzyme inhibitors and beta-blockers (27). Third, infarct size determined accurately in the acute setting may prove to be an adequate surrogate end point for the assessment of new therapies (28,29). For example, the efficacy of experimental therapies for acute coronary syndromes or acute MI could be evaluated without the need for "mega" trials with large sample sizes that use mortality as an end point. It is expected that the number of drug and device trials that employ cardiac magnetic resonance imaging (MRI) parameters as a primary end point will increase substantially in the future.

Thus, it is apparent that a diagnostic test capable of distinguishing between viable and nonviable myocardium independent of the level of contractile function in both the acute and chronic settings is essential in the clinical assessment of patients with ischemic heart disease. In this chapter we evaluate the ability of a contrast MRI technique—delayed contrast enhanced MRI (DE-MRI)—to fill this clinical role. We will start, however, with the basic definition of myocardial viability. Although the definition may appear to be self-evident, we will find that discrepancies between the results of DE-MRI and other clinical indexes of viability may arise because of assumptions concerning the definition of viability.

DEFINITION OF MYOCARDIAL VIABILITY

Before any technique used to identify myocardial viability can be evaluated, a definition of viability is required. The definition of viability is directly related to that of MI because infarction results in the loss of viability. A number of techniques are available in the clinical setting to determine whether or not infarction has occurred and if so, how much of the injured territory is not yet infarcted and can be salvaged. In a recent review article, Kaul (30) summarized clinical markers of infarct size and ranked them from least to most precise (Fig. 16.2). As discussed previously, observation of a wall-motion abnormality alone does not provide information regarding viability because both stunned and hibernating myocardium are dysfunctional. The electrocardiogram (ECG), although useful, is recognized as being insensitive to infarction because patients with smaller infarcts may demonstrate minimal ECG changes during the acute event and often will not have Q waves chronically. Serum markers such as creatine kinase (CK) and troponin I or T can be extremely useful but even these are associated with several limitations. For example, CK and troponin levels may exhibit differing time courses depending on whether or not reperfusion has occurred (31), and neither can be used to localize the infarction to a specific coronary artery territory.

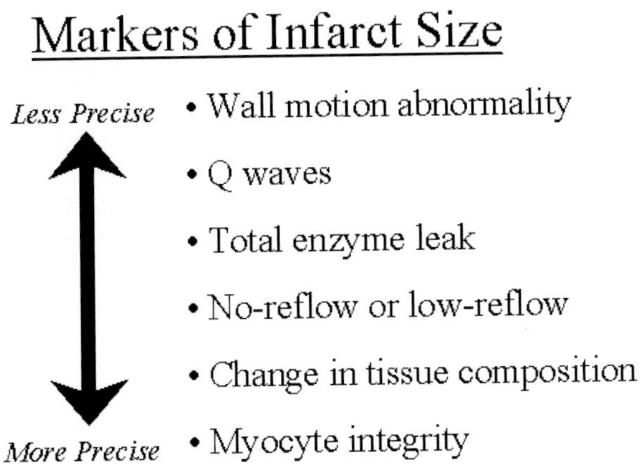

Markers of Infarct Size

Less Precise

- Wall motion abnormality
- Q waves
- Total enzyme leak
- No-reflow or low-reflow
- Change in tissue composition

More Precise
- Myocyte integrity

Figure 16.2. Clinical and physiological markers to determine the size of infarction. (Adapted from Kaul S. Assessing the myocardium after attempted reperfusion: should we bother? *Circulation* 1998;98(7):625–627, with permission.)

Perhaps most importantly, serum levels of CK are not elevated beyond the first few days and troponin levels are not elevated beyond the first 2 weeks following the ischemic event (32), precluding the detection of older infarcts.

According to Kaul (30), the most precise way to define infarction, and therefore the loss of viability, is to determine whether or not myocyte death has occurred. All ischemic events prior to cell death are at least in principle reversible; therefore, the further we deviate from a direct assessment of cell death, the more imprecise we become in defining infarction. Likewise, the most precise definition of myocardial viability is the presence of living myocytes. The presence or absence of living myocytes can be readily established in tissue specimens by light microscopy, electron microscopy, or by the use of histologic stains such as triphenyl tetrazolium chloride (TTC) (33). Testing for viability by microscopy or histologic staining, however, is obviously not practical in a clinical setting. Accordingly, a number of less precise definitions of viability that are based on parameters more easily measured in patients have been developed (Table 16.1).

In the literature, viability is often defined as improvement in contractile function after coronary revascularization. This definition is frequently the clinical "gold standard" to which imaging techniques are compared. Although convenient for clinical purposes, this definition can be inaccurate. If contractile function improves after revascularization, it is safe to assume that there is a significant amount of viability;

however, the converse is not true. In fact, analysis of transmural needle-biopsy specimens taken during CABG demonstrated that some regions that did *not* improve after revascularization *did* have a significant amount of viability. For example, Dakik et al (34) reported that the extent of viability was nearly 70% of total myocardium in their samples. Several factors may account for the absence of functional improvement after revascularization despite the presence of myocardial viability: (a) a single evaluation of ventricular function soon after revascularization may underestimate the true rate of functional recovery; (b) incomplete coronary revascularization, especially in patients with diffuse and extensive atherosclerosis; (c) viable regions that are tethered to regions of extensive scarring may attenuate the improvement in contractile performance of viable regions after revascularization; (d) new perioperative myocardial necrosis in regions that were viable prior to revascularization (35); and (e) partial viability—regional wall thickening may not improve in the presence of nontransmural scarring. A subendocardial (≤50% transmural extent) infarction may limit restoration of myocardial thickening after revascularization despite the presence of significant viability (36). Although of clinical relevance, owing to the aforementioned reasons, improvement in contractile performance after revascularization should not define the presence of myocardial viability.

Since the correct definition of viability is the presence of living myocytes, the ideal imaging method for assessing viability should be able to delineate infarcted tissue from viable tissue with high spatial resolution. Unfortunately, currently available techniques, such as single-photon emission computed tomography (SPECT), positron emission tomography (PET), and DSE, have various limitations. First, what is measured is not the direct presence and exact quantity of viable myocytes, but rather a physiologic parameter, such as contractile reserve or perfusion that has only an indirect relationship to viability. Second, there are technique-specific limitations, including partial volume effects due to poor spatial resolution (SPECT, PET), attenuation and scatter artifacts (SPECT), errors in registration between comparison images (DSE), and the occasional inability to visualize all parts of the LV myocardium (DSE). Third, all of these techniques interpret viability as an all-or-none phenomenon within a myocardial region since none can assess the transmural extent of viability across the ventricular wall. Figure 16.3 demonstrates the discrepancy that can arise due

TABLE 16-1	Common Clinical Definitions of Myocardial Viability

- Improvement in contraction after revascularization
- Improvement in contraction with low-dose dobutamine
- Preserved perfusion
- Preserved radionuclide tracer uptake
- Preserved glucose uptake
- Preserved wall thickness and/or thickening

Ideal Imaging Method

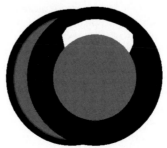

QUESTION:
Is the anterior wall viable or not-viable?

Figure 16.3. Cartoon showing infarction of the subendocardial half of the anterior wall (*white area*). See text for details.

to this limitation. In this particular example, assessment of the anterior wall using current clinical methods and definitions will be incorrect regardless of whether the anterior wall is determined to be viable or not viable since the correct assessment is that the subendocardial half of the wall is not viable and the epicardial half is viable.

SCOPE OF THE CHAPTER

This chapter focuses on the physiological and clinical interpretation of DE-MRI. The phenomenon of delayed hyperenhancement was first described over 20 years ago (37). Several excellent reviews of the literature concerning the interpretation of myocardial hyperenhancement before the development of the segmented inversion recovery sequence have been published, (38,39) and this literature is revisited here only briefly. We proceed by providing a comprehensive review of the technical aspects of DE-MRI, followed by a review of the original pathophysiological validation studies. We then demonstrate the clinical application of DE-MRI and compare this technique to other clinically available modalities used to assess myocardial viability. We finish by highlighting potential issues in image interpretation and provide a brief discussion on "novel" and emerging applications for which DE-MRI may be ideally suited.

DELAYED ENHANCEMENT MAGNETIC RESONANCE IMAGING

BACKGROUND

The primary action of most MRI contrast agents currently approved for use in humans is to shorten the longitudinal relaxation time (T_1). Accordingly, the goal of most MRI pulse sequences used for the purpose of examining contrast enhancement patterns is to make image intensities a strong function of T_1 (T_1-weighted images). Early approaches to acquiring T_1-weighted images of the heart often used ECG-gated spin-echo imaging in which one k-space line was acquired during each cardiac cycle. Because the duration of the cardiac cycle is comparable with the myocardial T_1 (~800 ms), the resulting images were T_1-weighted. Following the administration of gadolinium contrast, myocardial T_1 was shortened and image intensities increased. Using this approach, a number of investigators reported that as image intensities increased throughout the heart, regions associated with acute MI became particularly bright (hyperenhanced) on a timescale of minutes to tens of minutes after contrast administration (40–46). The use of ECG-gated spin-echo imaging, however, has several intrinsic limitations that adversely affect image quality. One such limitation is the need for relatively long acquisition times (minutes), which introduces artifacts caused by respiratory motion.

NEW TECHNIQUE

Since the early use of ECG-gated spin-echo imaging, a number of improvements have been made. One of the most im-

portant among these is the use of segmented k-space (47), in which multiple k-space lines are acquired after each cardiac cycle. As a result, imaging times are reduced to the point at which an entire image can be acquired during a single breath-hold (~8 s), thereby eliminating image artifacts caused by respiration. In addition, preparation of the magnetization before image acquisition with an inversion pulse significantly increases the degree of T_1-weighting in the images. Recently, a segmented inversion recovery pulse sequence was compared with nine other pulse sequences in a dog model of acute MI (48). Table 16.2 summarizes the literature in humans and in in vivo large animal models regarding the depiction of infarcted regions by gadolinium-enhanced MRI prior to the development of the segmented inversion recovery sequence. From 1986 to 1999, image intensities in "hyperenhanced" regions were generally 50% to 100% higher than normal regions. The use of a segmented inversion recovery pulse sequence with the inversion time set to null signal from normal myocardium increased this differential approximately 10-fold to 1,080% in animals and 485% in humans (labeled "New Technique" in Table 16.2).

OVERALL PROCEDURE

The procedure for DE-MRI is relatively simple (Fig. 16.4). It can be performed in a single brief examination, requires only a peripheral intravenous catheter that is placed before the patient enters the MRI scanner, and does not require pharmacologic or physiologic stress. After obtaining scout images to delineate the short- and long-axis views of the heart, we obtain cine images to provide a matched assessment of LV morphology and contractile function, and to aid in the detection of small subendocardial infarcts (to be discussed). Short-axis views (6-mm slice thickness with 4-mm gap to match contrast enhancement images) are taken every 10 mm from mitral valve insertion to LV apex along with two to three long-axis views in order to encompass the entire LV. The patient is then given a bolus of 0.10–0.15 mmol/kg intravenous gadolinium by hand injection. After a 10–15 min delay (timing issues will be discussed further), high spatial resolution delayed enhancement images of the heart are obtained at the same slice locations as the cine images using a segmented inversion recovery fast gradient echo (seg IR-FGE) pulse sequence. Figure 16.5 demonstrates cine and DE-MRI images from a typical patient scan. Each delayed enhancement image is acquired during an 8–10 s breath-hold, and the imaging time for the entire examination is generally 25–35 min.

PULSE SEQUENCE TIMING

The timing diagram for the seg IR-FGE pulse sequence is shown in Figure 16.6. Immediately after the onset of the R wave trigger, there is a delay or wait period (which is referred to as the trigger delay or TD) before a nonselective 180° hyperbolic secant adiabatic inversion pulse is applied. Following this inversion pulse, a second variable wait period (which is referred to as the inversion time or TI) occurs, corresponding to the time between the inversion pulse and the center of the data acquisition window (for linearly ordered k-space acquisition). The data acquisition window is

TABLE 16-2 Percentage Elevations in MR Signal Intensity of Infarcted Versus Nomal Myocardium and Voxel Sizes: Previous Studies Compared With New Technique

Year	Reference	Technique[a]	Breath Hold	Canine ΔI/R (%)[b]	Canine Voxel Size (mm³)	Human ΔI/R (%)[b]	Human Voxel Size (mm³)
1986	Rehr RB, et al (43)	Spin echo	No	80	NS		
1986	Tscholakoff D, et al[g]	Spin echo	No	70	NS		
1986	Eichstaedt HW, et al (41)	Spin echo	No			42[c]	29.3[d]
1988	de Roos A, et al[h]	Spin echo	No			60	29.3[d]
1989	de Roos A, et al[i]	Spin echo	No			36	29.3[d]
1990	van der Wall EE, et al (64)	Spin echo	No			32[c]	31.3[d]
1991	van Dijkman PR, et al (85)	Spin echo	No			31[c]	27.5
1991	Matheijssen NA, et al (42)	Spin echo	No			42	29.3[d]
1994	Fedele F, et al (86)	Spin echo	No			41[c]	29.3[d]
1995	Lima JA, et al (65)	MD-SPGRE	Yes			103[c]	33.3
1995	Judd RM, et al (62)	MD-SPGRE	Yes	123[e]	39.6		
1998	Ramani K, et al (87)	MD-SPGRE	Yes			58[e]	30.8
1999	Pereira RS, et al[j]	MD-SPGRE	Yes	79[e]	14.7		
1999	Rogers WJ, Jr, et al (66)	Single-shot inversion recovery GRE	Yes			39	54.9[f]
	Mean of previous studies			86	27.2	48	32.4
	New Technique	Segmented inversion-recovery GRE	Yes	1,080	6.2	485	16.8

MD-SPGRE, magnetization-driven spoiled gradient echo; NS, not stated; GRE, gradient recalled echo.
[a] All images were acquired in vivo at least 5 minutes after the administration of a United States Food and Drug Administration-approved MR imaging contrast agent.
[b] ΔI/R = percent elevation in MR signal intensityof infarcted myocardium compared with normal myocardium.
[c] Published data were reported as precontrast versus postcontrast values; values in Table 2 were calculated as follows: (postcontrast value—precontrast value)/precontrast value.
[d] Assuming a field of view of 320 mm.
[e] Estimated from data reported in graphical format.
[f] Assuming a rectangular (6/8) field of view.
[g] Tscholakoff D, Higgins CB, Sechtem U, et al. Occlusive and reperfused myocardial infarcts: effect of Gd-DTPA on ECG-gated MR imaging. *Radiology* 1986;160:515–519.
[h] de Roos A, Doornbos J, van der Wall EE, et al. MR imaging of acute myocardial infarction: value of Gd-DTPA. *AJR Am J Roentgenol* 1988;150:531–534.
[i] de Roos A, van Rossum AC, van der Wall E, et al. Reperfused and nonreperfused myocardial infarction: diagnostic potential of Gd-DTPA–enhanced MR imaging. *Radiology* 1989;172:717–720.
[j] Pereira RS, Prato FS, Sykes J, et al. Assessment of myocardial viability using MRI during a constant infusion of Gd-DTPA: further studies at early and late periods of reperfusion. *Magn Reson Med* 1999;42:60–68.
Adapted from Simonetti OP, Kim RJ, Fieno DS, et al. An improved MR imaging technique for the visualization of myocardial infarction. *Radiology* 2001;218:215–223.

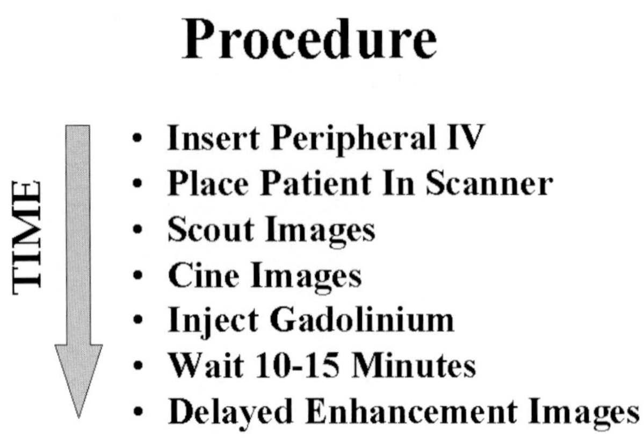

Procedure

TIME

- **Insert Peripheral IV**
- **Place Patient In Scanner**
- **Scout Images**
- **Cine Images**
- **Inject Gadolinium**
- **Wait 10-15 Minutes**
- **Delayed Enhancement Images**

Figure 16.4. The overall sequence of events in performing delayed-enhancement imaging.

generally 140 to 200 ms long, depending on the patient heart rate, and is placed during middiastole, when the heart is relatively motionless. A group of k-space lines are acquired during this acquisition window, where the flip angle used for radiofrequency excitation of each k-space line is shallow (20° to 30°) to retain regional differences in magnetization that result from the inversion pulse and TI delay. The number of k-space lines in the group is limited by the repetition time between each k-space line (8 to 9 ms) and the duration of middiastole. In the implementation shown on Figure 16.6, 23 lines of k-space are acquired during each data acquisition window, which occurs every other heart beat. With this implementation, typically a breath-hold duration of 12 cardiac

TYPICAL PATIENT SCAN

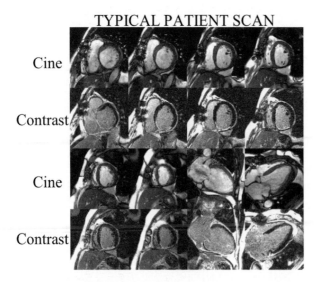

Cine

Contrast

Cine

Contrast

Figure 16.5. Images from a typical patient scan. Cine and delayed contrast-enhanced images are acquired at 6–8 short-axis locations and 2–3 long-axis locations during repeated breath-holds. Images are interpreted with cine images immediately adjacent to contrast images. This particular patient had a myocardial infarction caused by occlusion of the right coronary artery. Note hyperenhancement of the inferior wall. (From Kim RJ, Shah DJ, Mudd RM. How we perform delayed enhancement imaging. *J Cardiovasc Magn Reson* 2003;5(3):505–514, with permission.)

cycles is required to obtain all the k-space lines for the image matrix.

IMAGING PARAMETERS

The typical settings that we use for the seg IR-FGE sequence are shown in Table 16.3. The dose of gadolinium given is usually 0.10–0.15 mmol/kg. Previously, we have given doses as high as 0.3 mmol/kg in animals (48,49) and 0.2 mmol/kg in humans (48,50). More recently, we found that using doses as low as 0.10–0.15 mmol/kg still provides excellent image contrast between injured and normal myocardium and reduces the time required to wait between intravenous contrast administration and delayed enhancement imaging (51–54). Sufficient time is required in order to allow the blood pool signal in the LV cavity to decline and provide discernment between LV cavity and hyperenhanced myocardium. The field-of-view (FOV) in both read and phase-encoded directions is minimized to improve spatial resolution and minimize breath-hold time without resulting in phase aliasing or "wrap" artifact in the area of interest. For patients with heart rates less than 90 beats per minute, we typically acquire 23 lines of k-space data during the middiastolic portion of the cardiac cycle. For a repetition time of 8 ms, the data acquisition window is 184 ms in duration ($8 \times 23 = 184$). Since the middiastolic period of relative cardiac standstill is reduced in patients with faster heart rates, we decrease the number of segments (k-space lines) acquired per cardiac cycle in order to reduce the length of the imaging window. This eliminates blurring from cardiac motion during the k-space collection. In order to allow for adequate longitudinal relaxation between successive 180° inversion pulses, we typically image every other heartbeat (gating factor of 2). In our experience, an in-plane resolution of 1.2 to 1.8 mm by 1.2 to 1.8 mm with a slice thickness of 6 mm provides an ideal balance between adequate signal-to-noise while avoiding significant partial volume effects. As stated previously, the flip angle is kept shallow to retain the effects of the inversion prepulse, but it can be relatively greater (30°) if larger doses of gadolinium are given (0.2 mmol/kg) and the T_1 of myocardium is correspondingly shorter.

In patients who are unable to hold their breath for the duration required for the standard seg IR-FGE sequence, a number of options are available to reduce the breath-hold duration. Some simple strategies include: (a) minimizing the field-of-view in the phase-encode direction (FOV phase), (b) imaging with only the anterior coil elements (keeping the posterior or spine coils elements turned off), (c) allowing a smaller FOV phase than expected without resulting in wrap-around artifact over the heart, (d) increasing the number of k-space lines acquired per cardiac cycle (i.e., segments) (Table 16.3), and (e) reducing the phase resolution using a steady state free precession (SSFP) instead of FGE readout (resultant shorter TE and TR at the expense of a reduction in pure T_1 contrast effects). In some individuals, even with the approaches outlined here, there is still inadequate breath-holding. In this situation, the use of respiratory navigators or "single-shot" techniques may prove invaluable. Although there is a reduction in spatial and temporal resolution with single-shot methods, the IR-SSFP version

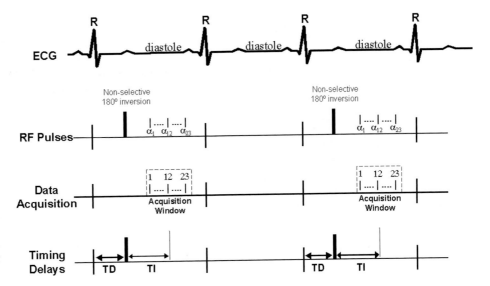

Figure 16.6. Timing diagram of two-dimensional segmented inversion recovery fast gradient echo pulse sequence. ECG, electrocardiogram; α, shallow flip angle excitation; RF, radiofrequency; TD, trigger delay; TI, inversion time delay. Note that in this implementation, 23 lines of k-space are acquired every other heartbeat. See text for further details. (From Kim RJ, Shah DJ, Mudd RM. How we perform delayed enhancement imaging. *J Cardiovasc Magn Reson* 2003;5(3):505–514, with permission.)

provides reasonable image quality in patients unable to hold their breath.

INVERSION TIME

Selecting the appropriate TI is extremely important for obtaining accurate imaging results. The TI is chosen to "null"

TABLE 16-3 Typical Parameters

Parameter	Typical Values
Gadolinium Dose	0.10–0.15 mmol/kg
Field of View	300–380 mm
In-Plane Voxel Size	1.2–1.8 × 1.2–1.8 mm
Slice Thickness	6 mm*
Flip Angle	20–30°
Segments†	13–31
TI (Inversion Time)	Variable
Bandwidth	90-250 Hz/pixel
TE (Echo Time)	3–4 msec
TR (Repetition Time)¶	8–9 msec
Gating Factor††	2
K-space Ordering	Linear
Fat Saturation	No
Asymmetric Echo	Yes
Gradient Moment Refocusing§	Yes

* Short axis slices acquired every 10 mm to achieve identical positions as the cine images.
† Fewer segments are used for higher heart rates. See text for details.
¶ TR is generally defined as the time between RF pulses, however, scanner manufacturers occasionally redefine the TR to represent the time from the ECG trigger (R wave) to the center or end of the data acquisition window (i.e., ~100 msecs less than the ECG R-R interval).
†† Image every other heart beat. See text for details.
§ Also known as gradient-moment nulling, gradient-moment rephrasing, or flow compensation. See text for details.

normal myocardium, the time at which the magnetization of normal myocardium reaches the zero crossing (Fig. 16.7A). It is at this point (or immediately just after) that the image intensity difference between infarcted and normal myocardium is maximized (Fig. 16.7C). If the TI is set too short, normal myocardium will be below the zero crossing and will have a negative magnetization vector at the time of k-space data acquisition. Since the image intensity corresponds to the magnitude of the magnetization vector, the image intensity of normal myocardium will increase as the TI becomes shorter and shorter, whereas the image intensity of infarcted myocardium will decrease until it reaches its own zero crossing (Fig. 16.7B). At this point, infarcted myocardium will be nulled and normal myocardium will be hyperenhanced. On the opposite extreme, if the TI is set too long, the magnetization of normal myocardium will be above zero and will appear gray (not "nulled"). Although areas of infarction will have high image intensity, the relative contrast between infarcted and normal myocardium will be reduced. In principle, the optimal TI at which normal myocardium is "nulled" must be determined by imaging iteratively with different inversion times. In practice, however, only one or two "test" images need to be acquired; with experience, one can estimate the optimal TI on the basis of the amount of contrast agent that is administered and the time after contrast agent administration. Figure 16.8 shows images of a patient with an anterior wall MI in whom the TI has been varied from too short to too long. Note that with the TI set moderately too short (Fig. 16.8B), the anterior wall has some regions that are hyperenhanced; however, the total extent of hyperenhancement is less than that seen when the TI is set correctly (Fig. 16.8C). This is due to the periphery of the infarcted region passing through a zero crossing, thereby affecting its apparent size (55). If the TI is set too long (Fig. 16.8D), although the contrast is reduced as previously stated, the total extent of hyperenhancement does not change. Lastly, if the TI is set far too short (Fig. 16.8A), infarct will be "nulled" and normal myocardium will hyperenhance. Thus, it is far better to err on the side of setting the TI too long rather than too short.

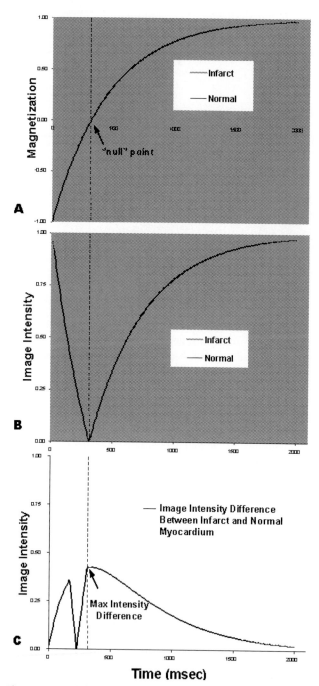

As stated previously, data are acquired every other heartbeat in order to allow for adequate longitudinal relaxation between successive inversion pulses. The time for recovery of 96% of the bulk magnetization is approximately 4 times the T_1 [$M(t) = M_0(1 - 2e^{-t/T1})$ or $M(4T_1) = M_0(1 - 2e^{-4})$]. For example, if the T_1 of normal myocardium after administration of gadolinium is 400 ms, then in order to achieve adequate longitudinal relaxation, there should be approximately 1,600 ms between successive inversion pulses or every other heartbeat imaging in patients with heart rates of 75 beats per minute (R-R interval = 800 ms). In this example, the optimal TI to null normal myocardium would be approximately 280 ms [TI(null) = ln(2)*T_1 = 0.69*T_1]. Occasionally, imaging is performed every third heartbeat (gating factor of 3) if the patient is tachycardic. Conversely, owing to limitations in breath-hold duration and/or bradycardia, every heartbeat imaging may be performed.

Fortunately, for those that are unfamiliar with inversion recovery relaxation curves, newer pulse sequences that allow phase-sensitive reconstruction of inversion recovery data may allow a nominal TI to be used rather than a precise null time for normal myocardium (56). These techniques, by restoring signal polarity, can provide consistent contrast between infarcted and normal myocardium over a wide range of inversion times and can eliminate the apparent reduction in infarct size that is seen on images acquired with inversion times that are too short (56). TI "scout" sequences also have been developed to aid in selecting the correct inversion time (57). In our experience, these sequences only provide a reasonable "first guess" at the correct TI since they can be off by as much as 40 to 50 ms. This discrepancy may be due to several reasons. For example, TI scout sequences generally do not account for the gating factor that is used in the seg IR-FGE sequence, which can lead to changes in the correct TI as described previously. Additionally, recovery of longitudinal magnetization is not identical for inversion recovery prepared SSFP (often used for TI scouting) (57) and inversion recovery prepared FGE sequences (58). In our laboratory, TI scout sequences are used infrequently.

IMAGING TIME AFTER CONTRAST ADMINISTRATION

In general, once the optimal TI has been determined, it does not require adjustment if all delayed enhancement images can be acquired within approximately 5 min. However, it is important to keep in mind that the gadolinium concentration within normal myocardium gradually washes out with time, and the TI will need to be adjusted upward if delayed enhancement imaging is performed over a long time span (>5 min). For example, Figure 16.9 demonstrates that the plasma concentration of gadolinium decreases exponentially with time following contrast administration (solid line). Because interstitial concentrations of Gd-DTPA in the myocardium depend primarily upon plasma concentrations, the correct TI needed to null normal myocardium can be estimated from basic physical principles (59). The dashed line in Figure 16.9 depicts the correct TI that is needed to account for the pharmacokinetics of the contrast agent. In this example (gadolinium dose of 0.125 mmol/kg), the correct TI to null normal myocardium at 30 min postcontrast will be 379 ms

Figure 16.7. **(A)** Inversion recovery curves of normal and infarcted myocardium assuming T1 of normal myocardium is 450 ms and infarcted myocardium is 250 ms. The time at which the magnetization of normal myocardium reaches the zero crossing is defined as the inversion time to "null" normal myocardium (312 ms in this example). **(B)** Image intensities resulting from an inversion prepulse with various inversion delay times. Note that image intensities correspond to the magnitude of the magnetization vector and cannot be negative. **(C)** Difference in image intensities between infarcted and normal myocardium as a function of inversion time. The optimal inversion time is when the maximum intensity difference occurs. (From Kim RJ, Shah DJ, Mudd RM. How we perform delayed enhancement imaging. *J Cardiovasc Magn Reson* 2003;5(3):505–514, with permission.)

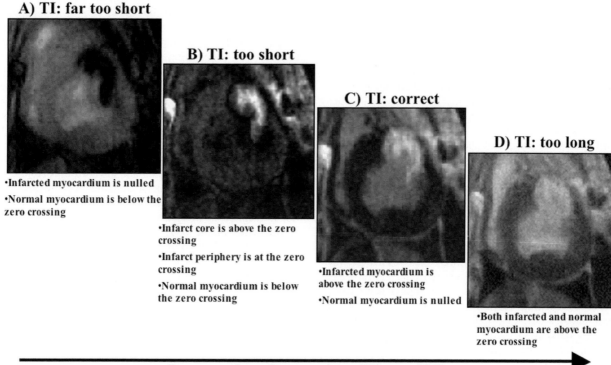

A) TI: far too short

•Infarcted myocardium is nulled
•Normal myocardium is below the zero crossing

B) TI: too short

•Infarct core is above the zero crossing
•Infarct periphery is at the zero crossing
•Normal myocardium is below the zero crossing

C) TI: correct

•Infarcted myocardium is above the zero crossing
•Normal myocardium is nulled

D) TI: too long

•Both infarcted and normal myocardium are above the zero crossing

Increasing Inversion Time (TI)

Figure 16.8. Delayed-enhancement images in a subject with an anterior wall myocardial infarction in which the TI has been varied from too short to too long. See text for details. (From Kim RJ, Shah DJ, Mudd RM. How we perform delayed enhancement imaging. *J Cardiovasc Magn Reson* 2003;5(3):505–514, with permission.)

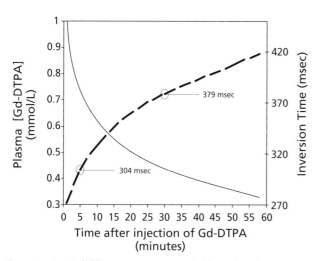

Figure 16.9. Solid line: Monoexponential fit to the plasma gadolinium concentration (*left-hand y axis*) as a function of time postcontrast administration extrapolated from data from Weinmann et al (76) in humans. **Dashed line:** MRI inversion time (*right-hand y axis*) to null normal myocardium calculated from the data of the solid line. **Open circles:** The calculated TI to null normal myocardium at 5 and 30 min postcontrast administration. (From Kim RJ, Shah DJ, Mudd RM. How we perform delayed enhancement imaging. *J Cardiovasc Magn Reson* 2003;5(3):505–514, with permission.)

as compared to 304 ms at 5 min. The basic premise here is not that one can calculate the correct TI for a given time point after contrast administration, but that the TI needs to be adjusted, sometimes significantly, if the imaging time is prolonged.

Recently, Oshinski et al (60) suggested that the "accurate determination of infarct size by delayed enhancement MRI requires imaging at specific times after gadolinium-DTPA injection." This conclusion was based on the observation that the size of the hyperenhanced regions decreased with increasing time after contrast administration. However, in this study, the TI was not adjusted to "null" normal myocardium but held constant throughout the 40 min of imaging postcontrast. In this situation, one is in effect choosing a TI that is further and further from the correct TI (too short) as the time after contrast administration increases. Mahrholdt et al (59) showed, in the setting of chronic infarction, that when the TI is adjusted appropriately to "null" normal myocardium, the size of hyperenhanced regions does not change if imaging is performed between 10 and 30 min postcontrast.

PATHOPHYSIOLOGIC VALIDATION

BACKGROUND

The clinical utility of DE-MRI is determined both by the quality of the images and their relationship to the underlying pathophysiology. While clinical studies clearly help to define the information available, direct comparison of the MR images to histologic tissue samples obtained from animals is a unique and important source of information. In principle, several species of animals can be employed for the study of myocardial contrast enhancement patterns. However, large animals such as the dog provide a practical advantage in that they can be studied on clinical scanners with the identical pulse sequences used for humans, thereby ensuring the clinical relevance of the findings.

In humans, the type and age of an ischemic injury are complex and often are only partially documented. Using animal models, however, several well-defined states of ischemic injury can be studied in a controlled setting. These states include acute infarction, chronic infarction, and severe but reversible ischemic injury. In this section, we review the data concerning MRI contrast enhancement patterns and their relationship to the underlying pathophysiology in animal models of these three pathologic states. Then we turn to studies performed in humans and determine if the concepts gleaned from the animal models can be applied successfully in the clinical setting. Since histopathologic correlations are rare in human studies, particular attention should be paid to the "gold standard" used to define MI and viability when reviewing the clinical literature. We end this section by discussing several potential scenarios in which DE-MRI results may be misinterpreted because of technical and or physiologic issues.

ANIMAL STUDIES

Acute Myocardial Infarction

Patterns of contrast enhancement have been described in the setting of acute infarction with and without reperfusion. Most, if not all, studies report that regions of acute infarction appear hyperenhanced in T_1-weighted images acquired more than a few minutes postcontrast (40–46,61–68). The exact relationship of the observed hyperenhanced regions to the underlying pathophysiology, however, has been a subject of debate in the past and deserves some additional consideration. Understanding the issues requires some background regarding the development of ischemic myocardial injury.

In the traditional view of ischemic myocardial injury, an "area at risk" (69) is defined as the territory with reduced blood flow following occlusion of a coronary artery. Following occlusion, myocardial contractile function falls almost immediately throughout the "area at risk" (70). Little or no cellular necrosis, however, is found until about 15 min after occlusion (71,72). After 15 min, a "wave front" of necrosis begins in the subendocardium and grows towards the epicardium over the next few hours (69,73). During this period, the size of the "area at risk" remains the same, but the size of the infarcted region within the "area at risk" increases. The interpretation of MRI hyperenhancement in the setting of acute infarction, therefore, requires a direct comparison of the MR images with the "area at risk" and the "area of infarction."

Both the "area at risk" and the "area of infarction" can only be precisely defined in histologic tissue sections. The "area at risk" can be identified experimentally with techniques involving microspheres (74) or blue dye (69),

whereas the "area of infarction" can be defined by staining with triphenyl tetrazolium chloride (TTC) (33). Understanding the relationship of MRI contrast enhancement patterns to the underlying pathophysiology depends importantly, therefore, on registration of the in vivo MR images to the postmortem tissue samples.

In practice, the accurate registration of in vivo MR images to histologic tissue sections is difficult for several reasons. First, the three-dimensional (3D) shape of both the "area at risk" and the "area of infarction" are very complex, and the details of their shapes are generally beyond the resolution of in vivo MRI. Second, after removal from the chest, the heart itself is easily deformed and almost impossible to cut along the exact plane used for imaging. As a result, tissue slices aligned by eye and cut by hand almost certainly will not be registered precisely enough to allow slice-by-slice comparisons of the detailed shapes of hyperenhanced regions observed in vivo by MRI with those defined histologically. In this setting, many investigators have avoided the image registration problem entirely by computing the percentage of the entire LV that is at risk or infarcted on the basis of the sum of regions identified in a series of slices, usually short-axis slices from base to apex. This "one point per animal" approach, however, effectively discards the much larger amount of information that could be obtained by careful image registration.

To address this issue in our laboratory we introduced the intermediate step of high-resolution ex vivo imaging. Immediately after the in vivo DE-MRI images were acquired, we removed the hearts, cooled them to 4°C, attached three MRI-visible registration markers, placed a balloon in the LV cavity (filled with deuterium to cause a proton signal void), and suspended the hearts in an extremity radiofrequency coil for high-resolution imaging. The absence of cardiac motion allowed us to acquire T_1-weighted images with spatial resolutions of $500 \times 500 \times 500$ μm. After imaging, the hearts were further cooled and made partially stiff by repeated immersion in -80°C ethanol and then sliced every 2 mm in a commercial rotating meat slicer along the same planes used for imaging (defined by the three MRI-visible markers). After this, each tissue slice was stained for myocyte necrosis with TTC (33) and compared with the MR images.

Figure 16.10 shows a comparison of MRI to histology in an animal with acute infarction using this approach. The "match" between TTC and MRI was extremely close, and even minute details such as "fingers" of necrosis defined by TTC were readily identified in the T_1-weighted MR images. This "match" held in a series of animals that were studied with acute infarction both with and without reperfusion (Fig. 16.11). On the basis of these findings, we concluded that in the setting of acute infarction, the spatial extent of hyperenhancement by MRI is identical to the spatial extent of myocardial necrosis (49).

The mechanisms at the cellular level responsible for hyperenhancement have not been fully elucidated. There is evidence that gadolinium concentrations are elevated in regions of acute infarction (68,75), and this observation would explain the shortened T_1 in these regions. Figure 16.12 describes one possible mechanism for hyperenhancement of acute infarction. Whole body data strongly suggest that in normal myocardial regions, gadolinium is excluded from the

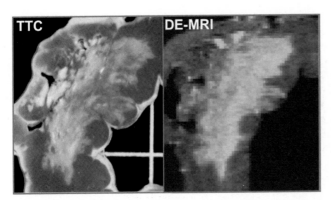

Figure 16.10. Comparison of ex vivo, high-resolution, delayed-enhanced MR images (*right*) with acute myocardial necrosis defined histologically by TTC staining (*left*). See text for details. TTC, triphenyl tetrozolium. (From Kim RJ, Fieno DS, Parrish TB, et al. Relationship of MRI delayed contrast enhancement to irreversible injury, infarct age, and contractile function. *Circulation* 1999; 100(19):1992–2002, with permission.)

myocyte intracellular space by intact sarcolemmal membranes (76,77). The hypothesis demonstrated in Figure 16.12 states that in acutely infarcted regions, the myocyte membranes are ruptured, allowing gadolinium to passively diffuse into the intracellular space. The result is an increased concentration of gadolinium at the tissue level and therefore hyperenhancement. Loss of sarcolemmal membrane integrity is thought to be very tightly related to cell death (70–72), and the idea that an event specific to cell death is related to hyperenhancement would explain the nearly one-to-one relationship of hyperenhancement to necrosis shown in Figure 16.10.

Chronic Myocardial Infarction

Unlike acute infarcts, which are characterized by necrotic myocytes, chronic infarcts are characterized by a dense col-

lagenous scar. Owing to these underlying structural differences, there is no reason a priori to believe that acute and chronic infarcts will appear similar in contrast-enhanced MR images. To address this issue, we scanned dogs 8 weeks after MI, when infarct healing had clearly progressed. Figure 16.13 shows an example of a dog with an 8-week-old infarct in which the hyperenhanced region observed in vivo is clearly associated with a dense collagenous scar (verified postmortem). Using the same technique of high-resolution ex vivo imaging described previously in the setting of acute infarction, the regions of hyperenhancement observed in the setting of chronic infarction also appeared to be identical in shape and size to the infarcted regions defined histologically (Fig. 16.11) (49). Furthermore, these data indicate that chronic infarcts systematically hyperenhance.

The mechanism of hyperenhancement in chronic infarcts remains to be elucidated. One potential mechanism is proposed in Figure 16.12. Although myocardial scar is characterized by a dense collagenous matrix, at a cellular level, the interstitial space between collagen fibers may be significantly greater than the interstitial space between densely packed living myocytes that are characteristic of normal myocardium. In this case, the concentration of gadolinium in scar would be greater than in normal myocardium because of the expanded volume of distribution of gadolinium. Higher concentrations of gadolinium would lower T_1, as in acute infarction, and the regions of scar would appear hyperenhanced by DE-MRI.

Reversible Ischemic Injury

Given that both acute and chronic myocardial infarcts exhibit hyperenhancement, the question of whether severe but reversible ischemic injury exhibits hyperenhancement takes on added importance. In our laboratory, we used two separate experimental approaches to examine this question. In the first approach, severe but reversible ischemic injury was in-

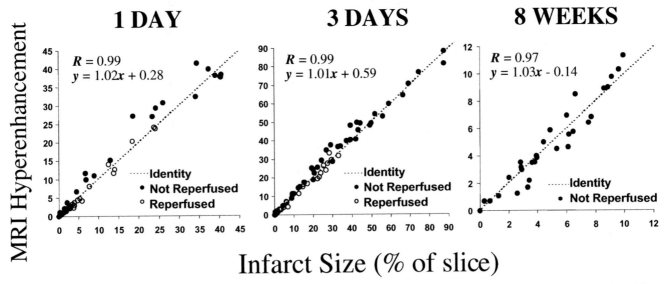

Figure 16.11. Comparison of hyperenhanced regions by MRI with infarct size measured by TTC at 1 day, 3 days, and 8 weeks with and without reperfusion. See text for details. TTC, triphenyl tetrozolium. (From Kim RJ, Fieno DS, Parrish TB, et al. Relationship of MRI delayed contrast enhancement to irreversible injury, infarct age, and contractile function. *Circulation* 1999;100(19):1992–2002, with permission.)

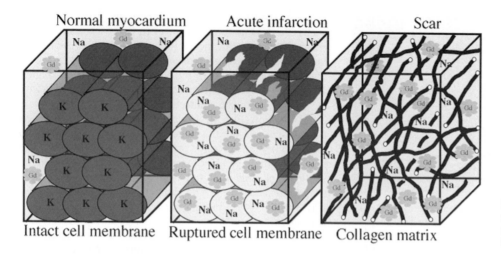

Normal myocardium — Intact cell membrane

Acute infarction — Ruptured cell membrane

Scar — Collagen matrix

Figure 16.12. Potential mechanisms of hyperenhancement in acute and chronic myocardial infarction. See text for details.

duced in the magnet and then delayed enhanced images were acquired. In the second approach, high-resolution ex vivo images were compared with the "area at risk but not infracted" defined histologically.

Figure 16.14 shows examples of the first approach (49). Under sterile conditions, two coronary arteries were manipulated. The first coronary artery was permanently ligated to cause myocardial infarction. The second coronary artery was instrumented with a reversible hydraulic occluder and a Doppler flow meter. The animals were then allowed to recover and were studied 3 days later. While in the magnet, regional wall motion was examined with cine MRI. The reversible occluder was then inflated for 15 min. During this period of occlusion, cine MRI was repeated to identify new wall-motion abnormalities to ensure that the region distal to the reversible occluder was within the imaging plane. After 15 min, the occluder was released, and flow was restored (verified by Doppler flow). The purpose of the 15-min occlusion was to induce severe but reversible ischemic injury (71,72). Cine MRI was then repeated a third time to document myocardial stunning. The colored bull's-eye plots in

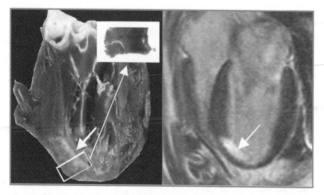

Figure 16.13. In vivo delayed contrast-enhanced images of a dog with an 8-week-old myocardial infarction (*right*). Despite replacement of necrotic myocytes with dense collagenous scar (revealed by trichrome staining of infarcted region) (*inset in left panel*), hyperenhancement is still observed. (From Kim RJ, Fieno DS, Parrish TB, et al. Relationship of MRI delayed contrast enhancement to irreversible injury, infarct age, and contractile function. *Circulation* 1999;100(19):1992–2002, with permission.)

Figure 16.14 correspond to wall thickening at this time. As can be seen in Figure 16.14, both the region associated with infarction (yellow arrows) and the region associated with severe but reversible ischemic injury (green arrows) show abnormal wall thickening. Gadolinium was then injected, and the images were inspected for hyperenhancement. The region of infarction exhibited hyperenhancement while the region of severe but reversible ischemic injury ("stunned" myocardium) did not. When these same animals were scanned 8 weeks later, wall thickening had returned to normal in the region of severe but reversible ischemic injury (49). Histologic examination (also at 8 weeks) revealed infarction in the territory subtended by the permanently occluded artery, but no evidence of infarction was found distal to the reversible occluder. These in vivo data support the view that severe but reversible ischemic injury does not result in hyperenhancement (49).

Figure 16.15 illustrates another approach to this question (78). In these experiments, TTC was used to define the "area of infarction" (middle left panel), and fluorescent microparticles injected into the left atrium during coronary artery occlusion were used to define the "area at risk" (bottom left panel). In this way, we could identify the region that was "at risk but not infracted," shown as zone 2. The top left panel shows the corresponding high resolution MRI image. On this image, it is clear that the "at risk but not infracted" myocardium (zone 2) does not exhibit hyperenhancement. Light microscopy of this region verified that normal myocyte architecture was present (middle right panel). Consistent with the data of Figure 16.14, the data of Figure 16.15 strongly support the view that severe but reversible ischemic injury does not result in hyperenhancement (78).

Further evidence that hyperenhancement is exclusively associated with irreversible injury is provided by Rehwald et al (79). Since MRI image intensities are highly dependent on the pulse sequence that is used, Rehwald et al directly examined regional gadolinium concentrations rather than image intensities in order to provide data that were independent of the MRI technique. To measure gadolinium concentrations over a range of myocardial injuries, electron probe x-ray microanalysis (EPXMA) was performed in animal models with reversible and irreversible injury. Infarcted regions were defined by antimyoglobin antibody or TTC stain-

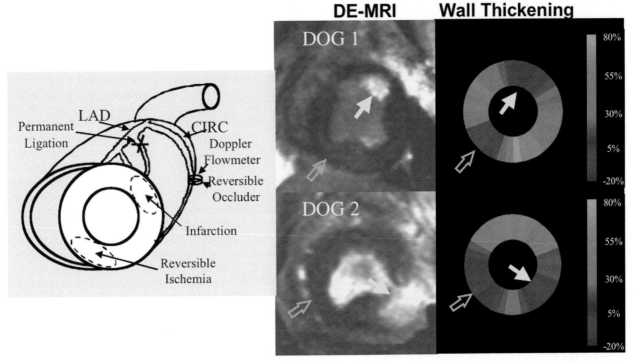

Figure 16.14. Stunned myocardium does not exhibit hyperenhancement. See text for details. (From Kim RJ, Fieno DS, Parrish TB, et al. Relationship of MRI delayed contrast enhancement to irreversible injury, infarct age, and contractile function. *Circulation* 1999; 100(19):1992–2002, with permission.)

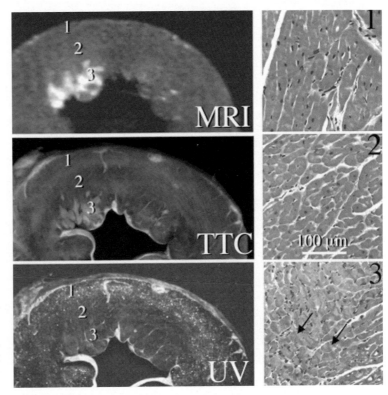

Figure 16.15. Comparison of MRI hyperenhancement (*left upper panel*), TTC staining (*left middle panel*), and the myocardium at risk (region without fluorescent microparticles) (*left lower panel*) in an animal with a 1-day-old reperfused infarction. Light microscopy views of region 1 (not at risk, not infarcted), region 2 (at risk but not infarcted), and region 3 (infarcted) are shown on the right panels. Arrows point to contraction bands. (From Fieno DS, Kim RJ, Chen EL, et al. Contrast-enhanced magnetic resonance imaging of myocardium at risk: distinction between reversible and irreversible injury throughout infarct healing. *J Am Coll Cardiol* 2000;36(6):1985–1991, with permission.)

ing. Regions at risk were defined by fluorescent microparticles administered during coronary occlusion. The results demonstrated that compared with normal regions, gadolinium concentration was increased in both acute and chronic infarction but not increased in "at risk but not infarcted" regions. The conclusion was that regional elevations in myocardial gadolinium concentrations are exclusively associated with irreversible ischemic injury.

The data of Figure 16.14 underscore that dissociation between wall thickening and delayed enhancement can occur in which wall thickening is impaired but hyperenhancement is not observed. In the setting of acute ischemic injury, this condition is related to the phenomenon of myocardial "stunning" (10,22), in which cell death has not occurred but contractile dysfunction persists for days or even weeks after a severe ischemic event. The data suggest that in the setting of an acute ischemic event, regions exhibiting contractile dysfunction can be subdivided into irreversibly and reversibly injured regions defined as those with and without hyperenhancement, respectively. This concept suggests that the presence or absence of hyperenhancement in regions of contractile dysfunction may be useful in the detection of myocardial salvage early after acute infarction. If correct, this approach would represent a new technique to define myocardial salvage in patients following acute infarction.

To test the hypothesis that DE-MRI can be used to index myocardial salvage, we initiated another study in which ani-

mals were imaged 3 days, 10 days, and 4 weeks after transient coronary artery occlusion (80). The hypothesis was that recovery of contractile dysfunction at 4 weeks could be predicted by DE-MRI at 3 days. Specific examples from that study are shown in Figure 16.16, in which each row represents a different animal. The first three columns show MRI data acquired at 3 days, whereas the data in columns four and five were acquired at 4 weeks. At 3 days, all three animals showed contractile dysfunction in the left anterior descending coronary artery (LAD) perfusion territory by cine MRI (columns 2 and 3). The first animal (row 1), however, showed nearly transmural hyperenhancement, the second animal (row 2) about 50% transmural hyperenhancement, and the third animal (row 3) almost no hyperenhancement. Four weeks later, contractile function did not improve in the first animal, improved partially in the second animal, and completely recovered in the third animal. A summary of the results from this study is shown in Figure 16.17. These data underscore that as predicted by the results of Figures 16.14 and 16.15, contrast enhancement patterns observed early after MI can be used to index the extent of myocardial salvage (80).

The mechanism for the lack of hyperenhancement in regions of severe but reversible ischemic injury may be directly related to the mechanism for hyperenhancement in acute infarcts (i.e., it may relate to the integrity of the myocyte membrane). Although severe but reversible ischemic

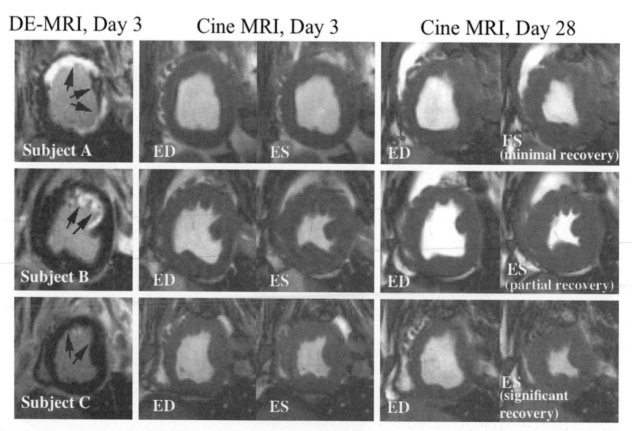

Figure 16.16. Contrast enhancement and wall thickening at 3 days (*columns 1–3*) compared to wall thickening at 28 days (*columns 5–6*) in three different animals (*rows*). See text for details. A full-motion version of this figure can be viewed on the internet at http://circ.ahajournals.org/cgi/content/full/102/14/1678/DC1/1. (From Hillenbrand HB, Kim RJ, Parker MA, et al. Early assessment of myocardial salvage by contrast-enhanced magnetic resonance imaging. *Circulation* 2000;102(14):1678–1683, with permission.)

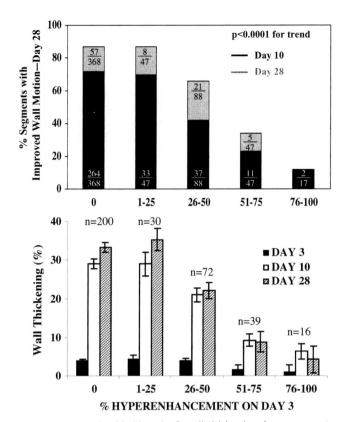

Figure 16.17. The likelihood of wall-thickening improvement (*upper panel*) and absolute wall thickening (*lower panel*) as a function of the transmural extent of hyperenhancement. Black and gray bars correspond to improvement by days 10 and 28, respectively. On the internet at http://circ.ahajournals.org/cgi/content/full/102/14/1678/DC1/1. (From Hillenbrand HB, Kim RJ, Parker MA, et al. Early assessment of myocardial salvage by contrast-enhanced magnetic resonance imaging. *Circulation* 2000; 102(14):1678–1683, with permission.)

injury has many effects on the myocyte, the sarcolemmal membrane remains intact (71,72), and therefore presumably continues to exclude the MRI contrast agent from the intracellular space. In this setting, the volume of distribution of the contrast agent in regions of severe but reversible ischemic injury would be expected to remain similar to that

in normal myocardium, and no hyperenhancement of these regions would be observed.

HUMAN STUDIES

Acute Myocardial Infarction

Simonetti et al (48) performed the first clinical study to evaluate segmented inversion recovery DE-MRI in the setting of acute MI. In this study, 18 consecutive patients were imaged 19 ± 7 days after acute MI documented by an appropriate rise (>2 times the upper limit of normal) and fall in CK-myocardial band (CK-MB) isoenzyme levels. Figure 16.18 shows representative images in three patients from this study. Starting from the left panel, infarction was due to occlusion of the LAD, left circumflex artery, and right coronary artery, respectively. Myocardial hyperenhancement is clearly visible in these patients in the appropriate infarct-related artery (IRA) perfusion territory. Similar results were observed in the other 15 patients. On average, hyperenhanced regions had image intensities that were 485 ± 43% higher than those in normal myocardial regions. As discussed previously, the degree of hyperenhancement was approximately 10-fold greater than that in previous reports (Table 16.2).

More recently, we evaluated a series of 24 patients who presented with their first MI (documented by cardiac enzymes) and were successfully reperfused (thrombolytics or angioplasty) (81). All patients underwent DE-MRI using the seg IR-FGE sequence within 7 days of their MI. There was a strong correlation between infarct size defined by DE-MRI and peak CK-MB values (Fig. 16.19). In a similar study, Beek et al (82) studied 30 patients 7 ± 3 days after a first-time reperfused acute MI. They found that 29 patients (97%) showed regional hyperenhancement, and in all 29, the area of hyperenhancement corresponded to the electrocardiographic infarct location. Ingkanisorn et al (83) studied 33 patients within 5 days after first-time acute MI. All patients had hyperenhancement despite the fact that many had small infarcts (troponin-I ≤9ng/mL). There was a good correlation between infarct size measured by DE-MRI and peak troponin-I levels in the 23 patients who were reperfused acutely (r = 0.83, p <0.001), whereas there was a poor correlation in the remaining 10 patients who were not (r = 0.28, p = NS). The results of these studies are consistent with the ani-

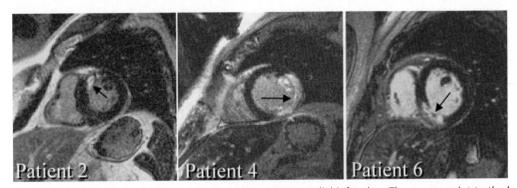

Figure 16.18. Short-axis DE-MRI images in three patients with acute myocardial infarction. The arrows point to the hyperenhanced region, which was in the appropriate infarct-related artery perfusion territory. (From Simonetti OP, Kim RJ, Fieno DS, et al. An improved MR imaging technique for the visualization of myocardial infarction. *Radiology* 2001;218(1):215–223, with permission.)

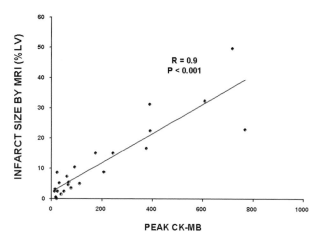

Figure 16.19. Relationship of infarct size by MRI to peak CK-MB. CK-MB, creatine kinase-myocardial band. (From Choi KM, Kim RJ, Gubernikoff G, et al. Transmural extent of acute myocardial infarction predicts long-term improvement in contractile function. *Circulation* 2001;104(10):1101–1107, with permission.)

mal studies previously discussed, and confirm that acute MI in humans hyperenhances and that the extent of hyperenhancement is an excellent metric for infarct size.

Chronic Myocardial Infarction

The studies of chronic infarction perhaps best demonstrate the importance of image quality in delayed contrast enhancement imaging. For example, Eichstaedt et al (41), Nishimura et al (84), and van Dijkman et al (85) all observed gadolinium hyperenhancement in patients with acute MI but found no hyperenhancement in patients with chronic infarction. These reports formed the basis for the initial widespread conclusion that chronic infarcts do not hyperenhance. More recently, Fedele et al (86) and Ramani et al (87) suggested that this conclusion is erroneous. They described hyperenhancement in patients with chronic CAD and a high clinical likelihood of chronic infarction. Unfortunately, biochemical evidence for infarction was not provided, the age of infarction was unknown, and differences in image intensity were modest, with hyperenhanced regions having on average less than 60% increase in image intensity over nonhyperenhanced regions.

Despite these conflicting results, we postulated that human chronic MI hyperenhances. This hypothesis was based on our experimental animal data demonstrating that collagenous scar hyperenhances in both ex vivo (Fig. 16.11) and in vivo imaging protocols (Fig. 16.13). To test this hypothesis, we enrolled patients at the time of acute infarction on the basis of abnormal CK release and then performed DE-MRI several months later after infarct healing (51). To assess the specificity of the findings, DE-MRI was also performed in patients with nonischemic cardiomyopathy and in healthy volunteers.

In the patients with chronic MI, we observed hyperenhancement in a variety of sizes, ranging from large, fully transmural hyperenhancement that extended over several short-axis slices to small, subendocardial hyperenhancement that was visible only in a single sector of a single view. Figure 16.20 shows typical images in three patients with large transmural hyperenhancement in different coronary ar-

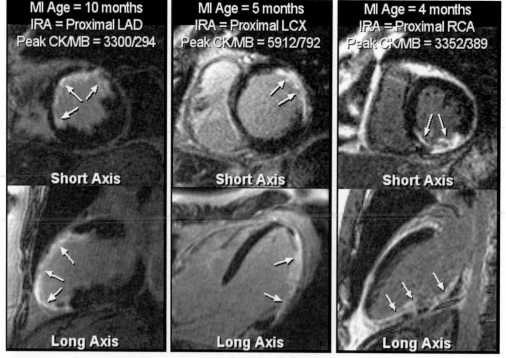

Figure 16.20. Typical short-axis and long-axis views of three patients with large transmural hyperenhancement in different coronary artery territories. (From Wu E, Judd RM, Vargas JD, et al. Visualisation of presence, location, and transmural extent of healed Q-wave and non-Q-wave myocardial infarction. *Lancet* 2001;357(9249):21–28, with permission.)

55. Judd RM, Kim RJ. Imaging time after Gd-DTPA injection is critical in using delayed enhancement to determine infarct size accurately with magnetic resonance imaging. *Circulation* 2002;106(2):e6; author reply.

56. Kellman P, Arai AE, McVeigh ER, et al. Phase-sensitive inversion recovery for detecting myocardial infarction using gadolinium-delayed hyperenhancement. *Magn Reson Med* 2002;47(2):372–383.

57. Chung YC, Lee VS, Laub G, et al. Inversion recovery cine trueFISP for optimizing TI in myocardial infarct imaging. *Proc Intl Soc Mag Reson Med* 2002;10:219.

58. Scheffler K, Hennig J. T(1) quantification with inversion recovery TrueFISP. *Magn Reson Med* 2001;45(4):720–723.

59. Mahrholdt H, Wagner A, Holly TA, et al. Reproducibility of chronic infarct size measurement by contrast-enhanced magnetic resonance imaging. *Circulation* 2002;106(18): 2322–2327.

60. Oshinski JN, Yang Z, Jones JR, et al. Imaging time after Gd-DTPA injection is critical in using delayed enhancement to determine infarct size accurately with magnetic resonance imaging. *Circulation* 2001;104(23):2838–2842.

61. Pereira RS, Prato FS, Wisenberg G, et al. The determination of myocardial viability using Gd-DTPA in a canine model of acute myocardial ischemia and reperfusion. *Magn Reson Med* 1996;36(5):684–693.

62. Judd RM, Lugo-Olivieri CH, Arai M, et al. Physiological basis of myocardial contrast enhancement in fast magnetic resonance images of 2-day-old reperfused canine infarcts. *Circulation* 1995;92(7):1902–1910.

63. de Roos A, van Rossum AC, van der Wall E, et al. Reperfused and nonreperfused myocardial infarction: diagnostic potential of Gd-DTPA—enhanced MR imaging. *Radiology* 1989; 172(3):717–720.

64. van der Wall EE, van Dijkman PR, de Roos A, et al. Diagnostic significance of gadolinium-DTPA (diethylenetriamine penta-acetic acid) enhanced magnetic resonance imaging in thrombolytic treatment for acute myocardial infarction: its potential in assessing reperfusion. *Br Heart J* 1990;63(1): 12–17.

65. Lima JA, Judd RM, Bazille A, et al. Regional heterogeneity of human myocardial infarcts demonstrated by contrast-enhanced MRI. Potential mechanisms. *Circulation* 1995;92(5): 1117–1125.

66. Rogers WJ Jr., Kramer CM, Geskin G, et al. Early contrast-enhanced MRI predicts late functional recovery after reperfused myocardial infarction. *Circulation* 1999;99(6):744–750.

67. Dendale P, Franken PR, Block P, et al. Contrast enhanced and functional magnetic resonance imaging for the detection of viable myocardium after infarction. *Am Heart J* 1998; 135(5 Pt 1):875–880.

68. Schaeffer S, Malloy CR, Katz J, et al. Gadolinium-DTPA-enhanced nuclear magnetic resonance imaging of reperfused myocardium identification of the myocardial bed at risk. *J Am Coll Cardiol* 1988;12:1064–1072.

69. Reimer KA, Jennings RB. The "wavefront phenomenon" of myocardial ischemic cell death. II. Transmural progression of necrosis within the framework of ischemic bed size (myocardium at risk) and collateral flow. *Lab Invest* 1979;40(6): 633–644.

70. Reimer KA, Jennings RB. Myocardial ischemia, hypoxia and infarction. In: Fozzard HA, et al, ed. *The heart and cardiovascular system.* 2nd ed. New York, NY: Raven Press; 1992: 1875–1973.

71. Jennings RB, Schaper J, Hill ML, et al. Effect of reperfusion late in the phase of reversible ischemic injury. Changes in cell volume, electrolytes, metabolites, and ultrastructure. *Circ Res* 1985;56(2):262–278.

72. Whalen DA, Hamilton DG, Ganote CE, et al. Effect of a transient period of ischemia on myocardial cells. I. Effects on cell volume regulation. *Am J Pathol* 1974;74(3):381–397.

73. Reimer KA, Lowe JE, Rasmussen MM, et al. The wavefront phenomenon of ischemic cell death. 1. Myocardial infarct size vs duration of coronary occlusion in dogs. *Circulation* 1977;56(5):786–794.

74. Kowallik P, Schulz R, Guth BD, et al. Measurement of regional myocardial blood flow with multiple colored microspheres. *Circulation* 1991;83(3):974–982.

75. Saeed M, Wendland MF, Masui T, et al. Dual mechanisms for change in myocardial signal intensity by means of a single MR contrast medium: dependence on concentration and pulse sequence. *Radiology* 1993;186:175–182.

76. Weinmann HJ, Brasch RC, Press WR, et al. Characteristics of gadolinium-DTPA complex: a potential NMR contrast agent. *AJR Am J Roentgenol* 1984;142(3):619–624.

77. Koenig SH, Spiller M, Brown RD 3rd, et al. Relaxation of water protons in the intra- and extracellular regions of blood containing Gd(DTPA). *Magn Reson Med* 1986;3(5):791–795.

78. Fieno DS, Kim RJ, Chen EL, et al. Contrast-enhanced magnetic resonance imaging of myocardium at risk: distinction between reversible and irreversible injury throughout infarct healing. *J Am Coll Cardiol* 2000;36(6):1985–1991.

79. Rehwald WG, Fieno DS, Chen EL, et al. Myocardial magnetic resonance imaging contrast agent concentrations after reversible and irreversible ischemic injury. *Circulation* 2002; 105(2):224–229.

80. Hillenbrand HB, Kim RJ, Parker MA, et al. Early assessment of myocardial salvage by contrast-enhanced magnetic resonance imaging. *Circulation* 2000;102(14):1678–1683.

81. Choi KM, Kim RJ, Gubernikoff G, et al. Transmural extent of acute myocardial infarction predicts long-term improvement in contractile function. *Circulation* 2001;104(10): 1101–1107.

82. Beek AM, Kuhl HP, Bondarenko O, et al. Delayed contrast-enhanced magnetic resonance imaging for the prediction of regional functional improvement after acute myocardial infarction. *J Am Coll Cardiol* 2003;42(5):895–901.

83. Ingkanisorn WP, Rhoads KL, Aletras AH, et al. Gadolinium delayed enhancement cardiovascular magnetic resonance correlates with clinical measures of myocardial infarction. *J Am Coll Cardiol* 2004;43(12):2253–2259.

84. Nishimura T, Kobayashi H, Ohara Y, et al. Serial assessment of myocardial infarction by using gated MR imaging and Gd-DTPA. *AJR Am J Roentgenol* 1989;153(4):715–720.

85. van Dijkman PR, van der Wall EE, de Roos A, et al. Acute, subacute, and chronic myocardial infarction: quantitative analysis of gadolinium-enhanced MR images. *Radiology* 1991;180(1):147–151.

86. Fedele F, Montesano T, Ferro-Luzzi M, et al. Identification of viable myocardium in patients with chronic coronary artery disease and left ventricular dysfunction: role of magnetic resonance imaging. *Am Heart J* 1994;128(3):484–489.

87. Ramani K, Judd RM, Holly TA, et al. Contrast magnetic resonance imaging in the assessment of myocardial viability in patients with stable coronary artery disease and left ventricular dysfunction. *Circulation* 1998;98(24):2687–2694.

88. Christian TF, Gibbons RJ, Gersh BJ. Effect of infarct location on myocardial salvage assessed by technetium-99m isonitrile. *J Am Coll Cardiol* 1991;17(6):1303–1308.

89. Effectiveness of intravenous thrombolytic treatment in acute myocardial infarction. Gruppo Italiano per lo Studio della

Streptochinasi nell'Infarto Miocardico (GISSI). *Lancet* 1986; 1(8478):397–402.

90. Randomised trial of intravenous streptokinase, oral aspirin, both, or neither among 17,187 cases of suspected acute myocardial infarction: ISIS-2. ISIS-2 (Second International Study of Infarct Survival) Collaborative Group. *Lancet* 1988; 2(8607):349–360.

91. Grines CL, Browne KF, Marco J, et al. A comparison of immediate angioplasty with thrombolytic therapy for acute myocardial infarction. The Primary Angioplasty in Myocardial Infarction Study Group. *N Engl J Med* 1993;328(10): 673–679.

92. Zijlstra F, de Boer MJ, Hoorntje JC, et al. A comparison of immediate coronary angioplasty with intravenous streptokinase in acute myocardial infarction. *N Engl J Med* 1993; 328(10):680–684.

93. Gersh BJ, Anderson JL. Thrombolysis and myocardial salvage. Results of clinical trials and the animal paradigm—paradoxic or predictable? *Circulation* 1993;88(1):296–306.

94. Gerber BL, Garot J, Bluemke DA, et al. Accuracy of contrast-enhanced magnetic resonance imaging in predicting improvement of regional myocardial function in patients after acute myocardial infarction. *Circulation* 2002;106(9):1083–1089.

95. Kitagawa K, Sakuma H, Hirano T, et al. Acute myocardial infarction: myocardial viability assessment in patients early thereafter comparison of contrast-enhanced MR imaging with resting (201)Tl SPECT. Single photon emission computed tomography. *Radiology* 2003;226(1):138–144.

96. Schvartzman PR, Srichai MB, Grimm RA, et al. Nonstress delayed-enhancement magnetic resonance imaging of the myocardium predicts improvement of function after revascularization for chronic ischemic heart disease with left ventricular dysfunction. *Am Heart J* 2003;146(3):535–541.

97. Bonow RO. Identification of viable myocardium. *Circulation* 1996;94(11):2674–2680.

98. Maes A, Flameng W, Nuyts J, et al. Histological alterations in chronically hypoperfused myocardium. Correlation with PET findings. *Circulation* 1994;90(2):735–745.

99. Polimeni PI. Extracellular space and ionic distribution in rat ventricle. *Am J Physiol* 1974;227(3):676–83.

100. Cerqueira MD, Weissman NJ, Dilsizian V, et al. Standardized myocardial segmentation and nomenclature for tomographic imaging of the heart: a statement for healthcare professionals from the Cardiac Imaging Committee of the Council on Clinical Cardiology of the American Heart Association. *Circulation* 2002;105(4):539–542.

101. Knuesel PR, Nanz D, Wyss C, et al. Characterization of dysfunctional myocardium by positron emission tomography and magnetic resonance: relation to functional outcome after revascularization. *Circulation* 2003;108(9):1095–1100.

102. Lee VS, Resnick D, Tiu SS, et al. MR imaging evaluation of myocardial viability in the setting of equivocal SPECT results with (99m)Tc sestamibi. Radiology 2004;230(1):191–7.

103. Baer FM, Theissen P, Schneider CA, et al. Dobutamine magnetic resonance imaging predicts contractile recovery of chronically dysfunctional myocardium after successful revascularization. *J Am Coll Cardiol* 1998;31(5):1040–1048.

104. Cwajg JM, Cwajg E, Nagueh SF, et al. End-diastolic wall thickness as a predictor of recovery of function in myocardial hibernation: relation to rest-redistribution T1-201 tomography and dobutamine stress echocardiography. *J Am Coll Cardiol* 2000;35(5):1152–1161.

105. Greaves SC, Zhi G, Lee RT, et al. Incidence and natural history of left ventricular thrombus following anterior wall acute myocardial infarction. *Am J Cardiol* 1997;80(4): 442–448.

106. Kim RJ, Choi KM, Judd RM. Assessment of myocardial viability by contrast enhancement. In: Higgins CB, deRoos A, eds. *Cardiovascular MRI & MRA*. Philadelphia: Lippincott Williams & Wilkins; 2003:209–237.

107. Rochitte CE, Lima JA, Bluemke DA, et al. Magnitude and time course of microvascular obstruction and tissue injury after acute myocardial infarction. *Circulation* 1998;98(10): 1006–1014.

108. Kloner RA, Ganote CE, Jennings RB. The "no-reflow" phenomenon after temporary coronary occlusion in the dog. *J Clin Invest* 1974;54(6):1496–508.

109. Ambrosio G, Weisman HF, Mannisi JA, et al. Progressive impairment of regional myocardial perfusion after initial restoration of postischemic blood flow. *Circulation* 1989;80(6): 1846–1861.

110. Ito H, Tomooka T, Sakai N, et al. Lack of myocardial perfusion immediately after successful thrombolysis. A predictor of poor recovery of left ventricular function in anterior myocardial infarction. *Circulation* 1992;85(5):1699–1705.

111. Ito H, Maruyama A, Iwakura K, et al. Clinical implications of the 'no reflow' phenomenon. A predictor of complications and left ventricular remodeling in reperfused anterior wall myocardial infarction. *Circulation* 1996;93(2):223–228.

112. McCrohon JA, Moon JC, Prasad SK, et al. Differentiation of heart failure related to dilated cardiomyopathy and coronary artery disease using gadolinium-enhanced cardiovascular magnetic resonance. *Circulation* 2003;108(1):54–59.

113. Bello D, Shah DJ, Farah GM, et al. Gadolinium cardiovascular magnetic resonance predicts reversible myocardial dysfunction and remodeling in patients with heart failure undergoing beta-blocker therapy. *Circulation* 2003;108(16): 1945–1953.

114. Schuster EH, Bulkley BH. Ischemic cardiomyopathy: a clinicopathologic study of fourteen patients. *Am Heart J* 1980; 100(4):506–512.

115. Boucher CA, Fallon JT, Johnson RA, et al. Cardiomyopathic syndrome caused by coronary artery disease. III: Prospective clinicopathological study of its prevalence among patients with clinically unexplained chronic heart failure. *Br Heart J* 1979;41(5):613–620.

116. Roberts WC, Siegel RJ, McManus BM. Idiopathic dilated cardiomyopathy: analysis of 152 necropsy patients. *Am J Cardiol* 1987;60(16):1340–1355.

117. Uretsky BF, Thygesen K, Armstrong PW, et al. Acute coronary findings at autopsy in heart failure patients with sudden death: results from the assessment of treatment with lisinopril and survival (ATLAS) trial. *Circulation* 2000;102(6):611–616.

118. Moon JC, McKenna WJ, McCrohon JA, et al. Toward clinical risk assessment in hypertrophic cardiomyopathy with gadolinium cardiovascular magnetic resonance. *J Am Coll Cardiol* 2003;41(9):1561–1567.

119. Mahrholdt H, Goedecke C, Wagner A, et al. Cardiovascular magnetic resonance assessment of human myocarditis: a comparison to histology and molecular pathology. *Circulation* 2004;109(10):1250–1258.

120. Shirani J, Freant LJ, Roberts WC. Gross and semiquantitative histologic findings in mononuclear cell myocarditis causing sudden death, and implications for endomyocardial biopsy. *Am J Cardiol* 1993;72(12):952–957.

121. Fuster V, Kim RJ. Frontiers in cardiovascular magnetic resonance. *Circulation* 2005. In Press.

122. Hurwitz JL, Josephson ME. Sudden cardiac death in patients with chronic coronary heart disease. *Circulation* 1992;85(1 Suppl):143–149.

123. Klem I, Weinsaft J, Heitner JF, et al. The utility of contrast enhanced MRI for screening patients at risk for malignant ventricular tachyarrhythmias. *J Cardiovasc Magn Reson* 2004;6(1):84.

17

Tissue Characterization of Ischemic Myocardial Injury

Norbert Watzinger, Maythem Saeed, and Charles B. Higgins

CLINICAL IMPLICATIONS

Coronary heart disease (CHD) is the most common cause of heart failure in industrialized countries. Despite recent advances in heart failure therapy, reversing its cause remains the best treatment option. This is accomplished in CHD by restoration of blood flow to dysfunctional myocardium usu-ally caused by thrombolysis, percutaneous transluminal coronary angioplasty (PTCA), or coronary artery bypass grafting (CABG). However, the success of these interventions largely depends on the presence and extent of viable myocardium. Viable areas will most likely benefit from revascularization, whereas restoration of blood flow in scar tissue does not lead to an improvement of ventricular function. Therefore, the exact determination of residual myocardial viability has a tremendous clinical impact on further decision making when patients present with recurrent angina, acute myocardial infarction (MI), or chronic left ventricular (LV) dysfunction.

Intensive work has been directed in the past decade toward the development of noninvasive imaging methods to identify and quantify myocardial injury and viability. Cardiac magnetic resonance imaging (MRI) is a relatively new and rapidly growing technique for examining patients with CHD (1,2) and assessing myocardial viability (3–6). Multiple MR strategies have been developed to characterize ischemic myocardial injury and to discriminate viable from nonviable zones. These involve (a) the assessment of regional wall thickness and systolic wall thickening at rest and during pharmacologic stress, (b) the use of contrast-enhanced MR techniques to assess myocardial perfusion and to identify regions with reversible and irreversible injury, and (c) MR spectroscopy to determine preserved myocardial metabolism. This chapter illustrates the multiple approaches to determine myocardial viability using MRI and focuses primarily on contrast-enhanced techniques to characterize ischemic myocardial injury.

HIBERNATION AND STUNNING

The pathophysiological understanding of myocardial ischemia and infarction has changed within the past decades. Previously, myocardial ischemia was viewed as an all-or-none process that caused myocardial necrosis when prolonged and severe, but only had transient effects when brief or mild. Thus, until the early 1980s, contractile dysfunction was exclusively attributed to myocardial cell death (7). Since then, it has been gradually recognized that areas of poor or no contractility are not always associated with myocardial necrosis. Instead, they may represent areas of potentially reversible damage that can improve spontaneously or after restoration of adequate perfusion (8).

The determination of viable myocardium has been a major focus in at least two circumstances (9–11): (a) in cases of chronic coronary artery disease at assessment of regional or global dysfunction and (b) in cases of acute myocardial ischemia followed by reperfusion therapy at the assessment of functional abnormality. Under these conditions, viable myocardium may be characterized as hibernating or stunned, whereas nonviable myocardium can be considered necrotic or scarred. In the clinical setting of CHD, all these states may coexist and differentiation is relevant with respect to patient treatment and outcome.

Hibernation describes a condition of persistently impaired myocardial function at rest due to chronic obstructive CHD that could be partially or completely restored by reestablishing adequate blood and oxygen supply (12). It has been postulated that hibernation results from a response to reduced myocardial blood flow at rest whereas cardiac function is downgraded to the extent that blood flow and function are once again at equilibrium (perfusion-contraction match). There is currently some controversy about this thesis, as newer data have demonstrated that hypoperfusion at rest is not always present (13), and that an impaired perfusion reserve resulting in inducible ischemia may also play an important role in myocardial hibernation (14). Although the underlying pathophysiologic mechanisms are not fully elucidated, the hallmark of hibernating myocardium is its capability of improving or regaining its normal contractile function after successful revascularization (15,16). The identification of myocardial hibernation is a real challenge to the clinician because it is thought to occur in up to 50% of all cases of ischemic cardiomyopathy (17). Moreover, a pooled analysis of more than 3,000 patients showed that the annual mortality rate in those with significant viable myocardium is more than fourfold higher when they were treated medically compared to those who underwent successful revascularization (18). On the other hand, patients with necrotic or scarred myocardium are unlikely to benefit from revascularization, which entails a greater risk in the presence of severely depressed LV function (19). Thus, accurate assessment of the presence and extent of hibernating myocardium allows a better estimation of the benefits of coronary revascularization procedures, and it is essential to guide the process of clinical decision-making in patients with LV dysfunction (20).

Recovery of contractile function following an acute ischemic insult may be delayed for some time despite the restoration of adequate blood flow (perfusion-contraction mismatch) (21). This condition is called *stunning* (22). It has been hypothesized that myocardial stunning consists of two components: one that develops during ischemia (ischemic injury) and one that develops after reperfusion (reperfusion injury) (23,24). Stunned myocardium usually recovers spontaneously after reperfusion, but transient myocardial dysfunction may persist for up to several days although coronary blood flow is normal (25). The severity

and duration of these postischemic changes depend on the length and intensity of ischemia, and also on the condition of the myocardium at the onset of the ischemic episode. The assessment of residual viability in reperfused MI or unstable angina is essential since the presence of viable myocardium in the ischemic zone is associated with recovery of function and a better outcome (26).

IMAGING TECHNIQUES

DIFFERENTIAL IMAGING TECHNIQUES FOR ASSESSING MYOCARDIAL VIABILITY

From a clinical standpoint, the utility of any diagnostic approach purported to identify viable myocardium can be ascertained accurately only by the occurrence of functional improvement after restoration of adequate perfusion (27). Recovery of function after revascularization is the best, but still imperfect, reference standard owing to difficulties in determining the completeness of revascularization and the possibility of restenosis within the time when contractility has not fully recovered (28). Moreover, it has to be assumed that the procedure itself does not lead to irreversible damage of a relevant portion of viable myocardium.

Currently, scintigraphic techniques and stress echocardiography are used predominantly to identify viable myocardium, each based on different hallmarks of viable tissue (29). Radionuclide tracers—such as ^{18}F-fluorodesoxyglucose (^{18}F-FDG), ^{201}thallium, and ^{99m}technetium sestamibi or tetrofosmin—have been used to characterize viable myocardium by preserved glucose utilization, cell membrane integrity, and intactness of mitochondria, respectively. Another characteristic of viable myocardium, preserved contractile reserve owing to inotropic stimulation, can be probed by low-dose (5 to 10 μg/kg/min) dobutamine echocardiography. All these imaging techniques have reported various sensitivities and specificities (Table 17.1) in predicting the clinical "gold standard"—improvement of regional function after successful revascularization (29). Overall, nuclear imaging has higher sensitivity but lower specificity than stress echocardiography for predicting the functional outcome after revascularization. Further drawbacks of single-photon emission tomography (SPECT) and positron emission tomography (PET) include the use of radioactivity, limited spatial resolution, inability to differentiate the transmural extent of myocardial injury, and the high costs and restricted availability of the latter. The disadvantages of stress echocardiography include limited visualization of basal lateral and inferior myocardial segments, predominantly in patients with poor acoustic windows, and its reliance on visual assessment of wall thickening. Moreover, the optimal display and interpretation of contractile response to pharmacologic stress require considerable technical aptitude, so that accuracy largely depends the expertise of centers and observers.

FUNDAMENTALS TO CHARACTERIZE ISCHEMIC MYOCARDIAL INJURY WITH MAGNETIC RESONANCE IMAGING

MRI has been used during the past 20 years to image the heart and coronary arteries, and its clinical applications con-

TABLE 17-1 Sensitivity and Specificity for Cardiac Imaging Techniques in Predicting the Gold Standard of Functional Recovery after Successful Revascularization

Ref #	Imaging Technique	No. of Pts	Sensitivity (%)	Specificity (%)
29[a]	^{18}F-FDG PET	332	88	73
29[a]	Rest-redistribution ^{201}Tl-SPECT	145	90	54
29[a]	Stress-redistribution-reinjection ^{201}Tl-SPECT	209	86	47
29[a]	^{99m}Tc-MIBI	207	83	69
29[a]	Low-dose dobutamine echocardiography	448	84	81
49	Stress MRI with myocardial tagging	10	89	93
51	MRI preserved EDWT ($\geq$5.5 mm)	43	92	56
51	MRI dobutamine-induced SWT ($\geq$2 mm)	43	89	94
104	Contrast-enhanced MRI: lack of late hyperenhancement	12	98	76

[a] Data from a metaanalysis.
^{18}F-FDG PET, ^{18}F-fluorodesoxyglucose positron emission tomography; ^{201}Tl-SPECT, [201]thallium single-photon emission computed tomography; ^{99m}Tc-MIBI, [99m]technetium sestamibi; EDWT, end-diastolic wall thickness; SWT, systolic wall thickening.
(From Watzinger N, Saeed M, Wendland MF, et al. Myocardial viability: magnetic resonance assessment of functional reserve and tissue characterization. *J Cardiovasc Magn Reson* 2001;3:195–208, with permission.)

tinue to evolve. Its versatile strengths are: noninvasiveness, inherent three-dimensional data acquisition without radiation exposure, excellent spatial resolution in the range of 1–2 mm, intrinsic soft-tissue contrast that can be exploited for tissue characterization, multitomographic imaging capabilities that allow acquisition of cardiac images in any plane, and sensitivity to cardiac wall motion and blood flow (30). Developments in MR hardware and software have increased the speed of image acquisition, and improved gating procedures have diminished motion-derived image degradation. Moreover, the newer fast imaging sequences, such as fast low-angle shot (FLASH) and echo-planar imaging, allow single or multiple image data sets to be acquired within a heart cycle and permit first-pass contrast profiles to be monitored on currently available clinical systems.

Substantial progress has taken place not only in MRI pulse sequence design but also in the development of MR contrast media. The combination of these advances has substantially improved the capability of contrast-enhanced MRI to characterize ischemic myocardial injury, including its ability to discriminate viable from nonviable zones. MR contrast media incorporate magnetic ions, such as gadolinium, manganese, iron, and dysprosium (31–33). Myocardial contrast is manipulated by combining the administration of agents that possess the desired contrast properties with the MR pulse sequence that is sensitive to the contrast medium. MR contrast media have been classified according to their effect on signal intensity of tissues in relationship to the major MR mechanism of this effect as follows: (a) positive enhancement (longitudinal relaxation) and (b) negative enhancement (transverse relaxation). MR contrast media can also be categorized according to their distribution in tissue into intravascular, extracellular, and intracellular. The distribution volumes of these agents in normal myocardium during equilibrium are 5% to 10% (equal to blood volume), 18% to 20% (equal to blood volume plus interstitial fluid volume), and 100% (equal to blood volume, interstitial volume, and cellular fluid). All MR contrast media currently approved for human use are nonspecific extracellular agents.

At the moment, several intravascular MR agents are under extensive clinical evaluation, mainly for the purpose of contrast-enhanced MR angiography, and some of them may be approved for human use in the near future.

In recent years, several promising approaches to assess myocardial viability by MRI have been proposed and tested in clinical or experimental studies (3–6), including the following:

1. Functional MRI to measure LV wall thickness and thickening before and after dobutamine stress.
2. Dynamic MRI to identify regions with abnormal wash-in/wash-out profiles.
3. Nonspecific extracellular MR contrast media to detect the breakdown of cellular membranes.
4. Necrosis-specific MR contrast media to determine the necrotic zone.
5. MRI to probe ionic transport across functional cellular membranes.

APPLICATIONS IN EXPERIMENTAL AND CLINICAL STUDIES

FUNCTIONAL MAGNETIC RESONANCE IMAGING TO EVALUATE MYOCARDIAL WALL THICKNESS AND THICKENING

The introduction of gradient-echo MRI made it possible to acquire images of the same plane at multiple time points throughout the cardiac cycle. The images can be viewed on a cinematic display so that cardiac motion can be visualized, as in echocardiography. Fast gradient-echo techniques with k-space segmentation allow the acquisition of a cine sequence during a breath-hold of approximately 15 s (34). Newer developments comprise sequences like steady state free precession (SSFP) (35), as well as elaborated data acquisition allowing real-time and cine high-resolution imaging within a few seconds (36,37). Gradient-echo MRI provides a naturally high level of contrast between intracavitary blood and myocardium and thus permits exact and reproducible determination of wall thickness and systolic wall thickening. The excellent delineation of the endocardium and epicardium facilitates a quantitative assessment of wall motion rather than the subjective evaluation commonly used in echocardiography (38). Accordingly, several clinical studies have shown that preserved wall thickness and systolic wall thickening measured with MRI are indicative of residual viability as defined by ^{201}Tl-SPECT or ^{18}F-FDG PET (39–41).

MRI, however, is not limited to observations of regional myocardial function at rest; it also can provide information about functional reserve in response to pharmacologic stress (42,43). Like stress echocardiography, MRI has been used to detect CHD (44–46) and viable myocardium (47–49) by analyzing the changes of global and regional function during inotropic stimulation with dobutamine. In comparison with ^{18}F-FDG PET, Baer et al (50) demonstrated that viable myocardium is characterized on MRI as regions with preserved end-diastolic wall thickness of 5.5 mm or more and dobutamine-elicited systolic wall thickening of at least 1 mm. Moreover, dobutamine-induced systolic wall thickening was found to be a better predictor of regional functional recovery after revascularization than preserved end-diastolic wall thickness (Table 17.1), whereas the presence of significantly reduced end-diastolic wall thickness reliably indicated irreversible myocardial damage (51). For more detailed information, the interested reader is referred to Chapters 14 and 15.

DYNAMIC MAGNETIC RESONANCE IMAGING TO IDENTIFY REGIONS WITH ABNORMAL WASH-IN/WASH-OUT PROFILES

Acute and subacute MI can be detected on unenhanced T2-weighted spin-echo images (52–54), but the visualization of infarction relies on the accumulation of free water within the infarcted region, which may take several hours to develop. In the early days after infarction, T2-weighted images tend to overestimate the area of necrosis because of the formation of edema within the infarcted region (52,55,56), whereas 3 weeks later, a good correlation is found between the true infarct size and the area of high signal intensity (57).

Although unenhanced MR techniques provide no information on tissue perfusion, contrast-enhanced MRI does. Thus, the administration of gadolinium-based extracellular compounds has considerably improved the characterization of myocardial injury and the distinction between viable and nonviable myocardium. It has been shown that after contrast injection, reversibly injured myocardium is indistinguishable from normal myocardium, whereas reperfused infarcted myocardium shows prominent hyperenhancement (hot-spot) on T1-weighted spin-echo images (58,59). In studies of animals with occlusive infarction, the infarcted zone was delineated by a rim of peripheral enhancement surrounding a central zone that did not show hyperenhancement in the first minutes after contrast injection (58,59). During the course of 1 hour, the central region slowly enhanced, which would

suggest a delayed wash-in of the contrast agent to the central zone.

More recently, ultrafast MRI techniques have become available. The high degree of temporal resolution of fast MRI made it possible to monitor the first-pass distribution of contrast agents (60,61) and to study dynamic contrast-enhancement patterns in ischemically injured myocardium (62,63). In an animal model of reperfused MI studied by Saeed et al (64), the first-pass arrival of contrast was delayed in infarcted myocardium; the delay was followed by a steady rise in signal to supranormal levels, whereas signal intensity in normal myocardium declined. A more pronounced manifestation of this phenomenon was reported by Lima et al (65) in a study of 22 patients with recent MI. Several days after reperfusion therapy, the patients were examined with a magnetization-driven gradient-echo pulse sequence (66) to monitor contrast distribution during the first 10 min after bolus administration. In 21 of 22 cases, an abnormal perfusion profile was observed within the infarcted region. It was characterized by a signal rise followed by a slower continued rise, whereas normal myocardium exhibited a rapid initial rise followed by a decline. Moreover, in 10 patients with large infarcts, an additional abnormal subregion could be identified. It was typically located in the subendocardium and exhibited a much slower initial signal rise, so that it appeared relatively hypointense during the first minutes after contrast injection. These regions were considered to represent no-reflow zones, a phenomenon that is caused by severe capillary damage or microvascular obstruction in the core of the infarcted region. Clinically, the pattern of hyperenhanced regions surrounding a hypoenhanced area at the center of the infarct was associated with coronary occlusion at angiography, Q waves on the electrocardiogram, and greater segmental dysfunction by echocardiography.

Next, these findings were corroborated in canine models of acute, reperfused MI and compared with results of histochemical staining (62,67–69). In infarcted tissue, two contrast enhancement patterns were observed, similar to those seen in patients. Some regions showed hypoenhancement on first-pass images that matched closely with thioflavin-negative regions at histomorphometry, indicating no reflow at the tissue level (62,67–69). Surrounding zones of hyperenhancement on delayed images obtained several minutes after contrast injection correlated well with necrotic myocardium defined by triphenyltetrazolium chloride (TTC) staining but tended to overestimate the extent of acute MI slightly (62,68). Using conventional T1-weighted spin-echo imaging after the administration of gadolinium diethylenetriamine pentaacetic acid (Gd-DTPA), several other groups reported similar findings in experimental models of acute MI. The results of these studies (56,70–74) suggested that areas of hyperenhancement on conventional spin-echo images regularly overestimate the extent of irreversible myocardial injury.

A few years ago, an advanced technique for visualization of MI after contrast administration was introduced using a breath-hold k-space segmented inversion recovery fast gradient-echo sequence (75,76). Preparation of the magnetization prior to image acquisition by an inversion prepulse suppresses the signal of normal myocardium and clearly increases the degree of T1-weighting in infarcted tissue. Compared to older techniques, image quality is considerably improved owing to elimination of respiratory motion and amplification of signal intensity. However, the setting of the optimal inversion time (typically set in a range of 200 to 350 ms) is critical for correctly sizing the hyperenhanced region. Because images are usually acquired in a time window of 10 to 30 min after contrast injection, this technique has been termed "late enhancement" or "delayed enhancement" MRI (see Chap. 16). Although delayed-contrast enhancement of infarcted tissue was observed more than a decade ago (53), its potential mechanisms have not been elucidated until recently. Rehwald et al (77) reported elevations of gadolinium concentration in irreversibly injured myocardium that appeared to be related to altered contrast kinetics (63), as well as increased accessibility and enlargement of the extracellular space (78–80).

Several studies (79–81) carefully validated the late-enhancement technique and concluded that the spatial extent of hyperenhancement in irreversible myocardial injury is identical to that of myocyte necrosis or scar in comparisons including ex vivo T1-weighted three-dimensional gradient-echo imaging and histochemical staining. This was in contradiction to previous research (56,70–74), which indicated that hyperenhancement on images acquired several minutes after contrast administration occurs not only in regions of cellular necrosis but also in the border zone of reversibly injured, viable myocardium surrounding the acute infarct (peri-infarction zone). Such a zone, however, can obviously not be visualized with the heavily T1-weighted pulse sequence applied for late-enhancement MRI, suggesting that selection of the imaging technique considerably influences the size of the hyperenhanced region. Moreover, it was assumed that partial volume effects might also have contributed to the contradictory findings in previous studies (79–81). A further issue was raised by other investigators (82–84), who observed a substantial change in the spatial extent of hyperenhancement with inversion-recovery imaging, depending on the timing of image acquisition after contrast injection. Whereas the enhanced region overestimated the infarcted region immediately after Gd-DTPA administration, it gradually receded over time to match the true infarct size. Nevertheless, accurate and reproducible measurements were obtained with late-enhancement MRI when images were acquired with the appropriate inversion time settings between 10 and 30 min after contrast administration (80,85).

Quite contrary to acute MI, several groups using conventional spin-echo imaging could not detect hyperenhancement in infarcts older than 3 to 4 weeks (86–89), but others could (90,91). With the introduction of more advanced MRI techniques, it became possible to show persistent contrast enhancement in healing and chronic infarcts (92) (Fig. 17.1). Because of the high degree of T1-weighting exerted by late-enhancement MRI, scarred myocardium could be visualized with minute details in canine models of chronic myocardial injury (79,81,93). Once acutely and chronically infarcted tissue could be differentiated from reversibly injured viable myocardium, the field was open for several clinical applications of contrast-enhanced MRI.

In the era of spin-echo imaging, only a few studies evaluated the transmural extent of MI to predict regional viability (94,95), whereas the majority of reports focused mainly on the presence and absence of hyperenhancement (86–88,96). However, newer imaging techniques offer improved image

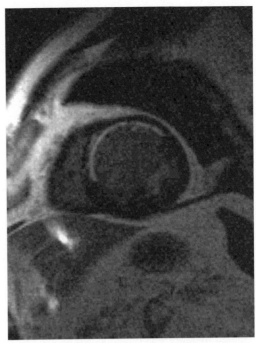

Figure 17.1. End-diastolic short-axis T1-weighted inversion-recovery turbo-FLASH (fast low-angle shot) image (repetition time/inversion time/echo time = 400/300/4 ms) obtained 20 min after the administration of 0.1 mmol of Gd-DTPA (gadolinium diethylenetriamine pentaacetic acid) per kilogram in a patient with a healed anterior myocardial infarction. Note the nontransmural hyperenhancement in the anteroseptal wall.

quality and higher spatial resolution, allowing for a transmural differentiation of contrast enhancement. Since myocardial necrosis in humans and various animals starts at the subendocardium, and with increasing duration of ischemia progresses toward the epicardium (97), it is important to determine the extent of nonviable and viable myocardium across the ventricular wall for prediction of functional recovery. Several studies in reperfused MI demonstrated that there is an inverse relationship between the transmural extent of late hyperenhancement and the likelihood of recovery of regional contractile function (98–103). Although any chosen cutoff value would be unphysiological and arbitrary, late hyperenhancement comprising more than 75% of LV wall thickness is highly predictive of lack of long-term improvement. Conversely, absence or minimal hyperenhancement of less than 25% correlates with recovery of regional wall motion. The amount of transmural enhancement has also prognostic implications in patients with chronic coronary artery and ischemic cardiomyopathy scheduled for coronary revascularization. Several studies (81,104–108), including more than 190 individuals, performed late-enhancement MRI before PTCA or CABG and assessed regional and global function several months thereafter. Consistently, it was observed that no or minimal hyperenhancement in dysfunctional segments is a powerful predictor of myocardial hibernation and residual viability. In addition, it was shown that late-enhancement MRI also has the capability of visualizing microinfarcts in patients with evidence of myocardial injury after coronary revascularization (107,109,110).

Since its introduction in 1999, the late-enhancement technique has been compared with several clinical tools to probe myocardial viability. The electrocardiogram, for instance, was shown to be an invalid method to assess the transmural extent of myocardial injury because the presence or absence of Q waves is determined by the total size rather than the transmurality of the underlying MI (111,112). Head-to-head comparisons between late-enhancement MRI and dobutamine-stress MRI in patients with LV dysfunction yielded excellent agreement for assessing hibernating myocardium (108,113). However, for segments with an intermediate extent of scar tissue (>25% and <75% transmurality), integration of both modalities may allow a more precise identification of segments with functional recovery. The results of SPECT (85,92,114–118) and PET imaging (106,119,120) also correlate well with those of contrast-enhanced MRI. Available data suggest that late-enhancement MRI has at least two major advantages over scintigraphic techniques: (a) superior spatial resolution, allowing detection of small and subendocardial infarcts, and (b) lack of photo attenuation from underlying soft tissue, resulting in higher accuracy, particularly for inferior wall segments. Most recently, late-enhancement imaging was implemented in several comprehensive MRI protocols to assess the presence of significant coronary artery stenosis in patients presenting with chest pain (121), acute coronary syndromes (122,123), and stable CHD (124).

In summary, contrast-enhanced MRI allows the visualization of the no-reflow zone and surrounding injured myocardium. Despite the restoration of epicardial blood flow, perfusion in the core of large infarcts may be limited at the tissue level because of injury to the microvasculature and subsequent obstruction by erythrocytes, neutrophils, and debris, a phenomenon known as "no reflow" (125). Since flow in the infarcted core is very low but not absent, these regions appear hypoenhanced on first-pass MR images but slowly over time become hyperenhanced. The presence of microvascular obstruction is associated with nonviability and greater regional dysfunction (62,65,67–69,95,100,126–129). Moreover, it has been shown that no reflow at the capillary level is a strong predictor of poor functional recovery, remodeling of the ventricle, and more frequent cardiovascular complications (67,69,130).

The interpretation of hyperenhancement on MR images has considerably changed in recent years due to advances in the MRI technique. Spin-echo imaging has repeatedly demonstrated that hyperenhanced regions include the infarcted area per se in addition to a portion of the area at risk (peri-infarction zone), so that the extent of necrosis is overestimated (56,70–74,131). Enhancement of the peri-infarction zone may be explained by residual flow via collateral vessels and the presence of interstitial edema (89). Healing or chronic infarcts, however, are irregularly visualized with conventional imaging techniques (86–88,90,91).

In recent years, late-enhancement imaging has rapidly assumed a prominent role in the assessment of myocardial injury (75,76). Published literature demonstrates that the spatial extent of late hyperenhancement is identical to that of necrotic or scarred myocardium, whereas reversibly injured viable myocardium within the jeopardized area remains indistinguishable from normal tissue (79–81). This new technique results in sharper and better delineation of hyperenhancement and allows discrimination between transmural and nontransmural spread of myocardial injury (98,99,132). Because acute and chronic infarcts generally cannot be differentiated from the appearance on late-enhancement images, a protocol combining T2-weighted and contrast-enhanced MRI can add important information to patients with nondiagnostic electrocardiograms or equivocal laboratory results (54).

In a comprehensive approach, several investigators combined first-pass and delayed MRI to characterize the extent and severity of myocardial injury in patients with recent MI (100,104,126,127,129). Improvement of systolic wall thickening after several weeks served as criterion of residual viability. Earlier studies (126,127) reported that regions displaying hypoenhancement during first pass did not show improvement in contractile function, whereas regions with normal first-pass signal followed by hyperenhancement on delayed images improved after several weeks. From that, it was concluded that segments with the latter pattern might represent predominantly viable myocardium. However, the MR sequence employed in these studies was one used primarily for perfusion protocols. Furthermore, imaging was completed within 10 min after contrast injection, which may not be sufficient enough time to reduce enhancement between edematous and normal tissue in the peri-infarction zone. Unlike that, newer research (100,104,129) using the typical late-enhancement settings indicates that the magnitude of functional recovery is inversely related to the transmural extent of regional hyperenhancement. With respect to that, the presence or absence of late hyperenhancement that reflects myocardial necrosis seems to be a more accurate parameter for predicting persistent dysfunction then early hypoenhancement, which solely corresponds to regions with microvascular obstruction, and thus underestimates the amount of irreversibly injured myocardium. Altogether, several factors must be considered when the results of all these studies that define myocardial viability from hyperenhanced regions are interpreted: (a) type of imaging sequence and its sensitivity to T1 changes, (b) dose of the contrast medium and timing of imaging after contrast administration, (c) transmural extent of the ischemic myocardial injury, (d) age of the infarct and flow in the infarct-related artery, (e) slice thickness and partial volume effects, (f) species-related differences in infarct pathology, and (g) the "reference standard" employed to infer myocardial viability.

NONSPECIFIC EXTRACELLULAR MAGNETIC RESONANCE CONTRAST MEDIA TO DETECT THE BREAKDOWN OF CELL MEMBRANES

In this approach, the degree of myocardial injury is determined by estimating the breakdown of cellular membranes within the ischemic zone with the use of nonspecific extracellular contrast media. These agents can increase or decrease signal intensity, depending on the type and concentration of the contrast medium in the tissue and the MR sequence employed. Relaxivity-enhancing media or T1-enhancing contrast agents, such as Gd-DTPA, usually increase the MR signal in tissue not excluded from blood supply on T1-weighted images, whereas susceptibility-enhancing media or T2*-enhancing agents, such as dysprosium-DTPA (Dy-DTPA), cause a signal loss with T2-sensitive imaging sequences. Both types of contrast media exit freely from the vascular space and are distributed rapidly in the extracellular space, but they are excluded from the intracellular compartment of cells with intact membranes.

After administration of Dy-DTPA, the decrease in signal intensity is a function of magnetic susceptibility and distribution within the tissue, a greater effect being associated with a more heterogeneous distribution. In normal myocardium, cell membranes act as a barrier and limit the distribution of contrast agents to the extracellular space, causing a heterogeneous distribution in tissue with attenuation of signal. Because loss of membrane selectivity is an indicator of cell death, it was hypothesized that alterations in the potency of susceptibility dependent signal loss are related to the severity of myocardial injury. In a rat model of reperfused MI, irreversibly injured regions that appeared hyperintense on Gd-DTPA-enhanced T1-weighted spin-echo images were also hyperintense on Dy-DTPA-enhanced T2-weighted spin-echo images (133). It was proposed that this effect is the result of a more homogeneous tissue distribution of dysprosium in the infarcted myocardium, signifying that the agent has entered the intracellular space. A subsequent study (134) in excised hearts corroborated this proposed mechanism. Geschwind et al (134) administered Gd-DTPA and Dy-DTPA in tandem to rats subjected to irreversible myocardial injury followed by reperfusion and performed spin-echo and gradient-echo imaging. Gd-DPTA was used to document the presence of flow and the delivery of contrast agent to the reperfused region, whereas Dy-DTPA was used to assess myocardial viability. Although Gd-DTPA caused a greater increase in the signal of reperfused infarcted myocardium, Dy-DTPA-bismethyamide (BMA) also delineated infarcted myocardium as a bright region. After imaging, the quantities of these agents present in reperfused infarcted and normal myocardium were measured by atomic absorption spectrometry. The tissue concentrations of both agents were greatly increased in infarcted versus normal myocardium. Thus, the authors concluded that the loss of magnetic susceptibility effect exerted by Dy-DTPA was caused by the failure of myocardial cells to exclude the compound from the intracellular space rather than by a reduced tissue concentration.

In another experimental model of acute MI, Diesbourg et al (78) demonstrated that within the first 5 min after bolus injection, the tissue concentration of T1-enhancing extracellular MR contrast media such as Gd-DTPA is determined primarily by blood flow, and after approximately 10 min is determined primarily by the agent's accessible space (fractional distribution volume, or fDV). Moreover, it is well known that Gd-DTPA produces considerably greater enhancement of irreversibly injured myocardium than of normal myocardium on images acquired several minutes after contrast injection (53,58,59). This observation also implies that a relatively larger quantity of contrast agent has distributed into the injured region. With the loss of cellular membrane integrity, virtually no barrier is present between extracellular and intracellular compartments. Consequently, the fDV of gadolinium chelates is expanded from approximately 20% in normal myocardium to nearly 100% in complete myocardial necrosis. As the fDV increases, the bulk tissue

concentration of extracellular contrast agents at the equilibrium phase also increases proportionally (77,78). Therefore, it was proposed that the calculation of the fDV in a region of interest encompassing a jeopardized myocardial region could provide a measure of the percentage of necrotic cells within this volume.

The concept of defining myocardial injury according to the distribution of extracellular MR contrast media into various myocardial compartments has been tested in several animal models (78,91,131,135–140). Using constant infusion, it was demonstrated that the partition coefficient (λ) of Gd-DTPA, which is proportional to the fDV, is maximal within the first week after reperfused MI and slowly decreases thereafter (91,136,140). Measured values of the partition coefficient by MRI agreed well with values determined ex vivo by radioactive counting of ^{111}In-DTPA but were inversely correlated with ^{201}Tl uptake as a marker of residual viability. Moreover, MRI allowed monitoring of the partition coefficient during the initial minutes of reperfusion, and an observed increase from normal to maximal values during the first 2 hours, suggested ongoing rupture of myocardial cells (91).

Using an echo-planar MRI technique, Wendland et al (138) measured the change in T1 relaxation rate ($\Delta R1$), which is proportional to the quantity of contrast medium within the tissue of interest after bolus administration of gadolinium chelates. They found a constant proportionality between the $\Delta R1$ values of myocardium and blood during the first 30 min after contrast injection, and a failure of increased doses of the agent to alter this proportionality was considered indicative of an approximately equilibrated state of distribution. The authors proposed that direct measurement of the T1 changes in myocardium and blood at this steady state provides an estimate of the fDV of the contrast agent, which can be calculated by the following formula: $\Delta R1$ myocardium/$\Delta R1$ blood $\times$ (1-hemotocrit). Subsequently, this hypothesis was tested in a rat model of reperfused myocardial infarction (131,135,137). Measured distribution volumes of gadolinium chelates were also compared with the results of ^{99m}Tc-DTPA autoradiography as an independent reference standard after sacrifice of the animals. Not surprisingly, a close agreement between both measurements was reported. In complete infarction, a fDV of approximately 90% suggests entrance of the indicators into nearly all myocardial cells. In animal models of graded myocardial injury, it was further shown that the fDV of extracellular contrast agents increases in relation to the duration of coronary occlusion (131,137) (Fig. 17.2). Additionally, it was found that cases subjected to 30 to 60 min of ischemia exhibited two regions of abnormally elevated count density at high-resolution ^{99m}Tc-DTPA autoradiography—a core of higher count density surrounded by a border zone of moderately increased count density (131,135). The fDV of ^{99m}Tc-DTPA and its surrogate Gd-DTPA were approximately two times greater than those in normal myocardium in the peri-infarction zone, but four times greater than those in normal myocardium in the infarcted core (Fig. 17.3). On electron microscopy, these regions contained moderately injured myocardium that comprised largely viable cells (56,131). Thus, it was inferred that this MRI approach has the potential to provide an estimate of the necrotic cell fraction and of potentially salvageable cells within the area at risk. This

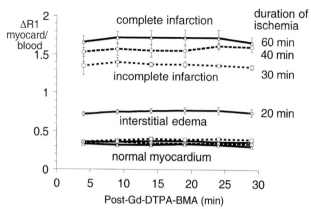

Figure 17.2. Plot of the effect of duration of ischemia on ΔR1 ratio in rats subjected to 20, 30, 40, and 60 min of coronary occlusion followed by 1 hour of reperfusion. During repetitive measurements, the ΔR1 ratios for myocardium/blood remain constant during the initial 30 min after injection of 0.2 mmol of Gd-DTPA-BMA per kilogram, which suggests a state close to equilibrium. This means that ΔR1 ratios represent partition coefficients (λ), which allows calculation of fractional distribution volume. Note the increase in ΔR1 ratio as a function of the severity of injury. ΔR1, relaxation rate; Gd-DTPA-BMA, gadolinium diethylenetriamine pentaacetic acid bismethyamide. (From Arheden H, Saeed M, Higgins CB, et al. Reperfused rat myocardium subjected to various durations of ischemia: estimation of the distribution volume of contrast material with echo-planar MR imaging. *Radiology* 2000;215:520–528, with permission.)

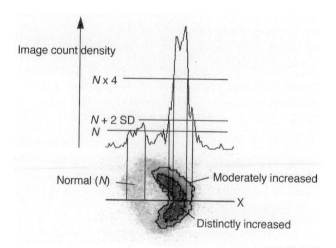

Figure 17.3. Profile of image count density through a section of an autoradiographic image of a 20-μm-thick slice from a rat subjected to 60 min of coronary artery occlusion followed by reperfusion. Several levels of image count density are seen: low count density (N) corresponding to normal myocardium, moderately increased count density (N + 2SD) in the rim corresponding to ischemic injury, and high count density (N × 4) in the core corresponding to severe ischemic injury. (From Arheden H, Saeed M, Higgins CB, et al. Measurement of the distribution volume of gadopentetate dimeglumine at echo-planar MR imaging to quantify myocardial infarction: comparison with ^{99m}Tc-DTPA autoradiography in rats. *Radiology* 1999;211:698–708, with permission.)

thesis is at odds with a recent report by Rehwald et al (77), who used electron probe x-ray microanalysis to examine the concentrations of gadolinium in a rabbit model of myocardial injury. They found that regional elevations of contrast agent concentrations are exclusively associated with irreversible ischemic injury defined by histochemical staining. Accordingly, in regions considered at risk but not infarcted, gadolinium concentrations were similar to that in remote myocardium. Moreover, in a canine model of stunned myocardium, the partition coefficient within reversibly injured stunned regions was not elevated above that of normal tissue (139). Further studies are needed to determine whether partially injured myocardium that surrounds the necrotic core is visible after Gd-DTPA administration or whether acute MI is an all-or-nothing process with respect to contrast-enhanced MRI.

Whereas the fDV or partition coefficient in acute infarction is elevated owing to loss of cell membrane integrity and interstitial edema, less information is available on healing or chronic infarcts characterized by collageneous tissue. It was shown that the partition coefficient (91,140) and the regional concentration of Gd-DTPA (77) are elevated up to several weeks after an acute ischemic event, resulting in increased signal intensity in infarcted regions. This is in line with observations made by other groups that reported hyperenhancement in chronic infarcts using rapid T1-weighted imaging (79,81,92). Although the exact mechanism of contrast enhancement in the nonacute setting remains to be fully elucidated, a possible explanation is provided by the fact that the extracellular compartment of collageneous scar is greater than that of normal myocardium with intact cells (141,142). Recent research supports these findings by measuring partition coefficients in humans with acute and chronic infarcts. Compared to normal myocardium, high and intermediate values were found in necrotic and scarred tissue, respectively, indicating expansion of the interstitial space to a different degree in these conditions (143). More importantly, quantification of partition coefficients also allowed differentiation between acutely and chronically infarcted regions.

Thus, the concept of using nonspecific extracellular MR contrast media to detect the breakdown of cellular membranes after ischemic injury is now proven. It seems conceivable that quantifying the partition coefficient or fDV of extracellular MR contrast agents provides valuable information for defining the age and severity of myocardial injury. However, whether this approach is sufficiently practical and reliable to be applied clinically remains to be determined.

NECROSIS-SPECIFIC MAGNETIC RESONANCE CONTRAST MEDIA TO DETERMINE THE NECROTIC ZONE

The development of MR contrast agents with a high specific affinity to irreversible damaged myocardium has been an elusive goal. Notable attempts include binding an indicator to antibodies specific for intracellular compounds (144) and using phosphonate-modified gadolinium chelates that interact with calcium deposits accumulating in necrotic tissue (145). All these efforts were discontinued due to concerns about agent toxicity.

Paramagnetic metalloporphyrins were originally developed as tumor-seeking contrast media because of their known tendency to accumulate in neoplastic tissue (146,147). However, the discovery that gadolinium mesoporphyrins, such as Gadophrin-2 and Gadophrin-3, are more necrosis-avid rather than tumor-selective opened up the field for new applications (148,149). In various animal models of reperfused MI, these agents provided strong and persistent enhancement of acutely infarcted tissue on conventional T1-weighted spin-echo images (72,150–153). The area demarcated by gadolinium mesoporphyrins revealed minute details of necrotic tissue that closely matched those defined by TTC histochemical staining. However, in larger animals with occlusive infarcts, less constant enhancement was observed (150,151,154,155). Moreover, chronically injured myocardium did not enhance with necrosis-specific contrast agents, presumably because there are no binding sites in scar tissue (156,157). Consequently, these agents might be useful for studying acute MI, infarct healing, and possibly for estimating infarct age in combination with Gd-DTPA-enhanced MRI.

To distinguish reversible from irreversibly injured myocardium, several investigators administered gadolinium mesoporphyrin and nonspecific extracellular MR contrast media in a double-contrast imaging protocol. Saeed et al (72) induced reversible and irreversible myocardial injury in rats and injected Gd-DTPA in addition to Gadophrin-2 at different time points after reperfusion. In animals with irreversibly injured myocardium, the size of Gadophrin-2-enhanced regions closely matched the size of infarction defined by histochemical staining. Conversely, the zone delineated by Gd-DTPA on conventional T1-weighted spin-echo images overestimated the true infarct size but was more closely related to the area at risk (Figs. 17.4 and 17.5). In a subsequent study (73), it was demonstrated that the gadolinium mesoporphyrin-enhanced region showed no wall thickening 24 hours after reperfusion, whereas the Gd-DTPA-enhanced area was characterized by moderately reduced function. It was concluded that the Gd-DTPA-enhanced region encompasses viable and nonviable portions and that the difference in size demarcated by the two compounds can be used to characterize the peri-infarction zone. A border zone surrounding the Gadophrin-2-enhanced necrotic area was also observed when Gadomer-17, an intravascular agent, was injected (158,159). However, comparisons between necrosis-specific and standard extracellular contrast media using the more advanced late-enhancement technique showed excellent agreement between the areas enhanced by both agents and true infarct size defined by TTC staining (156). Several possible explanations for these discrepant results seen with differential imaging techniques were discussed previously.

Although the exact mechanism is unknown, gadolinium mesoporphyrins bind to necrotic tissue and have the capability to visualize morphologic details, such nontransmural, subendocardial, and scattered infarcts. Enhancement persists from 40 min to more than 24 hours (83,148,153), allowing more flexible timing between contrast administration and

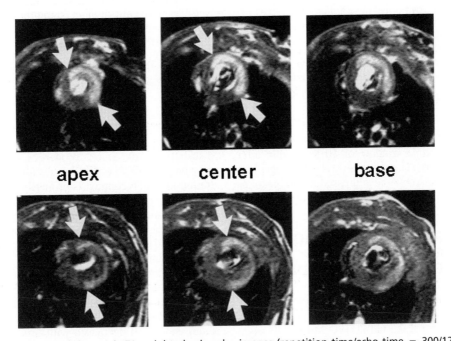

Figure 17.4. Multisection sets of short-axis T1-weighted spin-echo images (repetition time/echo time = 300/12 ms) at three levels (*apex, center,* and *base*) of the left ventricle in a rat heart subjected to reperfused irreversible myocardial injury. Images were obtained after the administration of Gd-DTPA 1 hour after reperfusion (*top row*), and after the administration Gadophrin-2 24 hours following reperfusion (*bottom row*). Both MR contrast media can delineate irreversibly injured myocardium as a hyperenhanced zone in comparison with normal myocardium. Note the smaller size of the hyperenhanced zone on gadolinium mesoporphyrin-enhanced images than on the images obtained after the administration of Gd-DTPA. The difference in the size of the hyperenhanced regions produced by the two compounds may represent salvageable peri-infarcted myocardium. Gd-DTPA, gadolinium diethylenetriamine pentaacetic acid; Gadophrin-2, gadolinium mesoporphyrin. (From Saeed M, Bremerich J, Wendland MF, et al. Reperfused myocardial infarction as seen with use of necrosis-specific versus standard extracellular MR contrast media in rats. *Radiology* 1999;213:247–257, with permission.)

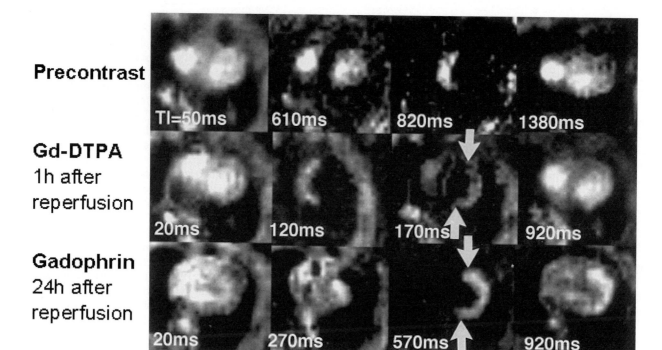

Figure 17.5. Axial inversion-recovery echo-planar MR images (repetition time/echo time = 7000/10 ms) obtained in a rat heart subjected to reperfused, irreversible myocardial injury. The images were obtained before the administration of contrast medium, after the administration of 0.3 mmol Gd-DTPA per kilogram, and after the administration of 0.05 mmol Gadophrin-2 per kilogram. These magnitude intensity images demonstrate that different regions of interest pass the null point of longitudinal magnetization recovery at different inversion time (TI) settings. On Gd-DTPA-enhanced images, reperfused irreversibly injured myocardium passes through the null point first at a TI of 120 ms because it has the highest Gd-DTPA content and the largest distribution volume. This was followed by left ventricular chamber blood at a TI of 170 ms, which contains less Gd-DTPA than infarcted myocardium but more than normal myocardium, and finally by normal myocardium. The reperfused, irreversibly injured myocardium passed through the null point at a TI of 270 ms because it has the highest Gadophrin-2 content, followed by left ventricular chamber blood and normal myocardium at a TI of 570 ms. The difference in T1 effect between the two contrast media is related to the injected dose, distribution volume, binding of the two agents, and the time of imaging after injection. Gd-DTPA, gadolinium diethylenetriamine pentaacetic acid; Gadophrin-2, gadolinium mesoporphyrin. (From Saeed M, Bremerich J, Wendland MF, et al. Reperfused myocardial infarction as seen with use of necrosis-specific versus standard extracellular MR contrast media in rats. *Radiology* 1999;213:247–257, with permission.)

imaging. This may be a true advantage over nonspecific agents, which provide reproducible infarct size measurements only within a time window of 10 to 30 min after contrast injection (83,85). However, several issues regarding toxicity and side effects must be addressed before gadolinium mesoporphyrins can be approved for clinical use.

ION TRANSPORT ACROSS FUNCTIONAL CELLULAR MEMBRANES TO CHARACTERIZE VIABLE MYOCARDIUM

Manganese dipyridoxyl diphosphate (Manganese-DPDP) is a hepatobiliary MR contrast agent approved in humans at a dose of 0.005 mmol/kg. Like Gd-DTPA, Mn-DPDP has a T1-shortening effect and nonspecific extracellular distribution properties. At high doses up to 0.4 mmol/kg, Mn-DPDP effectively delineated infarcted myocardium, allowed discrimination of occlusive and reperfused infarcts, and enabled distinction between reversibly and irreversibly injured myocardium (160–162). Further studies have shown that the manganese cation (Mn^{2+}) is slowly released from the ligand (163), quickly taken up via voltage-operated calcium channels, and retained in viable myocardial cells (164–166). Because intact Mn-DPDP and dissociated Mn^{2+} have distinct distributional and kinetic properties, it was proposed that it may be possible to obtain images after Mn-DPDP administration in which contrast is primarily provided by the intracellular uptake of Mn^{2+} released from the chelate (167). This was attempted in a study by Bremerich et al (168), in which three groups of rats were prepared with reperfused infarcts and given either 0.025, 0.05, or 0.1 mmol Mn-DPDP per kilogram. With inversion-recovery echo-planar imaging, $\Delta R1$ was measured successively for 60 min after contrast administration to monitor the accumulation of manganese in myocardial cells. The $\Delta R1$ values in normal myocardium increased linearly, whereas the values in infarcted myocardium and blood decreased with time, indicating clearance from this region. The enhancement caused by the slow accumulation of manganese in normal myocardium allowed delineation of infarcted regions on high-resolution inversion-recovery spin-echo images (Fig. 17.6). Compared with gadolinium-based agents, manganese-based contrast media provide differential contrast enhancement that is highly specific and less sensitive to timing for infarct size determination, since labeling of viable tissue persists for at least 1

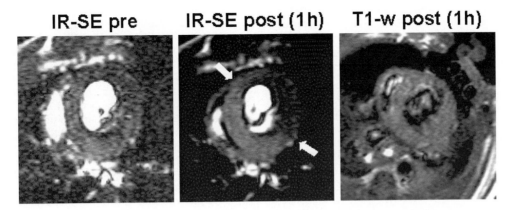

IR-SE pre   **IR-SE post (1h)**   **T1-w post (1h)**

Figure 17.6. Short-axis inversion-recovery spin-echo (repetition time/inversion time/echo time = 1000/500/12 ms) and conventional T1-weighted spin-echo (repetition time/echo time = 300/12 ms) images acquired before (left panel) and after (middle and right panels) contrast injection of 0.1 mmol Mn-DPDP per kilogram at the midventricular level. Note the dark appearance of the infarcted zone 1 hour after injection using inversion-recovery spin-echo imaging, whereas normal myocardium appears bright because of the uptake of paramagnetic Mn^{2+} ions. The nonviable zone is not visualized on unenhanced inversion-recovery spin-echo images and enhanced conventional T1-weighted spin-echo images. Mn-DPDP, manganese dipyridoxyl diphosphate. (From Watzinger N, Saeed M, Wendland MF, et al. Myocardial viability: magnetic resonance assessment of functional reserve and tissue characterization. *J Cardiovasc Magn Reson* 2001;3:195–208, with permission.)

hour (84). Moreover, it was shown that manganese-enhanced MRI can be used to define the spatial extent of stunned myocardium on the basis of a decline in manganese uptake by stunned cells (169,170). Although manganese-enhanced MRI has unique capabilities to assess myocardial viability, potential toxicity makes it difficult to envision its applications in humans.

An important indicator of myocyte death and lack of cell membrane integrity is loss of Na^+/K^+-ATPase function and intracellular-extracellular ion homeostasis. In normal myocardium, the intracellular sodium concentration is usually less than that in the extracellular space because of active transport across intact cell membranes. During ischemia, the intracellular sodium concentration rises and remains elevated in irreversible myocardial injury (171). Using sodium (^{23}Na) MRI in several experimental models, it was shown that regions of acutely or chronically infarcted myocardium are clearly visible as areas of increased signal (172–174). In the early phase of MI, the sodium content also seemed to depend on myocardial blood flow since slower sodium accumulation rates were observed in regions with microvascular obstruction (175). When coronary flow is entirely absent, the total sodium signal might not change, whereas the intracellular sodium concentration can rise. A newer technique helps to overcome this problem by enabling differentiation between intracellular and extracellular sodium resonances with the help of a chemical shift agent (176,177). Moreover, the feasibility of performing sodium MRI has recently been demonstrated in healthy volunteers (178) and in patients with acute and chronic MI (179,180).

tems facilitate comprehensive assessment of patients with CHD within a reasonable time (121,124). Compared to other established imaging techniques, cardiac MRI provides a unique tool to determine myocardial viability by interrogation of several interrelated hallmarks of viable cells. Owing to its capability to delineate acute and chronic infarcts with high accuracy, contrast-enhanced MRI may well become the new clinical imaging standard for the detection of irreversibly injured myocardium. Moreover, contrast-enhanced MRI can guide and monitor the effects of new treatments, such as gene therapy and stem cell delivery into damaged tissue (181,182). Diagnostic procedures and therapeutic interventions under fluoroscopy and MRI guidance are currently performed in cardiac facilities that often consist of adjoining MRI and angiographic units (183). Since a robust and uncomplicated technique for coronary MR angiography could denote the ultimate breakthrough, hopefully this goal will be achieved within the decade. In particular, intravascular contrast agents and imaging at higher field strengths may help to improve upon our current technology. In the future, cardiac MRI will also contribute to the assessment of atherosclerotic disease by characterization of plaque composition and vessel wall imaging (184,185). These ongoing developments, in conjunction with the general strengths of MRI—noninvasiveness, excellent spatial resolution, and tissue contrast—will certainly set a new standard for the assessment of myocardial viability. However, larger prospective randomized trials are warranted to determine the prognostic value and the cost-effectiveness of cardiac MRI in detecting reversible myocardial dysfunction as a means of guiding therapeutic interventions in patients with CHD and impaired LV function.

FUTURE PERSPECTIVE

Recent advances in MR hardware and software developments have resulted in improved image quality and shortened acquisition time; therefore, cardiac-dedicated MRI sys-

SUMMARY

MRI is a highly accurate method of characterizing reversible and irreversible myocardial injury and obtaining information

on residual myocardial viability. The various approaches used to achieve these important goals have been described. Preserved wall thickness and contractile reserve can be assessed by cine MRI qualitatively and quantitatively. Contrast-enhanced MRI provides information on tissue perfusion and cellular membrane function. Thorough assessment of all accepted parameters to characterize myocardial viability, such as structure, function, perfusion, and cellular integrity, can be readily performed with MRI. In this regard, cardiac MRI has the potential to replace or complement other commonly used techniques in the diagnostic armamentarium of physicians caring for patients with ischemic heart disease.

REFERENCES

1. Lipton MJ, Bogaert J, Boxt LM, et al. Imaging of ischemic heart disease. *Eur Radiol* 2002;12:1061–1080.
2. Pennell DJ, Sechtem UP, Higgins CB, et al. Clinical indications for cardiovascular magnetic resonance (CMR): Consensus Panel report. *Eur Heart J* 2004;25:1940–1965.
3. Wendland MF, Saeed M, Lund G, et al. Contrast-enhanced MRI for quantification of myocardial viability. *J Magn Reson Imaging* 1999;10:694–702.
4. Watzinger N, Saeed M, Wendland MF, et al. Myocardial viability: magnetic resonance assessment of functional reserve and tissue characterization. *J Cardiovasc Magn Reson* 2001;3:195–208.
5. Mahrholdt H, Wagner A, Judd RM, et al. Assessment of myocardial viability by cardiovascular magnetic resonance imaging. *Eur Heart J* 2002;23:602–619.
6. Shan K, Constantine G, Sivananthan M, et al. Role of cardiac magnetic resonance imaging in the assessment of myocardial viability. *Circulation* 2004;109:1328–1334.
7. Herman MV, Gorlin R. Implications of left ventricular asynergy. *Am J Cardiol* 1969;23:538–547.
8. Lewis SJ, Sawada SG, Ryan T, et al. Segmental wall motion abnormalities in the absence of clinically documented myocardial infarction: clinical significance and evidence of hibernating myocardium. *Am Heart J* 1991;121:1088–1094.
9. Birnbaum Y, Kloner RA. Myocardial viability. *West J Med* 1996;165:364–371.
10. Bax JJ, van Eck-Smit BL, van der Wall EE. Assessment of tissue viability: clinical demand and problems. *Eur Heart J* 1998;19:847–858.
11. Hendel RC, Chaudhry FA, Bonow RO. Myocardial viability. *Curr Probl Cardiol* 1996;21:145–221.
12. Rahimtoola SH. The hibernating myocardium. *Am Heart J* 1989;117:211–221.
13. Marinho NV, Keogh BE, Costa DC, et al. Pathophysiology of chronic left ventricular dysfunction. New insights from the measurement of absolute myocardial blood flow and glucose utilization. *Circulation* 1996;93:737–744.
14. Pagano D, Fath-Ordoubadi F, Beatt KJ, et al. Effects of coronary revascularisation on myocardial blood flow and coronary vasodilator reserve in hibernating myocardium. *Heart* 2001;85:208–212.
15. Tillisch J, Brunken R, Marshall R, et al. Reversibility of cardiac wall-motion abnormalities predicted by positron tomography. *N Engl J Med* 1986;314:884–888.
16. Underwood SR, Bax JJ, vom Dahl J, et al. Imaging techniques for the assessment of myocardial hibernation. Report of a Study Group of the European Society of Cardiology. *Eur Heart J* 2004;25:815–836.
17. Auerbach MA, Schoder H, Hoh C, et al. Prevalence of myocardial viability as detected by positron emission tomography in patients with ischemic cardiomyopathy. *Circulation* 1999;99:2921–2926.
18. Allman KC, Shaw LJ, Hachamovitch R, et al. Myocardial viability testing and impact of revascularization on prognosis in patients with coronary artery disease and left ventricular dysfunction: a meta-analysis. *J Am Coll Cardiol* 2002;39:1151–1158.
19. Mickleborough LL, Maruyama H, Takagi Y, et al. Results of revascularization in patients with severe left ventricular dysfunction. *Circulation* 1995;92:II73–79.
20. Haas F, Haehnel CJ, Picker W, et al. Preoperative positron emission tomographic viability assessment and perioperative and postoperative risk in patients with advanced ischemic heart disease. *J Am Coll Cardiol* 1997;30:1693–1700.
21. Heyndrickx GR, Millard RW, McRitchie RJ, et al. Regional myocardial functional and electrophysiological alterations after brief coronary artery occlusion in conscious dogs. *J Clin Invest* 1975;56:978–985.
22. Braunwald E, Kloner RA. The stunned myocardium: prolonged, postischemic ventricular dysfunction. *Circulation* 1982;66:1146–1149.
23. Kloner RA, Bolli R, Marban E, et al. Medical and cellular implications of stunning, hibernation, and preconditioning: an NHLBI workshop. *Circulation* 1998;97:1848–1867.
24. Galasko GI, Lahiri A. The non-invasive assessment of hibernating myocardium in ischaemic cardiomyopathy—a myriad of techniques. *Eur J Heart Fail* 2003;5:217–227.
25. Bolli R, Zhu WX, Thornby JI, et al. Time course and determinants of recovery of function after reversible ischemia in conscious dogs. *Am J Physiol* 1988;254:H102–114.
26. Berman DS. Use of 201Tl for risk stratification after myocardial infarction and thrombolysis. *Circulation* 1997;96:2758–2761.
27. Gropler RJ, Bergmann SR. Myocardial viability—what is the definition? *J Nucl Med* 1991;32:10–12.
28. Stillman AE, Wilke N, Jerosch-Herold M. Myocardial viability. *Radiol Clin North Am* 1999;37:361–378.
29. Bax JJ, Wijns W, Cornel JH, et al. Accuracy of currently available techniques for prediction of functional recovery after revascularization in patients with left ventricular dysfunction due to chronic coronary artery disease: comparison of pooled data. *J Am Coll Cardiol* 1997;30:1451–1460.
30. van der Wall EE, Vliegen HW, de Roos A, et al. Magnetic resonance techniques for assessment of myocardial viability. *J Cardiovasc Pharmacol* 1996;28(Suppl 1):S37–44.
31. Saeed M, Wendland MF, Watzinger N, et al. MR contrast media for myocardial viability, microvascular integrity and perfusion. *Eur J Radiol* 2000;34:179–195.
32. Schalla S, Higgins CB, Saeed M. Contrast agents for cardiovascular magnetic resonance imaging. Current status and future directions. *Drugs R D* 2002;3:285–302.
33. Edelman RR. Contrast-enhanced MR imaging of the heart: overview of the literature. *Radiology* 2004;232:653–668.
34. Atkinson DJ, Edelman RR. Cineangiography of the heart in a single breath hold with a segmented turboFLASH sequence. *Radiology* 1991;178:357–360.
35. Barkhausen J, Ruehm SG, Goyen M, et al. MR evaluation of ventricular function: true fast imaging with steady-state precession versus fast low-angle shot cine MR imaging: feasibility study. *Radiology* 2001;219:264–269.
36. Sodickson DK, Manning WJ. Simultaneous acquisition of spatial harmonics (SMASH): fast imaging with radiofrequency coil arrays. *Magn Reson Med* 1997;38:591–603.
37. Pruessmann KP, Weiger M, Scheidegger MB, et al. SENSE: sensitivity encoding for fast MRI. *Magn Reson Med* 1999;42:952–962.

38. van Rugge FP, van der Wall EE, Spanjersberg SJ, et al. Magnetic resonance imaging during dobutamine stress for detection and localization of coronary artery disease. Quantitative wall motion analysis using a modification of the centerline method. *Circulation* 1994;90:127–138.

39. Baer FM, Smolarz K, Jungehülsing M, et al. Chronic myocardial infarction: assessment of morphology, function, and perfusion by gradient echo magnetic resonance imaging and 99mTc-methoxyisobutyl-isonitrile SPECT. *Am Heart J* 1992; 123:636–645.

40. Perrone-Filardi P, Bacharach SL, Dilsizian V, et al. Regional left ventricular wall thickening. Relation to regional uptake of 18fluorodeoxyglucose and 201Tl in patients with chronic coronary artery disease and left ventricular dysfunction. *Circulation* 1992;86:1125–1137.

41. Lawson MA, Johnson LL, Coghlan L, et al. Correlation of thallium uptake with left ventricular wall thickness by cine magnetic resonance imaging in patients with acute and healed myocardial infarcts. *Am J Cardiol* 1997;80:434–441.

42. Pennell DJ, Underwood SR. Stress cardiac magnetic resonance imaging. *Am J Card Imaging* 1991;5:139–149.

43. Nagel E, Lorenz C, Baer F, et al. Stress cardiovascular magnetic resonance: consensus panel report. *J Cardiovasc Magn Reson* 2001;3:267–281.

44. Pennell DJ, Underwood SR, Manzara CC, et al. Magnetic resonance imaging during dobutamine stress in coronary artery disease. *Am J Cardiol* 1992;70:34–40.

45. Nagel E, Lehmkuhl HB, Bocksch W, et al. Noninvasive diagnosis of ischemia-induced wall motion abnormalities with the use of high-dose dobutamine stress MRI: comparison with dobutamine stress echocardiography. *Circulation* 1999;99: 763–770.

46. Hundley WG, Hamilton CA, Thomas MS, et al. Utility of fast cine magnetic resonance imaging and display for the detection of myocardial ischemia in patients not well suited for second harmonic stress echocardiography. *Circulation* 1999;100:1697–1702.

47. Dendale PA, Franken PR, Waldman GJ, et al. Low-dosage dobutamine magnetic resonance imaging as an alternative to echocardiography in the detection of viable myocardium after acute infarction. *Am Heart J* 1995;130:134–140.

48. Sechtem U, Baer FM, Voth E, et al. Stress functional MRI: detection of ischemic heart disease and myocardial viability. *J Magn Reson Imaging* 1999;10:667–675.

49. Sayad DE, Willett DL, Hundley WG, et al. Dobutamine magnetic resonance imaging with myocardial tagging quantitatively predicts improvement in regional function after revascularization. *Am J Cardiol* 1998;82:1149–1151

50. Baer FM, Voth E, Schneider CA, et al. Comparison of low-dose dobutamine-gradient-echo magnetic resonance imaging and positron emission tomography with [18F]fluorodeoxyglucose in patients with chronic coronary artery disease. A functional and morphological approach to the detection of residual myocardial viability. *Circulation* 1995;91: 1006–1015.

51. Baer FM, Theissen P, Schneider CA, et al. Dobutamine magnetic resonance imaging predicts contractile recovery of chronically dysfunctional myocardium after successful revascularization. *J Am Coll Cardiol* 1998;31:1040–1048.

52. Bouchard A, Reeves RC, Cranney G, et al. Assessment of myocardial infarct size by means of T2-weighted 1H nuclear magnetic resonance imaging. *Am Heart J* 1989;117:281–289.

53. Dulce MC, Duerinckx AJ, Hartiala J, et al. MR imaging of the myocardium using nonionic contrast medium: signal-intensity changes in patients with subacute myocardial infarction. *AJR Am J Roentgenol* 1993;160:963–970.

54. Abdel-Aty H, Zagrosek A, Schulz-Menger J, et al. Delayed enhancement and T2-weighted cardiovascular magnetic resonance imaging differentiate acute from chronic myocardial infarction. *Circulation* 2004;109:2411–2416.

55. Ryan T, Tarver RD, Duerk JL, et al. Distinguishing viable from infarcted myocardium after experimental ischemia and reperfusion by using nuclear magnetic resonance imaging. *J Am Coll Cardiol* 1990;15:1355–1364.

56. Choi SI, Jiang CZ, Lim KH, et al. Application of breath-hold T2-weighted, first-pass perfusion and gadolinium-enhanced T1-weighted MR imaging for assessment of myocardial viability in a pig model. *J Magn Reson Imaging* 2000;11: 476–480.

57. Wisenberg G, Prato FS, Carroll SE, et al. Serial nuclear magnetic resonance imaging of acute myocardial infarction with and without reperfusion. *Am Heart J* 1988;115:510–518.

58. Masui T, Saeed M, Wendland MF, et al. Occlusive and reperfused myocardial infarcts: MR imaging differentiation with nonionic Gd-DTPA-BMA. *Radiology* 1991;181:77–83.

59. Saeed M, Wendland MF, Takehara Y, et al. Reperfusion and irreversible myocardial injury: identification with a nonionic MR imaging contrast medium. *Radiology* 1992;182:675–683.

60. Atkinson DJ, Burstein D, Edelman RR. First-pass cardiac perfusion: evaluation with ultrafast MR imaging. *Radiology* 1990;174:757–762.

61. Manning WJ, Atkinson DJ, Grossman W, et al. First-pass nuclear magnetic resonance imaging studies using gadolinium-DTPA in patients with coronary artery disease. *J Am Coll Cardiol* 1991;18:959–965.

62. Judd RM, Lugo-Olivieri CH, Arai M, et al. Physiological basis of myocardial contrast enhancement in fast magnetic resonance images of 2-day-old reperfused canine infarcts. *Circulation* 1995;92:1902–1910.

63. Kim RJ, Chen EL, Lima JA, et al. Myocardial Gd-DTPA kinetics determine MRI contrast enhancement and reflect the extent and severity of myocardial injury after acute reperfused infarction. *Circulation* 1996;94:3318–3326.

64. Saeed M, Wendland MF, Yu KK, et al. Identification of myocardial reperfusion with echo planar magnetic resonance imaging. Discrimination between occlusive and reperfused infarctions. *Circulation* 1994;90:1492–1501.

65. Lima JA, Judd RM, Bazille A, et al. Regional heterogeneity of human myocardial infarcts demonstrated by contrast-enhanced MRI. Potential mechanisms. *Circulation* 1995;92: 1117–1125.

66. Judd RM, Reeder SB, Atalar E, et al. A magnetization-driven gradient echo pulse sequence for the study of myocardial perfusion. *Magn Reson Med* 1995;34:276–282.

67. Wu KC, Zerhouni EA, Judd RM, et al. Prognostic significance of microvascular obstruction by magnetic resonance imaging in patients with acute myocardial infarction. *Circulation* 1998;97:765–772.

68. Rochitte CE, Lima JA, Bluemke DA, et al. Magnitude and time course of microvascular obstruction and tissue injury after acute myocardial infarction. *Circulation* 1998;98: 1006–1014.

69. Gerber BL, Rochitte CE, Melin JA, et al. Microvascular obstruction and left ventricular remodeling early after acute myocardial infarction. *Circulation* 2000;101:2734–2741.

70. Nishimura T, Yamada Y, Hayashi M, et al. Determination of infarct size of acute myocardial infarction in dogs by magnetic resonance imaging and gadolinium-DTPA: comparison with indium-111 antimyosin imaging. *Am J Physiol Imaging* 1989;4:83–88.

71. Schaefer S, Malloy CR, Katz J, et al. Gadolinium-DTPA-enhanced nuclear magnetic resonance imaging of reperfused myocardium: identification of the myocardial bed at risk. *J Am Coll Cardiol* 1988;12:1064–1072.

72. Saeed M, Bremerich J, Wendland MF, et al. Reperfused myocardial infarction as seen with use of necrosis-specific versus standard extracellular MR contrast media in rats. *Radiology* 1999;213:247–257.

73. Saeed M, Lund G, Wendland MF, et al. Magnetic resonance characterization of the peri-infarction zone of reperfused myocardial infarction with necrosis-specific and extracellular nonspecific contrast media. *Circulation* 2001;103:871–876.

74. Lund GK, Higgins CB, Wendland MF, et al. Assessment of nicorandil therapy in ischemic myocardial injury by using contrast-enhanced and functional MR imaging. *Radiology* 2001;221:676–682.

75. Simonetti O, Kim RJ, Fieno DS, et al. An improved MR imaging technique for the visualization of myocardial infarction. *Radiology* 2001;218:215–223.

76. Kim RJ, Shah DJ, Judd RM. How we perform delayed enhancement imaging. *J Cardiovasc Magn Reson* 2003;5: 505–514.

77. Rehwald WG, Fieno DS, Chen EL, et al. Myocardial magnetic resonance imaging contrast agent concentrations after reversible and irreversible ischemic injury. *Circulation* 2002; 105:224–229.

78. Diesbourg LD, Prato FS, Wisenberg G, et al. Quantification of myocardial blood flow and extracellular volumes using a bolus injection of Gd-DTPA: kinetic modeling in canine ischemic disease. *Magn Reson Med* 1992;23:239–253.

79. Fieno DS, Kim RJ, Chen EL, et al. Contrast-enhanced magnetic resonance imaging of myocardium at risk: distinction between reversible and irreversible injury throughout infarct healing. *J Am Coll Cardiol* 2000;36:1985–1991.

80. Amado LC, Gerber BL, Gupta SN, et al. Accurate and objective infarct sizing by contrast-enhanced magnetic resonance imaging in a canine myocardial infarction model. *J Am Coll Cardiol* 2004;44:2383–2389.

81. Kim RJ, Fieno DS, Parrish TB, et al. Relationship of MRI delayed contrast enhancement to irreversible injury, infarct age, and contractile function. *Circulation* 1999;100: 1992–2002.

82. Oshinski JN, Yang Z, Jones JR, et al. Imaging time after Gd-DTPA injection is critical in using delayed enhancement to determine infarct size accurately with magnetic resonance imaging. *Circulation* 2001;104:2838–2842.

83. Ni Y, Pislaru C, Bosmans H, et al. Intracoronary delivery of Gd-DTPA and Gadophrin-2 for determination of myocardial viability with MR imaging. *Eur Radiol* 2001;11:876–883.

84. Flacke S, Allen JS, Chia JM, et al. Characterization of viable and nonviable myocardium at MR imaging: comparison of gadolinium-based extracellular and blood pool contrast materials versus manganese-based contrast materials in a rat myocardial infarction model. *Radiology* 2003;226:731–738.

85. Mahrholdt H, Wagner A, Holly TA, et al. Reproducibility of chronic infarct size measurement by contrast-enhanced magnetic resonance imaging. *Circulation* 2002;106:2322–2327.

86. Eichstaedt HW, Felix R, Dougherty FC, et al. Magnetic resonance imaging (MRI) in different stages of myocardial infarction using the contrast agent gadolinium-DTPA. *Clin Cardiol* 1986;9:527–535.

87. Nishimura T, Kobayashi H, Ohara Y, et al. Serial assessment of myocardial infarction by using gated MR imaging and Gd-DTPA. *AJR Am J Roentgenol* 1989;153:715–720.

88. van Dijkman PR, van der Wall EE, de Roos A, et al. Acute, subacute, and chronic myocardial infarction: quantitative analysis of gadolinium-enhanced MR images. *Radiology* 1991;180:147–151.

89. Saeed M, Wendland MF, Masui T, et al. Myocardial infarction: assessment with an intravascular MR contrast medium. Work in progress. *Radiology* 1991;180:153–160.

90. Fedele F, Montesano T, Ferro-Luzzi M, et al. Identification of viable myocardium in patients with chronic coronary artery disease and left ventricular dysfunction: role of magnetic resonance imaging. *Am Heart J* 1994;128:484–489.

91. Pereira RS, Prato FS, Sykes J, et al. Assessment of myocardial viability using MRI during a constant infusion of Gd-DTPA: further studies at early and late periods of reperfusion. *Magn Reson Med* 1999;42:60–68.

92. Ramani K, Judd RM, Holly TA, et al. Contrast magnetic resonance imaging in the assessment of myocardial viability in patients with stable coronary artery disease and left ventricular dysfunction. *Circulation* 1998;98:2687–2694.

93. Fieno DS, Hillenbrand HB, Rehwald WG, et al. Infarct resorption, compensatory hypertrophy, and differing patterns of ventricular remodeling following myocardial infarctions of varying size. *J Am Coll Cardiol* 2004;43:2124–2131.

94. Yokota C, Nonogi H, Miyazaki S, et al. Gadolinium-enhanced magnetic resonance imaging in acute myocardial infarction. *Am J Cardiol* 1995;75:577–581.

95. Dendale P, Franken PR, Block P, et al. Contrast enhanced and functional magnetic resonance imaging for the detection of viable myocardium after infarction. *Am Heart J* 1998;135: 875–880.

96. Van Rossum AC, Visser FC, Van Eenige MJ, et al. Value of gadolinium-diethylene-triamine pentaacetic acid dynamics in magnetic resonance imaging of acute myocardial infarction with occluded and reperfused coronary arteries after thrombolysis. *Am J Cardiol* 1990;65:845–851.

97. Reimer KA, Lowe JE, Rasmussen MM, et al. The wavefront phenomenon of ischemic cell death. 1. Myocardial infarct size vs duration of coronary occlusion in dogs. *Circulation* 1977;56:786–794.

98. Hillenbrand HB, Kim RJ, Parker MA, et al. Early assessment of myocardial salvage by contrast-enhanced magnetic resonance imaging. *Circulation* 2000;102:1678–1683.

99. Choi KM, Kim RJ, Gubernikoff G, et al. Transmural extent of acute myocardial infarction predicts long-term improvement in contractile function. *Circulation* 2001;104:1101–1107.

100. Gerber BL, Garot J, Bluemke DA, et al. Accuracy of contrast-enhanced magnetic resonance imaging in predicting improvement of regional myocardial function in patients after acute myocardial infarction. *Circulation* 2002;106:1083–1089.

101. Beek AM, Kuhl HP, Bondarenko O, et al. Delayed contrast-enhanced magnetic resonance imaging for the prediction of regional functional improvement after acute myocardial infarction. *J Am Coll Cardiol* 2003;42:895–901.

102. Mahrholdt H, Wagner A, Parker M, et al. Relationship of contractile function to transmural extent of infarction in patients with chronic coronary artery disease. *J Am Coll Cardiol* 2003;42:505–512.

103. Ingkanisorn WP, Rhoads KL, Aletras AH, et al. Gadolinium delayed enhancement cardiovascular magnetic resonance correlates with clinical measures of myocardial infarction. *J Am Coll Cardiol* 2004;43:2253–2259.

104. Sandstede JJ, Lipke C, Beer M, et al. Analysis of first-pass and delayed contrast-enhancement patterns of dysfunctional myocardium on MR imaging: use in the prediction of myocardial viability. *AJR Am J Roentgenol* 2000;174:1737–1740.

105. Schvartzman PR, Srichai MB, Grimm RA, et al. Nonstress delayed-enhancement magnetic resonance imaging of the myocardium predicts improvement of function after revascularization for chronic ischemic heart disease with left ventricular dysfunction. *Am Heart J* 2003;146:535–541.

106. Knuesel PR, Nanz D, Wyss C, et al. Characterization of dysfunctional myocardium by positron emission tomography and magnetic resonance: relation to functional outcome after revascularization. *Circulation* 2003;108:1095–1100.

107. Selvanayagam JB, Kardos A, Francis JM, et al. Value of delayed-enhancement cardiovascular magnetic resonance imaging in predicting myocardial viability after surgical revascularization. *Circulation* 2004;110:1535–1541.
108. Wellnhofer E, Olariu A, Klein C, et al. Magnetic resonance low-dose dobutamine test is superior to SCAR quantification for the prediction of functional recovery. *Circulation* 2004;109:2172–2174.
109. Ricciardi MJ, Wu E, Davidson CJ, et al. Visualization of discrete microinfarction after percutaneous coronary intervention associated with mild creatine kinase-MB elevation. *Circulation* 2001;103:2780–2783.
110. Steuer J, Bjerner T, Duvernoy O, et al. Visualisation and quantification of peri-operative myocardial infarction after coronary artery bypass surgery with contrast-enhanced magnetic resonance imaging. *Eur Heart J* 2004;25:1293–1299.
111. Wu E, Judd RM, Vargas JD, et al. Visualisation of presence, location, and transmural extent of healed Q-wave and non-Q-wave myocardial infarction. *Lancet* 2001;357:21–28.
112. Moon JC, De Arenaza DP, Elkington AG, et al. The pathologic basis of Q-wave and non-Q-wave myocardial infarction: a cardiovascular magnetic resonance study. *J Am Coll Cardiol* 2004;44:554–560.
113. Kaandorp TA, Bax JJ, Schuijf JD, et al. Head-to-head comparison between contrast-enhanced magnetic resonance imaging and dobutamine magnetic resonance imaging in men with ischemic cardiomyopathy. *Am J Cardiol* 2004;93:1461–1464.
114. Wagner A, Mahrholdt H, Holly TA, et al. Contrast-enhanced MRI and routine single photon emission computed tomography (SPECT) perfusion imaging for detection of subendocardial myocardial infarcts: an imaging study. *Lancet* 2003;361:374–379.
115. Lee VS, Resnick D, Tiu SS, et al. MR imaging evaluation of myocardial viability in the setting of equivocal SPECT results with (99m)Tc sestamibi. *Radiology* 2004;230:191–197.
116. Ansari M, Araoz PA, Gerard SK, et al. Comparison of late enhancement cardiovascular magnetic resonance and thallium SPECT in patients with coronary disease and left ventricular dysfunction. *J Cardiovasc Magn Reson* 2004;6:549–556.
117. Lund GK, Stork A, Saeed M, et al. Acute myocardial infarction: evaluation with first-pass enhancement and delayed enhancement MR imaging compared with 201Tl SPECT imaging. *Radiology* 2004;232:49–57.
118. Kitagawa K, Sakuma H, Hirano T, et al. Acute myocardial infarction: myocardial viability assessment in patients early thereafter comparison of contrast-enhanced MR imaging with resting (201)Tl SPECT. Single photon emission computed tomography. *Radiology* 2003;226:138–144.
119. Klein C, Nekolla SG, Bengel FM, et al. Assessment of myocardial viability with contrast-enhanced magnetic resonance imaging: comparison with positron emission tomography. Circulation 2002;105:162–167.
120. Kuhl HP, Beek AM, van der Weerdt AP, et al. Myocardial viability in chronic ischemic heart disease: comparison of contrast-enhanced magnetic resonance imaging with (18)F-fluorodeoxyglucose positron emission tomography. *J Am Coll Cardiol* 2003;41:1341–1348.
121. Kwong RY, Schussheim AE, Rekhraj S, et al. Detecting acute coronary syndrome in the emergency department with cardiac magnetic resonance imaging. *Circulation* 2003;107:531–537.
122. Chiu CW, So NM, Lam WW, et al. Combined first-pass perfusion and viability study at MR imaging in patients with non-ST segment-elevation acute coronary syndromes: feasibility study. *Radiology* 2003;226:717–722.
123. Plein S, Greenwood JP, Ridgway JP, et al. Assessment of non-ST-segment elevation acute coronary syndromes with cardiac magnetic resonance imaging. *J Am Coll Cardiol* 2004;44:2173–2181.
124. Plein S, Ridgway JP, Jones TR, et al. Coronary artery disease: assessment with a comprehensive MR imaging protocol—initial results. *Radiology* 2002;225:300–307.
125. Kloner RA, Ganote CE, Jennings RB. The "no-reflow" phenomenon after temporary coronary occlusion in the dog. *J Clin Invest* 1974;54:1496–1508.
126. Rogers WJ, Jr., Kramer CM, Geskin G, et al. Early contrast-enhanced MRI predicts late functional recovery after reperfused myocardial infarction. *Circulation* 1999;99:744–750.
127. Kramer CM, Rogers WJ, Mankad S, et al. Contractile reserve and contrast uptake pattern by magnetic resonance imaging and functional recovery after reperfused myocardial infarction. *J Am Coll Cardiol* 2000;36:1834–1840.
128. Gerber BL, Rochitte CE, Bluemke DA, et al. Relation between Gd-DTPA contrast enhancement and regional inotropic response in the periphery and center of myocardial infarction. Circulation 2001;104:998–1004.
129. Taylor AJ, Al-Saadi N, Abdel-Aty H, et al. Detection of acutely impaired microvascular reperfusion after infarct angioplasty with magnetic resonance imaging. *Circulation* 2004;109:2080–2085.
130. Ito H, Tomooka T, Sakai N, et al. Lack of myocardial perfusion immediately after successful thrombolysis. A predictor of poor recovery of left ventricular function in anterior myocardial infarction. *Circulation* 1992;85:1699–1705.
131. Arheden H, Saeed M, Higgins CB, et al. Reperfused rat myocardium subjected to various durations of ischemia: estimation of the distribution volume of contrast material with echo-planar MR imaging. *Radiology* 2000;215:520–528.
132. Kim RJ, Wu E, Rafael A, et al. The use of contrast-enhanced magnetic resonance imaging to identify reversible myocardial dysfunction. *N Engl J Med* 2000;343:1445–1453.
133. Saeed M, Wendland MF, Masui T, et al. Reperfused myocardial infarctions on T1- and susceptibility-enhanced MRI: evidence for loss of compartmentalization of contrast media. *Magn Reson Med* 1994;31:31–39.
134. Geschwind JF, Wendland MF, Saeed M, et al. AUR Memorial Award. Identification of myocardial cell death in reperfused myocardial injury using dual mechanisms of contrast-enhanced magnetic resonance imaging. *Acad Radiol* 1994;1:319–325.
135. Arheden H, Saeed M, Higgins CB, et al. Measurement of the distribution volume of gadopentetate dimeglumine at echo-planar MR imaging to quantify myocardial infarction: comparison with 99mTc-DTPA autoradiography in rats. *Radiology* 1999;211:698–708.
136. Pereira RS, Prato FS, Wisenberg G, et al. The determination of myocardial viability using Gd-DTPA in a canine model of acute myocardial ischemia and reperfusion. *Magn Reson Med* 1996;36:684–693.
137. Wendland MF, Saeed M, Arheden H, et al. Toward necrotic cell fraction measurement by contrast-enhanced MRI of reperfused ischemically injured myocardium. *Acad Radiol* 1998;5(Suppl 1):S42–44.
138. Wendland MF, Saeed M, Lauerma K, et al. Alterations in T1 of normal and reperfused infarcted myocardium after Gd-BOPTA versus GD-DTPA on inversion recovery EPI. *Magn Reson Med* 1997;37:448–456.
139. Thornhill RE, Prato FS, Pereira RS, et al. Examining a canine model of stunned myocardium with Gd-DTPA-enhanced MRI. *Magn Reson Med* 2001;45:864–871.
140. Thornhill RE, Prato FS, Wisenberg G, et al. Determining the extent to which delayed-enhancement images reflect the partition-coefficient of Gd-DTPA in canine studies of reper-

fused and unreperfused myocardial infarction. *Magn Reson Med* 2004;52:1069–1079.

141. Jugdutt BI, Amy RW. Healing after myocardial infarction in the dog: changes in infarct hydroxyproline and topography. *J Am Coll Cardiol* 1986;7:91–102.

142. Weber KT. Cardiac interstitium in health and disease: the fibrillar collagen network. *J Am Coll Cardiol* 1989;13:1637–1652.

143. Flacke SJ, Fischer SE, Lorenz CH. Measurement of the gadopentetate dimeglumine partition coefficient in human myocardium in vivo: normal distribution and elevation in acute and chronic infarction. *Radiology* 2001;218:703–710.

144. Weissleder R, Lee AS, Khaw BA, et al. Antimyosin-labeled monocrystalline iron oxide allows detection of myocardial infarct: MR antibody imaging. *Radiology* 1992;182:381–385.

145. Adzamli IK, Blau M, Pfeffer MA, et al. Phosphonate-modified Gd-DTPA complexes. III: The detection of myocardial infarction by MRI. *Magn Reson Med* 1993;29:505–511.

146. Hindre F, Le Plouzennec M, de Certaines JD, et al. Tetra-p-aminophenylporphyrin conjugated with Gd-DTPA: tumor-specific contrast agent for MR imaging. *J Magn Reson Imaging* 1993;3:59–65.

147. Nelson JA, Schmiedl U, Shankland EG. Metalloporphyrins as tumor-seeking MRI contrast media and as potential selective treatment sensitizers. *Invest Radiol* 1990;25(Suppl. 1):S71–73.

148. Ni Y, Marchal G, Yu J, et al. Localization of metalloporphyrin-induced "specific" enhancement in experimental liver tumors: comparison of magnetic resonance imaging, micro-angiographic, and histologic findings. *Acad Radiol* 1995;2:687–699.

149. Ni Y, Petre C, Miao Y, et al. Magnetic resonance imaging-histomorphologic correlation studies on paramagnetic metalloporphyrins in rat models of necrosis. *Invest Radiol* 1997;32:770–779.

150. Ni Y, Marchal G, Herijgers P, et al. Paramagnetic metalloporphyrins: from enhancers of malignant tumors to markers of myocardial infarcts. *Acad Radiol* 1996;3(Suppl. 2):S395–397.

151. Herijgers P, Laycock SK, Ni Y, et al. Localization and determination of infarct size by Gd-Mesoporphyrin enhanced MRI in dogs. *Int J Card Imaging* 1997;13:499–507.

152. Pislaru SV, Ni Y, Pislaru C, et al. Noninvasive measurements of infarct size after thrombolysis with a necrosis-avid MRI contrast agent. *Circulation* 1999;99:690–696.

153. Choi SI, Choi SH, Kim ST, et al. Irreversibly damaged myocardium at MR imaging with a necrotic tissue-specific contrast agent in a cat model. *Radiology* 2000;215:863–868.

154. Marchal G, Ni Y, Herijgers P, et al. Paramagnetic metalloporphyrins: infarct avid contrast agents for diagnosis of acute myocardial infarction by MRI. *Eur Radiol* 1996;6:2–8.

155. Choi SH, Lee SS, Choi SI, et al. Occlusive myocardial infarction: investigation of bis-gadolinium mesoporphyrins-enhanced T1-weighted MR imaging in a cat model. *Radiology* 2001;220:436–440.

156. Barkhausen J, Ebert W, Debatin JF, et al. Imaging of myocardial infarction: comparison of magnevist and gadophrin-3 in rabbits. *J Am Coll Cardiol* 2002;39:1392–1398.

157. Watzinger N, Lund GK, Higgins CB, et al. The potential of contrast-enhanced magnetic resonance imaging for predicting left ventricular remodeling. *J Magn Reson Imaging* 2002;16:633–640.

158. Jeong AK, Choi SI, Kim DH, et al. Evaluation by contrast-enhanced MR imaging of the lateral border zone in reperfused myocardial infarction in a cat model. *Korean J Radiol* 2001;2:21–27.

159. Lee SS, Goo HW, Park SB, et al. MR imaging of reperfused myocardial infarction: comparison of necrosis-specific and intravascular contrast agents in a cat model. *Radiology* 2003;226:739–747.

160. Saeed M, Wagner S, Wendland MF, et al. Occlusive and reperfused myocardial infarcts: differentiation with Mn-DPDP-enhanced MR imaging. *Radiology* 1989;172:59–64.

161. Pomeroy OH, Wendland M, Wagner S, et al. Magnetic resonance imaging of acute myocardial ischemia using a manganese chelate, Mn-DPDP. *Invest Radiol* 1989;24:531–536.

162. Saeed M, Wendland MF, Takehara Y, et al. Reversible and irreversible injury in the reperfused myocardium: differentiation with contrast material-enhanced MR imaging. *Radiology* 1990;175:633–637.

163. Gallez B, Bacic G, Swartz HM. Evidence for the dissociation of the hepatobiliary MRI contrast agent Mn-DPDP. *Magn Reson Med* 1996;35:14–19.

164. Chauncey DM, Jr., Schelbert HR, Halpern SE, et al. Tissue distribution studies with radioactive manganese: a potential agent for myocardial imaging. *J Nucl Med* 1977;18:933–936.

165. Hunter DR, Haworth RA, Berkoff HA. Cellular manganese uptake by the isolated perfused rat heart: a probe for the sarcolemma calcium channel. *J Mol Cell Cardiol* 1981;13:823–832.

166. Brurok H, Schjott J, Berg K, et al. Effects of MnDPDP, DPDP—, and MnCl2 on cardiac energy metabolism and manganese accumulation. An experimental study in the isolated perfused rat heart. *Invest Radiol* 1997;32:205–211.

167. Wendland MF. Applications of manganese-enhanced magnetic resonance imaging (MEMRI) to imaging of the heart. *NMR Biomed* 2004;17:581–594.

168. Bremerich J, Saeed M, Arheden H, et al. Normal and infarcted myocardium: differentiation with cellular uptake of manganese at MR imaging in a rat model. *Radiology* 2000;216:524–530.

169. Wendland MF, Krombach GA, Higgins CB, et al. Contrast enhanced MRI of stunned myocardium using Mn-based MRI contrast media. *Acad Radiol* 2002;9:S341–342.

170. Krombach GA, Saeed M, Higgins CB, et al. Contrast-enhanced MR delineation of stunned myocardium with administration of MnCl(2) in rats. *Radiology* 2004;230:183–190.

171. Pike MM, Kitakaze M, Marban E. 23Na-NMR measurements of intracellular sodium in intact perfused ferret hearts during ischemia and reperfusion. *Am J Physiol* 1990;259:H1767–1773.

172. Cannon PJ, Maudsley AA, Hilal SK, et al. Sodium nuclear magnetic resonance imaging of myocardial tissue of dogs after coronary artery occlusion and reperfusion. *J Am Coll Cardiol* 1986;7:573–579.

173. Kim RJ, Lima JA, Chen EL, et al. Fast 23Na magnetic resonance imaging of acute reperfused myocardial infarction. Potential to assess myocardial viability. *Circulation* 1997;95:1877–1885.

174. Horn M, Weidensteiner C, Scheffer H, et al. Detection of myocardial viability based on measurement of sodium content: A (23)Na-NMR study. *Magn Reson Med* 2001;45:756–764.

175. Rochitte CE, Kim RJ, Hillenbrand HB, et al. Microvascular integrity and the time course of myocardial sodium accumulation after acute infarction. *Circ Res* 2000;87:648–655.

176. Weidensteiner C, Horn M, Fekete E, et al. Imaging of intracellular sodium with shift reagent aided (23)Na CSI in isolated rat hearts. *Magn Reson Med* 2002;48:89–96.

177. Jansen MA, Van Emous JG, Nederhoff MG, et al. Assessment of myocardial viability by intracellular 23Na magnetic resonance imaging. *Circulation* 2004;110:3457–3464.

178. Parrish TB, Fieno DS, Fitzgerald SW, et al. Theoretical basis for sodium and potassium MRI of the human heart at 1.5 T. *Magn Reson Med* 1997;38:653–661.

179. Sandstede JJ, Pabst T, Beer M, et al. Assessment of myocardial infarction in humans with (23)Na MR imaging: comparison with cine MR imaging and delayed contrast enhancement. *Radiology* 2001;221:222–228.

180. Sandstede JJ, Hillenbrand H, Beer M, et al. Time course of 23Na signal intensity after myocardial infarction in humans. *Magn Reson Med* 2004;52:545–551.

181. Kraitchman DL, Heldman AW, Atalar E, et al. In vivo magnetic resonance imaging of mesenchymal stem cells in myocardial infarction. *Circulation* 2003;107:2290–2293.

182. Wollert KC, Meyer GP, Lotz J, et al. Intracoronary autologous bone-marrow cell transfer after myocardial infarction: the BOOST randomised controlled clinical trial. *Lancet* 2004; 364:141–148.

183. Weber OM, Schalla S, Martin AJ, et al. Interventional cardiac magnetic resonance imaging. *Semin Roentgenol* 2003;38: 352–357.

184. Fayad ZA, Fuster V, Nikolaou K, et al. Computed tomography and magnetic resonance imaging for noninvasive coronary angiography and plaque imaging: current and potential future concepts. *Circulation* 2002;106:2026–2034.

185. Fayad ZA. MR imaging for the noninvasive assessment of atherothrombotic plaques. *Magn Reson Imaging Clin N Am* 2003;11:101–113.

18

Coronary Magnetic Resonance Angiography: Technical Approaches

Oliver Weber and Matthias Stuber

Coronary artery disease is one of the major causes of morbidity and mortality in the Western world. The current gold standard for the diagnosis of coronary disease is selective x-ray coronary angiography. In the United States (1) and Europe, more than 1,000,000 of these diagnostic procedures are performed each year. X-ray coronary angiography is used to define coronary anatomy and guide patient therapy. However, x-ray coronary angiography is expensive and invasive, exposes both patient and operator to potentially harmful ionizing radiation, and carries a small risk for serious complications. Furthermore, a significant minority of patients undergoing x-ray angiography are found not to have significant disease (2) but remain exposed to the costs and risks of this invasive procedure. Thus, a more cost-effective, noninvasive approach for defining luminographic disease is urgently needed.

Multidetector computed tomography (MDCT) has recently gained great popularity for coronary angiography. Three-dimensional (3D) data sets can be obtained during intravenous injection of contrast media in a single breath-hold. The diagnostic accuracy for the detection of significant stenoses is promising (3), but MDCT also exposes the patients to ionizing radiation and considerable volumes of iodinated contrast agents. Furthermore, coronary MDCT yields unsatisfactory image quality in a considerable number of patients. Artifacts render the images nondiagnostic for as many as 25% of all coronary segments investigated (3). Major problems are associated with cardiac, respiratory, or patient motion, as well as with beam-hardening effects caused by metallic implants or severe calcifications (4).

Coronary magnetic resonance angiography (MRA) combines several advantages and great potential. It is noninvasive and can survey the heart in arbitrary image planes, and it does not involve the use of possibly harmful ionizing radiation or iodinated contrast media. In addition to providing a high degree of spatial resolution, magnetic resonance (MR) is not associated with any known short- or long-term side effects. The utility of MRA for visualizing the coronary anatomy has been investigated since the late 1980s (5,6). Although no coronary stenoses were identified in these early studies, demonstrations of the potential of magnetic resonance imaging (MRI) to assess the anatomy of the coronary vessels triggered intense and ongoing interest in the field.

Successful coronary MRA data acquisition is technically demanding because of the small caliber and tortuosity of the coronary arteries and the presence of signal from surrounding epicardial fat and myocardium. In addition, cardiac and respiratory motion affects the position of the coronary arteries by a multiple of their diameter. Efficient strategies to suppress motion must therefore be applied. Furthermore, enhancement of the contrast between the coronary vessel lumen and the surrounding tissue (myocardium, epicardial fat) is mandatory for a successful visualization of the coronary anatomy.

The general approaches described in this chapter are available on current state-of-the-art cardiac MR units from all vendor platforms, but some nuances may be vendor-specific (e.g., navigator implementation). Established and advanced coronary MRA methods are reviewed. Specific strategies for motion suppression and contrast enhancement are discussed, and representative image material is displayed.

TECHNICAL CONSIDERATIONS

The bulk of research studies and methods development in coronary MRA has been conducted on 1.5 Tesla (T) whole-body systems. However, high-quality coronary MRA data have also been obtained at a lower field strength on 0.5 T systems (7–9), as well as more recently on high-field 3.0 T systems (10,11).

SUPPRESSION OF MOTION ARTIFACTS

The heart is subject to intrinsic and extrinsic motion. Intrinsic myocardial motion is the rhythmic contraction and relaxation during the R-R interval. Extrinsic myocardial motion is bulk motion of the heart induced by respiration. Both extrinsic and intrinsic myocardial motion may greatly exceed the coronary artery diameter and so cause blurring and ghosting of the coronary vessels on images. Therefore, strategies that minimize the adverse effects of both motion components are needed.

Suppression of Intrinsic Myocardial Motion

For submillimeter coronary MRA, the image data cannot be collected during a single R-R interval. Therefore, the coronary MRA data acquisition must be synchronized with the cardiac cycle, and k-space segmentation must be applied (Fig. 18.1). For segmented k-space techniques, an accurate electrocardiographic (ECG) synchronization is mandatory. Less robust peripheral pulse detection methods yield inferior results. Even though ECG triggering is superior to peripheral pulse detection, reliable R-wave detection in the presence of a strong static magnetic field (causing the "hydrodynamic effect") and switching magnetic field gradients is technically challenging. A four-lead vector ECG approach has been shown to provide more robust ECG triggering than three-lead recording (12), especially at higher magnetic field strengths.

During the cardiac cycle, the coronary arteries can move more than 1 cm, a multiple of their own diameter (Fig. 18.2). The displacement of the right coronary artery (RCA) is larger than that of the left anterior descending (LAD) or the left circumflex (LCX) artery. The coronary arteries are relatively quiescent for short periods after completion of ventricular systole and, for a longer period, at middiastole (13,14). To

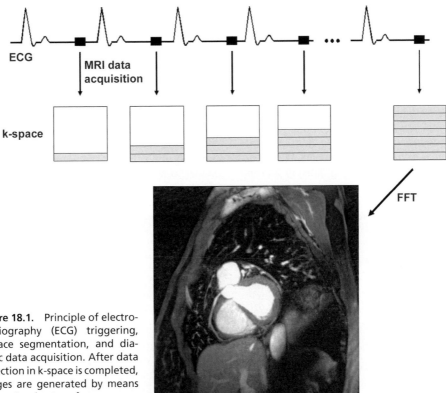

Figure 18.1. Principle of electro-cardiography (ECG) triggering, k-space segmentation, and diastolic data acquisition. After data collection in k-space is completed, images are generated by means of fast Fourier transform.

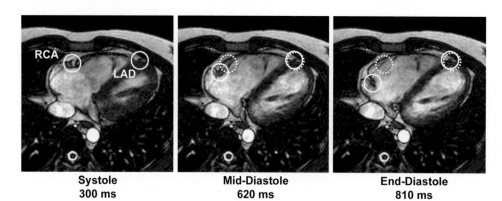

Systole
300 ms

Mid-Diastole
620 ms

End-Diastole
810 ms

Figure 18.2. Three frames (of 40 frames covering the R-R interval) of an axial steady state free precession (SSFP) cine magnetic resonance imaging (MRI) illustrate motion of right coronary artery (RCA) and left anterior descending (LAD) coronary artery. The RCA undergoes more pronounced motion than the LAD. In middiastole, both vessels are quiescent for a short interval (in this subject, ~160 ms). For optimal coronary magnetic resonance angiography (MRA), an acquisition window during minimal motion should be chosen (i.e., trigger delay of 620 ms in this subject). Position at systole (*dashed circles*).

minimize motion artifacts in the images, the coronary MRA data should be acquired during a period of minimal myocardial motion. Middiastole offers a longer acquisition opportunity and represents a period of rapid coronary blood flow resulting in inflow of unsaturated spins, a major mechanism of contrast in many bright-blood (gradient-echo) sequences. Both duration and time point after R-wave of the quiescent phases are strongly subject-specific (14). For optimal results, subject-specific trigger delays and optimal acquisition windows may thus have to be defined by visual inspection of cine images or more advanced automated approaches (15).

Suppression of Extrinsic Myocardial Motion

Breath-hold Techniques

Among the major difficulties encountered in coronary MRA is the bulk cardiac motion associated with respiration (Fig. 18.3). Early compensation of respiratory motion consisted of breath-holding (16). Two-dimensional (2D) breath-hold coronary MRA relied on the acquisition of contiguous parallel images, with the goal of surveying the proximal segments of the coronary arteries during serial breath-holds (17). More recently, 3D breath-hold techniques for coronary MRA were also implemented (18–20) and showed promising prelimi-

nary results (21). Breath-hold approaches offer the advantage of rapid imaging and are technically easy to implement in compliant patients.

However, breath-hold strategies have several practical limitations. Major patient and operator involvement is required for serial breath-holds. Patients with cardiac or pulmonary disease frequently have difficulty sustaining adequate breath-holds, particularly when the duration exceeds 5 to 10 s. For sufficient anatomic coverage, a considerable number of serial breath-holds are often needed. Alternative breath-holding techniques, including serial brief breath-holds (22) and coached breath-holding with visual or audible feedback (23–25), have been used to minimize respiratory motion artifacts and patient inconvenience, but these are practical only for highly motivated subjects. Even with cooperative patients, breath-holding may be problematic. With a sustained breath-hold, cranial diaphragmatic drift, which is often substantial (~1 cm), may occur (16,26–28). During serial breath-holds, the diaphragmatic and cardiac positions frequently vary by up to 1 cm, so that image registration errors result (29). Misregistration causes apparent gaps between the segments of the visualized coronary arteries, which can be misinterpreted as signal voids from coronary stenoses. Finally, breath-holds of reasonable duration (15 s) severely limit the options for improving spatial resolution, signal-to-noise ratio (SNR), and volume coverage.

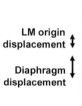

LM origin
displacement

Diaphragm
displacement

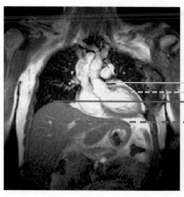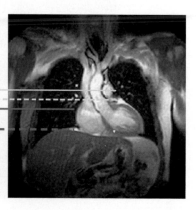

Figure 18.3. End-expiratory (*left*) and end-inspiratory (*right*) coronal single-shot SSFP images, from a series of images acquired during free breathing. Images demonstrate the extent of craniocaudal diaphragm motion (*dark gray lines*) and associated motion of the left main coronary origin (*light gray lines*). Positions in expiration (*solid lines*); positions in inspiration (*dashed lines*).

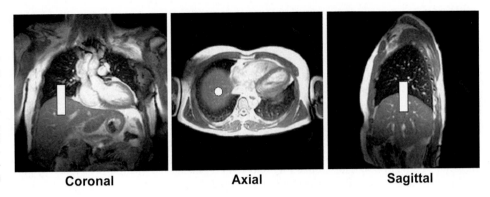

Figure 18.4. Free-breathing, single-shot scout images in three orthogonal planes show navigator placement on the right hemidiaphragm. For optimal detection of the lung–liver interface, the navigator should be placed through the top of the right hemidiaphragm dome, its length covering the full range of diaphragm motion.

Coronal   **Axial**   **Sagittal**

Signal Averaging and Respiratory Belts

Initial free-breathing coronary MRA approaches used signal averaging to minimize motion artifacts (30,31). This averaging approach is reasonable for relatively low (>1–2 mm) spatial resolutions, but inadequate for reliable detection of stenoses. As an alternative early free-breathing approach, thoracic respiratory belts were used to monitor chest wall expansion and thereby gate image acquisition to the end-expiratory position. Results were promising in comparison with breath-holding (28,32). Enhancements included respiratory feedback monitoring (25). However, respiratory belt gating is often not reliable, and a time delay between chest wall expansion and diaphragmatic motion may occur, introducing motion artifacts to the images. Subsequently, more accurate and flexible MR navigators have replaced belt gating.

Free-breathing Navigator Approaches

The use of free breathing with respiratory navigators, first proposed by Ehman and Felmlee (32), serves to overcome the time constraints and cooperation imposed by breath-hold approaches. Free-breathing navigator methods are particularly well suited for prolonged 3D coronary MRA approaches, which combine the benefits of thin, adjacent slices with the submillimeter spatial resolution afforded by an improved SNR. The use of navigator gating has received considerable attention, and implementations vary from rela-

tively simple retrospective gating based on a single right-diaphragm navigator (33) to complex prospective affine motion correction based on multiple navigator signals (34). In principle, the MR navigator monitors the motion of an interface such as the lung-diaphragm interface (Fig. 18.4) or the lung-myocardium interface. Data are accepted only when the selected interface falls within a user-defined window (usually 3–7 mm) positioned around the end-expiratory level of the interface (Fig. 18.5). Although the need for patient cooperation and operator involvement is reduced with navigator/free-breathing methods, diaphragmatic drift and patient motion remain relevant issues (28,35). They may be taken into account by manual or automated adjustment of the position of the acceptance window.

Navigator Localization and Geometry

Navigators can be positioned at any interface that accurately reflects respiratory motion, including the dome of the right hemidiaphragm (24,31,36), the left hemidiaphragm, and the anterior chest wall, or directly through the anterior free wall of the left ventricle (28,37). Navigators have been implemented as two intersecting planes (38,39) and as 2D selective pencil beam excitations (40). Although the intersecting planes are easier to implement, they may compromise magnetization in the volume of interest. In contrast, 2D selective pencil beam excitations can be implemented with the use of shallow radio frequency (RF) excitation angles, so that they only minimally affect the magnetization in the region of

Figure 18.5. Free-breathing navigator display, as visualized in real-time on the scanner console. The x-axis represents time; the y-axis shows the magnetic resonance (MR) signal of the navigator pencil beam. During a preparation phase, the end-expiratory position of the lung–liver interface is determined. A 5-mm gating window is then automatically calculated, and subsequent acquisitions are only accepted if the detected interface position is within this window. Typical navigator efficiency is approximately 50% for a 5-mm gating window.

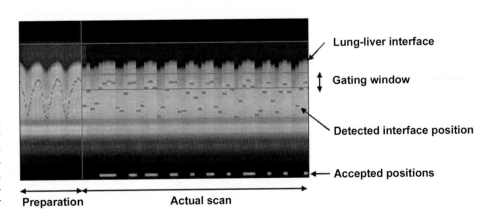

→ **Lung-liver interface**

↕ **Gating window**

→ **Detected interface position**

← **Accepted positions**

← **Preparation** →   ← **Actual scan** →

interest. Studies suggest that cardiac motion related to respiration is predominantly in the superior-inferior axis (41,42) and that most single-navigator locations yield similar image quality (28,37). The right hemidiaphragm is therefore the preferred location for the navigator because of the relative ease of identifying the interface from a series of coronal, sagittal, and transverse scout images (Fig. 18.4).

Navigator Gating. The gating process can be retrospective or prospective. In retrospective gating, actual MRA data are recorded with the respiratory position they are acquired in. After completion of data acquisition, only data segments acquired in a narrow acceptance window are used for the reconstruction of the MRA images. To ensure availability of all data segments at an acceptable respiratory position, k-space must be oversampled several times. In prospective gating, data segments are stored only if they are acquired in an acceptable respiratory position. Otherwise, the pulse sequence is played out (to maintain steady state), but data are not recorded. Exactly one copy of each data segment is thus acquired at an acceptable position, making this approach more efficient than retrospective gating. With navigator gating (without tracking), a 3-mm end-expiratory diaphragmatic window is typically used, and data are collected on average from one third of R-R intervals (33% navigator efficiency) (28).

Navigator Gating and Tracking. From several MR studies, it was noted that the dominant impact of respiration on cardiac position is in the superior-inferior direction (41,42). The correction factor between diaphragm displacement and craniocaudal displacement of the RCA and left coronary artery (LCA) was early on reported to be approximately 0.6 and 0.7, respectively (41). Newer results suggest that the actual factors might be smaller and show considerable intersubject variability and that motion along the other two axes might not be negligible (42). Nevertheless, a great number of successful studies were performed with a factor of 0.6 in craniocaudal direction only. Knowledge of this relationship offers the opportunity for prospective navigator gating with real-time tracking of the imaged volume position (36). This facilitates the use of wider gating windows and shortens scan time through increased navigator efficiency. The correction of the imaged volume position is obtained by a prospective run-time adaptation of the frequency of the slice-selective RF excitation and/or of the demodulator phase and frequency. With real-time tracking, a 5-mm diaphragmatic gating window is often used with a navigator efficiency close to 50% (43). Coronary MRA with real-time navigator tracking has been shown to minimize registration errors (in comparison with breath-holding), and image quality is maintained or improved in both 2- and 3D approaches (28,37).

A more elaborate tracking algorithm was recently proposed (34) to account for not only craniocaudal translation but also translation in the other two directions, as well as rotation, scaling, and shear transformation (summarized as affine transformation). Transformation parameters are determined in a low-resolution dynamic scan during free breathing, with simultaneous recording of one to three navigator signals. During the high-resolution coronary scan, the imaged volume is then prospectively adapted to compensate motion. The affine motion model offers the potential to in-

crease the navigator acceptance window and thus to increase the scan efficiency.

Navigator Tracking Alone. Limitations of breath-hold techniques include diaphragmatic drift and inconsistent end-expiratory positions between serial breath-holds. To overcome these limitations, breath-hold coronary MRA has been combined with navigator tracking (44,45). With these techniques, coronary MRA data can be acquired in serial breath-holds, and adverse effects of diaphragmatic drift during or between serial breath-holds can be minimized. Breath-holding with tracking during acquisition of central k-lines and subsequent free-breathing with gating and tracking during acquisition of outer k-space data were also successfully combined to accelerate data acquisition or for use in combination with contrast media (46).

Advanced Navigator Techniques. Sophisticated navigator algorithms have been implemented to collect important k-space profiles more efficiently based on the navigator-detected interface position. Implementations of such k-space-reordered techniques include motion adaptive gating (47); the diminishing variant algorithm (48); phase ordering with automated window selection (49); and the zonal motion adaptive reordering technique (50).

Adaptive Averaging. Preliminary data for a novel respiratory suppressive approach that does not use ECG gating, breath-holds, or navigator gating have suggested that it may prove useful, particularly for patients with an irregular heart rhythm or irregular breathing pattern. With real-time imaging and adaptive averaging (51), cross correlation is used to identify automatically those real-time imaging frames in which a coronary vessel is present and to determine the location of the vessel within each frame. This information is then used for selective averaging of frames to increase the SNR and spatial resolution. The robustness of this technique in patients with coronary disease remains to be demonstrated.

Navigators, Prepulses, and Imaging Sequences. Most of the navigator concepts described can be freely combined with prepulses and 2- or 3D imaging sequences (Fig. 18.6). It has been found that navigator accuracy is improved by preceding it with a fat-saturation pulse because of reduced effect of the excitation sidebands. To provide optimal fat suppression during acquisition of the coronary MR data, a second fat-suppression pulse immediately preceding data acquisition is beneficial. Because the navigator data are intended to reflect the position of the heart during the subsequent acquisition period, a short delay between the navigator and the data acquisition block and rapid navigator analysis is crucial (52). Some prepulses preceding the navigator excitation, such as nonselective inversion or dual-inversion pulses, compromise navigator detection of the interface position. Countermeasures such as local reinversion of the magnetization after the inversion or dual-inversion prepulses (Nav-Restore) were developed and successfully applied (53).

CONTRAST ENHANCEMENT

The coronary arteries are surrounded by both epicardial fat and myocardium. For successful visualization of the coro-

Trigger delay

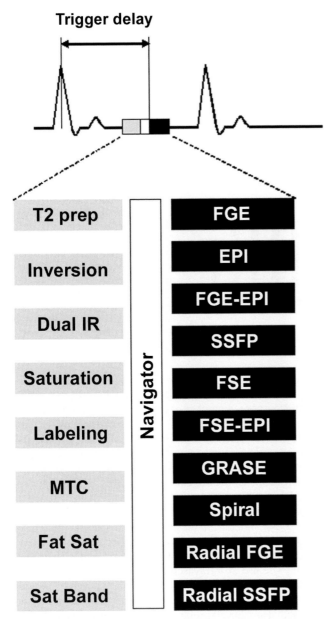

Figure 18.6. Modular blocks used for navigator-controlled coronary MRA. ECG triggering is used for the suppression of intrinsic motion. Contrast is generated by prepulses (*gray boxes*), such as T2 preparation, inversion, dual inversion, saturation, spin labeling, magnetic transfer contrast, fat saturation, or local saturation bands. Some of these contrast mechanisms may be combined with the administration of contrast media. Candidate imaging sequences (*black boxes*) include fast gradient echo, echo planar imaging, fast gradient-echo planar imaging, SSFP, fast spin echo, fast spin-echo planar imaging, gradient and spin echo, spiral imaging, radial fast gradient echo, and radial SSFP. In addition, all sequences can theoretically be combined with parallel imaging techniques.

nary arteries, a high level of contrast between the coronary lumen and the surrounding tissue is desirable. The contrast between the coronary blood-pool and the surrounding tissue can be manipulated by using the inflow effect (unsaturated protons entering the imaging field between successive RF

pulses), by the application of MR prepulses (endogenous contrast enhancement), or by the administration of contrast agents (exogenous contrast enhancement) with or without preparatory pulses. Preparatory pulses such as fat saturation (54), magnetization transfer contrast (30), T2 preparation (55,56), local saturation bands, and inversion (57,58) and dual-inversion (59) prepulses were all shown to enhance contrast in coronary MRA.

Endogenous Contrast Enhancement

Fat Saturation in Bright-blood Coronary Magnetic Resonance Angiography

In most subjects, the coronary arteries are surrounded by epicardial fat. Fat has a relatively short T1 (250 ms at 1.5 T) and a resultant MR signal intensity similar to that of flowing blood. Fat saturation prepulses are used to suppress signal from surrounding fat selectively to allow visualization of the underlying coronary arteries. This is often accomplished with a frequency-selective prepulse that minimizes the fat signal and thereby allows visualization of the coronary vessels. In the case of spiral imaging, a spectral-spatial RF excitation pulse may be used, which selectively excites water (60) exclusively in the imaging slice.

Signal from the Myocardium in Bright-blood Coronary Magnetic Resonance Angiography

The coronary arteries run in close proximity to the epimyocardium. The relatively similar T1 relaxation values of myocardium and coronary blood (850 and 1,200 ms, respectively, at 1.5 T) complicate the differentiation of the coronary arteries for 3D coronary MRA because blood exchange (inflow effect) is reduced between successive RF excitations as compared to 2D acquisitions. Different methods can be used to enhance the contrast between the coronary arteries and myocardium. The most promising ones are prepulses such as T2 preparation (55,56) and magnetization transfer contrast (30). Because the T2 relaxation times of coronary arterial blood (250 ms) and myocardium (50 ms) are substantially different, the application of a T2 preparation prepulse serves to suppress myocardial signal, with relative preservation of the signal from coronary arterial blood (Fig. 18.7). As an added benefit, the signal of deoxygenated blood in the cardiac veins, which has a T2 of 35 ms, is also suppressed when T2 preparation is used (56). Thus, with the use of fat saturation and T2 preparation (or magnetization transfer contrast) prepulses, the coronary lumen appears bright, and the signal intensity of the surrounding tissue (including fat, myocardium, and veins) is reduced (Fig. 18.8).

Signal from the Myocardium and Epicardial Fat in Black-blood Coronary Magnetic Resonance Angiography

In black-blood coronary MRA, a signal-enhanced myocardium and a signal-attenuated coronary lumen are desirable. For this purpose, a dual-inversion prepulse consisting of a nonselective inversion followed by a slice-selective inversion is used to reestablish the initial magnetization of the myocardium at the slice of interest (61). For black-blood

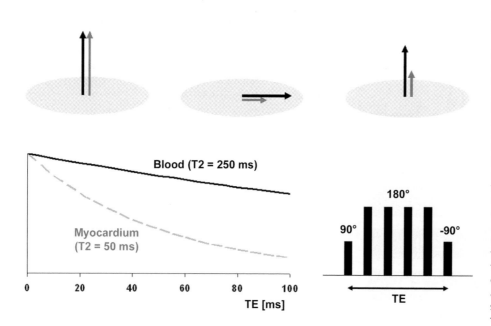

Figure 18.7. Principle of T2 preparation for T2 contrast enhancement between arterial blood (T2 = 250 ms) and myocardium (T2 = 50 ms). T2 affects only magnetization in the xy-plane, but not magnetization along the z-axis (the direction of the main magnetic field). An initial 90-degree pulse rotates the equilibrium M_z magnetization of blood (*black*) and myocardium (*gray*) into the xy-plane, where it is subject to T2 decay. Because of its longer T2 time, the magnetization of arterial blood undergoes slower decay. After a number of refocusing 180-degree pulses, the magnetization is rotated back along the z-axis and is now available for the subsequent imaging part. Because less magnetization is available for the myocardium, it will show up darker in the MR images than the blood.

coronary MRA, a high signal from the myocardium and epicardial fat is necessary to maximize the contrast between the signal-attenuated coronary blood pool and the surrounding tissue. Therefore, no fat saturation is used in this approach (59).

Exogenous Contrast Enhancement

Bright-blood, time-of-flight coronary MRA methods depend heavily on the inflow of unsaturated protons/blood into the imaging plane. If, however, flow is slow, saturation effects will cause a loss of signal. Furthermore, vessel wall, plaque, and thrombus can have signal intensities similar to that of coronary blood (62). In contrast-enhanced MRA, enhancement of the blood signal is based primarily on the intravascular T1 relaxation rate and therefore may allow for true lumen imaging. With the use of MR contrast agents, the T1 relaxa-

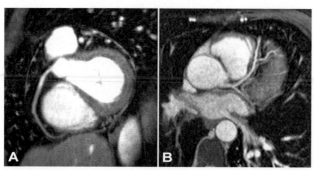

Figure 18.8. Curved reformats of double-oblique, T2-prepared coronary MRA of the right **(A)** and left **(B)** system. A prospective navigator with gating and tracking was used to image 20 overlapping slices during free breathing. In-plane resolution is 0.7 × 1.0 mm², and slice thickness is 3 mm. Note the reduced signal of the great cardiac vein because of the short T2 time of venous blood.

tion of blood can be markedly shortened to increase the contrast-to-noise ratio (CNR) for coronary MRA (57,58,63–65). For this purpose, a number of extracellular and intravascular contrast agents are available. Because extracellular agents quickly extravasate into the extravascular space, their use requires rapid first-pass imaging and therefore breath-hold techniques (18). However, first-pass coronary MRA with extravascular contrast agents is limited by the need for repeated injections of contrast when more than one slab is imaged. With each subsequent injection, the CNR becomes lower as the signal from the extracellular space continuously increases (because of a progressively decreasing T1 due to accumulation of contrast agent) after initial contrast administration. The use of intravascular agents has the inherent advantage of allowing image acquisition for longer periods of time. Thus, non-breath-hold schemes can be used, and repeated scans have similar CNRs without the need for repeated injections (58). When intravascular contrast agents are used in conjunction with navigator technology, 3D, free-breathing, high-resolution coronary MRA data acquisition is possible (58), resulting in improved CNR compared with non–contrast-enhanced approaches.

SPATIAL RESOLUTION

The spatial resolution requirements for coronary MRA depend on whether the goal is simply to identify the ostial takeoff and proximal course of the coronary artery (as in suspected cases of congenital anomalous coronary arteries) or to identify focal stenoses. Figure 18.9 displays an x-ray coronary angiogram at 0.3-mm spatial resolution, along with simulated resolutions of 0.5, 1.0, and 2.0 mm. At resolutions of 0.5 and 1.0 mm, the focal coronary stenoses are readily detectable, whereas at in-plane resolutions more than 1.0 mm, focal stenoses are not discernible. Thus, a spatial resolu-

less, the increase in SNR makes spiral imaging a promising approach, particularly for MRA of the proximal segments.

Contrast-enhanced Coronary MRA

With contrast-enhanced MRA, enhancement of the blood signal is based primarily on the intravascular T1 relaxation rate and therefore may allow true lumen imaging also in the presence of turbulent flow. Exogenous MR contrast agents can be subcategorized into extracellular and intravascular (blood-pool) agents. Extracellular paramagnetic contrast agents (gadolinium chelates) have been used for first-pass coronary MRA (18,19,88,89). The effective T1 relaxation rate depends on the relaxivity of gadolinium and its local concentration, with prominent but transient shortening of the blood T1 relaxation (T1 of 1,200 ms at 1.5 T) to less than 100 ms during first passage of the bolus. Rapid vascular equilibration and extravasation into the extravascular space (and decreasing the myocardial T1) subsequently take place. To identify the timing of the peak gadolinium concentration (minimal T1), a test dose may be administered during dynamic imaging at the aortic root (88).

Under development are several intravascular MR contrast agents that afford longer scan times with free-breathing and navigator technology. By applying a nonselective 180-degree inversion pulse, image acquisition can be timed to occur when the longitudinal magnetization of myocardium crosses the null point (58,90,91). CNR improvements in the range of 60% to 160%, and SNR improvements in the range of 20% to 60%, over conventional (T2-prepared) methods were reported (Fig. 18.18). Taylor et al (92) performed 2D segmented k-space gradient-echo imaging with a contrast

agent consisting of ultrasmall superparamagnetic iron oxide particles. The agent effectively decreased the T1 relaxation rate of blood to less than 100 ms for more than 2 hours and provided superior SNR and CNR in comparison with noncontrast methods. Intravascular agents remain under investigation at this time.

Coronary MRA Spin-labeling Methods

Conventional coronary MRA methods display the coronary blood pool along with the surrounding structures, including the coronary vessel wall, myocardium, ventricular and atrial blood pool, and great vessels. This representation of the coronary anatomy is not directly analogous to the information provided by selective x-ray coronary angiography, in which only the coronary lumen displayed by the radiopaque contrast agent is seen. Analogous luminographic data was obtained with MRI by means of selective tagging of blood in the aortic root using a 2D selective "pencil" inversion pulse (93). After a wash-in time of 300 to 600 ms, the labeled blood entered the proximal coronary vessels and was imaged with a 2- to 3-cm-thick slab in either the transverse or oblique projection. The entire acquisition occurred during a 24-s breath-hold. This principle was reexamined in a free-breathing, navigator-gated and -corrected 3D interleaved segmented spiral approach (94). The technique enables a 3D luminographic display of the coronary tree under various viewing angles (Fig. 18.19). For visualization of the data, no user-assisted postprocessing is required. Although dependent on blood-flow velocity, such an approach may be an alternative for assessing the proximal coronary arteries and antegrade blood flow through intracoronary stents.

T2 preparation

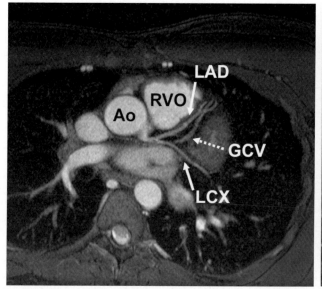

Blood pool agent

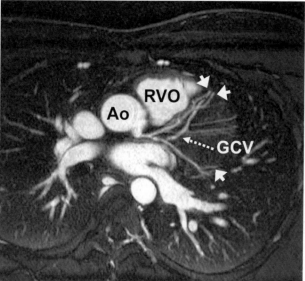

Figure 18.18. Multiplanar reformatted images of T2-prepared (*left*) and intravascular contrast agent-enhanced (*right*) acquisitions obtained in the same volunteer. The combination of the contrast agent and 3D inversion-recovery MRA improves visibility of the coronary arteries and the great cardiac vein (GCV), and depicts additional small-diameter branches of the LCA (*short arrows*). Ao, aorta; RVO, right ventricular outflow tract. (From Huber ME, Paetsch I, Schnackenburg B, et al. Performance of a new gadolinium-based intravascular contrast agent in free-breathing inversion-recovery 3D coronary MRA. *Magn Reson Med* 2003;49:115–121, with permission.)

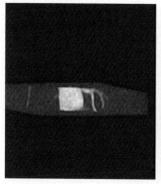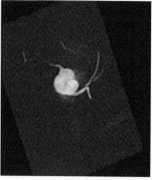

Figure 18.19. Two orthogonal views of 3D visualizations of the LCA system after spin labeling in the aortic root. The complete absence of surrounding tissue signal enables 3D visualization without need for user-directed postprocessing. (From Stuber M, Bornert P, Spuentrup E, et al. Selective three-dimensional visualization of the coronary arterial lumen using arterial spin tagging. *Magn Reson Med* 2002;47:322–329, with permission.)

BLACK-BLOOD CORONARY MRA

Two-dimensional Spin-echo Coronary MRA

Early attempts to image the coronary arteries included the use of conventional ECG-gated spin-echo coronary MRA. On these images, the signal of the blood pool appeared dark, whereas that of the surrounding tissue, including myocardium and epicardial fat, was bright. Although occasionally successful in identifying coronary ostia, this approach was not reliable for assessing anomalous vessels or disease. In one of the earliest studies, an ECC-gated spin-echo technique was able to visualize portions of the native coronary arteries in only 7 (30%) of 23 subjects (5). Subsequently, a similar methodology was used in six patients who had undergone x-ray coronary angiography (6). Even though the data were acquired during ventricular systole, respiratory motion was not suppressed, and the data were acquired over several minutes, the origin of the left main coronary artery was seen in all six subjects and the ostium of the RCA in four of the six subjects. No stenoses were visualized in either report. Subsequently, bright-blood gradient-echo techniques came into greater use and made it possible to visualize proximal to middle portions of the coronary arteries in healthy and diseased states.

Two- and Three-dimensional Fast Spin-echo Black-blood Coronary MRA

Although used successfully for the detection of coronary stenoses (80), bright-blood sequences are prone to overestimate lesions because of artificial darkening caused by focal turbulent flow (95). The vessel luminal diameter may therefore be underestimated, and results appear biased in comparison with those of conventional x-ray angiography. On the other hand, the signal intensity of thrombus, vessel wall, and various components of plaque may appear high on bright-blood coronary MRA (62), obscuring focal stenoses. A black-blood spin-echo-based coronary MRA technique that exclusively displays the coronary blood pool may offer ad-

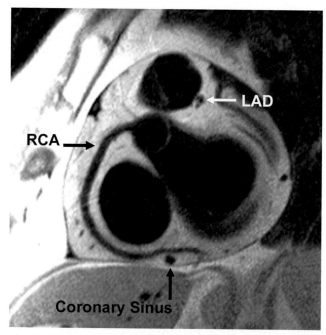

Figure 18.20. Free-breathing black-blood 2D coronary MR angiogram acquired with a fast spin-echo sequence. View shows RCA in-plane, and cross sections of LAD and coronary sinus. (From Stuber M, Botnar RM, Kissinger KV, et al. Free-breathing black-blood coronary MR angiography: initial results. *Radiology* 2001; 219:278–283, with permission.)

vantages in coronary MRA. Methods based on spin-echo imaging also have the potential for enhancing CNR in comparison with gradient-echo approaches.

Submillimeter black-blood coronary MRA images have been acquired successfully with the use of ECC-triggered navigator-gated free-breathing dual-inversion 2D (59) and 3D fast spin-echo MRA (53) (Fig. 18.20). Black-blood methods appear to be particularly advantageous for patients with metallic implants, such as vascular clips, markers, and sternal wires. These metallic objects are a source of local magnetic field inhomogeneities. The size of the artifacts is increased with gradient-echo bright-blood coronary MRA but minimized with black-blood approaches.

CORONARY MRA: FUTURE PERSPECTIVE

Current research in coronary MRA is focused on the clinical assessment of many of the advanced methods described in this chapter. The goal is to provide a novel noninvasive test that makes it possible to screen for major disease of the proximal and middle coronary arteries. Despite many advances during the past decade, the SNR and speed of data acquisition still must be improved for routine coronary MRA. Research and development of novel methods is therefore ongoing. Although beyond the scope of this chapter, cardiac MR also has the potential to image the coronary vessel wall noninvasively and to detect subclinical atherosclerotic plaque, so that new insights may be acquired on the development and progress of subclinical atherosclerosis.

STENTS

The number of patients with cardiac disease who undergo percutaneous revascularization with intracoronary stents deployment is increasing. Stents are metallic implants that locally distort the magnetic field, and they may appear as signal voids on MR images. As a consequence, the direct assessment of stent patency with MR is not practical. In comparison with gradient-echo approaches, techniques based on fast spin-echo imaging may minimize such artifacts; however, no large patient studies have been reported. The stent geometry, material, and orientation with respect to the main magnetic field are variables that cannot be controlled and that substantially influence the appearance of artifacts (96–98). Recently, MR-compatible stents were developed (99,100), demonstrating complete absence of artifacts and full visualization within the stent, potentially solving the problem in the future.

INTERVENTIONAL CORONARY MRA

With the availability of short-bore MR imagers with real-time imaging capability and interactive user interfaces, interventional MRI has gained considerable interest during recent years (101). Coronary artery catheterization (102), selective contrast injection (103) (Fig. 18.21), and coronary angioplasty and stent placement (104) under real-time MR guidance were all successfully demonstrated in experimental models. However, the benefit of interventional coronary

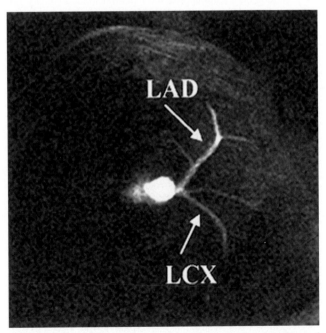

Figure 18.21. LCA system imaged during selective injection of diluted contrast media in the left main coronary artery after catheterization under MRI guidance. A thick-slice (3 cm), magnetization-prepared SSFP sequence was used. LAD, LCX, and several marginal arteries are well depicted. (From Green JD, Omary RA, Schirf BE, et al. Catheter-directed contrast-enhanced coronary MR angiography in swine using magnetization-prepared True-FISP. *Magn Reson Med* 2003;50:1317–1321, with permission.)

MRA will have to be defined in comparison with that of conventional x-ray coronary angiography.

HIGH-FIELD-STRENGTH CORONARY MRA

In recent years, high-field MR imagers (mostly 3T systems) have become more widely available for cardiac applications. The potential increase in SNR (linearly proportional to the field strength) promises further progress in many cardiac applications, including coronary MRA. However, increased susceptibility effects between tissue borders, compromised RF penetration, and an increased hydrodynamic effect hampering ECG triggering are all major concerns. Nevertheless, first results of cardiac MRI in general, and coronary MRA in particular (10,11,105), at higher field strengths look promising.

IMAGING OF THE CORONARY VESSEL WALL

In a healthy person, the thickness of the proximal coronary artery wall is less than 1 mm. Therefore, the requirements for techniques to suppress motion and enhance the contrast between coronary vessel wall, epicardial fat, myocardium, and coronary blood pool are even more stringent in imaging the coronary vessel wall than in coronary MRA. However, with the advanced techniques of motion suppression and contrast enhancement discussed in this chapter, several groups have successfully imaged the coronary vessel wall (106–108).

SUMMARY

State-of-the-art coronary MRA methodologies allow a successful suppression of intrinsic and extrinsic myocardial motion. At the same time, the contrast between the coronary blood pool and the surrounding tissue can be enhanced with the use of either exogenous or endogenous mechanisms of contrast enhancement. These techniques enable the visualization of the coronary arteries with submillimeter in-plane spatial resolution. The utility of coronary MRA for assessing native coronary artery stenosis is still the focus of intense clinical investigation. Several competing approaches have been described and are currently being evaluated for the diagnosis of coronary artery disease in native coronary arteries and coronary artery bypass grafts. Technical and methodologic advances, in concert with a more experienced application of knowledge, will make further improvements in visualizing the coronary arteries with MRI possible.

REFERENCES

1. American Heart Association. *Heart disease and stroke statistics—2004 update.* Dallas, TX: American Heart Association; 2003.
2. Budoff MJ, Georgiou D, Brody A, et al. Ultrafast computed tomography as a diagnostic modality in the detection of coro-

nary artery disease: a multicenter study. *Circulation* 1996; 93:898–904.

3. Schoenhagen P, Halliburton SS, Stillman AE, et al. Noninvasive imaging of coronary arteries: current and future role of multi-detector row CT. *Radiology* 2004;232:7–17.

4. Choi HS, Choi BW, Choe KO, et al. Pitfalls, artifacts, and remedies in multi-detector row CT coronary angiography. *Radiographics* 2004;24:787–800.

5. Lieberman JM, Botti RE, Nelson AD. Magnetic resonance imaging of the heart. *Radiol Clin North Am* 1984;22: 847–858.

6. Paulin S, von Schulthess GK, Fossel E, et al. MR imaging of the aortic root and proximal coronary arteries. *AJR Am J Roentgenol* 1987;148:665–670.

7. Bornert P, Jensen D. Coronary artery imaging at 0.5 T using segmented 3D echo planar imaging. *Magn Reson Med* 1995; 34:779–785.

8. Yang GZ, Gatehouse PD, Keegan J, et al. Three-dimensional coronary MR angiography using zonal echo planar imaging. *Magn Reson Med* 1998;39:833–842.

9. Jhooti P, Keegan J, Gatehouse PD, et al. 3D coronary artery imaging with phase reordering for improved scan efficiency. *Magn Reson Med* 1999;41:555–562.

10. Stuber M, Botnar RM, Fischer SE, et al. Preliminary report on in vivo coronary MRA at 3 Tesla in humans. *Magn Reson Med* 2002;48:425–429.

11. Huber ME, Kozerke S, Pruessmann KP, et al. Sensitivity-encoded coronary MRA at 3T. *Magn Reson Med* 2004;52: 221–227.

12. Fischer SE, Wickline SA, Lorenz CH. Novel real-time R-wave detection algorithm based on the vectorcardiogram for accurate gated magnetic resonance acquisitions. *Magn Reson Med* 1999;42:361–370.

13. Hofman MB, Wickline SA, Lorenz CH. Quantification of in-plane motion of the coronary arteries during the cardiac cycle: implications for acquisition window duration for MR flow quantification. *J Magn Reson Imaging* 1998;8:568–576.

14. Johnson KR, Patel SJ, Whigham A, et al. Three-dimensional, time-resolved motion of the coronary arteries. J Cardiovasc Magn Reson 2004;6:663–673.

15. Wang Y, Watts R, Mitchell I, et al. Coronary MR angiography: selection of acquisition window of minimal cardiac motion with electrocardiography-triggered navigator cardiac motion prescanning—initial results. *Radiology* 2001;218: 580–585.

16. Edelman RR, Manning WJ, Burstein D, et al. Coronary arteries: breath-hold MR angiography. *Radiology* 1991;181: 641–643.

17. Manning WJ, Edelman RR. Magnetic resonance coronary angiography. *Magn Reson Q* 1993;9:131–151.

18. Goldfarb JW, Edelman RR. Coronary arteries: breath-hold, gadolinium-enhanced, three-dimensional MR angiography. *Radiology* 1998;206:830–834.

19. Wielopolski PA, van Geuns RJ, de Feyter PJ, et al. Breath-hold coronary MR angiography with volume-targeted imaging. *Radiology* 1998;209:209–219.

20. Stuber M, Botnar RM, Danias PG, et al. Breathhold three-dimensional coronary magnetic resonance angiography using real-time navigator technology. *J Card Magn Reson* 1999;1: 233–238.

21. van Geuns RJ, Wielopolski PA, de Bruin HG, et al. MR coronary angiography with breath-hold targeted volumes: preliminary clinical results. *Radiology* 2000;217:270–277.

22. Doyle M, Scheidegger MB, de Graaf RG, et al. Coronary artery imaging in multiple 1-sec breath holds. *Magn Reson Imaging* 1993;11:3–6.

23. Liu YL, Riederer SJ, Rossman PJ, et al. A monitoring, feedback, and triggering system for reproducible breath-hold MR imaging. *Magn Reson Med* 1993;30:507–511.

24. Wang Y, Grimm RC, Rossman PJ, et al. 3D coronary MR angiography in multiple breath-holds using a respiratory feedback monitor. *Magn Reson Med* 1995;34:11–16.

25. Wang Y, Christy PS, Korosec FR, et al. Coronary MRI with a respiratory feedback monitor: the 2D imaging case. *Magn Reson Med* 1995;33:116–121.

26. Taylor AM, Jhooti P, Keegan J, et al. Magnetic resonance navigator echo diaphragm monitoring in patients with suspected diaphragm paralysis. *J Magn Reson Imaging* 1999;9: 69–74.

27. Holland AE, Goldfarb JW, Edelman RR. Diaphragmatic and cardiac motion during suspended breathing: preliminary experience and implications for breath-hold MR imaging. *Radiology* 1998;209:483–489.

28. McConnell MV, Khasgiwala VC, Savord BJ, et al. Comparison of respiratory suppression methods and navigator locations for MR coronary angiography. *AJR Am J Roentgenol* 1997;168:1369–1375.

29. Danias PG, Stuber M, Botnar RM, et al. Navigator assessment of breath-hold duration: impact of supplemental oxygen and hyperventilation. *AJR Am J Roentgenol* 1998;171:395–397.

30. Li D, Paschal CB, Haacke EM, et al. Coronary arteries: three-dimensional MR imaging with fat saturation and magnetization transfer contrast. *Radiology* 1993;187:401–406.

31. Oshinski JN, Hofland L, Mukundan S Jr., et al. Two-dimensional coronary MR angiography without breath holding. *Radiology* 1996;201:737–743.

32. Ehman RL, Felmlee JP. Adaptive technique for high-definition MR imaging of moving structures. *Radiology* 1989;173: 255–263.

33. Post JC, van Rossum AC, Hofman MB, et al. Three-dimensional respiratory-gated MR angiography of coronary arteries: comparison with conventional coronary angiography. *AJR Am J Roentgenol* 1996;166:1399–1404.

34. Manke D, Nehrke K, Bornert P. Novel prospective respiratory motion correction approach for free-breathing coronary MR angiography using a patient-adapted affine motion model. *Magn Reson Med* 2003;50:122–131.

35. Taylor AM, Jhooti P, Wiesmann F, et al. MR navigator-echo monitoring of temporal changes in diaphragm position: implications for MR coronary angiography. *J Magn Reson Imaging* 1997;7:629–636.

36. Sachs TS, Meyer CH, Hu BS, et al. Real-time motion detection in spiral MRI using navigators. *Magn Reson Med* 1994; 32:639–645.

37. Stuber M, Botnar RM, Danias PG, et al. Submillimeter three-dimensional coronary MR angiography with real-time navigator correction: comparison of navigator locations. *Radiology* 1999;212:579–587.

38. Korin HW, Ehman RL, Riederer SJ, et al. Respiratory kinematics of the upper abdominal organs: a quantitative study. *Magn Reson Med* 1992;23:172–178.

39. Li D, Kaushikkar S, Haacke EM, et al. Coronary arteries: three-dimensional MR imaging with retrospective respiratory gating. *Radiology* 1996;201:857–863.

40. Hardy CJ, Cline HE. Broadband nuclear magnetic resonance pulses with two-dimensional spatial selectivity. *J Appl Phys* 1989;66:1513.

41. Wang Y, Riederer SJ, Ehman RL. Respiratory motion of the heart: kinematics and the implications for the spatial resolution in coronary imaging. *Magn Reson Med* 1995;33: 713–719.

42. Keegan J, Gatehouse P, Yang GZ, et al. Coronary artery motion with the respiratory cycle during breath-holding and free-breathing: implications for slice-followed coronary artery imaging. *Magn Reson Med* 2002;47:476–481.

43. Danias PG, McConnell MV, Khasgiwala VC, et al. Prospective navigator correction of image position for coronary MR angiography. *Radiology* 1997;203:733–736.

44. Stuber M, Botnar RM, Kissinger KV, et al. 3D real-time navigator corrected black-blood coronary MRA. *J Cardiovasc Magn Reson* 1999;1:340.

45. Shea SM, Kroeker RM, Deshpande V, et al. Coronary artery imaging: 3D segmented k-space data acquisition with multiple breath-holds and real-time slab following. *J Magn Reson Imaging* 2001;13:301–307.

46. Huber ME, Oelhafen ME, Kozerke S, et al. Single breath-hold extended free-breathing navigator-gated three-dimensional coronary MRA. *J Magn Reson Imaging* 2002;15:210–214.

47. Weiger M, Bornert P, Proksa R, et al. Motion-adapted gating based on k-space weighting for reduction of respiratory motion artifacts. *Magn Reson Med* 1997;38:322–333.

48. Sachs TS, Meyer CH, Irarrazabal P, et al. The diminishing variance algorithm for real-time reduction of motion artifacts in MRI. *Magn Reson Med* 1995;34:412–422.

49. Jhooti P, Gatehouse PD, Keegan J, et al. Phase ordering with automatic window selection (PAWS): a novel motion-resistant technique for 3D coronary imaging. *Magn Reson Med* 2000;43:470–480.

50. Huber ME, Hengesbach D, Botnar RM, et al. Motion artifact reduction and vessel enhancement for free-breathing navigator-gated coronary MRA using 3D k-space reordering. *Magn Reson Med* 2001;45:645–652.

51. Hardy CJ, Saranathan M, Zhu Y, et al. Coronary angiography by real-time MRI with adaptive averaging. *Magn Reson Med* 2000;44:940–946.

52. Spuentrup E, Manning WJ, Botnar RM, et al. Impact of navigator timing on free-breathing submillimeter 3D coronary magnetic resonance angiography. *Magn Reson Med* 2002;47:196–201.

53. Stuber M, Botnar RM, Spuentrup E, et al. Three-dimensional high-resolution fast spin-echo coronary magnetic resonance angiography. *Magn Reson Med* 2001;45:206–211.

54. Manning WJ, Li W, Boyle NG, et al. Fat-suppressed breath-hold magnetic resonance coronary angiography. *Circulation* 1993;87:94–104.

55. Brittain JH, Hu BS, Wright GA, et al. Coronary angiography with magnetization-prepared T2 contrast. *Magn Reson Med* 1995;33:689–696.

56. Botnar RM, Stuber M, Danias PG, et al. Improved coronary artery definition with T2-weighted, free-breathing, three-dimensional coronary MRA. *Circulation* 1999;99:3139–3148.

57. Li D, Dolan RP, Walovitch RC, et al. Three-dimensional MRI of coronary arteries using an intravascular contrast agent. *Magn Reson Med* 1998;39:1014–1018.

58. Stuber M, Botnar RM, Danias PG, et al. Contrast agent-enhanced, free-breathing, three-dimensional coronary magnetic resonance angiography. *J Magn Reson Imaging* 1999;10:790–799.

59. Stuber M, Botnar RM, Kissinger KV, et al. Free-breathing black-blood coronary MR angiography: initial results. *Radiology* 2001;219:278–283.

60. Meyer CH, Pauly JM, Macovski A, et al. Simultaneous spatial and spectral selective excitation. *Magn Reson Med* 1990;15:287–304.

61. Edelman RR, Chien D, Kim D. Fast selective black blood MR imaging. *Radiology* 1991;181:655–660.

62. Jara H, Yu BC, Caruthers SD, et al. Voxel sensitivity function description of flow-induced signal loss in MR imaging: implications for black-blood MR angiography with turbo spin-echo sequences. *Magn Reson Med* 1999;41:575–590.

63. Hofman MB, Henson RE, Kovacs SJ, et al. Blood pool agent strongly improves 3D magnetic resonance coronary angiography using an inversion pre-pulse. *Magn Reson Med* 1999;41:360–367.

64. Stillman AE, Wilke N, Li D, et al. Ultrasmall superparamagnetic iron oxide to enhance MRA of the renal and coronary arteries: studies in human patients. *J Comput Assist Tomogr* 1996;20:51–55.

65. Taylor AM, Panting JR, Keegan J, et al. Safety and preliminary findings with the intravascular contrast agent NC100150 injection for MR coronary angiography. *J Magn Reson Imaging* 1999;9:220–227.

66. Botnar RM, Stuber M, Kissinger KV, et al. Free-breathing 3D coronary MRA: the impact of "isotropic" image resolution. *J Magn Reson Imaging* 2000;11:389–393.

67. Stuber M, Botnar RM, Danias PG, et al. Double-oblique free-breathing high resolution three-dimensional coronary magnetic resonance angiography. *J Am Coll Cardiol* 1999;34:524–531.

68. Weber OM, Martin AJ, Higgins CB. Whole-heart steady-state free precession coronary artery magnetic resonance angiography. *Magn Reson Med* 2003;50:1223–1228.

69. Sodickson DK, Manning WJ. Simultaneous acquisition of spatial harmonics (SMASH): fast imaging with radiofrequency coil arrays. *Magn Reson Med* 1997;38:591–603.

70. Pruessmann KP, Weiger M, Scheidegger MB, et al. SENSE: sensitivity encoding for fast MRI. *Magn Reson Med* 1999;42:952–962.

71. Madore B, Glover GH, Pelc NJ. Unaliasing by Fourier-encoding the overlaps using the temporal dimension (UNFOLD), applied to cardiac imaging and fMRI. *Magn Reson Med* 1999;42:813–828.

72. Griswold MA, Jakob PM, Heidemann RM, et al. Generalized autocalibrating partially parallel acquisitions (GRAPPA). *Magn Reson Med* 2002;47:1202–1210.

73. Sodickson DK, Stuber M, Botnar RM, et al. Accelerated coronary MRA in volunteers and patients using double-oblique 3D acquisitions with SMASH. *Proc ISMRM* 1999;2:1249.

74. Hardy CJ, Darrow RD, Saranathan M, et al. Large field-of-view real-time MRI with a 32-channel system. *Magn Reson Med* 2004;52:878–884.

75. Etienne A, Botnar RM, Van Muiswinkel AM, et al. "Soap-Bubble" visualization and quantitative analysis of 3D coronary magnetic resonance angiograms. *Magn Reson Med* 2002;48:658–666.

76. Oppelt A, Graumann R, Barfuss H, et al. FISP-a new fast MRI sequence. *Electromedica* 1986;54:15–18.

77. Mansfield P. Real-time echo-planar imaging by NMR. *Br Med Bull* 1984;40:187–190.

78. Meyer CH, Hu BS, Nishimura DG, et al. Fast spiral coronary artery imaging. *Magn Reson Med* 1992;28:202–213.

79. Burstein D. MR imaging of coronary artery flow in isolated and in vivo hearts. *J Magn Reson Imaging* 1991;1:337–346.

80. Kim WY, Danias PG, Stuber M, et al. Coronary magnetic resonance angiography for the detection of coronary stenoses. *N Engl J Med* 2001;345:1863–1869.

81. Deshpande VS, Shea SM, Laub G, et al. 3D magnetization-prepared true-FISP: a new technique for imaging coronary arteries. *Magn Reson Med* 2001;46:494–502.

82. Weber OM, Pujadas S, Martin AJ, et al. Free-breathing, three-dimensional coronary artery magnetic resonance angiography: comparison of sequences. *J Magn Reson Imaging* 2004;20:395–402.

83. Weber OM, Martin AJ, Higgins CB. Whole-heart coronary MR angiography using a magnetization-prepared SSFP sequence. *J Cardiovasc Magn Reson* 2003;5:23–24.

84. McKinnon GC. Ultrafast interleaved gradient-echo-planar imaging on a standard scanner. *Magn Reson Med* 1993;30:609–616.

85. Botnar RM, Stuber M, Danias PG, et al. A fast 3D approach for coronary MRA. *J Magn Reson Imaging* 1999;10:821–825.

86. Bornert P, Aldefeld B, Nehrke K. Improved 3D spiral imaging for coronary MR angiography. *Magn Reson Med* 2001;45: 172–175.

87. Bornert P, Stuber M, Botnar RM, et al. Direct comparison of 3D spiral vs. Cartesian gradient-echo coronary magnetic resonance angiography. *Magn Reson Med* 2001;46:789–794.

88. Zheng J, Li D, Bae KT, et al. Three-dimensional gadolinium-enhanced coronary magnetic resonance angiography: initial experience. *J Cardiovasc Magn Reson* 1999;1:33–41.

89. Green JD, Schirf BE, Omary RA, et al. Projection imaging of the right coronary artery with an intravenous injection of contrast agent. *Magn Reson Med* 2004;52:699–703.

90. Huber ME, Paetsch I, Schnackenburg B, et al. Performance of a new gadolinium-based intravascular contrast agent in free-breathing inversion-recovery 3D coronary MRA. *Magn Reson Med* 2003;49:115–121.

91. Dirksen MS, Kaandorp TA, Lamb HJ, et al. Three-dimensional navigator coronary MRA with the aid of a blood pool agent in pigs: improved image quality with inclusion of the contrast agent first-pass. *J Magn Reson Imaging* 2003;18: 502–506.

92. Taylor AM, Keegan J, Jhooti P, et al. A comparison between segmented k-space FLASH and interleaved spiral MR coronary angiography sequences. *J Magn Reson Imaging* 2000; 11:394–400.

93. Wang SJ, Hu BS, Macovski A, et al. Coronary angiography using fast selective inversion recovery. *Magn Reson Med* 1991;18:417–423.

94. Stuber M, Bornert P, Spuentrup E, et al. Selective three-dimensional visualization of the coronary arterial lumen using arterial spin tagging. *Magn Reson Med* 2002;47:322–329.

95. Evans AJ, Blinder RA, Herfkens RJ, et al. Effects of turbulence on signal intensity in gradient echo images. *Invest Radiol* 1988;23:512–518.

96. Klemm T, Duda S, Machann J, et al. MR imaging in the presence of vascular stents: A systematic assessment of artifacts for various stent orientations, sequence types, and field strengths. *J Magn Reson Imaging* 2000;12:606–615.

97. Lenhart M, Volk M, Manke C, et al. Stent appearance at contrast-enhanced MR angiography: in vitro examination with 14 stents. *Radiology* 2000;217:173–178.

98. Hug J, Nagel E, Bornstedt A, et al. Coronary arterial stents: safety and artifacts during MR imaging. *Radiology* 2000;216: 781–787.

99. Buecker A, Spuentrup E, Ruebben A, et al. Artifact-free in-stent lumen visualization by standard magnetic resonance angiography using a new metallic magnetic resonance imaging stent. *Circulation* 2002;105:1772–1775.

100. Buecker A, Spuentrup E, Ruebben A, et al. New metallic MR stents for artifact-free coronary MR angiography: feasibility study in a swine model. *Invest Radiol* 2004;39:250–253.

101. Weber OM, Schalla S, Martin AJ, et al. Interventional cardiac magnetic resonance imaging. *Semin Roentgenol* 2003;38: 352–357.

102. Omary RA, Green JD, Schirf BE, et al. Real-time magnetic resonance imaging-guided coronary catheterization in swine. *Circulation* 2003;107:2656–2659.

103. Green JD, Omary RA, Schirf BE, et al. Catheter-directed contrast-enhanced coronary MR angiography in swine using magnetization-prepared True-FISP. *Magn Reson Med* 2003; 50:1317–1321.

104. Spuentrup E, Ruebben A, Schaeffter T, et al. Magnetic resonance-guided coronary artery stent placement in a swine model. *Circulation* 2002;105:874–879.

105. Kaul MG, Stork A, Bansmann PM, et al. Evaluation of balanced steady-state free precession (TrueFISP) and K-space segmented gradient echo sequences for 3D coronary MR angiography with navigator gating at 3 Tesla. *Rofo* 2004;176: 1560–1565.

106. Fayad ZA, Fuster V, Fallon JT, et al. Noninvasive in vivo human coronary artery lumen and wall imaging using black-blood magnetic resonance imaging. *Circulation* 2000;102: 506–510.

107. Botnar RM, Stuber M, Kissinger KV, et al. Noninvasive coronary vessel wall and plaque imaging with magnetic resonance imaging. *Circulation* 2000;102:2582–2587.

108. Kim WY, Stuber M, Bornert P, et al. Three-dimensional black-blood cardiac magnetic resonance coronary vessel wall imaging detects positive arterial remodeling in patients with nonsignificant coronary artery disease. *Circulation* 2002;106: 296–299.

19

Coronary Artery Imaging—Clinical Applications

Evan Appelbaum, Thomas H. Hauser, Susan B. Yeon, René M. Botnar, and Warren J. Manning

Despite decades of progress in both prevention and early diagnosis, coronary artery disease (CAD) remains the leading cause of mortality for both men and women in the United States and throughout the Western world (1). For over 40 years, invasive x-ray coronary angiography has been the "gold standard" for the diagnosis of significant ($\geq$50% diameter stenosis) CAD with over a million diagnostic x-ray coronary angiograms performed annually in the United States (1) and higher volumes in Europe and Japan. Although numerous noninvasive tests are available to help discriminate among those with and without significant angiographic disease, studies continue to demonstrate that 25% to 40% of patients referred for elective x-ray coronary angiography are found to have no significant stenoses (2). Despite the absence of disease, these patients remain subjected to the cost, inconvenience, and potential morbidity of invasive x-ray angiography (3,4). In addition, data suggest that in selected high risk populations, the incidence of subclinical stroke associated with diagnostic cardiac catheterization may exceed 20% (5). Because surgical revascularization of left main (LM) and multivessel proximal coronary disease has the greatest impact on patient mortality, and >90% of coronary segments undergoing intervention fall within the proximal/middle segments (6,7), it would be desirable to have a noninvasive method to directly visualize the proximal/middle native coronary vessels for the accurate identification/exclusion of LM/multivessel CAD.

Over the last decade, coronary magnetic resonance imaging (MRI) has evolved as a potential replacement for diagnostic x-ray angiography among patients with suspected anomalous coronary artery disease and coronary artery aneurysms, and has currently reached sufficient maturity, such that it may obviate the need for invasive x-ray angiography when performed at experienced centers. The technical aspects related to coronary MRI acquisition have been reviewed in Chapter 18.

This chapter will review the published clinical data for coronary MRI in the assessment of anomalous coronary artery disease, coronary artery aneurysms, native coronary artery stenosis, and coronary artery bypass graft disease.

Since the mid-1980s, numerous investigators have contributed to our current understanding of the clinical assessment of coronary MRI in comparison with x-ray angiography. The largest body of published clinical experience has used electrocardiogram-triggered (ECG-) two-dimensional (2D) or three-dimensional (3D) segmented k-space gradient-echo approaches, with increasing reports using the "whole heart" steady-state free precession (SSFP), intravascular contrast, and 3T methods.

MAGNETIC RESONANCE IMAGING OF NORMAL CORONARY ARTERIES

Conventional ECG-triggered spin-echo MRI was intermittently successful at imaging the native coronary arteries (8,9), but it was the relatively low spatial resolution (1.5×2.0 mm) breath-hold, 2D segmented k-space gradient echo approach described in humans by Edelman (10) that first offered a robust approach for imaging the native coronary arteries. As implemented across numerous vendor platforms, the LM, left anterior descending (LAD), and right coronary artery (RCA) are visualized in the nearly all compliant subjects (Table 19.1) (11–16). Early reports had reduced (67% to 77%) success for imaging of the left circumflex coronary artery (LCX), a finding likely related to the use of an anterior surface coil (with reduced signal from the posteriorly directed LCX). Improved (>95%) success has been reported with the now routine use of anterior and posterior thoracic phased array coils. Despite relatively limited spatial resolution, normal proximal coronary artery diameter is similar to values obtained by x-ray angiography and pathology (17,18). Currently, both targeted 3D segmented k-space gradient echo and whole-heart SSFP coronary MRI methods have been the dominant imaging approaches with reported successful visualization of all of the major vessels in nearly every subject (Table 19.1) (19,20). In addition to improved visualization of the origin of the native coronary arteries, another distinct advantage of the 3D approaches is increased contiguous visualization of length/distal segments, as compared with 2D methods. With 3D coronary MRI, similar success (as measured by length of coronary artery seen) is found among healthy adults and patients with angiographic coronary artery disease (21).

ANOMALOUS CORONARY ARTERY IDENTIFICATION

The ability of coronary MRI to reliably identify the major coronary arteries led to its early adoption for the identification and characterization of anomalous coronary artery disease. Though unusual (<1% of the general population) (22,23) and most often benign, congenital coronary anomalies in which the anomalous segment courses anterior to the aorta and posterior to the pulmonary artery are a well-recognized cause of myocardial ischemia and sudden cardiac death, especially among adolescents and young adults (24). These adverse events commonly occur during or immediately following intense exercise and are thought to be related to compression of the anomalous segment, vessel kinking, or the presence of eccentric stenoses (24). Projection x-ray angiography had traditionally been the imaging test of choice for the diagnosis and characterization of these anomalies. However, the presence of an anomalous vessel is sometimes only suspected after the invasive procedure, particularly in a case where there was unsuccessful engagement or visualization of a coronary artery. In addition, the declining use of a pulmonary artery catheter during routine x-ray coronary angiography has made characterization of the anterior versus posterior trajectory of the anomalous vessels more difficult to discern.

Coronary MRI has several advantages in the diagnosis of coronary anomalies. In addition to being noninvasive and not requiring ionizing radiation (an important consideration among adolescents and younger adults) or iodinated contrast agents, coronary MRI provides a definitive 3D "road map" of the mediastinal structures. With 3D coronary MRI, one can subsequently acquire and/or reconstruct an image in arbitrary single and double oblique orientations (Fig. 19.1).

TABLE 19-1	Successful Visualization of the Native Coronary Arteries Using 2D and 3D Segmented K-Space Gradient Echo Coronary Magnetic Resonance Imaging

Investigator	Technique	Resp Comp	# of Sub	RCA	LM	LAD	LCX
Manning (12)	2D GRE	BH	25	100%	96%	100%	76%
Pennell (11)	2D GRE	BH	26	95%	95%	91%	76%
Duerinckx (13)	2D GRE	BH	20	100%	95%	86%	77%
Sakuma (14)	2D GRE cine	BH	18	100%	100%	100%	67%
Masui (15)	2D GRE	BH	13	85%	92%	100%	92%
Davis (16)	2D GRE	BH	33[a]	100%	100%	100%	100%
Li (92)	3D GRE	Mult averages	14	100%	100%	86%	93%
Post (43)	3D GRE	Retro Nav G	20	100%	100%	100%	100%
Wielopolski (93)	3D Seg EPI	BH	32	100%	100%	100%	100%
Botnar (20)	3D GRE	Pro Nav G/C	13	97%	100%	100%	97%
Weber (19)	3D SSFP	Pro Nav G/C	12	100%	100%	100%	100%

[a] Including 18 heart transplant recipients.
GRE, gradient echo; BH, breath-hold; LAD, left anterior descending coronary artery; LCX, left circumflex coronary artery; LM, left main coronary artery; RCA, right coronary artery; Res Comp, respiratory compensation; Sub, subjects.

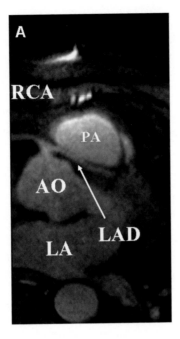

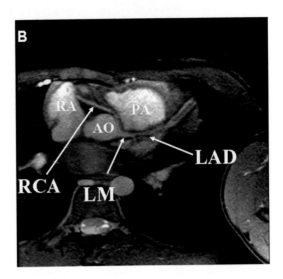

Figure 19.1. Free-breathing 3D coronary MRI using T2 prepulse navigator gating with real-time motion correction. **(A)** Transverse orientation depicting a malignant-type anomalous LAD originating from the RCA and traversing between the aortic root and the pulmonary artery. **(B)** Transverse image in another patient with a malignant-type anomalous origin of the RCA from the left coronary cusp. Ao, aorta; PA, pulmonary artery; LA, left atrium; RA, right atrium.

Early reports of coronary MRI to visualize anomalous coronary arteries included case report confirmation of x-ray angiographic data (25,26). Subsequently, there have been at least six published series (27–32) of patients who underwent a blinded comparison of coronary MRI data with x-ray angiography (Table 19.2). These early coronary MRI studies often used a 2D breath-hold, ECG-triggered segmented k-space gradient echo approach (25–28,30–32). These 2D coronary MRI studies have uniformly reported excellent accuracy, including several studies in which coronary MRI was determined to be superior to x-ray angiography (30,31). Most centers now use 3D coronary MRI because of superior reconstruction capabilities with similar excellent results (29) (Table 19.3). As a result, clinical coronary MRI is now the preferred test for young patients in whom anomalous disease is suspected or known anomalous disease needs to be further clarified, or if the patient has another cardiac anomaly associated with coronary anomalies (e.g., tetralogy of Fallot).

In a somewhat analogous fashion, 2D breath-hold coronary MRI has also been used to define the altered coronary artery orientation in the cardiac transplant population (16). Among cardiac transplant recipients, coronary MRI has documented a 25-degree anterior (clockwise) ostial rotation, likely explaining the more complex coronary engagement during x-ray angiography.

CORONARY ARTERY ANEURYSMS/ KAWASAKI'S DISEASE

Though coronary artery aneurysms are relatively uncommon, recent studies indicate an important role for coronary MRI for assessment of this condition. The vast majority of acquired coronary aneurysms in children and younger adults are a result of mucocutaneous lymph node syndrome (Kawasaki's disease), a generalized vasculitis of unknown etiology, usually occurring in children under 5 years old. Infants and children with this syndrome may show evidence of myocarditis and/or pericarditis, with nearly 20% developing coronary artery aneurysms. These aneurysms are the source of both short- and long-term morbidity and mortality (33). Approximately half of the children with coronary aneurysms during the acute phase of the disease will have angiographically normal-appearing vessels 1 or 2 years later (33,34). For afflicted young children, transthoracic echocardiography is usually adequate for diagnosing and following these aneurysms, but transthoracic echocardiography is often inadequate after adolescence and in obese children. These patients are therefore often referred for serial x-ray coronary angiography. Data from a series of adolescents and young adults with coronary artery aneurysms (Figs. 19.2 and 19.3)

TABLE 19-2	Anomalous Coronary Magnetic Resonance Imaging	
Investigator	# Patients	Correctly Classified Anomalous Vessels
McConnell (27)	15	14 (93%)
Post (30)	19	19 (100%)[a]
Vliegen (31)	12	11 (92%)[b]
Taylor (28)	25	24 (96%)
Bunce (29)	26	26 (100%)[c]
Razmi (32)	12	12 (100%)

[a] Including 3 patients originally misclassified by x-ray angiography.
[b] Including 5 patients unable to be classified by x-ray angiography.
[c] Including 11 patients unable to be classified by x-ray angiography.

			For ≥50% Diameter	
Investigator Stenosis	# Subjects	# Vessels (%)	Sensitivity	Specificity
Retrospective Navigator Gating				
Post (43)	20	21 (27%)	38% (0–57)	95% (85–100)
Muller (45)	35		83%[a]	94%[a]
Woodard (44)	10	10 (100%)	70%	
Sandstede (94)	30	30 (100%)	81%[b]	89%[b]
Van Geuns (46)	32		50% (50–55)[c]	91% (73–95)[c]
Huber (47)	40	20 (50%)	73% (25–100)	50% (25–82)
Sardanelli (48)	42	40% of segments	82% (57–100) 90% proximal	89% (72–100) 90% proximal
Prospective Navigators with Real-Time Motion Correction				
Bunce (49)	34		88%	72%
Moustapha (50)	25		92%	55%
Sommer (51)	112		90% (proximal) 74% 88% (good qual.)	92% (proximal) 63% 91% (good qual.)
Bogaert (52)	19		85–92%	50%–83%
Plein (53)	10		75%	85%
Osgun (95)	14	TFE SSFP	91% 76%	57% 85%

TABLE 19-3 Free-breathing 3D K-Space Segmented Gradient Echo Coronary Magnetic Resonance Imaging Using Retrospective and Prospectice Navigators for Identification of Focal Greater or Equal to 50% Diameter Coronary Stenoses

[a] Excluding 5 patients for "lack of cooperation" and 15 segments for being uninterpretable.
[b] Based on 23 (77%) with high quality scans.
[c] Based on 74% of coronary artery segments analyzable by MRI.

defined on x-ray angiography have confirmed the high accuracy of coronary MRI for both the identification and the characterization (diameter, length) of these aneurysms (Fig. 19.4) (35,36). Though no longitudinal studies have been reported, it is likely that coronary aneurysms can now be effectively followed with serial coronary MRI examinations, an approach particularly beneficial for young patients for whom repeated exposure to ionizing radiation is often a concern. Good correlation between coronary MRI and x-ray coronary angiography has also been reported for ectatic coronary arteries (distinct from Kawasaki's disease) among adults (37).

CORONARY MAGNETIC RESONANCE IMAGING FOR IDENTIFICATION OF NATIVE VESSEL CORONARY STENOSES

Although data support a broad clinical role for coronary MRI in the assessment of suspected anomalous coronary artery disease (and coronary artery bypass graft patency—see later), data are currently in evolution regarding clinical coronary MRI for routine identification of coronary artery stenoses among patients presenting with chest pain under consideration for x-ray angiography, and no efficacy data have

been reported regarding "screening coronary" MRI in high risk populations. However, based on data published from a multicenter study, for populations in which the concern is LM or multivessel disease, coronary MRI approaches are appropriate (38).

Gradient echo sequences depict flow in the coronary lumen, with rapidly moving laminar blood flow appearing "bright" and areas of stagnant flow and/or focal turbulence appearing "dark" because of local saturation (stagnant flow) or dephasing (turbulence) (Fig. 19.5). Areas of focal stenoses produce varying severity of "signal void" in the coronary MRI with the severity of the signal loss related to the angiographic stenosis (Fig. 19.6) (39). However, gradient echo coronary MRI may sometimes be misleading. If there is slow blood flow distal to a stenosis, there may be complete loss of signal in the segment distal to the lesion, despite the absence of a total occlusion. Similarly, because lumen signal is insensitive to the direction of blood flow, a total occlusion with adequate retrograde (or antegrade collateral blood flow) to the distal segment may result in signal in the lumen distal to the occlusion. SSFP sequences are less dependent on blood flow for signal intensity, but the overall depiction of stenoses is similar.

Because of time constraints of a breath-hold, 2D breath-hold coronary MRI has relatively limited in-plane spatial resolution, but the technique has successfully demonstrated

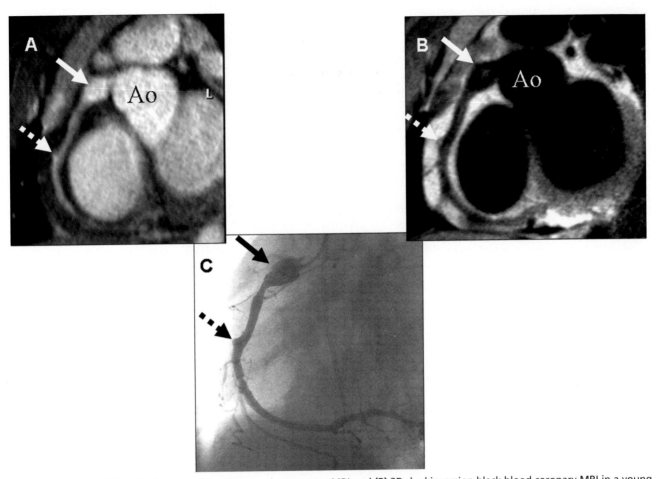

Figure 19.2. **(A)** Oblique 3D free-breathing T2 prepulse coronary MRI and **(B)** 3D dual inversion black blood coronary MRI in a young adult with RCA coronary artery aneurysms (*arrows*) as a result of Kawasaki disease with **(C)** the corresponding x-ray angiogram. Flow-related signal within the aneurysms is homogeneous, with no evidence of thrombosis. Ao, aorta. (From Greil GF, Stuber M, Botnar RM, et al. Coronary magnetic resonance angiography in adolescents and young adults with Kawasaki disease. *Circulation* 2002;105(8): 908–911, with permission.)

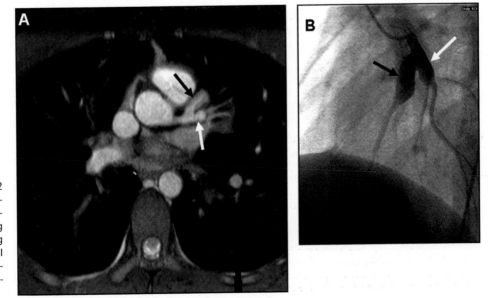

Figure 19.3. **(A)** Transverse 3D T2 prepulse coronary MRI of a subject with a left coronary artery aneurysm and **(B)** corresponding x-ray angiogram, demonstrating good correlation of coronary MRI findings (*black arrow*, LAD aneurysm; *white arrow*, LCX aneurysm).

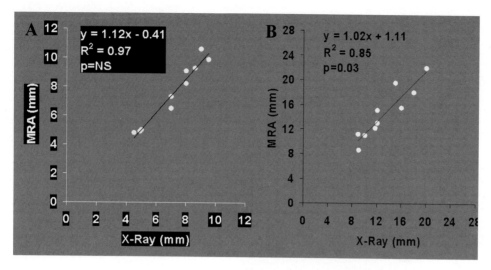

Figure 19.4. Correlation of coronary artery aneurysm length **(A)** and diameter **(B)** as determined by coronary x-ray angiography and coronary MRI. (Adapted from Greil GF, Stuber M, Botnar RM, et al. Coronary magnetic resonance angiography in adolescents and young adults with Kawasaki disease. *Circulation* 2002;105(8): 908–911, with permission.)

proximal coronary stenoses in several clinical studies (Table 19.4) (13,39–42). When reported, the distance from the vessel origin to the focal stenosis on coronary MRI correlates closely with x-ray angiography (Fig. 19.7) (39). However, there has been wide variation in reported sensitivity and specificity of this approach, differences that are likely the result of technical issues/methodology—including the wide variation in patient selection, presence of arrhythmias, prevalence of disease and technical (MR vendor, echo time, receiver coils, timing of the acquisition, acquisition duration, breath-hold maneuvers) issues, and the need for somewhat exhausting 20- to 40-second breath-holds to complete a study. To date, no multicenter 2D coronary MRI study using a uniform hardware, software, and scanning protocol has been reported.

With the increasing availability of MR navigators, many cardiac magnetic resonance (CMR) imaging centers have migrated to a free-breathing targeted 3D gradient echo or "whole heart" SSFP coronary MRI for ease in patient acceptance (free breathing) and for improved signal-to-noise ratio (SNR) with facilitated multiplanar reconstructions. As with 2D gradient echo methods, a focal stenosis/turbulence appears as a signal void along the course of the vessel (Fig. 19.8). Data from several single center sites have now been published using both retrospective navigators and prospective navigators with real-time correction in combination with targeted 3D k-space segmented gradient echo (Table 19.4). Early studies using *retrospective* diaphragmatic navigators used relatively prolonged acquisition times (260 milliseconds per R-R interval) (43–45), whereas more recent reports have used acquisition intervals of <120 milliseconds (46–48). These single center reports were encouraging with overall sensitivity and specificity of up to 90% for proximal coronary disease (48).

Subsequently, single-center targeted 3D k-space segmented gradient echo studies using more sophisticated pro-

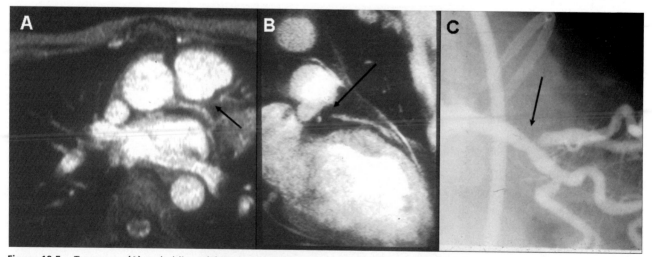

Figure 19.5. Transverse **(A)** and oblique **(B)** 2D breath-hold coronary MRI. In panel *A*, a 45-year-old woman with atypical chest pain demonstrates a signal void (*arrows*) in the proximal LAD. The more distal LAD and diagonal vessel are also visualized, as well as the proximal LCX. Panel *C* demonstrates the corresponding right anterior oblique (*RAO*) caudal x-ray angiogram (*XRA*), confirming the tight ostial LAD stenosis (*arrow*) seen by MRI.

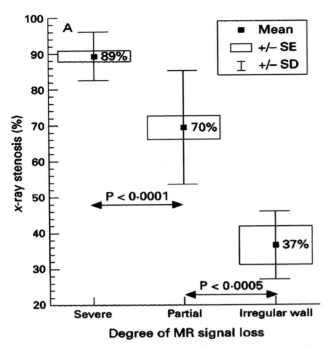

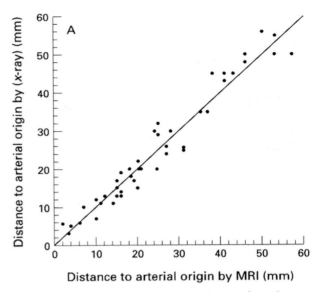

Figure 19.6. Breath-hold 2D segmented k-space gradient echo coronary MRI comparison of focal MR signal loss versus x-ray coronary artery diameter stenosis. Note the strong correlation between the severity of signal loss by coronary MRI and the degree of x-ray angiographic stenosis. (From Pennell DJ, Bogren HG, Keegan J, et al. Assessment of coronary artery stenosis by magnetic resonance imaging. *Heart* 1996;75(2):127–133, with permission.)

Figure 19.7. Scatterplot comparing the distance from the coronary origin to the stenosis as measured by x-ray and magnetic resonance coronary angiography. (From Danias PG, McConnell MV, Khasgiwala VC, et al. Prospective navigator correction of image position for coronary MR angiography. *Radiology* 1997; 203(3):733–736, with permission.)

spective diaphragmatic navigators with real-time motion correction have shown improved results, especially for the proximal coronary segments and in subjects with high image-quality scans (Table 19.4) (49–53). An international multicenter, free-breathing 3D volume targeted coronary MRI study of 109 patients without prior x-ray angiography, using common hardware and software, demonstrated high sensitivity (though only modest specificity) and high negative predictive value of coronary MRI for the identification of coronary disease (as defined as ≥50% diameter stenosis by quantitative coronary angiography) (Table 19.5) (38).

The sensitivity and negative predictive value were particularly high for the identification of left main or multivessel disease, demonstrating a clinical role for coronary MRI for this subset. Accordingly, we have found coronary MRI to be especially valuable for patients who present with a dilated cardiomyopathy/congestive heart failure in the absence of clinical infarction to determine the etiology (ischemic versus nonischemic) (54). For this group, more conventional noninvasive tests often have suboptimal diagnostic accuracy, with coronary MRI also being superior to delayed enhancement CMR methods (54).

The widespread recognition of the benefits of SSFP cine MR for superior SNR and contrast-to-noise ratio (CNR), with decreased dependence on inflow of unsaturated protons, has led to excitement regarding SSFP coronary MRI. Despite

TABLE 19-4	Two-Dimensional Breath-Hold Coronary Magnetic Resonance Imaging for Identification of Greater or Equal to 50% Diameter Focal Coronary Stenoses			
Investigator	# Subjects	# Vessels (%)	Sensitivity	Specificity
Manning (40)	39	52 (35%)	90% (71–100)	92% (78–100)
Duerinckx (13)	20	27 (34%)	63% (0–73)	– (37–82)
Pennel (39)	39	55 (35%)	85% (75–100)	
Post (41)	35	35 (28%)	63% (0–100)	89% (73–96)
Nitatori (42)	57[a]		87%	94%
	13[b]		43%	90%

[a] With ≥90% diameter stenosis.
[b] With 50%–75% diameter stenosis.

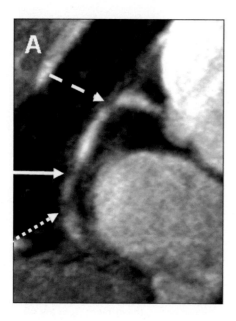

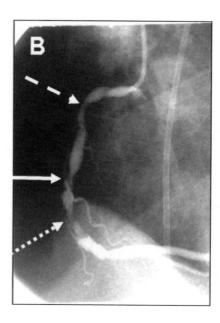

Figure 19.8. **(A)** Free-breathing 3D T2 prepulse coronary MRI with navigator gating and real-time motion correction and **(B)** corresponding x-ray angiography (XRA) in a patient with proximal (*dashed arrow*) and mid-RCA stenoses (*solid and dotted arrows*). (From Stuber M, Botnar RM, Danias PG, et al. Double-oblique free-breathing high resolution three-dimensional coronary magnetic resonance angiography. *J Am Coll Cardiol* 1999;34(2):524–531, with permission.)

inferior in-plane spatial resolution (typically 1.2 mm × 1.2 mm), single center data, using free-breathing, navigator gated, and corrected whole-heart SSFP among patient series, are particularly impressive for reconstruction (Fig. 19.9) and suggest superior accuracy for this approach (55–57) with sensitivities of 80% to 90% and specificity exceeding 90% (Fig. 19.10). An approach that uses the affine prospective navigator algorithm (compensates for motion in both the inferior-superior and the anterior-posterior orientations) offers theoretical advantages (56), but no direct comparison with a single diaphragmatic navigator is available. An early comparative study of k-space segmented gradient echo versus SSFP did confirm the expected improvement of SNR and CNR but no benefit with regard to accuracy for identification of CAD (58).

Comparative data for noncontrast and contrast enhanced coronary MRA in patients are currently sparse. Conventional extracellular gadolinium-based agents appear to offer minimal benefit. Considerable interest in intravascular agents has been boosted by early reports demonstrating increased CNR,

both using MS-325 (EPIX Pharmaceuticals, Cambridge, MA) (59) and Gadomer-17 (Schering, Berlin, Germany) (60). In small series, overall sensitivity and specificity of free-breathing navigator corrected Gadomer-17 coronary MRI was 80% and 93%, respectively, and similar to that of noncontrast single center studies (Fig. 19.11).

High (3 T) field coronary MRI offers the theoretical benefit of a doubling of SNR. In practice, the SNR gain is more modest owing to lack of optimization of surface coils, shimming, and so forth. Only preliminary comparative data re-

TABLE 19-5	Free-Breathing 3D Navigator Coronary Magnetic Resonance Imaging: Multicenter Trial Results	
	Patients	**Left Main/3VD**
Sensitivity	93%	100%
Specificity	58%	85%
Prevalence	42%	15%
Positive Predictive Value	70%	54%
Negative Predictive Value	81%	100%

Adapted from Kim WY, Danias PG, Stuber M, et al. Coronary magnetic resonance angiography for the detection of coronary stenoses. *N Engl J Med* 2001;345(26):1863–1869, with permission.

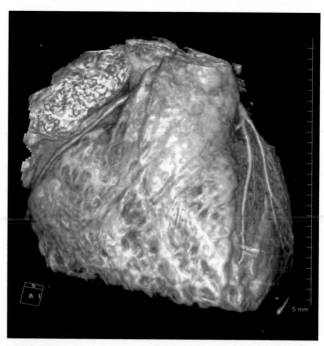

Figure 19.9. Three-dimensional reconstruction of a whole-heart SSFP coronary MRI following computer-assisted image segmentation enables major coronary vessels to be visualized. (Courtesy of Oliver Weber, PhD.)

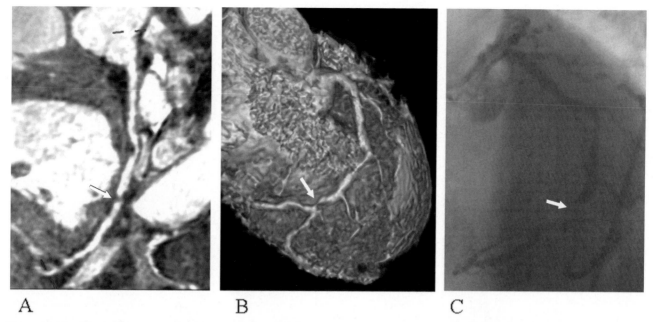

A   B   C

Figure 19.10. Whole heart coronary MR angiography (TR/TE = 4.6/2.3 milliseconds, navigator-gated 3D steady-state free precession sequence with fat saturation and T2 preparation) in a 54-year-old man with LCX stenosis (*arrow*). **(A)** Curved multiplanar reformatted image of the LCX artery. **(B)** Three-dimensional volume rendering image of the LCX artery. **(C)** Catheter angiography. (Courtesy of Hajime Sakuma, Mir, Japan.)

garding the clinical use of 3-T coronary MRI have been reported. These suggest superior SNR but similar sensitivity and specificities of 82% and 89% to 88%, respectively, for detection of significant CAD (Fig. 19.12) (61).

INTRACORONARY STENTS

Improvements in long-term patency rates for percutaneous coronary interventions using conventional and drug-eluting intracoronary stents have resulted in their widespread use in over 80% of the growing number of percutaneous coronary artery revascularizations. Typically made from high-grade stainless steel, preliminary data demonstrate no short- or long-term adverse events for patients who undergo "early" CMR scanning after stent implantation (62,63), but the presence of stents does pose imaging problems. Although the attractive force and local heating are negligible both at 1.5 T (64–69) and 3 T (70), the local susceptibility effects lead to substantial signal voids/artifacts at the site of the stent (Fig. 19.13). The size of the artifact is dependent on both

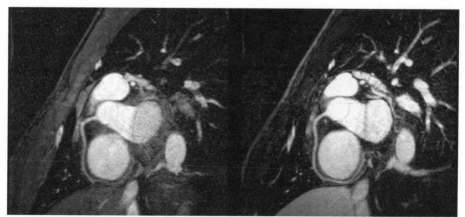

Figure 19.11. Free breathing, navigator echo gated segmented 3D turboflash coronary MRA showing the RCA of a healthy volunteer. Images were taken with endogenous contrast (*left*) using a T2prep magnetization preparation scheme, and after administration of 0.075 mmol/kg of B-22956 (*right*) using an Inversion Recovery preparation pulse. Note the much better delineation of distal portions of the RCA after contrast. High vascular containment of this contrast agent allows for an efficient nulling of myocardial signal, resulting in a 100% increase in vessel-myocardium contrast after B-22956. (Reprinted with permission from Paetsch I, Huber ME, Bornstedt A, et al. Improved three-dimensional free-breathing coronary magnetic resonance angiography using gadocoletic acid (B-22956) for intravascular contrast enhancement. *J Magn Reson Imaging* 2004;20:288–293.)

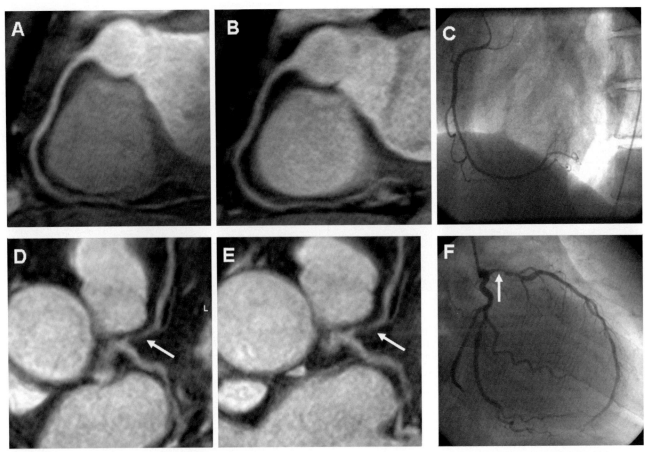

Figure 19.12. Comparison of multiplanar reformatted coronary MRI at **(A,D)** 3.0 T and at **(B,E)** 1.5 T and **(C,F)** corresponding x-ray angiogram in patients **(A–C)** with no hemodynamically significant stenosis of the RCA, including atherosclerotic wall irregularities but no hemodynamically relevant coronary artery stenosis and **(D–F)** in a patient with a proximal stenosis (*arrow*) of the LAD. At both field strengths there is good correlation between coronary MRI and the x-ray angiogram. (Images courtesy of Torsten Sommer, MD, PhD.)

the stent material [increased with stainless steel and less with titanium stents (71,72) and the MR sequence (larger with gradient echo sequences). A novel MR-lucent stent has also been reported (73) (Fig. 19.14). The signal void/artifact precludes direct evaluation of intrastent and peristent coronary integrity, although assessment of blood flow/direction proximal and distal to the stent using MR flow methods or spin-labeling methods may provide indirect evidence of a patency by documentation of antegrade flow.

MAGNETIC RESONANCE IMAGING FOR CORONARY ARTERY BYPASS GRAFT ASSESSMENT

Until the advent of intracoronary stents a decade ago, coronary artery bypass graft surgery was among the most common procedures performed in the United States. Unfortunately, early (<1 month) vein graft occlusion occurs in up to 10% of patients because of mechanical issues, and an accelerated atherosclerotic process often leads to late (5 to 10 years) stenoses/occlusion in the majority of grafts (74,75).

In comparison with the native coronary arteries, reverse saphenous vein and internal mammary artery grafts are relatively easy to image (in the absence of adjacent vascular clips) because of their relatively stationary position during the cardiac and respiratory cycle and their larger lumen. Furthermore, their predictable and less convoluted course has allowed imaging of bypass grafts, even with conventional MR techniques.

With schematic knowledge of the origin and touchdown site of each graft, conventional free-breathing ECG-gated 2D spin-echo (74–77) and 2D gradient-echo (78–81) MR in the transverse plane both have been used to reliably assess bypass graft patency (Fig. 19.15) (Tables 19.6 and 19.7). Patency is generally determined by visualizing a patent graft lumen in at least two contiguous transverse levels along its expected course (presence of flow appearing as signal void for spin-echo techniques and bright signal for gradient-echo approaches). If signal consistent with flow is identified in the area of the graft lumen on two levels, it is likely to be patent. If a patent lumen is seen at only one level (e.g., for spin-echo techniques, a signal void is seen at only one level), a graft is considered "indeterminate." If a patent graft lumen is not seen at any level, the graft is considered occluded. Combining spin-echo and gradient-echo imaging in the same

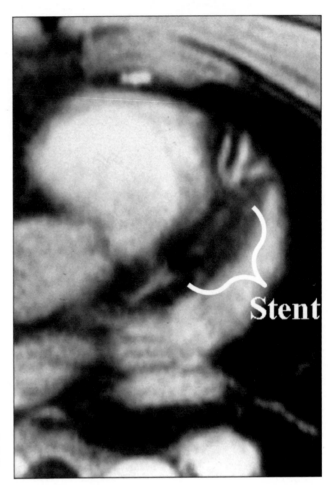

Figure 19.13. Transverse, 2D breath-hold gradient-echo coronary MRI at the level of the LAD in a patient with a patent stent. Note the signal void (*black marker*) corresponding to the site of the stent. (Courtesy of Christopher Kramer, MD.)

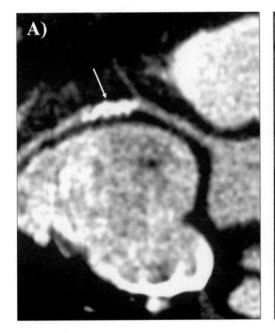

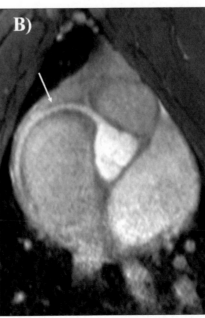

Figure 19.14. MR-lucent stent: **(A)** Multidetector CT (MDCT) with Aachen Resonance prototype MR stent in the RCA. **(B)** Three-dimensional coronary MRI in the same animal. Note the absence of local susceptibility effects on the MR image. (Courtesy of Arno Buecker, MD.)

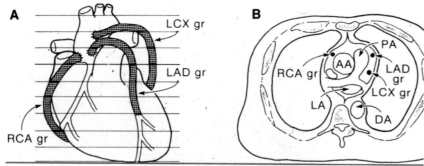

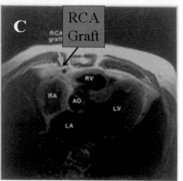

Figure 19.15. (A) Coronal and **(B)** transverse schematic of the anatomic location of coronary artery bypass grafts (*CABG; RCA gr, LAD gr, LCX gr*) originating from the aortic root (*AA*) and anastomosing with the distal native coronary arteries with location of contiguous transverse slices. **(C)** Transverse ECG-gated conventional spin-echo coronary MRI image demonstrating flow (*white arrow*) in an anatomic area corresponding to the RCA vein graft indicating graft patency at that level. (From Rubinstein RI, Askenase AD, Thickman D, et al. Magnetic resonance imaging to evaluate patency of aortocoronary bypass grafts. *Circulation* 1987;76(4): 786–791, with permission.)

TABLE 19-6	Free-Breathing, Electrocardiogram-Triggered "Whole Heart" 3D SSFP Coronary Magnetic Resonance Imaging for Identification of Focal Greater or Equal to 50% Diameter Coronary Stenoses

| | | | For ≥50% Diameter Stenosis | |
Investigator	# Subjects	Prev CAD (%)	Sensitivity (%)	Specificity (%)
Ichikawa (55)	92		94	94
Jahnke (56)	32	50	79	91

TABLE 19-7	Sensitivity, Specificity, and Accuracy of Coronary Magnetic Resonance Imaging for Assessment of Coronary Artery Bypass Graft Patency

Investigator	Technique	# Grafts	Patency (%)	Sens (%)	Spec (%)	Accuracy (%)
White (77)	2D Spin-echo	72	69	86	59	78
Rubenstein (91)	2D Spin-echo	47	62	90	72	83
Jenkins (96)	2D Spin-echo	41	63	89	73	83
Galjee (79)	2D Spin-echo	98	74	98	85	89
White (78)	2D GRE	28	50	93	86	89
Aurigemma (80)	2D GRE	45	73	88	100	91
Galjee (79)	2D GRE	98	74	98	88	96
Engelman (81)	2D GRE	55	100 (IMA)	100		100
			66 (SVG)	92	85	89
Molinari (82)	3D GRE	51	76.5	91	97	96
Bunce (85)	3D SSFP	56 SVG	82	84	45	78
		23 IMA	96			
Wintersperger (84)	CE-3D GRE	39	87	97	100	97
Vrachliotis (83)	CE-3D GRE	45	67	93	97	95

IMA, internal mammary artery; SVG, saphenous vein graft; Sens, sensitivity; Spec, specificity.

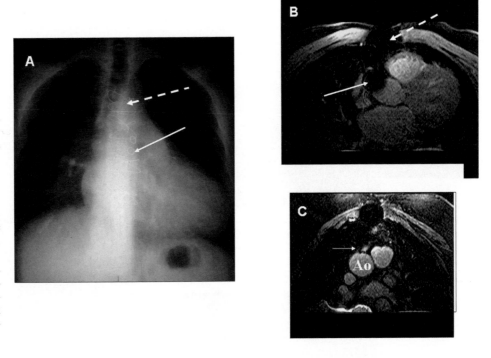

Figure 19.16. (A) Posterior-anterior (*PA*) chest x-ray in a patient with coronary artery bypass grafts. Note the sternal wires (*dashed arrow*) as well as the coronary artery bypass graft markers (*solid arrow*). (B) Transverse coronary MRI in the same patient. Note the large local artifacts (signal voids) related to the sternal wires (*dashed arrow*) and bypass graft markers (*solid arrows*). The size of the artifacts are related to the type of graft marker used. (C) Barium and tantalum markers (*arrow*) result in the smallest artifacts. The size of the artifacts are also somewhat less with spin-echo/black blood MRI, as compared with gradient-echo imaging.

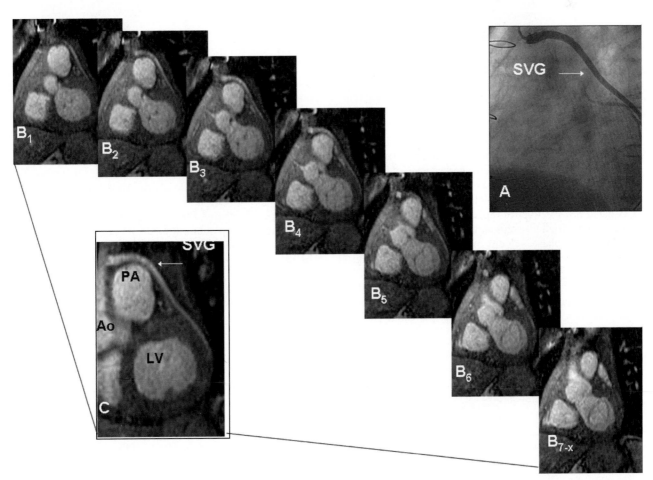

Figure 19.17. (A) X-ray angiogram (*XRA*) of widely patent saphenous vein graft (*SVG*) to the obtuse marginal branch (*OM*) of the left circumflex coronary artery. (B1–7) Individual slices of the 3D MRI in the oblique coronal plane. (C) MPR of the 3D scan demonstrates the widely patent vein graft. (From Langerak SE, Vliegen HW, de Roos A, et al. Detection of vein graft disease using high-resolution magnetic resonance angiography. *Circulation* 2002;105(3):328–333, with permission.)

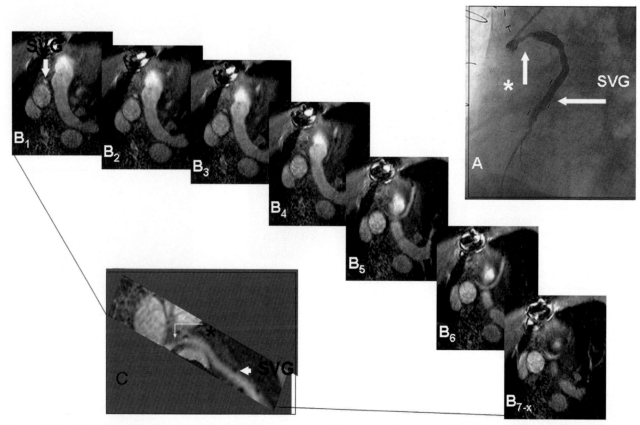

Figure 19.18. **(A)** X-ray angiogram (*XRA*) of saphenous vein graft (*SVG*) to the left anterior descending (*LAD*) coronary artery with a 56% proximal stenosis (*). **(B1–7)** Individual slices of the MRI obtained in the oblique plane. **(C)** MPR of the 3D scan demonstrating the loss of graft lumen (tapering graft contour) corresponding to the x-ray angiographic stenosis (*arrow*). (From Langerak SE, Vliegen HW, de Roos A, et al. Detection of vein graft disease using high-resolution magnetic resonance angiography. *Circulation* 2002;105(3): 328–333, with permission.)

patient does not appear to improve accuracy (79). Both 3D noncontrast (82) and contrast-enhanced coronary MRI have also been described for the assessment of graft patency (83,84), with slightly improved results. The accuracy of ECG-gated SSFP sequences appears to be similar to that of spin-echo and gradient-echo approaches (85). Data suggest that the use of phase velocity mapping for assessment of coronary artery bypass graft flow may be superior to graft imaging (86,87).

A practical limitation of coronary MRI bypass graft assessment is related to local signal loss/artifacts because of nearby metallic objects (hemostatic clips, ostial stainless

steel graft markers, sternal wires, coexistent prosthetic valves and supporting struts or rings, and graft stents) (Figs. 19.13 and 19.16). The inability to identify severely diseased yet patent grafts is also a hindrance to clinical use and acceptance. Langerak (88) has reported on the use of free-breathing T2 prep submillimeter 3D coronary MRI for assessment of saphenous vein graft stenoses (Figs. 19.17 and 19.18). Very good agreement occurred between quantitative x-ray angiography for assessment of both graft occlusion and graft stenoses (Table 19.8). This group has also advocated assessment of rest and adenosine stress coronary artery flow assessment, using phase velocity MR techniques (86,87).

TABLE 19-8	Diagnostic Accuracy of Coronary Magnetic Resonance Imaging for Saphenous Vein Graft Disease	
	Sensitivity (%)	**Specificity (%)**
Graft occlusion	83 (36–100)	100 (92–100)
Graft stenosis ≥50%	82 (57–96)	88 (72–97)
Graft stenosis ≥70%	73 (39–94)	80 (64–91)

Adapted from Langerak SE, Vliegen HW, de Roos A, et al. Detection of vein graft disease using high-resolution magnetic resonance angiography. *Circulation* 2002;105(3):328–333, with permission.

SUMMARY

Over the past decade, coronary MRI has been transformed from a laboratory curiosity to a clinically useful imaging tool in selected populations—including the identification/ characterization of anomalous coronary arteries, serial assessment of children and young adults with coronary artery aneurysms, and the assessment of coronary artery bypass graft patency. Coronary MRI also appears to be clinically valuable for assessment of native vessel stenosis in selected patients, especially those patients presenting with a dilated cardiomyopathy/congestive heart failure with suspected left main/multivessel disease. A normal coronary MRI in this population strongly suggests a nonischemic cardiomyopathy.

REFERENCES

1. American Heart Association. *Heart disease and stroke statistics—2003 update.* Dallas, TX: 2003.
2. Budoff MJ, Georgiou D, Brody A, et al. Ultrafast computed tomography as a diagnostic modality in the detection of coronary artery disease: a multicenter study. *Circulation* 1996; 93(5):898–904.
3. Johnson LW, Lozner EC, Johnson S, et al. Coronary arteriography 1984–1987: a report of the Registry of the Society for Cardiac Angiography and Interventions. I. Results and complications. *Cathet Cardiovasc Diagn* 1989;17(1):5–10.
4. Davidson CJ, Mark DB, Pieper KS, et al. Thrombotic and cardiovascular complications related to nonionic contrast media during cardiac catheterization: analysis of 8,517 patients. *Am J Cardiol* 1990;65(22):1481–1484.
5. Omran H, Schmidt H, Hackenbroch M, et al. Silent and apparent cerebral embolism after retrograde catheterisation of the aortic valve in valvular stenosis: a prospective, randomised study. *Lancet* 2003;361(9365):1241–1246.
6. Kelle S, Hug J, Koehler U, et al. Potential intrinsic error of non-invasive coronary angiography. *J Cardiovasc Magn Reson* 2005;7(2):401–407.
7. Rizzo MJ, Moynihan J, Ryan K, et al. Distance from the ostium to the culprit coronary lesions: implications for new non-invasive coronary imaging techniques. *Circulation* 1997;96: I–306.
8. Paulin S, von Schulthess GK, Fossel E, et al. MR imaging of the aortic root and proximal coronary arteries. *Am J Roentgenol* 1987;148(4):665–670.
9. Lieberman JM, Botti RE, Nelson AD. Magnetic resonance imaging of the heart. *Radiol Clin North Am* 1984;22(4):847–858.
10. Edelman RR, Manning WJ, Burstein D, et al. Coronary arteries: breath-hold MR angiography. *Radiology* 1991;181(3): 641–643.
11. Pennell DJ, Keegan J, Firmin DN, et al. Magnetic resonance imaging of coronary arteries: technique and preliminary results. *Br Heart J* 1993;70(4):315–326.
12. Manning WJ, Li W, Boyle NG, et al. Fat-suppressed breath-hold magnetic resonance coronary angiography. *Circulation* 1993;87(1):94–104.
13. Duerinckx AJ, Urman MK. Two-dimensional coronary MR angiography: analysis of initial clinical results. *Radiology* 1994;193(3):731–738.
14. Sakuma H, Caputo GR, Steffens JC, et al. Breath-hold MR cine angiography of coronary arteries in healthy volunteers: value of multiangle oblique imaging planes. *Am J Roentgenol* 1994;163(3):533–537.
15. Masui T, Isoda H, Mochizuki T, et al. MR angiography of the coronary arteries. *Radiat Med* 1995;13(1):47–50.
16. Davis SF, Kannam JP, Wielopolski P, et al. Magnetic resonance coronary angiography in heart transplant recipients. *J Heart Lung Transplant* 1996;15(6):580–586.
17. Botnar RM, LT, Kissinger KV, et al. Improved motion compensation in coronary MRA [abstract]. *Proc Int Soc Magn Reson Med* 2004.
18. Scheidegger MB, Hess OM, Boesiger P. Validation of coronary artery MR angiography: comparison of measured vessel diameters with quantitative contrast angiography [abstract]. *Soc Magn Reson* 1994:497.
19. Weber OM, Martin AJ, Higgins CB. Whole-heart steady-state free precession coronary artery magnetic resonance angiography. *Magn Reson Med* 2003;50(6):1223–1228.
20. Botnar RM, Stuber M, Danias PG, et al. Improved coronary artery definition with T2-weighted, free-breathing, three-dimensional coronary MRA. *Circulation* 1999;99(24):3139–3148.
21. Stuber M, Botnar RM, Danias PG, et al. Double-oblique free-breathing high resolution three-dimensional coronary magnetic resonance angiography. *J Am Coll Cardiol* 1999;34(2): 524–531.
22. Engel HJ, Torres C, Page HL Jr. Major variations in anatomical origin of the coronary arteries: angiographic observations in 4,250 patients without associated congenital heart disease. *Cathet Cardiovasc Diagn* 1975;1(2):157–169.
23. Chaitman BR, Lesperance J, Saltiel J, et al. Clinical, angiographic, and hemodynamic findings in patients with anomalous origin of the coronary arteries. *Circulation* 1976;53(1):122–131.
24. Cheitlin MD, De Castro CM, McAllister HA. Sudden death as a complication of anomalous left coronary origin from the anterior sinus of Valsalva, a not-so-minor congenital anomaly. *Circulation* 1974;50(4):780–787.
25. Doorey AJ, Wills JS, Blasetto J, et al. Usefulness of magnetic resonance imaging for diagnosing an anomalous coronary artery coursing between aorta and pulmonary trunk. *Am J Cardiol* 1994;74(2):198–199.
26. Machado C, Bhasin S, Soulen RL. Confirmation of anomalous origin of the right coronary artery from the left sinus of Valsalva with magnetic resonance imaging. *Chest* 1993;104(4): 1284–1286.
27. McConnell MV, Ganz P, Selwyn AP, et al. Identification of anomalous coronary arteries and their anatomic course by magnetic resonance coronary angiography. *Circulation* 1995; 92(11):3158–3162.
28. Taylor AM, Thorne SA, Rubens MB, et al. Coronary artery imaging in grown up congenital heart disease: complementary role of magnetic resonance and x-ray coronary angiography. *Circulation* 2000;101(14):1670–1678.
29. Bunce NH, Lorenz CH, Keegan J, et al. Coronary artery anomalies: assessment with free-breathing three-dimensional coronary MR angiography. *Radiology* 2003;227(1):201–208.
30. Post JC, van Rossum AC, Bronzwaer JG, et al. Magnetic resonance angiography of anomalous coronary arteries. A new gold standard for delineating the proximal course? *Circulation* 1995;92(11):3163–3171.
31. Vliegen HW, Doornbos J, de Roos A, et al. Value of fast gradient echo magnetic resonance angiography as an adjunct to coronary arteriography in detecting and confirming the course of clinically significant coronary artery anomalies. *Am J Cardiol* 1997;79(6):773–776.
32. Razmi RM, Meduri A, Chun W, et al. Coronary magnetic resonance angiography (CMRA): the gold standard for determining the proximal course of anomalous coronary arteries [abstract]. *J Am Coll Cardiol* 2001;37:380.

33. Akagi T, Rose V, Benson LN, et al. Outcome of coronary artery aneurysms after Kawasaki disease. *J Pediatr* 1992;121(5 Pt 1):689–694.

34. Kato H, Ichinose E, Yoshioka F, et al. Fate of coronary aneurysms in Kawasaki disease: serial coronary angiography and long-term follow-up study. *Am J Cardiol* 1982;49(7): 1758–1766.

35. Greil GF, Stuber M, Botnar RM, et al. Coronary magnetic resonance angiography in adolescents and young adults with Kawasaki disease. *Circulation* 2002;105(8):908–911.

36. Mavrogeni S, Papadopoulos G, Douskou M, et al. Magnetic resonance angiography is equivalent to x-ray coronary angiography for the evaluation of coronary arteries in Kawasaki disease. *J Am Coll Cardiol* 2004;43(4):649–652.

37. Mavrogeni S, Manginas A, Papadakis E, et al. Correlation between magnetic resonance angiography (MRA) and quantitative coronary angiography (QCA) in ectatic coronary vessels. *J Cardiovasc Magn Reson* 2004;6:17–23.

38. Kim WY, Danias PG, Stuber M, et al. Coronary magnetic resonance angiography for the detection of coronary stenoses. *N Engl J Med* 2001;345(26):1863–1869.

39. Pennell DJ, Bogren HG, Keegan J, et al. Assessment of coronary artery stenosis by magnetic resonance imaging. *Heart* 1996;75(2):127–133.

40. Manning WJ, Li W, Edelman RR. A preliminary report comparing magnetic resonance coronary angiography with conventional angiography. *N Engl J Med* 1993;328(12):828–832.

41. Post JC, van Rossum AC, Hofman MB, et al. Clinical utility of two-dimensional magnetic resonance angiography in detecting coronary artery disease. *Eur Heart J* 1997;18(3):426–433.

42. Nitatori T, Yokoyama K, Hachiya J, et al. Comparison of 2D coronary MR angiography with conventional angiography—difference in imaging accuracy according to the severity of stenosis. *Asian Oceania J Radiol* 1998;3:15–19.

43. Post JC, van Rossum AC, Hofman MB, et al. Three-dimensional respiratory-gated MR angiography of coronary arteries: comparison with conventional coronary angiography. *Am J Roentgenol* 1996;166(6):1399–1404.

44. Woodard PK, Li D, Haacke EM, et al. Detection of coronary stenoses on source and projection images using three-dimensional MR angiography with retrospective respiratory gating: preliminary experience. *Am J Roentgenol* 1998;170(4): 883–888.

45. Muller MF, Fleisch M, Kroeker R, et al. Proximal coronary artery stenosis: three-dimensional MRI with fat saturation and navigator echo. *J Magn Reson Imaging* 1997;7(4):644–651.

46. van Geuns RJ, de Bruin HG, Rensing BJ, et al. Magnetic resonance imaging of the coronary arteries: clinical results from three dimensional evaluation of a respiratory gated technique. *Heart* 1999;82(4):515–519.

47. Huber A, Nikolaou K, Gonschior P, et al. Navigator echo-based respiratory gating for three-dimensional MR coronary angiography: results from healthy volunteers and patients with proximal coronary artery stenoses. *Am J Roentgenol* 1999; 173(1):95–101.

48. Sardanelli F, Molinari G, Zandrino F, et al. Three-dimensional, navigator-echo MR coronary angiography in detecting stenoses of the major epicardial vessels, with conventional coronary angiography as the standard of reference. *Radiology* 2000; 214(3):808–814.

49. Bunce N, Rahman S, Jhooti P, et al. The assessment of coronary artery disease by combined magnetic resonance coronary arteriography and perfusion [abstract]. *J Cardiovasc Magn Reson* 2001;3:118.

50. Moustapha AI, Proctor M, Muthupillai R, et al. Coronary magnetic resonance angiography using a free breathing, T2 weighted, three-dimensional gradient echo sequence with navigator respiratory and ECG gating can be used to detect coronary artery disease [abstract]. *J Am Coll Cardiol* 2001;37:380.

51. Sommer T, Hackenbroch M, Hofer U, et al. Submillimeter 3D coronary MR angiography with real-time navigator correction inn 112 patients with suspected coronary artery disease [abstract]. *J Cardiovasc Magn Reson* 2002;4:28.

52. Bogaert J, Kuzo R, Dymarkowski S, et al. Coronary artery imaging with real-time navigator three-dimensional turbo-field-echo MR coronary angiography: initial experience. *Radiology* 2003;226(3):707–716.

53. Plein S, Ridgway JP, Jones TR, et al. Coronary artery disease: assessment with a comprehensive MR imaging protocol—initial results. *Radiology* 2002;225(1):300–307.

54. Hauser TH, Yeon S, Appelbaum E, et al. Discrimination of ischemic vs. non-ischemic cardiomyopathy among patients with heart failure using combined coronary MRI and delayed enhancement MR. *J Cardiovasc Magn Reson* 2005;7:94.

55. Ichikawa Y, Sakuma H, Makino K, et al. Diagnostic accuracy of whole heart coronary magnetic resonance angiography for the detection of significant coronary stenoses in patients with suspected coronary artery disease. *J Cardiovasc Magn Reson* 2005;7:60.

56. Jahnke C, Paetsch I, Nehrke K, et al. Rapid and complete coronary arteries tree visualization with magnetic resonance imaging. *J Cardiovasc Magn Reson* 2005;7:221.

57. Cheng L, Guan Y, Guaricci A, et al. Manifestation of coronary stenoses on breath-hold steady state free precession sequences: retrospectively compared to conventional x-ray coronary angiography. *J Cardiovasc Magn Reson* 2005;7:117.

58. Maintz D, Aepfelbacher FC, Kissinger KV, et al. Coronary MR angiography: comparison of quantitative and qualitative data from four techniques. *Am J Roentgenol* 2004;182(2): 515–521.

59. Stuber M, Botnar RM, Danias PG, et al. Contrast agent-enhanced, free-breathing, three-dimensional coronary magnetic resonance angiography. *J Magn Reson Imaging* 1999; 10(5):790–799.

60. Herborn CU, Schmidt M, Bruder O, et al. MR coronary angiography with SH L 643 A: initial experience in patients with coronary artery disease. *Radiology* 2004;233(2):567–573.

61. Hackenbroch M, Meyer C, Schmiedel A, et al. Coronary MRA at 3.0 tesla compared to 1.5 tesla: initial results in patients with suspected coronary artery disease. *J Cardiovasc Magn Reson* 2005;7(1):6–7.

62. Syed MA, Murphy M, Arai AE. Safety of magnetic resonance imaging in the first few days after primary angioplasty/stenting for acute myocardial infarction. *Circulation* 2004;110:17.

63. Patel MR, Honeycutt E. Clinical safety of cardiac MRI prior to discharge in patients with acute myocardial infarction and coronary artery stenting with both bare metal and drug-eluting stents. *J Cardiovasc Magn Reson* 2005;7:50.

64. Strohm O, Kivelitz D, Gross W, et al. Safety of implantable coronary stents during 1H-magnetic resonance imaging at 1.0 and 1.5 T. *J Cardiovasc Magn Reson* 1999;1(3):239–245.

65. Kramer CM, Rogers WJ Jr, Pakstis DL. Absence of adverse outcomes after magnetic resonance imaging early after stent placement for acute myocardial infarction: a preliminary study. *J Cardiovasc Magn Reson* 2000;2(4):257–261.

66. Gerber TC, Fasseas P, Lennon RJ, et al. Clinical safety of magnetic resonance imaging early after coronary artery stent placement. *J Am Coll Cardiol* 2003;42(7):1295–1298.

67. Hug J, Nagel E, Bornstedt A, et al. Coronary arterial stents: safety and artifacts during MR imaging. *Radiology* 2000; 216(3):781–787.

68. Scott NA, Pettigrew RI. Absence of movement of coronary stents after placement in a magnetic resonance imaging field. *Am J Cardiol* 1994;73(12):900–901.

69. Shellock FG, Shellock VJ. Metallic stents: evaluation of MR imaging safety. *Am J Roentgenol* 1999;173(3):543–547.

70. Schmiedel A. MR imaging at 3.0 tesla and coronary artery stents. Ex vivo evaluation of magnetic attraction forces and heating [abstract]. *J Cardiovasc Magn Reson* 2003;5:17–18.

71. Spuentrup E, Ruebben A, Schaeffter T, et al. Magnetic resonance—guided coronary artery stent placement in a swine model. *Circulation* 2002;105(7):874–879.

72. Maintz D, Botnar RM, Fischbach R, et al. Coronary magnetic resonance angiography for assessment of the stent lumen: a phantom study. *J Cardiovasc Magn Reson* 2002;4(3):359–367.

73. Spuentrup E, Ruebben A, Mahnken AH, et al. Artifact-free coronary MR angiography and coronary vessel wall imaging in the presence of a new metallic coronary MRI stent. *Circulation,* 2005;111:1019–1026.

74. Goldman S, Copeland J, Moritz T, et al. Saphenous vein graft patency 1 year after coronary artery bypass surgery and effects of antiplatelet therapy. Results of a Veterans Administration Cooperative Study. *Circulation* 1989;80(5):1190–1197.

75. Fitzgibbon GM, Kafka HP, Leach AJ, et al. Coronary bypass graft fate and patient outcome: angiographic follow-up of 5,065 grafts related to survival and reoperation in 1,388 patients during 25 years. *J Am Coll Cardiol* 1996;28(3):616–626.

76. van Geuns RJ, Wielopolski PA, de Bruin HG, et al. MR coronary angiography with breath-hold targeted volumes: preliminary clinical results. *Radiology* 2000;217(1):270–277.

77. White RD, Caputo GR, Mark AS, et al. Coronary artery bypass graft patency: noninvasive evaluation with MR imaging. *Radiology* 1987;164(3):681–686.

78. White RD, Pflugfelder PW, Lipton MJ, et al. Coronary artery bypass grafts: evaluation of patency with cine MR imaging. *Am J Roentgenol* 1988;150(6):1271–1274.

79. Galjee MA, van Rossum AC, Doesburg T, et al. Value of magnetic resonance imaging in assessing patency and function of coronary artery bypass grafts. An angiographically controlled study. *Circulation* 1996;93(4):660–666.

80. Aurigemma GP, Reichek N, Axel L, et al. Noninvasive determination of coronary artery bypass graft patency by cine magnetic resonance imaging. *Circulation* 1989;80(6):1595–1602.

81. Engelmann MG, Knez A, von Smekal A, et al. Non-invasive coronary bypass graft imaging after multivessel revascularisation. *Int J Cardiol* 2000;76(1):65–74.

82. Molinari G, Sardanelli F, Zandrino F, et al. Value of navigator echo magnetic resonance angiography in detecting occlusion/patency of arterial and venous, single and sequential coronary bypass grafts. *Int J Card Imaging* 2000;16(3):149–160.

83. Vrachliotis TG, Bis KG, Aliabadi D, et al. Contrast-enhanced breath-hold MR angiography for evaluating patency of coronary artery bypass grafts. *Am J Roentgenol* 1997;168(4):1073–1080.

84. Wintersperger BJ, Engelmann MG, von Smekal A, et al. Patency of coronary bypass grafts: assessment with breath-hold contrast-enhanced MR angiography—value of a non-electro-cardiographically triggered technique. *Radiology* 1998;208(2):345–351.

85. Bunce NH, Lorenz CH, John AS, et al. Coronary artery bypass graft patency: assessment with true ast imaging with steady-state precession versus gadolinium-enhanced MR angiography. *Radiology* 2003;227(2):440–446.

86. Langerak SE, Kunz P, Vliegen HW, et al. MR flow mapping in coronary artery bypass grafts: a validation study with Doppler flow measurements. *Radiology* 2002;222(1):127–135.

87. Langerak SE, Vliegen HW, Jukema JW, et al. Value of magnetic resonance imaging for the noninvasive detection of stenosis in coronary artery bypass grafts and recipient coronary arteries. *Circulation* 2003;107(11):1502–1508.

88. Langerak SE, Vliegen HW, de Roos A, et al. Detection of vein graft disease using high-resolution magnetic resonance angiography. *Circulation* 2002;105(3):328–333.

89. Danias PG, McConnell MV, Khasgiwala VC, et al. Prospective navigator correction of image position for coronary MR angiography. *Radiology* 1997;203(3):733–736.

90. Rubinstein RI, Askenase AD, Thickman D, et al. Magnetic resonance imaging to evaluate patency of aortocoronary bypass grafts. *Circulation* 1987;76(4):786–791.

91. Li D, Paschal CB, Haacke EM, et al. Coronary arteries: three-dimensional MR imaging with fat saturation and magnetization transfer contrast. *Radiology* 1993;187(2):401–406.

92. Wielopolski PA, van Geuns RJ, de Feyter PJ, et al. Breath-hold coronary MR angiography with volume-targeted imaging. *Radiology* 1998;209(1):209–219.

93. Sandstede JJ, Pabst T, Beer M, et al. Three-dimensional MR coronary angiography using the navigator technique compared with conventional coronary angiography. *Am J Roentgenol* 1999;172(1):135–139.

94. Ozgun M, Hoffmeier A, Quante M, et al. Comparison of spoiled TFE and Balanced TFE coronary MR angiography [abstract]. *J Cardiovasc Magn Reson* 2004;6:268–269.

95. Jenkins JP, Love HG, Foster CJ, et al. Detection of coronary artery bypass graft patency as assessed by magnetic resonance imaging. *Br J Radiol* 1988;61(721):2–4.

20

Coronary Blood Flow Measurements

Hajime Sakuma and Charles B. Higgins

Selective coronary angiography has been used to evaluate coronary artery disease. However, an assessment of the anatomic severity of a coronary stenosis does not adequately determine the functional significance of the lesion (1,2). Quantitative coronary angiography, which was designed to minimize variability in interpretation, cannot reliably predict the physiologic significance of a stenosis of intermediate severity (3). An assessment of the functional significance of a stenosis is particularly important in lesions with intermediate severity because the interpretation of such lesions significantly influence therapeutic decisions in patients with coronary artery disease. The functional significance of a coronary arterial stenosis can be evaluated by measuring the coronary flow reserve, which is the ratio of maximal hyperemic coronary flow to the baseline coronary flow (4,5). In the presence of normal epicardial coronary artery and normal myocardial microcirculation, the adminis-

tration of a vasodilator (e.g., dipyridamole and adenosine) induces approximately a three- to fourfold increase in coronary blood flow. In patients with significant stenoses in the coronary arteries, however, compensatory dilatation takes place in the downstream microcirculation to maintain myocardial blood flow. Thus, the ability to augment coronary blood flow during pharmacologic stress is attenuated in patients with significant coronary arterial stenosis.

The evaluation of blood flow velocity and flow velocity reserve with an intracoronary Doppler guidewire allows a functional assessment of the severity of a stenosis. A study in which an intracoronary Doppler guidewire was used showed that the sensitivity, specificity, and overall predictive accuracy of the coronary flow velocity reserve were 94%, 95%, and 94%, respectively, when stress thallium-201 single-photon emission computed tomography was used as a gold standard (6). Another study demonstrated that a coronary flow velocity reserve below 2.0 by the Doppler technique had a sensitivity of 92% and specificity of 82% for predicting the presence of a significant stenosis in the coronary artery on selective coronary angiography (7). However, intracoronary flow velocity measurement with a Doppler guidewire is invasive and available only during cardiac catheterization.

Fast phase-contrast cine magnetic resonance imaging (MRI) is an emerging application of MRI that can provide noninvasive assessments of blood flow and flow reserve in human coronary arteries. Several studies have demonstrated the usefulness of this technique in detecting coronary arterial restenosis after percutaneous revascularization procedures and in assessing patency and stenosis in coronary artery bypass conduits. In addition, magnetic resonance (MR) measurement of the coronary sinus blood flow allows the noninvasive assessment of global myocardial blood flow. This chapter reviews the current status and potential clinical applications of MR measurements of blood flow and flow reserve in the coronary artery during coronary artery bypass grafting (CABG).

21

Cardiovascular Magnetic Resonance and Computed Tomography of Coronary Artery Bypass Grafts

Liesbeth P. Salm, Jeroen J. Bax, Joanne D. Schuijf, Hildo J. Lamb, J. Wouter Jukema,
Ernst E. van der Wall, and Albert de Roos

Coronary artery bypass grafting (CABG) is a commonly performed surgical procedure for alleviating symptoms and prolonging survival for patients with ischemic heart disease. Bypass graft disease is a common consequence, requiring x-ray coronary angiography for diagnosis. Coronary angiography is an invasive procedure that includes x-ray exposure, hospitalization, and a small risk of complications, including arrhythmias, coronary artery dissection, and cardiac death. A noninvasive diagnostic method for the assessment of bypass graft anatomy and function is of great benefit. This chapter reviews the research that has been performed in evaluating bypass grafts noninvasively using cardiovascular magnetic resonance (CMR) and computed tomography (CT).

CARDIOVASCULAR MAGNETIC RESONANCE OF CORONARY ARTERY BYPASS GRAFTS

ANATOMY ASSESSMENT: ANGIOGRAPHY

During the past decades, a considerable amount of effort has been invested to achieve noninvasive visualization of the coronary arteries and bypass grafts with MRI. The relatively larger size, straight course, and immobility during the cardiac cycle of coronary bypass grafts allowed the evaluation of graft patency even in the earliest studies, whereas assessment of the coronary arteries could not be achieved at that stage. In these initial investigations, two-dimensional (2D) spin-echo and gradient-echo techniques were applied to acquire successive axial slices during repetitive breath-holds (1–8). With the spin-echo technique, absence of signal at different levels was considered to indicate the presence of a patent graft because in normal grafts, rapid blood movement is present. To obtain adequate contrast, however, sufficient flow between the graft lumen and the wall is needed, whereas the presence of metallic clips, stents, or calcifications may result in a signal void that can be mistaken for graft stenosis or occlusion. In contrast, flowing blood is depicted as a bright signal during imaging with gradient MR techniques. As shown in Table 21.1, both acquisition techniques have been evaluated in several studies with conventional angiography as the standard of reference, demonstrating sensitivities and specificities varying from 71% to 100%

TABLE 21-1 Detection of Occlusion in Vein and Arterial Grafts by Magnetic Resonance Angiography Compared with Invasive Angiography

Author	Patients	Grafts	Graft Type	Magnetic Resonance Technique	Assessable Grafts (%)	Sensitivity (%)	Specificity (%)
White et al (4)	25	72	Vein	2-D SE	90	72	91
Rubinstein et al (6)	20	47	Vein	2-D SE	100	72	90
Jenkins et al (3)	22	45	Vein	2-D SE	100	73	89
Frija et al (2)	28	52	Vein and arterial	2-D SE	100	71	97
White el at (5)	10	28	Vein and arterial	2-D GE	100	86	93
Aurigemma et al (1)	20	45	Vein and arterial	2-D GE	100	100	88
Vanninen et al (7)	8	8	GEA	2-D GE	100	100	100
Galjee et al (8)	47	84	Vein	2-D SE	92	84	98
				2-D GE	92	88	98
Weighted Mean 2D					95	81	94
Kessler et al (11)	8	21	Vein and arterial	3-D NAV	90	100	87
Engelmann et al (9)	16	55	Vein and arterial	3-D CE	100	85	95
Vrachliotis et al (14)	15	45	Vein and arterial	3-D CE	98	93	97
Wintersperger et al (15)	27	76	Vein and arterial	3-D CE	100	81	95
Kalden et al (10)	22	59	Vein and arterial	3-D CE	100	93	93
Molinari et al (13)	18	51	Vein and arterial	3-D NAV	96	92	97
Langerak et al (12)	38	56	Vein	3-D NAV	100	83	98
Wittlinger et al (16)	34	82	Vein and arterial	3-D NAV	90	78	96
Bunce et al (17)	34	79	Vein and arterial	3-D CE	100	73	85
Weighted Mean 3D					96	85	94

CE, contrast-enhanced; GE, gradient-echo; GEA, gastroepiploic artery; HASTE, half-Fourier acquisition single-shot turbo spin-echo; NAV, navigator; SE, spin-echo; SSFP, steady state free precession.

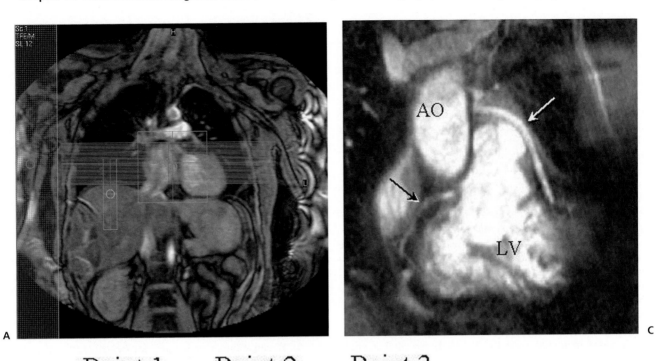

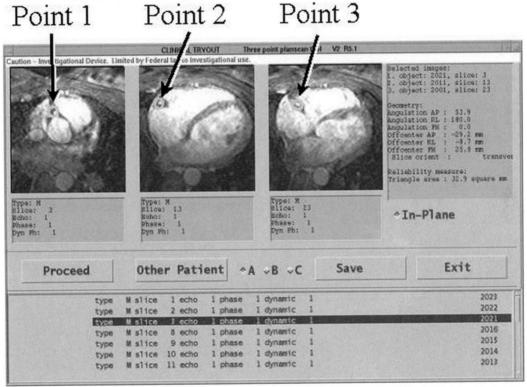

Figure 21.1. Typical magnetic resonance (MR) acquisition protocol. **(A)** Typical plan-scan for cardiovascular magnetic resonance (CMR) angiography. Axial imaging volume (*horizontal lines*); volume used for localized shimming (*large box*); position in the right hemidiaphragm of the respiratory navigator (*rectangular box*); position of a saturation band for suppression of image artifacts (*left box*). **(B)** With the use of axial scout images, the three-point plan-scan is used to select three points in space, one at the origin of the coronary artery or bypass graft, one at the most distal point, and one in the middle of the first two points. From this information, an imaging plane is automatically calculated in plane with the coronary artery or bypass graft of interest. **(C)** CMR angiography of a patient with a bypass of the left coronary system (*white arrow*) and a visible native right coronary artery (*black arrow*). This imaging approach can be used clinically to assess bypass graft patency. AO, aorta; LV, left ventricle. (Courtesy of H.J. Lamb.)

and 89% to 100%, respectively. Pooled analysis of these eight studies (with 180 patients and 381 grafts) revealed a weighted mean sensitivity and specificity of 81% and 94%, with inclusion of 95% of grafts. Despite these promising results in the distinction between patent and occluded grafts, these 2D techniques were still limited by their low signal-to-noise ratio and low spatial resolution. Substantial progress in image quality was achieved by the development of three dimensional (3D) imaging techniques, allowing the acquisition of volume slabs containing several thin slices and imaging with high spatial resolution. To improve patient comfort, navigator techniques have been developed that permit real-time monitoring of diaphragm motion and thus free-breathing during data acquisition. In addition, improved enhancement of blood/muscle contrast can be expected by the administration of intravascular contrast agents. An example of a typical MR acquisition protocol with navigator respiratory gating is depicted in Figure 21.1. In Figure 21.2 a resulting 3D reconstruction is shown, and an example of a patent bypass graft as confirmed by conventional angiography is provided in Figure 21.3.

Pooled analysis of nine studies using 3D techniques, with more than 200 patients included, revealed a slight increase in weighted sensitivity from 81% to 85%, with no loss in specificity (Fig. 21.4) (9–17). Sensitivity and specificity for the different types of grafts (as reported in seven studies) are shown in Figure 21.5. No difference in diagnostic accuracy for detection of graft occlusion was noted between arterial and venous grafts. In particular, the sensitivity and specificity of arterial grafts were 85% and 95% compared with 86% and 93% in venous grafts (9,10,12–14,16,17). These studies illustrate the potential of MRI to evaluate graft patency in clinical routine. Its safe and noninvasive nature in combination with the high specificity (~94%) and negative predictive value (~96%) suggests that in patients presenting with recurrent symptoms after bypass grafting, MRI may function as a first-line investigation tool to rule out graft occlusion before more invasive diagnostic procedures.

However, few attempts thus far have been made to evaluate graft stenosis in addition to assessment of patency. Langerak and colleagues observed a sensitivity and specificity of 82% and 88% for the detection of ≥50% luminal narrowing in venous bypass grafts (12). In contrast, a discouraging sensitivity of 38% was reported by Kalden et al (10). Because the presence of graft stenosis rather than total

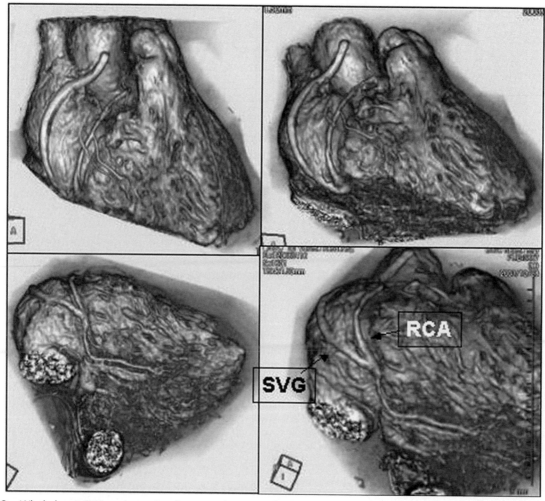

Figure 21.2.   Whole-heart CMR angiography of a venous bypass graft to the right coronary artery at different rotation angles. (Courtesy of Dr. H. Sakuma.)

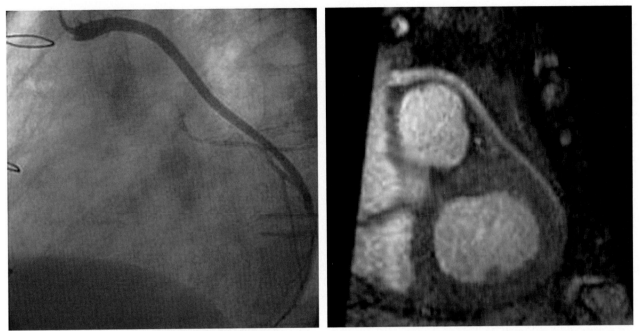

Figure 21.3. MR angiogram of a vein graft (*right*) in comparison with a coronary angiogram (*left*). Multiplanar reformat reconstruction of a free-breathing, three-dimensional (3D), navigator-gated sequence used for acquisition of the MR angiogram.

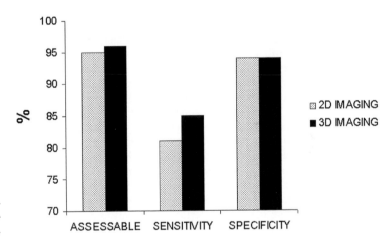

Figure 21.4. Sensitivities and specificities of two-dimensional (2D) and 3D MR angiography (MRA) acquisition techniques (data based on references 1–17).

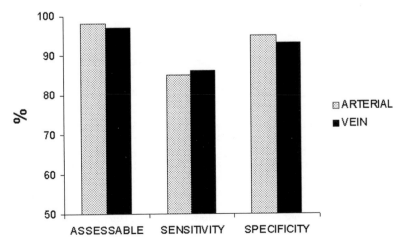

Figure 21.5. Performance of 3D MRA in arterial and vein grafts (data based on references 9,10, 12–14,16,17).

occlusion of the graft may be the cause of recurrent complaints, the value of MR angiography (MRA) to evaluate graft stenosis needs to be further explored before routine use of the technique is feasible. In addition, recurrent anginal complaints may also be attributable to progression of coronary artery disease in native coronary vessels, and assessment in these vessels is still severely hampered by the current spatial and temporal resolution. A possible solution to this limitation may lie in the combination of MRA with MR flow mapping, because the latter provides a functional measurement of the entire vascular tree beyond the level of the flow measurement. Moreover, because the functional graft status is not directly related to the degree of luminal narrowing, improved diagnostic accuracy and management may be expected by such a combined approach.

FUNCTIONAL ASSESSMENT: FLOW VELOCITY

A vessel narrowing, visualized by means of angiography, may or may not impair flow through that vessel (18,19). The assessment of blood flow through coronary arteries and bypass grafts has gained wide attention. To evaluate the hemodynamic impairment of a lesion, flow is measured at rest and during pharmacologically induced stress, for instance, with adenosine or dipyridamole (20). By dividing the flow value during stress by the flow value at rest, the coronary flow reserve (CFR) is calculated (21,22). Flow-limiting stenoses cause a compensatory vasodilatation at rest to maintain sufficient blood flow to the myocardium. As a consequence, the vessel cannot respond adequately to an increase in absolute blood flow by vasodilatation during pharmacologically induced stress, and CFR will be reduced. At first, blood flow was determined by means of Doppler flow transducers at open-chest procedures (18,21–25), limiting extensive use of CFR in clinical practice. When the diameter of intravascular catheter-based Doppler ultrasonographic devices could be reduced to 0.018 inch, it became feasible to measure the velocity of the blood flow and calculate the coronary flow velocity reserve (CFVR) for coronary arteries in patients during catheterization. Blood flow correlated well with Doppler-derived velocity of blood flow both in vitro and in vivo (26–28). Invasive Doppler-derived CFVR has proven its potential in numerous clinical applications, such as in identifying hemodynamic significant stenoses in native coronary arteries and vein grafts (29,30), in the functional assessment of stenoses of intermediate severity (31), in the determination of the need for and the outcome after coronary intervention (32–34), and in the prediction of restenosis (35).

With the use of MR, blood flow velocity can be measured using phase-contrast, velocity-encoded sequences (36). To use such a sequence accurately, an imaging plane perpendicular to the target vessel has to be selected by means of survey images. Throughout the cardiac cycle, the acquisition yields anatomic modulus images, paired with phase images, in which every pixel contains a different velocity value. Volume flow (in milliliters/min) can be obtained by calculating the integrated volumetric flow rate of all pixels in the vessel lumen per heartbeat and multiply it with the heart rate. To display the flow pattern, a flow rate-versus-time graph can be presented. Alternatively, the central peak velocity (in centimeters per second) can be obtained by selecting several pixels in the vessel center. Figure 21.6 depicts a typical example of an MR velocity mapping examination in a vein graft.

Early Magnetic Resonance Studies in Vein Grafts

For vein grafts, feasibility to quantify flow and characterize the flow pattern noninvasively by MR was demonstrated

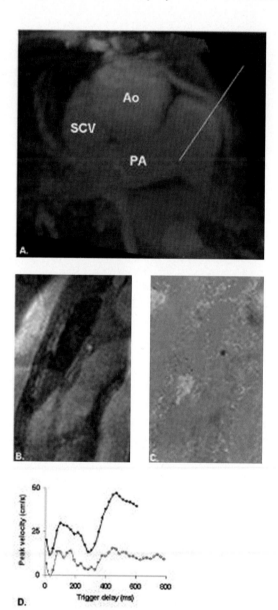

Figure 21.6. MR flow velocity study. Survey image visualizing a vein graft in plane **(A)**. A plane perpendicular to the graft is selected, and modulus and phase images are acquired **(B,C)**. The graft is pictured as a white (black) spot in the center of the image. In every image in the cardiac cycle 4 pixels in the center of the graft are selected to obtain a velocity curve **(D)**. The MR flow velocity acquisition is repeated during adenosine-induced stress to obtain the stress velocity curve (*black graph*). Ao, aorta; PA, pulmonary artery; SCV, supracaval vein.

(37,38). To establish feasibility, an attempt to measure flow in 49 vein grafts with ≤50% luminal stenosis at coronary angiography in 27 patients was made (38). In 84% of grafts, flow could be measured adequately. In another early study, 23 vein grafts in 18 patients were studied to distinguish normal from dysfunctional grafts by MR with flow mapping plus coronary angiography as the gold standard (39). They found that graft flow <20 mL/min and a loss of the biphasic flow pattern, typical for bypass grafts, would indicate a dysfunctional graft. In addition to comparing spin-echo with cine gradient-echo MR assessment of vein graft patency, Galjee et al (40) investigated vein graft function by phase-velocity imaging. In 62 of the 73 angiographically patent grafts (85%), adequate biphasic flow profiles could be obtained. A significant difference in flow between single grafts and sequential grafts to three vascular regions was demonstrated. These early vein graft flow studies were limited by the use of a gradient-echo sequence with limited spatial resolution ($1.9 \times 1.2 \times 5$ mm^3) and no compensation for respiratory motion on 0.5 to 0.6 Tesla (T) magnets.

Early Magnetic Resonance Studies in Arterial Grafts

Feasibility to quantify flow in native and grafted internal mammary arteries (IMAs) was demonstrated in 10 volunteers and 15 patients using a free-breathing gradient-echo sequence on a 1.5 T MR scanner (41). Patients had recently undergone IMA grafting; no control angiography of the arterial grafts was performed. A large intersubject variation of IMA graft flow (range 28–164 mL/min) was observed. Mean flow and peak velocity were lower in IMA grafts compared with native IMAs. In a different feasibility study, respiratory motion was compensated using a breath-hold segmented k-space gradient-echo sequence to quantify velocity in native and grafted IMAs (42). IMA grafts were investigated within 6 months after CABG; no control angiography was available. Comparison with a free-breathing technique in native IMAs demonstrated a higher peak velocity using the breath-hold sequence because of elimination of respiratory motion artifacts and averaging of velocities. This sequence allowed imaging time to decrease from approximately 4 minutes at free-breathing to a 20-s breath-hold. By means of a view-sharing reconstruction, an effective temporal resolution of 64 ms could be maintained, allowing an acquisition of 7 to 13 temporal phases in a cardiac cycle.

Angiographically Controlled Magnetic Resonance Studies in Vein and Arterial Grafts

To evaluate the diagnostic value of MR flow velocity in bypass grafts, several angiographically controlled studies were performed. In addition to investigating the accuracy of contrast-enhanced MRA in the evaluation of bypass grafts postoperatively, Brenner et al (43) performed additional MR velocity mapping of the grafts. Only 65% of the 247 obtained MR velocity images could be evaluated

because of metal clip artifacts in IMA grafts. Concerning the MR velocity measurements, they concluded that this technique was not qualified for the detection of bypass graft stenoses.

With the use of breath-hold sequences, flow measurements at rest and during pharmacologically induced stress with determination of CFR in bypass grafts could be achieved. Langerak et al (44) validated a breath-hold turbo-field echo-planar imaging sequence by demonstrating a good correlation with a free-breathing technique for aortic and native IMA flow in volunteers. This sequence was subsequently used to measure flow at rest and during adenosine-induced stress in 2 arterial and 18 vein grafts, which were patent at coronary angiography. A significant increase at adenosine-induced stress for flow and velocity parameters was observed, and CFR (mean 2.7 ± 1.1 for single grafts) could be calculated. In another study, MR-derived velocity measurements correlated well with invasive Doppler-derived velocity measurements in 27 grafts (26 veins/1 arterial graft) (45). A significant difference between grafts with <50% stenosis and ≥50% stenosis was demonstrated for MR-derived average peak velocity during adenosine-induced stress (20.2 ± 0.4 vs. 12.2 ± 0.4 cm/s) and diastolic peak velocity during adenosine-induced stress (35.3 ± 0.3 vs. 25.6 ± 0.3 cm/s). Measurements obtained at rest did not show a significant difference between grafts with <50% stenosis and ≥50% stenosis. The detection of ≥70% angiographic stenosis in IMA grafts by breath-hold MR flow velocity at rest and during dipyridamole-induced stress was investigated (46). In 24 early postoperative patients, successful MR flow measurements were performed in the mid-IMA graft. At CABG surgery, titanium clips were used to avoid metal artifacts at MR imaging. A significant difference between grafts with <70% and ≥70% stenosis was demonstrated for baseline mean blood flow (79.8 ± 38.2 mL/min vs. 16.9 ± 5.5 m/min) and the diastolic-to-systolic velocity ratio (1.88 ± 0.96 vs. 0.61 ± 0.44). Threshold values of 35 mL/min for baseline mean flow and 1.0 for diastolic-to-systolic velocity ratio was proposed to separate IMA grafts with <70% and ≥70% stenosis. Respective sensitivity and specificity were 86% (95% confidence interval [CI]: 49.5%–98.7%) and 94% (95% CI: 79.2%–99.5%) for the threshold value of baseline mean flow, and 86% (95% CI: 48.6%–99.2%) and 88% (95% CI: 72.9%–93.8%) for the threshold value of diastolic-to-systolic velocity ratio. CFR did not differ significantly between IMA grafts with <70% and ≥70% stenosis.

The value of MR flow in the prediction of vein graft disease was assessed (47). Forty vein grafts in 21 patients were examined by contrast-enhanced MRA and breath-hold gradient-echo MR flow at rest and during adenosine-induced stress and coronary angiography. An algorithm was formulated combining baseline flow <20 mL/min or CFR <2 to detect grafts or runoffs with a significant stenosis (≥50%) or a myocardial infarction in the graft vascular territory, yielding a sensitivity of 78% with a specificity of 80%. The algorithm was designed to exclude normal-functioning vein grafts from further invasive examinations. A different approach for the detection of stenotic vein and arterial grafts or recipient vessels by MR with velocity mapping was also developed (48). In this study,

166 grafts were examined by breath-hold MR velocity at rest and during adenosine-induced stress, controlled by coronary angiography. In 80% of grafts, full MR examination was successful. Single and sequential vein and arterial grafts were separately analyzed. Marginal logistic regression was used to predict the probability for the presence of ≥50% or ≥70% stenosis per graft type using multiple MR velocity parameters, including CFVR. Sensitivity and specificity for detecting single vein grafts or recipient vessels with ≥50% and ≥70% stenosis were 94% (95% CI: 86%–100%) and 63% (95% CI: 48%–79%), and 96% (95% CI: 87%–100%) and 92% (95% CI: 84%–100%), respectively; for detecting ≥50% and ≥70% stenosis in sequential vein grafts these values were 91% (95% CI: 78%–100%) and 82% (95% CI: 64%–100%), and 94% (95% CI: 83%–100%) and 71% (95% CI: 52%–91%), respectively. A proposed cutoff point for separating <70% and ≥70% stenosis in single vein grafts was 1.43 for CFVR. Not enough stenoses in arterial grafts were present to formulate an adequate logistic regression model for those grafts.

These studies show that MR flow velocity assessment has high potential to become a valuable, diagnostic tool in predicting patency and even the presence or absence of a significant stenosis in both vein and IMA grafts in clinical practice. Future studies should focus on an integration of bypass graft and native coronary artery MR flow velocity assessment, by which an absence of significant stenosis can be predicted with high accuracy to avoid unnecessary invasive coronary angiographic examinations.

Applied Studies Using Magnetic Resonance Flow Velocity in Bypass Grafts

Some studies were conducted using MR flow velocity as a tool to evaluate a certain procedure (surgical or percutaneous intervention) or noninvasive modality. Miller et al (49) used a comprehensive approach of breath-hold contrast-enhanced MRA, non-breath-hold MR flow quantification at rest, and MR cardiac function assessment to evaluate the status of IMA grafts after minimally invasive direct CABG surgery. The protocol was successfully completed in six patients postoperatively. Patency of the grafts was accurately assessed by this MR approach, compared with coronary angiography. To evaluate the value of color-Doppler echography and MRA with navigator-gated flow measurements to assess bypass graft patency postoperatively, a comparison with intraoperative flow measurements was performed (50). Only IMA grafts could be evaluated with color Doppler. They found that both modalities were useful to assess IMA graft patency after surgery, but MR flow measurements had the best correlation with intraoperative flow measurements. In one study, the success of percutaneous interventions in 15 veins was evaluated by breath-hold MR flow, and reference values for rest and adenosine-stress MR flow and velocity parameters were formulated using data of 39 single and 20 sequential vein grafts with <50% stenosis (51). Significant improvements by MR flow after a percutaneous intervention were observed for baseline (before, 9.2 ± 6.6 cm/s; after, 12.9 ± 7.9 cm/s) and adenosine-induced stress (before, 12.9

± 6.3 cm/s; after, 27.1 ± 13.9 cm/s) mean velocity. CFVR did not significantly improve after an intervention (before, 2.4 ± 1.4; after, 2.6 ± 0.9) as a result of an equal recovery of both baseline and stress mean velocity. Reference values confirmed a significant difference between single and sequential vein graft values, underscoring the need to evaluate these grafts separately. Because a MR velocity map can be analyzed to evaluate both flow and velocity, the diagnostic accuracy of the flow and velocity analysis approach was investigated using velocity maps of 80 single vein grafts (52). A similar diagnostic accuracy was demonstrated for the flow (92%) and velocity analysis (93%) in the detection of ≥70% stenosis. Velocity analysis seemed to be the preferred method, because it is less time-consuming compared with flow analysis.

The functional significance of a bypass graft stenosis was evaluated by single-photon emission computed tomography (SPECT), breath-hold MR velocity at rest and during adenosine-induced stress, and coronary angiography (53). In 18 of 20 grafts (90%) with a normal myocardial perfusion as determined by SPECT, preserved CFVR (≥2.0) was observed, whereas a reduced CFVR was noted in 19 of 26 grafts (69%) with abnormal perfusion on SPECT. Accordingly, agreement between SPECT perfusion imaging and MR velocity assessment was 80% (κ = 0.61). In relation to invasive coronary angiography the following was observed: In grafts with a stenosis <50% and normal perfusion on SPECT, normal CFVR was observed in 86%, whereas reduced CFVR was observed in 78% of grafts with a stenosis ≥50% and abnormal perfusion. All grafts with a stenosis ≥50% and normal perfusion, suggesting no hemodynamic significance of the stenosis, had normal CFVR. Finally, reduced CFVR was observed in 33% of grafts with a stenosis <50% and abnormal perfusion (suggestive of microvascular disease).

FUNCTIONAL ASSESSMENT: LEFT VENTRICULAR FUNCTION, CONTRAST-ENHANCEMENT, VIABILITY

Few studies have been performed evaluating patients after CABG surgery by a functional MR examination. In one study, global and regional left ventricular (LV) function by 3D MR served as the gold standard for the assessment of LV function by 99m-technetium-sestamibi gated SPECT in patients post-CABG surgery (54). After cardiac surgery, exaggerated systolic anteromedial translation of the entire heart within the chest has been observed, enhancing difficulties in assessing regional wall motion (especially in the septum). They demonstrated that an automated software algorithm (55,56) for the assessment of LV function by SPECT agreed well compared with MR functional assessment in this particular group of patients.

Several studies focused on evaluating myocardial injury by contrast-enhanced MR during off-pump and on-pump CABG surgery. Conventional on-pump surgery uses a cardiopulmonary bypass and aortic cross-clamping, which may lead to a systemic inflammatory response syndrome with multiorgan dysfunction (57) and myocardial damage as the result of ischemia (58). Selvanayagam et al (59) randomized 60 patients to either off-pump or on-pump CABG surgery and examined those patients before and after surgery by contrast-enhanced MR. Troponin I measurements were also obtained, which correlated with mean mass of new myocardial hyperenhancement. The authors found that off-pump CABG resulted in a significantly better LV function early after surgery; however, it did not reduce the incidence or extent of irreversible myocardial injury. Correlation of elevated biochemical markers (creatinine kinase-MB, troponin I and T) after CABG with the amount of perioperatively infarcted myocardium was confirmed in another study (60). A 6-month follow-up, contrast-enhanced MR examination was then performed in the same patient group to assess the diagnostic value of MR contrast enhancement in predicting viability, and to assess late regional wall motion recovery (61). A strong correlation between the transmural extent of hyperenhancement and regional function recovery at 6 months was demonstrated, revealing contrast-enhanced MR as a powerful predictor of myocardial damage after CABG surgery.

COMPUTED TOMOGRAPHY OF CORONARY ARTERY BYPASS GRAFTS

CT has been intensively investigated in its ability and value to visualize bypass grafts noninvasively. Early studies were using conventional CT scanners to assess bypass graft patency postoperatively, in comparison with coronary angiography. Repeated axial images were acquired at multiple levels of the graft. If the contrast agent was able to visualize the graft at two levels at least, a graft was scored as patent (62,63). This technique required an intravenous bolus of 20 to 50 mL contrast agent per image and therefore burdened the patient with a relatively large quantity of x-ray radiation. Then, CT scanners could be programmed to acquire multiple axial images after one bolus injection of contrast agent (dynamic scanning), allowing faster acquisition of images (64–70). Scans could be repeated after a 1- to 4-s interval, and per bolus injection four to six sequenced scans could be obtained. Diagnostic accuracy for this technique to detect bypass graft patency ranged from 45% to 95%. Ultrafast CT scanning allowed acquisition of one axial image in 50 ms, and repeating of scans after 8 ms (71–73). Total image acquisition time was 10 to 30 heartbeats, using electrocardiograph (ECG) triggering. Sensitivity to detect bypass graft patency using this technique was 93% to 96%, with a specificity of 89% to 100%. With spiral CT scanning the complete heart could be scanned in one breath-hold acquisition of 24 to 30 s (9,74–76). Optimal in-plane spatial resolution using this technique was 0.29 mm^2. Reported diagnostic accuracy for the detection of graft patency was 96% for vein grafts and 88% for arterial grafts (76). Then, it became feasible to use four detectors in a single spiral CT acquisition, allowing detection of graft patency with very high accuracy: 98% to 100% for vein grafts and 97% to 100% for arterial grafts (77–83).

Another approach in assessing bypass graft patency is to estimate the graft blood flow. The contrast clearance curve of a contrast bolus injection is evaluated by cine CT (84). This technique was tested in patients, showing a good agreement with observations at coronary angiography ($\kappa = 0.75$) (85).

In addition to assessment of bypass graft patency, the extent of graft disease may be evaluated by CT. With four-detector row CT technology, adequate stenosis assessment of all grafts was prevented by motion artifacts, metal clip artifacts, or beam hardening from calcium deposits (81–83). Table 21.2 shows the percentage of graft segments that could be analyzed and the sensitivity, specificity, and diagnostic accuracy in detecting significant stenoses in patent bypass grafts. Bypass grafts have been examined by 16-detector row spiral CT, allowing a scanning range of the proximal IMA insertion to the heart apex. By using retrospective ECG gating and a segmental reconstruction algorithm, images with an in-plane spatial resolution of up to 0.35 mm^2 can be acquired in a single breath-hold (86,87). In Figure 21.7, a typical 16-slice multislice computed tomography (MSCT) protocol is explained, whereas the different image displays that are available for evaluation of the MSCT angiograms are shown in Figure 21.8.

In comparison with coronary angiography, the 16-detector row CT technique was demonstrated to detect bypass

| TABLE 21-2 | Accuracy of Multislice Spiral Computed Tomography in the Detection of Significant Stenoses ($\geq$50% Luminal Narrowing) in Bypass Grafts, Controlled by Coronary Angiography |

Author	Number of Patients	Number of Grafts	Graft Type	Assessable Grafts (%)	Sensitivity (%)	Specificity (%)
Ropers et al (83)	65	124	Vein and arterial	62	75	92
Nieman et al (82)	24	39	Vein	95	83	90
Marano et al (81)	57	92	Vein and arterial	67	80	96
Martuscelli et al (89)	96	278	Vein and arterial	88	90	100
Salm et al (92)	25	67	Vein and arterial	–	100	95
Weighted Mean		600		80	84	95

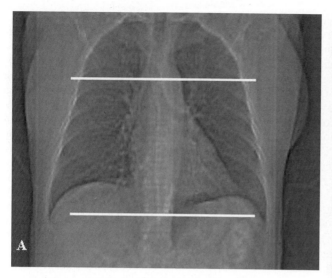

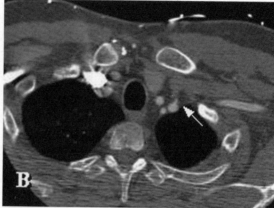

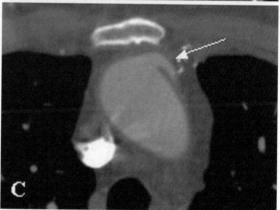

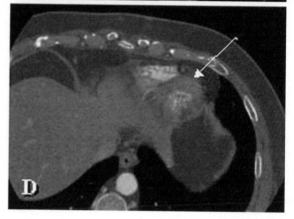

Figure 21.7. Typical 16-slice multislice computed tomography (MSCT) acquisition protocol. **(A)** Typical coronary computed tomographic angiography (CTA) protocol starts with correct supine patient positioning, positioning of intravenous line, placement of three electrocardiograph (ECG) leads, and patient instruction concerning breath-holding. First, a scanogram for overview is acquired **(A)**. Approximate cranial and caudal imaging margins (*white lines*) to acquire a second noncontrast localizer with prospective ECG triggering (30–40 slices, 3-mm slice thickness, 120 kV at 200 mA). **(B)** On the basis of the second localizer, the exact cranial and caudal margins are defined. These margins are depending on the clinical setting, for example, for CTA of arterial graft, such as the left internal mammary artery (IMA) graft, a higher cranial slice is needed **(B**, *arrow*) than for CTA of venous grafts **(C**, *arrow*). The actual contrast-enhanced helical acquisition should be planned from 1 cm above the defined cranial margin to 1 cm below the caudal margin (i.e., the apex of the heart) **(D**, *arrow*). **(C)** For optimal timing of the contrast arrival in the coronary arteries and bypass grafts, automated bolus tracking is applied by placement of a region of interest in the ascending aorta (*continues*).

graft stenosis of 50% to 100% with a sensitivity of 96% and specificity of 95% (88). In another study, ≥50% angiographic stenoses in patent grafts were detected with a sensitivity of 90% with a specificity of 100% (89). Diagnostic accuracy to detect graft patency was 100%.

Multidetector row CT was used to preoperatively assess the surgical site before totally endoscopic CABG, and the results were correlated with findings at coronary angiography and during surgery (90). Multidetector row CT demonstrated extended information about the coronary target site and is recommended as a planning tool before complex cardiac surgery, such as endoscopic bypass grafting or minimally invasive direct CABG.

Retrospective ECG gating allows reconstruction of CT images at 0% to 90% during the cardiac cycle. The best reconstruction interval to view CABGs anastomosed to the right coronary artery and branches was shown to be at 50%, whereas grafts anastomosed to the left anterior descending or circumflex artery (or branches) were best viewed at 60% to 70% of the cardiac cycle (91).

As illustrated in Figure 21.9, multidetector row CT technology allows a very accurate evaluation of vein and arterial bypass graft patency. Also, significant stenosis in bypass grafts may be assessed by MDCT. CT technology is rapidly evolving, with 32- and 64-detector row technology being readily available. A simultaneous assessment of native coronary arteries, CABGs, and recipient vessels noninvasively by MDCT may soon be a part of daily clinical practice.

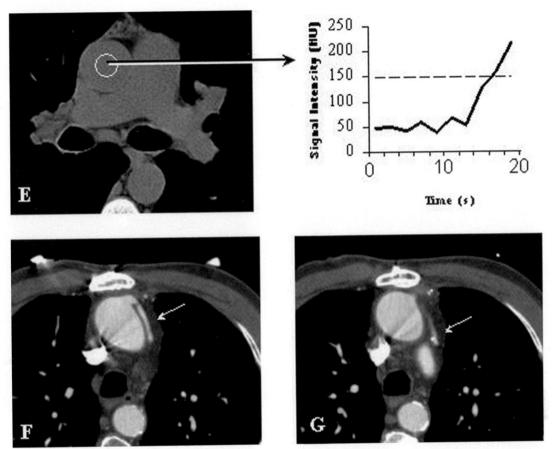

Figure 21.7. (*continued*) **(E)** After the signal intensity reaches a predefined threshold (see graph), the final CTA scan starts automatically. Two levels are shown from the resulting CTA of a venous coronary artery bypass graft (CABG) (**F,G**, *arrows*). CTA was performed with retrospective ECG gating (0.5-mm slice thickness, 120 kV at 250 mA, pitch and rotation time depending on heart rate).

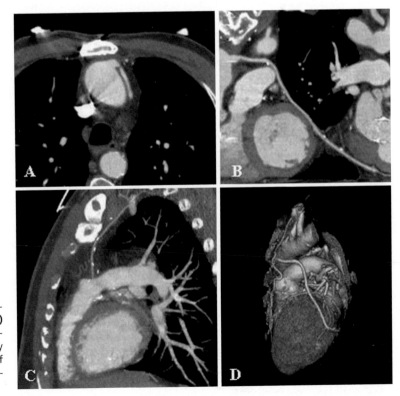

Figure 21.8. For the evaluation of MSCT angiograms, several imaging displays can be used. **(A)** Original axial slice. **(B)** Curved multiplanar reconstruction of a venous graft. **(C)** Maximum intensity projection of an arterial graft. **(D)** For an overview of the coronary arteries and bypass grafts, 3D volume-rendered reconstructions can be useful.

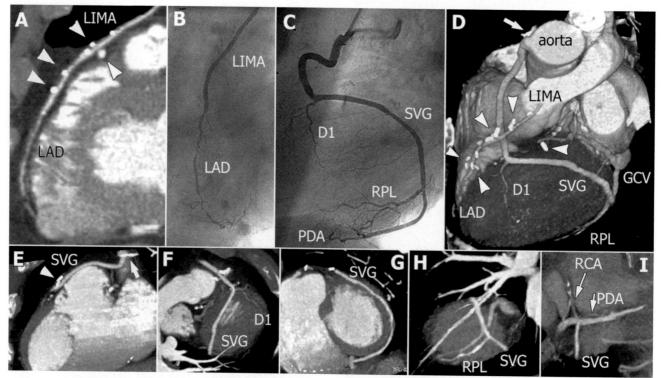

Figure 21.9. Arterial and venous bypass grafts. Images obtained with contrast-enhanced multidetector row CT angiography (**A,E–I,** maximum intensity projections; **D,** 3D volume rendering) and corresponding conventional angiography (**B,C**) show a left IMA graft (LIMA) connected to the left anterior descending coronary artery (LAD). Saphenous vein graft (SVG) runs from the aorta to the diagonal branch (*D1*), with consecutive jumps to the posterolateral branch (RPL) and posterior descending coronary artery (PDA). Surgical clips (*arrowheads*) and bypass indicator (*arrow* in **D,E**) appear as bright structures. Location of labeled right coronary and posterior descending coronary arteries (*arrows* in **I**). GCV, great cardiac vein; RCA, right coronary artery. (Reproduced with permission from *Radiology*.)

SUMMARY

CMR and CT have made rapid progress in the last two decades in detecting patency/occlusion and eventually stenoses in CABG. Other applications of CMR and CT include pre- and postoperative assessment of the CABG procedure. Future studies should focus on integrating assessment of native coronary arteries and bypass grafts as a full noninvasive evaluation before coronary angiography.

REFERENCES

1. Aurigemma GP, Reichek N, Axel L, et al. Noninvasive determination of coronary artery bypass graft patency by cine magnetic resonance imaging. *Circulation* 1989;80(6):1595–1602.
2. Frija G, Schouman-Claeys E, Lacombe P, et al. A study of coronary artery bypass graft patency using MR imaging. *J Comput Assist Tomogr* 1989;13(2):226–232.
3. Jenkins JP, Love HG, Foster CJ, et al. Detection of coronary artery bypass graft patency as assessed by magnetic resonance imaging. *Br J Radiol* 1988;61(721):2–4.
4. White RD, Caputo GR, Mark AS, et al. Coronary artery bypass graft patency: noninvasive evaluation with MR imaging. *Radiology* 1987;164(3):681–686.
5. White RD, Pflugfelder PW, Lipton MJ, et al. Coronary artery bypass grafts: evaluation of patency with cine MR imaging. *AJR Am J Roentgenol* 1988;150(6):1271–1274.
6. Rubinstein RI, Askenase AD, Thickman D, et al. Magnetic resonance imaging to evaluate patency of aortocoronary bypass grafts. *Circulation* 1987;76(4):786–791.
7. Vanninen RL, Vainio PA, Manninen HI, et al. Gastroepiploic artery as an in situ coronary artery bypass graft: evaluation of MRI and colour Doppler ultrasound in follow-up. *Scand J Thorac Cardiovasc Surg* 1995;29(1):7–10.
8. Galjee MA, van Rossum AC, Doesburg T, et al. Value of magnetic resonance imaging in assessing patency and function of coronary artery bypass grafts. An angiographically controlled study. *Circulation* 1996;93(4):660–666.
9. Engelmann MG, Knez A, von Smekal A, et al. Non-invasive coronary bypass graft imaging after multivessel revascularisation. *Int J Cardiol* 2000;76(1):65–74.
10. Kalden P, Kreitner KF, Wittlinger T, et al. Assessment of coronary artery bypass grafts: value of different breath-hold MR imaging techniques. *AJR Am J Roentgenol* 1999;172(5):1359–1364.
11. Kessler W, Achenbach S, Moshage W, et al. Usefulness of respiratory gated magnetic resonance coronary angiography in assessing narrowings > or = 50% in diameter in native coronary arteries and in aortocoronary bypass conduits. *Am J Cardiol* 1997;80(8):989–993.
12. Langerak SE, Vliegen HW, de Roos A, et al. Detection of vein graft disease using high-resolution magnetic resonance angiography. *Circulation* 2002;105(3):328–333.

13. Molinari G, Sardanelli F, Zandrino F, et al. Value of navigator echo magnetic resonance angiography in detecting occlusion/patency of arterial and venous, single and sequential coronary bypass grafts. *Int J Card Imaging* 2000;16(3):149–160.

14. Vrachliotis TG, Bis KG, Aliabadi D, et al. Contrast-enhanced breath-hold MR angiography for evaluating patency of coronary artery bypass grafts. *AJR Am J Roentgenol* 1997;168(4):1073–1080.

15. Wintersperger BJ, Engelmann MG, von Smekal A, et al. Patency of coronary bypass grafts: assessment with breath-hold contrast-enhanced MR angiography—value of a non-electrocardiographically triggered technique. *Radiology* 1998;208(2):345–351.

16. Wittlinger T, Voigtlander T, Kreitner KF, et al. Non-invasive magnetic resonance imaging of coronary bypass grafts. Comparison of the haste- and navigator techniques with conventional coronary angiography. *Int J Cardiovasc Imaging* 2002;18(6):469–477.

17. Bunce NH, Lorenz CH, John AS, et al. Coronary artery bypass graft patency: assessment with true fast imaging with steady-state precession versus gadolinium-enhanced MR angiography. *Radiology* 2003;227(2):440–446.

18. White CW, Wright CB, Doty DB, et al. Does visual interpretation of the coronary arteriogram predict the physiologic importance of a coronary stenosis? *N Engl J Med* 1984;310(13):819–824.

19. Topol EJ, Nissen SE. Our preoccupation with coronary luminology. The dissociation between clinical and angiographic findings in ischemic heart disease. *Circulation* 1995;92(8):2333–2342.

20. Uren NG, Melin JA, De Bruyne B, et al. Relation between myocardial blood flow and the severity of coronary-artery stenosis. *N Engl J Med* 1994;330(25):1782–1788.

21. Gould KL, Lipscomb K, Hamilton GW. Physiologic basis for assessing critical coronary stenosis. Instantaneous flow response and regional distribution during coronary hyperemia as measures of coronary flow reserve. *Am J Cardiol* 1974;33(1):87–94.

22. Gould KL, Kirkeeide RL, Buchi M. Coronary flow reserve as a physiologic measure of stenosis severity. *J Am Coll Cardiol* 1990;15(2):459–474.

23. Gould KL, Lipscomb K. Effects of coronary stenoses on coronary flow reserve and resistance. *Am J Cardiol* 1974;34(1):48–55.

24. Bittar N, Kroncke GM, Dacumos GC Jr., et al. Vein graft flow and reactive hyperemia in the human heart. *J Thorac Cardiovasc Surg* 1972;64(6):855–860.

25. Wilson RF, White CW. Does coronary artery bypass surgery restore normal maximal coronary flow reserve? The effect of diffuse atherosclerosis and focal obstructive lesions. *Circulation* 1987;76(3):563–571.

26. Doucette JW, Corl PD, Payne HM, et al. Validation of a Doppler guide wire for intravascular measurement of coronary artery flow velocity. *Circulation* 1992;85(5):1899–1911.

27. Sudhir K, Hargrave VK, Johnson EL, et al. Measurement of volumetric coronary blood flow with a Doppler catheter: validation in an animal model. *Am Heart J* 1992;124(4):870–875.

28. Labovitz AJ, Anthonis DM, Cravens TL, et al. Validation of volumetric flow measurements by means of a Doppler-tipped coronary angioplasty guide wire. *Am Heart J* 1993;126(6):1456–1461.

29. Ofili EO, Labovitz AJ, Kern MJ. Coronary flow velocity dynamics in normal and diseased arteries. *Am J Cardiol* 1993;71(14):3d–9d.

30. White CW. Clinical applications of Doppler coronary flow reserve measurements. *Am J Cardiol* 1993; 71(14):10d–16d.

31. Kern MJ, Donohue TJ, Aguirre FV, et al. Assessment of angiographically intermediate coronary artery stenosis using the Doppler flowire. *Am J Cardiol* 1993;71(14):26d–33d.

32. Segal J. Applications of coronary flow velocity during angioplasty and other coronary interventional procedures. *Am J Cardiol* 1993;71(14):17d–25d.

33. Serruys PW, De Bruyne B, Carlier S, et al. Randomized comparison of primary stenting and provisional balloon angioplasty guided by flow velocity measurement. Doppler Endpoints Balloon Angioplasty Trial Europe (DEBATE) II Study Group. *Circulation* 2000;102(24):2930–2937.

34. Nishida T, Di Mario C, Kern MJ, et al. Impact of final coronary flow velocity reserve on late outcome following stent implantation. *Eur Heart J* 2002;23(4):331–340.

35. Albertal M, Regar E, Van Langenhove G, et al. Value of coronary stenotic flow velocity acceleration in prediction of angiographic restenosis following balloon angioplasty. *Eur Heart J* 2002;23(23):1849–1853.

36. Lotz J, Meier C, Leppert A, et al. Cardiovascular flow measurement with phase-contrast MR imaging: basic facts and implementation. *Radiographics* 2002;22(3):651–671.

37. van Rossum AC, Galjee MA, Doesburg T, et al. The role of magnetic resonance in the evaluation of functional results after CABG/PTCA. *Int J Card Imaging* 1993;9(Suppl 1):59–69.

38. Galjee MA, van Rossum AC, Doesburg T, et al. Quantification of coronary artery bypass graft flow by magnetic resonance phase velocity mapping. *Magn Reson Imaging* 1996;14(5):485–493.

39. Hoogendoorn LI, Pattynama PM, Buis B, et al. Noninvasive evaluation of aortocoronary bypass grafts with magnetic resonance flow mapping. *Am J Cardiol* 1995;75(12):845–848.

40. Galjee MA, van Rossum AC, Doesburg T, et al. Value of magnetic resonance imaging in assessing patency and function of coronary artery bypass grafts. An angiographically controlled study. *Circulation* 1996;93(4):660–666.

41. Debatin JF, Strong JA, Sostman HD, et al. MR characterization of blood flow in native and grafted internal mammary arteries. *J Magn Reson Imaging* 1993;3(3):443–450.

42. Sakuma H, Globits S, O'Sullivan M, et al. Breath-hold MR measurements of blood flow velocity in internal mammary arteries and coronary artery bypass grafts. *J Magn Reson Imaging* 1996;6(1):219–222.

43. Brenner P, Wintersperger B, von Smekal A, et al. Detection of coronary artery bypass graft patency by contrast enhanced magnetic resonance angiography. *Eur J Cardiothorac Surg* 1999;15(4):389–393.

44. Langerak SE, Kunz P, Vliegen HW, et al. Improved MR flow mapping in coronary artery bypass grafts during adenosine-induced stress. *Radiology* 2001;218(2):540–547.

45. Langerak SE, Kunz P, Vliegen HW, et al. Magnetic resonance flow mapping in coronary artery bypass grafts: a validation study with Doppler flow measurements. *Radiology* 2002;222(1):127–135.

46. Ishida N, Sakuma H, Cruz BP, et al. MR flow measurement in the internal mammary artery-to-coronary artery bypass graft: comparison with graft stenosis at radiographic angiography. *Radiology* 2001;220(2):441–447.

47. Bedaux WL, Hofman MB, Vyt SL, et al. Assessment of coronary artery bypass graft disease using cardiovascular magnetic resonance determination of flow reserve. *J Am Coll Cardiol* 2002;40(10):1848–1855.

48. Langerak SE, Vliegen HW, Jukema JW, et al. Value of magnetic resonance imaging for the noninvasive detection of stenosis in coronary artery bypass grafts and recipient coronary arteries. *Circulation* 2003;107(11):1502–1508.

49. Miller S, Scheule AM, Hahn U, et al. MR angiography and flow quantification of the internal mammary artery graft after minimally invasive direct coronary artery bypass. *AJR Am J Roentgenol* 1999;172(5):1365–1369.

50. Walpoth BH, Muller MF, Genyk I, et al. Evaluation of coronary bypass flow with color-Doppler and magnetic resonance imaging techniques: comparison with intraoperative flow measurements. *Eur J Cardiothorac Surg* 1999;15(6):795–802.

51. Langerak SE, Vliegen HW, Jukema JW, et al. Vein graft function improvement after percutaneous intervention: evaluation with MR flow mapping. *Radiology* 2003;228(3):834–841.

52. Salm LP, Langerak SE, Vliegen HW, et al. Blood flow in coronary artery bypass vein grafts: volume versus velocity at cardiovascular MR imaging. *Radiology* 2004;232(3):915–920.

53. Salm LP, Bax JJ, Vliegen HW, et al. Functional significance of stenoses in coronary artery bypass grafts Evaluation by single-photon emission computed tomography perfusion imaging, cardiovascular magnetic resonance, and angiography. *J Am Coll Cardiol* 2004;44(9):1877–1882.

54. Tadamura E, Kudoh T, Motooka M, et al. Use of technetium-99m sestamibi ECG-gated single-photon emission tomography for the evaluation of left ventricular function following coronary artery bypass graft: comparison with three-dimensional magnetic resonance imaging. *Eur J Nucl Med* 1999;26(7):705–712.

55. Germano G, Kiat H, Kavanagh PB, et al. Automatic quantification of ejection fraction from gated myocardial perfusion SPECT. *J Nucl Med* 1995;36(11):2138–2147.

56. Germano G, Erel J, Kiat H, et al. Quantitative LVEF and qualitative regional function from gated thallium-201 perfusion SPECT. *J Nucl Med* 1997;38(5):749–754.

57. Ascione R, Lloyd CT, Underwood MJ, et al. Inflammatory response after coronary revascularization with or without cardiopulmonary bypass. *Ann Thorac Surg* 2000;69(4):1198–1204.

58. Taggart DP. Biochemical assessment of myocardial injury after cardiac surgery: effects of a platelet activating factor antagonist, bilateral internal thoracic artery grafts, and coronary endarterectomy. *J Thorac Cardiovasc Surg* 2000;120(4):651–659.

59. Selvanayagam JB, Petersen SE, Francis JM, et al. Effects of off-pump versus on-pump coronary surgery on reversible and irreversible myocardial injury: a randomized trial using cardiovascular magnetic resonance imaging and biochemical markers. *Circulation* 2004;109(3):345–350.

60. Steuer J, Bjerner T, Duvernoy O, et al. Visualisation and quantification of peri-operative myocardial infarction after coronary artery bypass surgery with contrast-enhanced magnetic resonance imaging. *Eur Heart J* 2004;25(15):1293–1299.

61. Selvanayagam JB, Kardos A, Francis JM, et al. Value of delayed-enhancement cardiovascular magnetic resonance imaging in predicting myocardial viability after surgical revascularization. *Circulation* 2004;110(12):1535–1541.

62. Albrechtsson U, Stahl E, Tylen U. Evaluation of coronary artery bypass graft patency with computed tomography. *J Comput Assist Tomogr* 1981;5(6):822–826.

63. Daniel WG, Dohring W, Stender HS, et al. Value and limitations of computed tomography in assessing aortocoronary bypass graft patency. *Circulation* 1983;67(5):983–987.

64. Brundage BH, Lipton MJ, Herfkens RJ, et al. Detection of patent coronary bypass grafts by computed tomography. A preliminary report. *Circulation* 1980;61(4):826–831.

65. Guthaner DF, Brody WR, Ricci M, et al. The use of computed tomography in the diagnosis of coronary artery bypass graft patency. *Cardiovasc Intervent Radiol* 1980;3(1):3–8.

66. Godwin JD, Califf RM, Korobkin M, et al. Clinical value of coronary bypass graft evaluation with CT. *AJR Am J Roentgenol* 1983;140(4):649–655.

67. Wilson PC, Gutierrez O, Moss A. Early evaluation of coronary artery bypass grafts: CT or selective angiography. *Eur J Radiol* 1984;4(1):22–27.

68. Foster CJ, Sekiya T, Brownlee WC, et al. Computed tomographic assessment of coronary artery bypass grafts. *Br Heart J* 1984;52(1):24–29.

69. Muhlberger V, Knapp E, zur Nedden D. Predictive value of computed tomographic determination of the patency rate of aortocoronary venous bypasses in relation to angiographic results. *Eur Heart J* 1990;11(5):380–388.

70. Kahl FR, Wolfman NT, Watts LE. Evaluation of aortocoronary bypass graft status by computed tomography. *Am J Cardiol* 1981;48(2):304–310.

71. Bateman TM, Gray RJ, Whiting JS, et al. Prospective evaluation of ultrafast cardiac computed tomography for determination of coronary bypass graft patency. *Circulation* 1987;75(5):1018–1024.

72. Stanford W, Rooholamini M, Rumberger J, et al. Evaluation of coronary bypass graft patency by ultrafast computed tomography. *J Thorac Imaging* 1988;3(2):52–55.

73. Stanford W, Brundage BH, MacMillan R, et al. Sensitivity and specificity of assessing coronary bypass graft patency with ultrafast computed tomography: results of a multicenter study. *J Am Coll Cardiol* 1988;12(1):1–7.

74. Tello R, Costello P, Ecker C, et al. Spiral CT evaluation of coronary artery bypass graft patency. *J Comput Assist Tomogr* 1993;17(2):253–259.

75. Ueyama K, Ohashi H, Tsutsumi Y, et al. Evaluation of coronary artery bypass grafts using helical scan computed tomography. *Catheter Cardiovasc Interv* 1999;46(3):322–326.

76. Engelmann MG, von Smekal A, Knez A, et al. Accuracy of spiral computed tomography for identifying arterial and venous coronary graft patency. *Am J Cardiol* 1997;80(5):569–574.

77. Yoo KJ, Choi D, Choi BW, et al. The comparison of the graft patency after coronary artery bypass grafting using coronary angiography and multi-slice computed tomography. *Eur J Cardiothorac Surg* 2003;24(1):86–91.

78. Ko YG, Choi DH, Jang YS, et al. Assessment of coronary artery bypass graft patency by multislice computed tomography. *Yonsei Med J* 2003;44(3):438–444.

79. Burgstahler C, Kuettner A, Kopp AF, et al. Non-invasive evaluation of coronary artery bypass grafts using multi-slice computed tomography: initial clinical experience. *Int J Cardiol* 2003;90(2–3):275–280.

80. Willmann JK, Weishaupt D, Kobza R, et al. Coronary artery bypass grafts: ECG-gated multi-detector row CT angiography—influence of image reconstruction interval on graft visibility. *Radiology* 2004;232(2):568–577.

81. Marano R, Storto ML, Maddestra N, et al. Non-invasive assessment of coronary artery bypass graft with retrospectively ECG-gated four-row multi-detector spiral computed tomography. *Eur Radiol* 2004;14(8):1353–1362.

82. Nieman K, Pattynama PM, Rensing BJ, et al. Evaluation of patients after coronary artery bypass surgery: CT angiographic assessment of grafts and coronary arteries. *Radiology* 2003;229(3):749–756.

83. Ropers D, Ulzheimer S, Wenkel E, et al. Investigation of aortocoronary artery bypass grafts by multislice spiral computed tomography with electrocardiographic-gated image reconstruction. *Am J Cardiol* 2001;88(7):792–795.

84. Rumberger JA, Feiring AJ, Hiratzka LF, et al. Quantification of coronary artery bypass flow reserve in dogs using cine-computed tomography. *Circ Res* 1987;61(5 Pt 2):117–123.

85. Tello R, Hartnell GG, Costello P, et al. Coronary artery bypass graft flow: qualitative evaluation with cine single-detector row CT and comparison with findings at angiography. *Radiology* 2002;224(3):913–918.

86. Dewey M, Lembcke A, Enzweiler C, et al. Isotropic half-millimeter angiography of coronary artery bypass grafts with 16-slice computed tomography. *Ann Thorac Surg* 2004;77(3): 800–804.

87. Gurevitch J, Gaspar T, Orlov B, et al. Noninvasive evaluation of arterial grafts with newly released multidetector computed tomography. *Ann Thorac Surg* 2003;76(5):1523–1527.

88. Schlosser T, Konorza T, Hunold P, et al. Noninvasive visualization of coronary artery bypass grafts using 16-detector row computed tomography. *J Am Coll Cardiol* 2004;44(6): 1224–1229.

89. Martuscelli E, Romagnoli A, D'Eliseo A, et al. Evaluation of venous and arterial conduit patency by 16-slice spiral computed tomography. *Circulation* 2004;110(20):3234–3238.

90. Herzog C, Dogan S, Diebold T, et al. Multi-detector row CT versus coronary angiography: preoperative evaluation before totally endoscopic coronary artery bypass grafting. *Radiology* 2003;229(1):200–208.

91. Willmann JK, Weishaupt D, Kobza R, et al. Coronary artery bypass grafts: ECG-gated multi-detector row CT angiography—influence of image reconstruction interval on graft visibility. *Radiology* 2004;232(2):568–577.

22

Computed Tomography Imaging of Coronary Calcification

William Stanford and Brad H. Thompson

Coronary heart disease (CHD) affects millions of individuals annually. It is the number-one killer of Americans. This year, an estimated 650,000 Americans will have a new heart attack, and, of these, 500,000 will die. Only 50% of patients who experience an acute myocardial infarction will have a history of heart disease. Because 80% of CHD mortality occurs in individuals aged less than 65 years, it also represents a major socioeconomic problem, with costs approximating $326 billion per year, thus making CHD the single most expensive component of the country's total health care expenditures (1).

Although epidemiologic studies have identified numerous cardiac risk factors, traditional risk factors alone predict only two thirds of patients who will eventually succumb to heart disease (2). In fact, approximately one third of the 500,000 individuals dying annually of cardiac disease have no identifiable Framingham risk factors that would predict a future "hard" cardiac event (3). Thus, it is important to develop screening methodologies that can both quantitatively measure the severity of coronary vascular disease and accurately predict future risk. Because coronary calcification correlates with the severity of the disease and has potential as an indicator of increased risk, numerous investigators have examined the role of computed tomography (CT) coronary calcium quantification as an accurate, cost-effective screening methodology for evaluating CHD.

ATHEROSCLEROTIC PLAQUE HISTOLOGY

Coronary arteriosclerosis is a complex and unpredictable process thought to be related to biochemical, genetic, and environmental factors. Because traditional risk factors, such as smoking, age, gender, obesity, hypertension, hyperlipidemia, and diabetes mellitus, are thought to be linked to an increased overall risk for developing atherosclerosis, these assessments are important; however, they do a relatively poor job in predicting individual risk for CHD. Regardless of the presence or absence of specific risk factors, the development of arteriosclerosis remains an inevitable part of aging (1).

Atherosclerosis begins early in life. The earliest atherosclerotic lesion (type I lesion) is characterized by the accumulation of lipid-laden macrophages (foam cells) within the intima of arterial walls. With further accumulations of both intra- and extracellular lipids, type II (fatty streak) and type III (preatheroma) lesions develop. These latter lesions may be grossly visible and often contain small foci of calcium on histologic examination. Although these lesions are hemodynamically innocuous and potentially reversible, they represent lesions that can progress to the more clinically important type IV and V lesions (4).

Both type IV and type V lesions (atheroma) are well-developed plaques characterized by intramural collections of both cholesterol and phospholipids and known as the lipid core. These lipid collections are often covered by a thin, fibrous cap (fibroatheroma). These lesions often coexist without associated significant luminal narrowing and, therefore, are often underestimated and undetected by angiography. In fact, up to two thirds of patients with acute myocardial infarctions or unstable angina may have only minimal angiographic narrowing at the site of the occlusion (5,6). Similarly, myocardial perfusion studies that attempt to identify the hemodynamic effects of stenoses may be normal, and, thus, traditional screening examinations and risk-factor assessments often underestimate an individual's risk for sudden cardiac death.

Because they are predisposed to spontaneous rupture, type IV and V lesions, often referred to as "vulnerable plaques," are responsible for most of the morbidity and mortality from coronary artery disease (CAD) (4). Why plaques rupture is unclear, but the process is likely multifactorial and related to biomechanical stresses and localized plaque inflammation (5).

Once the fibrous cap ruptures, the lipid core is exposed to blood and an acute thrombogenic reaction frequently ensues. This thrombosis and subsequent recanalization may result in partial narrowing or complete occlusion with the narrowing manifested clinically by episodes of ischemia and/or silent infarction. If a high degree of stenosis were present at the site of rupture, total vascular occlusion is often likely, and this may account for many of the sudden cardiac deaths seen annually (5).

With repeated plaque rupture, type IV and V lesions become transformed into type VI lesions, which are considered histologically "complicated" plaques that are characterized by fibromuscular tissue deposition occurring from plaque repair and healing. With repeated injury and healing, type VI lesions may slowly grow in size to produce significant arterial narrowing (6). Thus, type VI lesions have a greater prevalence in patients with chronic and/or stable angina, and, as such, they are commonly detected by traditional diagnostic techniques that screen for the hemodynamic effects of stenoses (7).

The presence of calcium during plaque development makes these lesions identifiable by fluoroscopy and CT. In fact, Rumberger et al (8) showed that calcium can be identifiable by CT when plaque area measures 5 to 10 mm^2 per 3-mm segment.

IMPORTANCE OF MEASURING CORONARY CALCIUM

Strong correlations have been found between quantitative measurements of coronary artery calcium (CAC) and pathologic measurements of plaque area and volume (8–11). Qualitative measurements of coronary calcification performed by fluoroscopy have similarly shown a strong relationship between calcium mass and histologic mass (11), as well as between the amount of coronary calcification and the severity of the CAD (12). Furthermore, it has been established that as quantities of coronary plaque calcium increase, so does the likelihood of hemodynamically significant stenoses (13). Thus, heavy concentrations of vascular calcium suggest a greater likelihood of hemodynamically significant stenoses, which, as mentioned, is typical of patients with stable angina. Supporting this was an article by Kragel et al (14), who reported that atherosclerotic plaques associated with significant narrowing often contain more calcium than do nonobstructive plaques. As such, patients with coronary calcium in excess of the mean for age or gender have up to a 90% specificity in detecting hemodynamically significant coronary stenosis (15,16). In addition, autopsy studies have shown that large CAC burdens correlate with greater likelihoods of significant arterial luminal narrowing, especially when distributed over multiple vessels. One such study was by Mautner et al (17), who examined 1,298 segments from 50 heart specimens and observed that 93% of arteries with stenoses greater than 75% had CAC. Conversely, only 14% of arteries with stenoses less than 25% were associated with calcium. A number of studies have shown that heavier CAC burdens were strongly associated with significant stenoses on angiography and overall poorer patient outcomes (10,19–21). However, calcium measurements derived from CT do not predict site-specific stenoses. Therefore, these CAC measurements cannot be used to predict either the site or the severity of the stenoses (22,23).

COMPUTED TOMOGRAPHY SCREENING FOR CORONARY CALCIUM

CT is an extremely sensitive imaging modality with which to detect coronary calcium; thus, CT exhibits greater detection rates than either fluoroscopy or digital radiography (24). Furthermore, the fast temporal and excellent spatial resolution of the newer CT scanners can accurately localize calcific deposits within the coronary arterial tree. Because CAC has been shown to be a proven marker for CAD, numerous investigators have attempted to validate the accuracy of CAC measurements to detect CHD. To date, many of these validation studies have been performed using electron-beam CT (EBCT) (13,18,25–29), but helical CT (HCT) is playing an ever-increasing role (30–37).

ELECTRON-BEAM COMPUTED TOMOGRAPHY

The unique design of the EBCT scanner has many advantages in coronary artery imaging. Its excellent temporal resolution has afforded EBCT a niche role in the qualitative and quantitative assessment of cardiac morphology and function. In contrast with conventional CT, EBCT produces images of the heart in near real-time and does so with excellent spatial and temporal resolution. Having no moving parts, other than the patient table, EBCT has acquisition times from 100 ms down to 32 ms, which when coupled with its inherent superior spatial resolution initially made EBCT the gold standard in CAC detection and quantification.

Unlike conventional CT scanners with rotating x-ray tubes, EBCT scanners possess an electron gun that generates electrons, which are electromagnetically focused on tungsten target rings. The photons generated from the sweep of the target rings then pass through the patient onto two parallel, solid-state detector rings located within the scanner gantry above the patient. In the volume-scan mode, each sweep of the target rings requires 100 ms. From it, slice thicknesses from 1.5 to 10 mm and pixel sizes from 0.25 to 0.6 mm can be generated (38), depending on the field of view used. A common voxel size is 1.03 mm^3 (35-cm reconstruction circle).

With the volume-scanning mode, a 40-slice, 100-ms study of the entire coronary arterial tree can usually be completed within 20 to 30 seconds. In an effort to further decrease heart motion, imaging has incorporated electrocardiography (ECG) gating. The EBCT image acquisitions are commonly triggered from ECG gating at 60% to 80% of the RR interval, which corresponds with peak diastole (Fig. 22.1). An entire coronary calcium study delivers an effective radiation dose of approximately 0.7 mSv (39).

HELICAL COMPUTED TOMOGRAPHY

Recent advances in HCT scanner technology have improved the ability of these scanners to perform cardiac imaging, particularly coronary calcium assessment (Fig. 22.2). New multidetector-row configurations, coupled with progressively shorter scan times and ECG gating, have significantly expanded the cardiac applications of HCT scanners. These technologic advances have helped narrow the performance gap that once existed between EBCT and HCT (31).

Although fixed scan times for the newer-generation HCT scanners (330–500 ms) are still significantly slower than EBCT and are considerably slower than the time required to absolutely freeze cardiac motion (<10 ms), they still are sufficiently fast to perform single breath-hold CAC scans (36). HCT algorithms with 180-degree interpolation in the nonhelical, sequential single-slice mode not only effectively decrease acquisition times but also improve the z-axis resolution. This, in turn, has helped eliminate many of the slice misregistration problems that plagued older scanners. The introduction of multidetector-row scanners (4-, 8-, 16-, 32- and 64-detector-row scanners) has additionally improved z-axis coverage per revolution, further decreasing scan and examination times. Images with 33-ms temporal resolution can now be produced with 64-detector-row scanners.

Helical scanners obtain images using either sequential, "single-slice" or helical sequences. Although helical acquisitions are inherently faster and can interrogate the heart in larger blocks, they tend to be associated with more radiation exposure.

ELECTROCARDIOGRAPHY GATING

The absence of ECG gating can produce slice misregistration artifacts, which when coupled with slower scan times may cause smearing of calcium deposits and an overall suboptimal image. This deficiency has been largely corrected with the development and incorporation of ECG-gating software. As a result, ECG gating has improved overall examination performance by decreasing calcium score variability and improving CAC measurement accuracy.

ECG gating can be implemented with either sequential (single-slice) mode or helical acquisitions, and can be performed with either prospective or retrospective sequences. The latter algorithm requires the retrospective analysis of the entire data set to identify diastolic images. Prospective multidetector CT (MDCT) ECG-gated protocols performed with sequential scanning closely resemble EBCT acquisitions. In both, an ECG trigger point is set to coincide with diastole (usually 60%–80% of the RR interval). Prospectively gated sequential acquisitions often result in slightly longer examination times, which are necessary to allow incremental scanner couch movement to occur between each acquisition. Depending on heart rate, sequential scanning can extend imaging times beyond what can be accomplished with a single breath hold, thereby necessitating two separate studies to complete the image data set. Unfortunately, splitting the acquisition into two separate components can introduce slice overlap, as well as breathing and slice misregistration artifacts; however, the new 16- to 64-slice detector-row scanners have pretty much eliminated this problem.

Retrospective ECG-gated studies, which are associated with larger data sets, may require additional time investments for postprocessing. Retrospectively gated studies are also associated with significant increases in radiation exposure to the patient, compared with prospective MDCT acquisitions and EBCT (39); however, newer modulation techniques have reduced this exposure by 40% to 50% (40).

REPRODUCIBILITY ISSUES

To assess for disease progression, CT measurements must be accurate and reproducible. Although studies that have examined interscan variability between EBCT and helical scanners report excellent correlations ($r \approx 0.99$) (34–37), individual scanner variability can be problematic, particularly in regard to the ability of CT to consistently identify small foci of calcium. Bielak et al (41) reported that lesions with areas less than 3.09 mm^2 were detected on the second

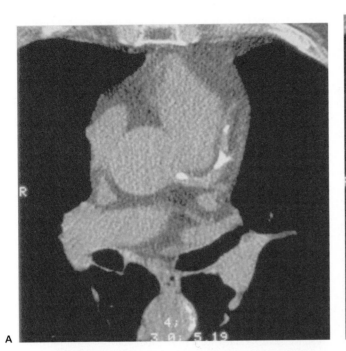

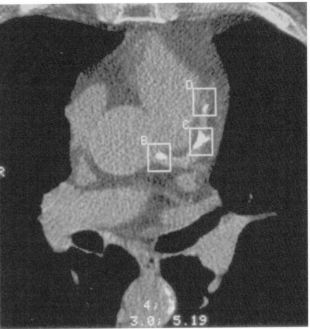

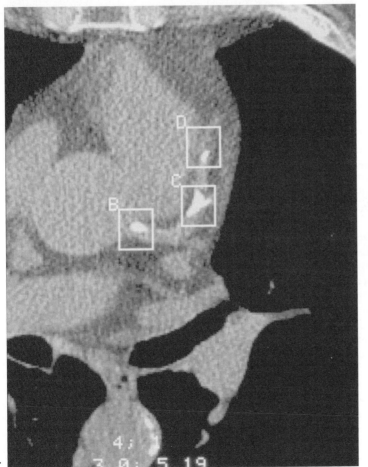

R	PEAK	BVA(130)	
A	488	28.687	MM2
B	774	26.856	MM2
C	817	52.490	MM2
D	519	12.207	MM2
E	229	9.766	MM2
F	359	7.935	MM2

Figure 22.1. **(A)** Electron-beam computed tomography (EBCT) image showing calcium as white areas in left main and left anterior descending coronary arteries. **(B)** Same subject as in **(A)**, with regions of interest placed around the calcium deposits. **(C)** Calcium score of each region of interest shows peak attenuation in Hounsfield units (peak) and calcification area in mm². Lesions were scored at a base value of +130 Hounsfield units [Base value area (130)].

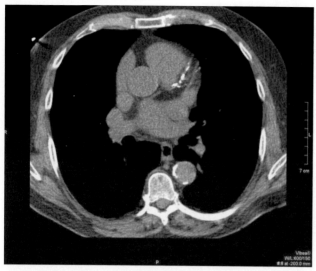

Figure 22.2. Sixteen-slice multidetector CT (MDCT) image showing calcium deposits in the left main, left anterior descending, diagonal, and proximal circumflex coronary arteries.

scan only 50% of the time. With smaller lesions, the reproducibility is even poorer. They found that the difference in the absolute calcium score between sequential scans could be as large as 200% (41) in patients with mean total calcium scores less of than 20. Variabilities of repeated EBCT scans have approximated 22% (30), 29% (21), 37% (42), and 49% (43,44), whereas four-slice gated MDCT variabilities have approximated 25% for overlapping images and 45% for Agatston scoring without overlap (45).

Interscan variability between EBT and HCT has been shown to be approximately 15%; interreader variability has been shown to be approximately 3%; and intrareader variability has been shown to be less than 1% (43,46–49). Other studies have shown interscan variabilities of 20% to 36% for volume scoring and 14% to 43% for Agatston scoring (50–52).

Factors primarily responsible for the poor interscan variability are slice misregistration resulting from cardiac and respiratory motion, noncontiguous acquisition of image data (image gaps), image noise, changes in scanner calibration, cardiac arrhythmias/ECG triggering problems, and patient motion. These problems can be minimized by changing either the attenuation threshold or the slice thickness or by averaging several measurements of the same lesion (41). In an attempt to decrease this variability, many screening sites have implemented duplicate scanning. With dual scanning, Shields et al (53) reported a reliability coefficient of 0.99 in 50 subjects who underwent dual CAC scanning, and Hernigou et al (54) reported an inter-examination error rate of 7.2% using sequential scanning. Also, Bielak et al (41) reported that with the use of regression methodology to assess for nonuniform differences, the transformed calcific area between two scans was highly correlative (intraclass correlation coefficient, 0.98; $p <0.001$).

The use of volumetric plaque measurement (48) is also a useful technique to improve reproducibility, as is the incorporation of phantoms as part of the examination. The latter helps in scanner calibration and determination of calcium mass (55,56). Volumetric and calcium mass measurements

are increasingly being used at many of the sites that perform CAC screening (57,58).

SCORING SOFTWARE

Several software scoring packages, which enable operators to quickly perform CAC quantitative measurements, are commercially available. In these packages, coronary calcification thresholds are generally set at 2 to 3 or more contiguous pixels with CT attenuations of +130 Hounsfield units. The +130 Hounsfield unit threshold was chosen because it is approximately 2 standard deviations higher than the attenuation of blood and has been found to correlate with plaque histologic measurements (17,59). The total calcium burden is commonly reported as the Agatston calcium score (59), which is calculated by multiplying the lesion area (millimeters squared) by a weighted attenuation coefficient corresponding with the measured peak CT attenuation or by the volume and mass scores. Calcium scores are recognized to provide a quantitative measurement of calcium burden and disease severity, either for individual vessels or for the entire heart (total calcium score). These values can then be compared with normalized scores, based on age- and gender-matched controls, and used in assessing both initial disease severity and determining disease progression. The calcium volume score and calcium mass score are increasingly being used in reporting calcium burden.

CALCIFICATION AS AN INDICATOR OF CORONARY STENOSIS

Coronary artery calcification shows promise as an indicator of stenosis. It has been shown that as coronary calcification increases, so does the likelihood of finding one or more significant (>50%) stenoses somewhere in the coronary arterial tree (13).

Mautner et al (17) compared the amount of calcification detected on EBCT examinations with the percent of blockage as determined histomorphometrically. In 1,426 segments of coronary arteries from patients with histories of symptomatic CAD, EBCT calcium was present in 41%; compared with 24% in 1,535 segments from asymptomatic patients with CAD, only 4% of control subjects had calcium. The sensitivity of EBCT for detecting calcium in a coronary artery was 94%, the specificity was 76%, the positive predictive value was 84%, and the negative predictive value was 90%. These investigators concluded that the EBCT calcium score seemed to be an effective predictor of the presence of CAD. In this study, the symptomatic CAD group was defined as having a history of angina or myocardial infarction or an angiographic narrowing greater than 75% in at least one coronary artery. The asymptomatic group had at least one segmental narrowing greater than 75%, but no symptoms, and the control group had no symptoms and no narrowing greater than 75%.

Studies reporting sensitivities and specificities for EBCT calcium as an indicator of significant stenosis are shown in Table 22.1 (25).

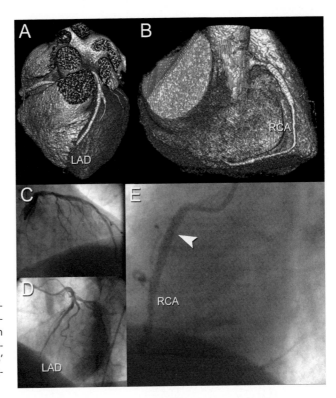

Figure 23.11. Coronary stents. Patient with previous percutaneous coronary intervention (PCI) of the RCA and LAD. **(A,B)** 3D volume rendering images show the coronary CTA (64-slice CT with 0.6-mm detector width and 330-ms gantry rotation time) appearance of the stents in the RCA and LAD. **(A,B)** Presence of the stents' struts on the coronary CTA image. **(C–E)** Corresponding conventional coronary angiograms.

to promote this technique as a reliable alternative to invasive diagnostic coronary angiography. Misinterpretation of the presence and severity of a coronary stenosis because of the presence of coronary calcium seriously limits the reliability of the technique. Persistent arrhythmia (e.g., atrial fibrillation) precludes CT coronary imaging. Fast heart rates (>70 beats/min) often result in poor image quality and are the reason why most investigators recommend the use of β-blockers to reduce the heart rate before the CT investigation.

Highly attenuating materials, such as surgical clips or heavy calcification, cause "blooming" artifacts that create or exaggerate the apparent severity of a stenosis. Imaging of coronary stents with CT causes significant "artificial" enlargement of the stent struts and obscurity of the in-stent lumen.

Coronary CTA is a technique that requires considerable training and still remains operator-dependent (26). This will be partially solved with the introduction of scanners characterized by improved performance and of software able

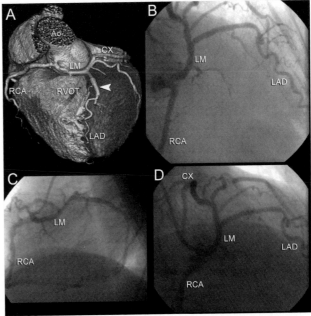

Figure 23.12. Anomaly of the coronary artery origin post-PCI. **(A)** 3D volume rendering image of the coronary CTA (64-slice CT with 0.6-mm detector width and 330-ms gantry rotation time) showing the anatomy of the proximal coronary artery tree with a left main coronary artery originating from the right coronary sinus and running between the Ao and the main pulmonary artery trunk (RVOT). The patient previously underwent PCI for a significant stenosis (*arrowhead* in **A**) on the LAD coronary artery. **(B–D)** Several different projections of conventional coronary angiography of the same patient. Ao, Aortic root; CX, left circumflex coronary artery; LAD, left anterior descending coronary artery; LM, left main coronary artery; RCA, right coronary artery; RVOT, right ventricular outflow tract).

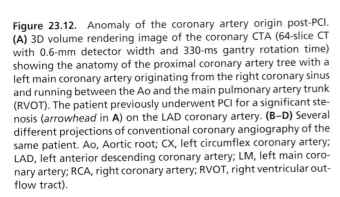

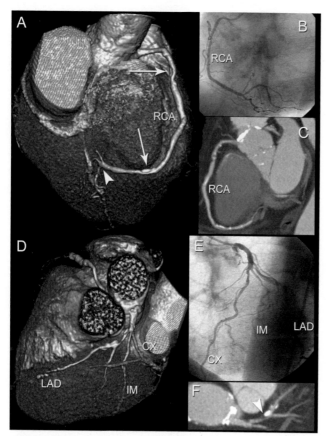

Figure 23.13. Coronary artery angiography: correlation between conventional coronary angiography and CT angiography. Patient with stable angina undergoing 64-slice CT with 0.6-mm detector width and 330-ms gantry rotation time. **(A)** RCA of the patient appears diffusely diseased (*arrows*), particularly in middle and distal segment, without significant stenoses in the 3D volume rendering image until the crux (*arrowhead*). Conventional coronary angiograms confirm the finding **(B)**. The same information is extracted from the thick slab maximum intensity projection image performed parallel to the right atrioventricular groove **(C)**. At coronary CTA, left coronary artery **(D)** and LAD, in particular, show diffuse disease with a significant stenosis at the level of proximal LAD. The finding is confirmed by conventional coronary angiography **(E)**. **(F)** Mixed plaque (calcific and noncalcific tissue) that determines the significant obstruction of the LAD (*arrowhead*).

to provide a more reproducible diagnostic yield including quantification of the degree of coronary stenoses.

Of great concern is the rather high radiation exposure associated with CT scanning. The effective doses of 4-slice CT coronary angiography are reported to be 6.7 to 10.9 mSv for male patients and 8.1 to 13.0 mSv for female patients (48,49). It is expected that the effective radiation dose will be higher with the use of 16- and 64-slice CT scanners. The use of prospective x-ray tube modulation, a feature that reduces the radiation exposure during coronary CTA in up to 50% in patients with low (<60 beats/min) heart rates, makes this technique more sensible to arrhythmia and does not allow reconstruction of high-resolution data sets during the end-systolic phase. These limitations may have a significant impact on the diagnostic accuracy of coronary CTA to detect significant stenoses. In general, this feature should only be applied in young patients with a lower likelihood

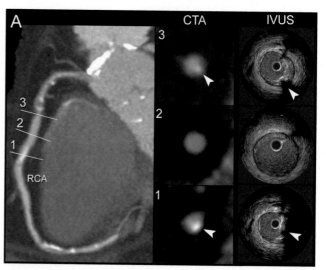

Figure 23.14. Coronary plaque imaging: correlation between coronary CTA and intravascular ultrasound (IVUS). Same patient as in Figure 23.9. IVUS pullback was performed in the proximal RCA. The panoramic maximum intensity projection image **(A)** through the right atrioventricular grove shows the position of the orthogonal cuts used for comparison (i.e., 1–3) between coronary CTA (*left*) and IVUS (*right*). The pullback started at position number 1 and shows an eccentric plaque predominantly calcified. At coronary CTA this plaque appears as a hyperattenuating region within the vessel wall (*arrowhead*) that determines shadowing of the ultrasound. At position number 2 the vessel has a normal configuration on both CT and IVUS. At position number 3, there is a predominantly noncalcified plaque featuring a calcific nodule. At CT this plaque appears as a hypoattenuating region within the vessel wall surrounding a small rounded hyperattenuating region (*arrowhead*). On IVUS the same plaque appears as an eccentric thickening of the vessel wall with a small area of ultrasound shadowing.

of the presence of significant coronary stenoses and a regular heart rate less than 60 beats/min.

SUMMARY

CT coronary angiography has emerged as a significant breakthrough noninvasive modality to diagnose coronary artery stenoses. Further studies in various patient groups with a high likelihood of coronary stenoses should be performed to establish the role of coronary CT in clinical cardiology.

REFERENCES

1. Flohr TG, Schoepf UJ, Kuettner A, et al. Advances in cardiac imaging with 16-section CT systems. *Acad Radiol* 2003;10: 386–401.
2. Flohr T, Stierstorfer K, Raupach R, et al. Performance evaluation of a 64-slice CT system with z-flying focal spot. *Rofo* 2004;176:1803–1810.
3. de Feyter PJ, Krestin GP, Cademartiri F, et al. *Computed tomography of the coronary arteries.* London and New York: Taylor & Francis, A Martin Dunitz Book; 2005.
4. Nieman K, Oudkerk M, Rensig BJ, et al. Coronary angiography with multislice computed tomography. *Lancet* 2001;357: 599–603.

5. Achenbach S, Giesler T, Ropers D, et al. Detection of coronary artery stenoses by contrast-enhanced, retrospectively electrocardiographically-gated, multislice spiral computed tomography. *Circulation* 2001;103:2535–2538.
6. Knez A, Becker CR, Leber A, et al. Usefulness of multislice spiral computed tomography angiography for determination of coronary artery stenoses. *Am J Cardiol* 2001;88:1191–1194.
7. Nieman K, Rensing BJ, van Geuns RJ, et al. Non-invasive coronary angiography with multislice spiral computed tomography: impact of heart rate. *Heart* 2002;88:470–474.
8. Kopp AF, Schroeder S, Kuettner A, et al. Non-invasive coronary angiography with high resolution multidetector-row computed tomography. Results in 102 patients. *Eur Heart J* 2002; 23:1714–1725.
9. Vogl TJ, Abolmaali ND, Diebold T, et al. Techniques for the detection of coronary atherosclerosis: multi-detector row CT coronary angiography. *Radiology* 2002;223:212–220.
10. Giesler T, Baum U, Ropers D, et al. Noninvasive visualization of coronary arteries using contrast-enhanced multidetector CT: influence of heart rate on image quality and stenosis detection. *AJR Am J Roentgenol* 2002;179:911–916.
11. Nieman K, Cademartiri F, Lemos PA, et al. Reliable noninvasive coronary angiography with fast submillimeter multislice spiral computed tomography. *Circulation* 2002;106:2051–2054.
12. Ropers D, Baum U, Pohle K, et al. Detection of coronary artery stenoses with thin-slice multi-detector row spiral computed tomography and multiplanar reconstruction. *Circulation* 2003; 107:664–666.
13. Kuettner A, Kopp AF, Schroeder S, et al. Diagnostic accuracy of multidetector computed tomography coronary angiography in patients with angiographically proven coronary artery disease. *J Am Coll Cardiol* 2004;43:831–839.
14. Kuettner A, Trabold T, Schroeder S, et al. Noninvasive detection of coronary lesions using 16-detector multislice spiral computed tomography technology: initial clinical results. *J Am Coll Cardiol* 2004;44:1230–1237.
15. Martuscelli E, Romagnoli A, D'Eliseo A, et al. Accuracy of thin-slice computed tomography in the detection of coronary stenoses. *Eur Heart J* 2004;25:1043–1048.
16. Mollet NR, Cademartiri F, Nieman K, et al. Multislice spiral computed tomography coronary angiography in patients with stable angina pectoris. *J Am Coll Cardiol* 2004;43:2265–2270.
17. Hoffmann U, Moselewski F, Cury RC, et al. Predictive value of 16-slice multidetector spiral computed tomography to detect significant obstructive coronary artery disease in patients at high risk for coronary artery disease: patient-versus segment-based analysis. *Circulation* 2004;110:2638–2643.
18. Kuettner A, Beck T, Drosch T, et al. Diagnostic accuracy of noninvasive coronary imaging using 16-detector slice spiral computed tomography with 188 ms temporal resolution. *J Am Coll Cardiol* 2005;45:123–127.
19. Mollet NR, Cademartiri F, Krestin GP, et al. Improved diagnostic accuracy with 16-row multi-slice computed tomography coronary angiography. *J Am Coll Cardiol* 2005;45:128–132.
20. Cademartiri F, Mollet NR, Lemos PA, et al. Impact of coronary calcium score on diagnostic accuracy for the detection of significant coronary stenosis with multislice computed tomography angiography. *Am J Cardiol* 2005;95:1225–1227.
21. Cademartiri F, Mollet NR, Runza G, et al. Improving diagnostic accuracy of multislice computed tomography coronary angiography in patients with mild heart rhythm irregularities using ECG-editing. *Am J Roentgenol* (in press).
22. Halliburton SS, Stillman AE, Flohr T, et al. Do segmented reconstruction algorithms for cardiac multi-slice computed tomography improve image quality? *Herz* 2003;28:20–31.
23. Dewey M, Laule M, Krug L, et al. Multisegment and halfscan reconstruction of 16-slice computed tomography for detection of coronary artery stenoses. *Invest Radiol* 2004;39:223–229.
24. Cademartiri F, Mollet N, van der Lugt A, et al. Non-invasive 16-row multislice CT coronary angiography: usefulness of saline chaser. *Eur Radiol* 2004;14:178–183.
25. Cademartiri F, Nieman K, van der Lugt A, et al. Intravenous contrast material administration at 16-detector row helical CT coronary angiography: test bolus versus bolus-tracking technique. *Radiology* 2004;233:817–823.
26. Cademartiri F, Mollet N, Lemos PA, et al. Standard versus user-interactive assessment of significant coronary stenoses with multislice computed tomography coronary angiography. *Am J Cardiol* 2004;94:1590–1593.
27. Juergens KU, Grude M, Maintz D, et al. Multi-detector row CT of left ventricular function with dedicated analysis software versus MR imaging: initial experience. *Radiology* 2004;230: 403–410.
28. Grude M, Juergens KU, Wichter T, et al. Evaluation of global left ventricular myocardial function with electrocardiogram-gated multidetector computed tomography: comparison with magnetic resonance imaging. *Invest Radiol* 2003;38:653–661.
29. Dirksen MS, Bax JJ, de Roos A, et al. Usefulness of dynamic multislice computed tomography of left ventricular function in unstable angina pectoris and comparison with echocardiography. *Am J Cardiol* 2002;90:1157–1160.
30. Dirksen MS, Jukema JW, Bax JJ, et al. Cardiac multidetector-row computed tomography in patients with unstable angina. *Am J Cardiol* 2005;95:457–461.
31. Ropers D, Ulzheimer S, Wenkel E, et al. Investigation of aorto-coronary artery bypass grafts by multislice spiral computed tomography with electrocardiographic-gated image reconstruction. *Am J Cardiol* 2001;88:792–795.
32. Nieman K, Pattynama PM, Rensing BJ, et al. Evaluation of patients after coronary artery bypass surgery: CT angiographic assessment of grafts and coronary arteries. *Radiology* 2003; 229:749–756.
33. Yoo KJ, Choi D, Choi BW, et al. The comparison of the graft patency after coronary artery bypass grafting using coronary angiography and multi-slice computed tomography. *Eur J Cardiothorac Surg* 2003;24:86–91; discussion 91.
34. Martuscelli E, Romagnoli A, D'Eliseo A, et al. Evaluation of venous and arterial conduit patency by 16-slice spiral computed tomography. *Circulation* 2004;110:3234–3238.
35. Schlosser T, Konorza T, Hunold P, et al. Noninvasive visualization of coronary artery bypass grafts using 16-detector row computed tomography. *J Am Coll Cardiol* 2004;44:1224–1229.
36. Maintz D, Juergens KU, Wichter T, et al. Imaging of coronary artery stents using multislice computed tomography: in vitro evaluation. *Eur Radiol* 2003;13:830–835.
37. Cademartiri F, Mollet N, Nieman K, et al. Images in cardiovascular medicine. Neointimal hyperplasia in carotid stent detected with multislice computed tomography. *Circulation* 2003;108:e147.
38. Schuijf JD, Bax JJ, Jukema JW, et al. Feasibility of assessment of coronary stent patency using 16-slice computed tomography. *Am J Cardiol* 2004;94:427–430.
39. Mollet NR, Cademartiri F. Images in cardiovascular medicine. In-stent neointimal hyperplasia with 16-row multislice computed tomography coronary angiography. *Circulation* 2004; 110:e514.
40. Mollet NR, Hoye A, Lemos PA, et al. Value of preprocedure multislice computed tomographic coronary angiography to predict the outcome of percutaneous recanalization of chronic total occlusions. *Am J Cardiol* 2005;95:240–243.
41. Cademartiri F, Nieman K, Raaymakers RH, et al. Non-invasive demonstration of coronary artery anomaly performed using 16-slice multidetector spiral computed tomography. *Ital Heart J* 2003;4:56–59.

42. Horisaki T, Yamashita T, Yokoyama H, et al. Three-dimensional reconstruction of computed tomographic images of anomalous origin of the left main coronary artery from the pulmonary trunk in an adult. *Am J Cardiol* 2003;92:898–899.

43. Lessick J, Kumar G, Beyar R, et al. Anomalous origin of a posterior descending artery from the right pulmonary artery: report of a rare case diagnosed by multidetector computed tomography angiography. *J Comput Assist Tomogr* 2004;28:857–859.

44. Cademartiri F, Mollet N, Nieman K, et al. Images in cardiovascular medicine. Right coronary artery arising from the left circumflex demonstrated with multislice computed tomography. *Circulation* 2004;109:e185–186.

45. Schroeder S, Kopp AF, Baumbach A, et al. Noninvasive detection and evaluation of atherosclerotic coronary plaques with multislice computed tomography. *J Am Coll Cardiol* 2001;37:1430–1435.

46. Leber AW, Knez A, Becker A, et al. Accuracy of multidetector spiral computed tomography in identifying and differentiating the composition of coronary atherosclerotic plaques: a comparative study with intracoronary ultrasound. *J Am Coll Cardiol* 2004;43:1241–1247.

47. Achenbach S, Ropers D, Hoffmann U, et al. Assessment of coronary remodeling in stenotic and nonstenotic coronary atherosclerotic lesions by multidetector spiral computed tomography. *J Am Coll Cardiol* 2004;43:842–847.

48. Hunold P, Vogt FM, Schmermund A, et al. Radiation exposure during cardiac CT: effective doses at multi-detector row CT and electron-beam CT. *Radiology* 2003;226:145–152.

49. Morin RL, Gerber TC, McCollough CH. Radiation dose in computed tomography of the heart. *Circulation* 2003;107:917–922.

24

Atherosclerotic Plaque Imaging

Michael J. Lipinski, Venkatesh Mani, Marc Sirol, and Zahi A. Fayad

ATHEROSCLEROTIC PLAQUES

Atherosclerosis, a systemic disease of the vessel wall that occurs in the aorta, carotid, coronary, and peripheral arteries, is the primary cause of heart disease and stroke (1) and accounts for 50% of all deaths in Western societies. The main components of atherosclerotic plaque are: (a) fibrous elements such as connective tissue, extracellular matrix (includ-

ing collagen), proteoglycans, and fibronectin elastic fibers, (b) lipids such as crystalline cholesterol, cholesteryl esters, and phospholipids, and (c) inflammatory cells such as monocyte-derived macrophages, T-lymphocytes, and smooth-muscle cells (2). The occurrence of these components in varying proportions in different plaques gives rise to a spectrum of lesions (1,3,4). Furthermore, the characteristics of "high-risk" or "vulnerable" plaque vary depending on the arterial region (i.e., coronaries, carotids, or aorta) in which it is located.

CORONARY ARTERY VULNERABLE PLAQUES

Atherosclerotic plaques prone to rupture in the coronary arteries, so-called "vulnerable" plaques, tend to have a thin (~65 μm to 150 μm) fibrous cap and a large lipid core. Acute coronary syndromes often result from the rupture of modestly stenotic plaques (3,4) often not visible by x-ray angiography (3). According to the criteria of the American Heart Association Committee on Vascular Lesions, the different lesion types depend in part on stage or phase of progression (1,4). The coronary "vulnerable" types IV and Va lesions (phase 2) and the "complicated" type VI lesion (phase 4) are the most relevant to acute coronary syndrome. Types IV and Va lesions, although not necessarily stenotic at angiography, frequently have increased density of resident macrophages that release proteolytic enzymes such as metalloproteinases (2,5) that degrade the fibrous cap and increase the risk of plaque rupture. Type IV lesions consist of extracellular lipid intermixed with fibrous tissue that is covered by a fibrous cap, whereas type Va lesions possess a predominantly extracellular lipid core covered by a thin fibrous cap. Disruption of a type IV or Va lesion leads to the formation of thrombus or "complicated" type VI lesions. The lipid core is made highly thrombogenic by the presence of tissue factor (1,6). The type VI lesion that results in acute coronary syndrome, rather than being characterized by a small mural thrombus, consists of an occlusive thrombus.

As demonstrated by serial angiographic studies, moderately stenotic type IV and Va coronary lesions might account for as many as two-thirds of patients who develop unstable angina or myocardial infarction (7,8). While a greater percentage of severely stenotic lesions progress to total occlusion then minimally stenosed lesions (10% to 23% of lesions >50% progress, while <3% of lesions <50% progress) (9), the majority of atherosclerotic lesions in the coronary arteries are minimally stenosed (10). These relatively nonstenotic plaques with large lipid cores are vulnerable and at high risk for rupture and thrombosis; the caps are often thinnest at the shoulder regions, where macrophages (11) and mast cells (12) accumulate, and disruption is a frequent occurrence (5). In contrast, the most severely stenotic plaques at angiography, which have a high content of smooth muscle cells and collagen and little lipid, are less susceptible to rupture.

CAROTID ARTERY HIGH-RISK PLAQUES

In contrast to vulnerable plaques in the coronary arteries, which are characterized by a high lipid content and thin fibrous cap, high-risk plaques in the carotid arteries are severely stenotic. We use the term *high-risk* rather than the classic term *vulnerable* because *vulnerable* implies the presence of a lipid-rich core. Indeed, high-risk carotid plaques are not necessarily lipid-rich but rather heterogeneous, and are very rich in fibrous tissue. These plaques often become symptomatic due to an intramural hematoma or dissection that likely develops secondary to the impact of blood during systole against a resistant area of stenosis (13). Because the carotid arteries are superficial and not subject to significant motion, they are much easier to image than the coronary arteries (14). This is also true of the peripheral vessels (i.e., in the lower extremities), in which the pathobiology is similar to that in the carotid arteries. However, more information is available about the imaging of carotid plaque than of peripheral vascular lesions.

AORTIC VULNERABLE PLAQUES

Studies performed at autopsy (15) and with transesophageal echocardiography (TEE) (16) have shown that atherosclerosis in the thoracic aorta is a significant marker for coronary disease. In fact, parameters such as aortic wall thickness, luminal irregularities, and plaque composition are strong predictors of future vascular events (17). Thus, with the use of TEE, the French Aortic Plaque Study (FAPS) investigators found a significantly increased risk for all vascular events (stroke, myocardial infarction, peripheral embolism, and cardiovascular death) in patients who had noncalcified aortic plaques with a thickness of more than 4 mm (17). These noncalcified, frequently lipid-laden plaques (American Heart Association types IV and Va) (17), which are relatively easy to assess and characterize by magnetic resonance imaging (MRI), are similar to the "vulnerable" coronary plaques that are prone to rupture and thrombosis.

TECHNIQUES

The direct visualization of atherosclerotic plaques should enhance our understanding of the natural history of this disease. Several invasive imaging techniques, such as x-ray angiography, intravascular ultrasonography, angioscopy, and optical coherence tomography, in addition to noninvasive imaging techniques, such as surface B-mode ultrasonography and ultrafast computed tomography, can be used to assess atherosclerotic vessels. Most of the standard techniques identify the luminal diameter or stenosis, wall thickness, and plaque volume. However, none of these imaging methods can completely characterize the composition of the atherosclerotic plaque and, therefore, have inadequate sensitivity and specificity to identify vulnerable or high-risk plaques (18).

High-resolution MR has emerged as the potential leading noninvasive imaging modality for characterizing atherosclerotic plaque in vivo. With improvements in imaging technology, the ability of MR to delineate these vessels has significantly improved (19–24). MR differentiates plaque components on the basis of biophysical and biochemical parameters, such as chemical composition and concentration, water content, physical state, molecular motion, and diffusion (25). MR provides a method of imaging without the need for ionizing radiation that can be repeated sequentially over time. Dedicated pulse sequences have become more readily available for time-efficient multislice imaging (19,20,22,26). Over time, a diverse array of black-blood MRI techniques (27,28) has developed into practical tools for the arterial imaging and evaluation of atherosclerosis.

In black-blood MR, images are commonly acquired using a rapid acquisition with relaxation enhancement (RARE) sequence with double inversion recovery (DIR) pulses (27) to provide good contrast between the lumen and vessel wall. DIR modules consist of two 180° radiofrequency (RF) pulses. Magnetization in the whole volume is inverted by the first nonselective RF pulse, while magnetization in the slab of interest is subsequently restored by the second selective RF pulse. The application of these two preparatory RF pulses causes spins outside the slab of interest to be inverted, with no effect on spins within the slab. Image acquisition begins following a time delay (TI) necessary for magnetization of inverted blood flowing into the imaging slice to reach null point (27). Recently, DIR techniques have been modified for multislice black-blood imaging (19,20,22,26). The use of black-blood MRI to directly image atherosclerotic plaques provides the unique opportunity of measuring plaque and wall changes due to atherosclerotic disease with high accuracy, taking into account the intrinsic variations of the diseased arterial wall. One technique for multislice black-blood imaging that was recently developed is the rapid extended coverage (REX) method (20). This method allows for imaging up to 20 times faster than the conventionally used single-slice black-blood DIR technique. An example of black-blood multislice imaging of the aorta using the REX sequence is shown in Figure 24.1. Images of the carotid artery from the same patient showing complex atherosclerotic plaque are shown in Figure 24.2.

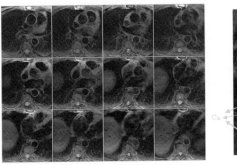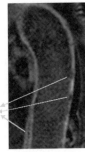

Candycane

Figure 24.1. Twelve axial images of the thoracic aorta of a 68-year-old patient with a history of coronary artery disease showing atherosclerotic plaque in the vessel wall. Proton density-weighted images obtained using the REX sequence is shown. The corresponding candy cane (*longitudinal section*) image of aorta shows areas of calcification in aortic wall. REX, rapid extended coverage. (Courtesy of Venkatesh Mani, Mount Sinai School of Medicine, New York.)

APPLICATIONS

MAGNETIC RESONANCE EX VIVO PLAQUE STUDIES

The initial work on the application of MR techniques to characterize plaque focused on lipid assessment with nuclear MR spectroscopy and chemical shift imaging (29–36). Unfortunately, the concentration of lipid in plaque is very low in comparison with that of water, and these techniques suffered from poor signal-to-noise ratio (SNR) (29,33,37). Therefore, it has been difficult to apply them in vivo, thus leading current studies to focus on MRI of water protons.

MAGNETIC RESONANCE MULTICONTRAST PLAQUE IMAGING

Following an ex vivo MRI study of iliac artery specimens by Kaufman et al (38), Herfkens et al (39) performed the

first in vivo imaging study of human aortic atherosclerosis. Only the anatomic or morphologic features of the atherosclerotic lesions, such as wall thickening and luminal narrowing, were assessed.

Following improvements in MR techniques (e.g., faster imaging and detection coils), high resolution and contrast imaging became possible, and studies were undertaken to identify the different components of plaque with multicontrast MR generated by T1, T2, and proton density weightings (18). The characterization of atherosclerotic plaque by MR is based on the signal intensities and morphologic appearance of plaque on T1-weighted, proton density-weighted, and T2-weighted images, as previously validated (14,37, 40–45).

The fibrous tissues of plaque, consisting of extracellular matrix elaborated by smooth muscle cells, are associated with a short T1. This T1 shortening (increased signal intensity on T1-weighted images) is the consequence of specific interactions between protein and water (46).

Plaque lipids consist primarily of unesterified cholesterol and cholesteryl esters, and are associated with a short T2 (37). The short T2 (decreased signal intensity of T2-weighted images) of the lipid components is in part a consequence of the micellar structure of lipoproteins, their denaturation by oxidation, or an exchange between cholesteryl esters and water molecules (both from the fatty chain or the cholesterol ring), with a further interchange between free and bound water (37,47,48). Perivascular fat, mainly composed of triglycerides, differs in appearance on MR images from atherosclerotic plaque lipids (49). The signal intensities of the calcified regions of plaque, which consist primarily of calcium hydroxyapatite, are low on MR images because of their low proton density and diffusion-mediated susceptibility effects (38,50).

The MR appearance and evolution of thrombus or hemorrhage in the central nervous system (51), pelvis (52), and aorta (53,54) has been studied. The identification of hemorrhage with MRI depends on the structure of hemoglobin and its oxidation state. At various stages blood clots contain different products (i.e., oxyhemoglobin, deoxyhemoglobin, methemoglobin, and hemosiderin/ferritin). Each of these has a set of specific MR relaxation properties (T1 and T2) that produce different signal intensities (55–59). Blood shortens the T1 and T2 of water. Presumably, T1 shortening is caused by the formation of methemoglobin (which is paramagnetic) from hemoglobin, whereas T2 shortening is caused by magnetic susceptibility. In this regard, ferritin-rich or hemosiderin-rich mature thrombus is associated with marked signal loss on T2-weighted images.

We analyzed 22 human carotid endarterectomy specimens with ex vivo MR and performed histopathologic examinations (60). Sixty-six cross-sectional multicontrast MR images were matched with corresponding histopathology. The overall sensitivity and specificity for each component were very high, and calcification, fibrous tissue, lipid core, and thrombus were readily identified. Diffusion imaging, which probes the motion of the water molecules, was found to be useful for thrombus detection, as has been demonstrated previously (61). Recent efforts have been made to determine the sensitivity and specificity of MRI for detection of human coronary lesions. Nikolaou et al (62) demonstrated recently that ex vivo MRI detected 23

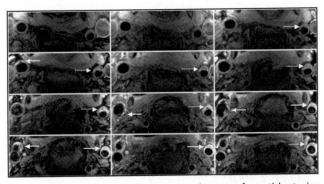

Figure 24.2. Axial magnetic resonance images of carotid arteries in a 68-year-old patient with history of coronary artery disease. The 12 consecutive axial slices are acquired using the REX sequence. The proton density-weighted images obtained show complex atherosclerotic plaque in the carotid wall. The white arrows indicate plaque. REX, rapid extended coverage. (Courtesy of Venkatesh Mani, Mount Sinai School of Medicine, New York.)

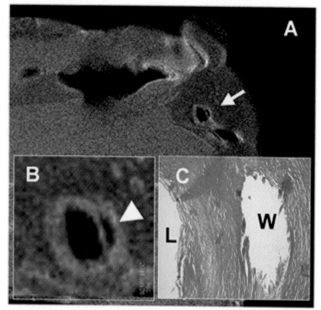

Figure 24.3. Ex vivo images of a human heart, with a fibrocalcified in the left anterior descending coronary artery (LAD), corresponding to a type Vb atherosclerotic lesion according to the classification of the American Heart Association (AHA). MRI T2-weighted image **(A)**, with magnified inlet **(B)** using a fast spin-echo technique. Image shows vessel wall thickening and complete signal loss in the area of the calcification (*arrow, arrowhead*). Corresponding histopathologic section **(C)** with a calcification in the area of the media, calcium is washed out (*W*) during the preparation process. L, lumen of the coronary artery. (From Nikolaou K, Becker CR, Muders M, Loehrs U, et al. High resolution magnetic resonance and multislice CT imaging of coronary artery plaques in human ex vivo coronary arteries. *Radiology* 2001;221: 503, with permission.)

atherosclerotic plaques of 28 plaques that were identified based on histopathology. The images in this study had an in-plane resolution of 195 μm with a 3-mm slice thickness. An example of the image quality achievable is demonstrated in Figure 24.3.

Once multicontrast imaging has been performed, the atherosclerotic plaques can be characterized automatically using various techniques. One such technique is the spatially enhanced k-means cluster analysis. Itskovich et al demonstrated the use of this technique on ex vivo human coronary artery specimens (63).

IN VIVO MAGNETIC RESONANCE IMAGING EXPERIMENTAL STUDIES

MR has been used to study plaques in several animal models, including mice (64), rats (65), rabbits (66), pigs (67), and nonhuman primates (68). In atherosclerotic rabbits, we validated the ability of MRI to quantify lipid-rich and fibrous components of lesions. The plaques were induced in the thoracic and abdominal aorta by a combination of atherogenic diet and double-balloon denudation (69). Fast spin-echo sequences were obtained with an in-plane resolution of 0.35 mm, and a slice thickness of 3-mm proton density-weighted and T2-weighted images were obtained. A signifi-

cant correlation between MRI and histology was observed in the analysis of lipid-rich and fibrous areas.

In two separate serial studies (70,71) MRI demonstrated significant regression of aortic plaque in vivo in atherosclerotic rabbits that underwent cholesterol lowering. After aortic balloon injury and feeding of a high-cholesterol diet, one group of rabbits was continued on the atherogenic diet (atherosclerosis progression), and another group was placed on a normal chow, low-cholesterol diet (atherosclerosis regression). A significant reduction in vessel wall area and mean wall thickness was observed in the dietary regression group, and an increase was seen in the dietary progression group. A significant reduction in the lipid-rich component of plaques was also observed in the dietary regression group, and an increase in the dietary progression group. A small, nonsignificant increase in the fibrous plaque components was noted in the dietary regression group, but there was a significant decrease in the fibrous composition of lesions in the progression group. A significant correlation was found between MR and histopathology for atherosclerotic burden and plaque composition (70).

In another serial MRI study, hepatic hydroxymethylglutaryl coenzyme A (HMG CoA) reductase inhibitors (statins) and a novel class of agents, the acylcholesterol acyltransferase (ACAT) inhibitors, showed beneficial effects in Watanabe rabbits (72). The combination of statins and ACAT inhibitors induced a significant regression of previously established atherosclerotic lesions.

In the rabbit model of aortic atherosclerosis we also showed that MRI could be used to document arterial remodeling (73). With conventional MR systems (i.e., 1.5 T), an in-plane spatial resolution of 300 μm or more can be achieved with sufficient SNR and contrast-to-noise ratio for in vivo imaging of the vessel wall. To study small structures, such as the abdominal aorta of mice (<1 mm in luminal diameter), it is necessary to increase the SNR by using high magnetic field scanners equipped with small RF coils and strong magnetic field gradients (64). Using a 9.4-T (89 mm) bore system we studied atherosclerosis in live animals (64). The achievable in-plane spatial resolution with MR microscopy was approximately 50 μm to 97 μm, and the slice thickness was 500 μm. Using transgenic apolipoprotein E knockout mice, we showed an excellent agreement between MR microscopy and histologic findings for aortic plaque size, shape, and characteristics. We recently extended this study to follow the rapid progression of atherosclerosis in animals with lesions of varying severity (74). High-resolution MRI and MR microscopy might allow convenient and noninvasive quantitative assessment of serial changes in atherosclerosis in different animal models of disease progression and regression (75).

IN VIVO MAGNETIC RESONANCE IMAGING STUDIES OF HUMAN CAROTID ARTERY PLAQUE

MR has been used to study atherosclerotic plaque in human carotid (14,76), aortic (77), peripheral (78), and coronary (79) artery disease. In vivo images of advanced lesions in carotid arteries have been obtained from patients referred for endarterectomy (14). The carotid arteries, with a superficial location and relative absence of motion, present less of a technical challenge for imaging than do vessels such as the aorta and coronary arteries. Short T2 components were quantified in vivo before surgery, and values were correlated with values obtained in vitro after surgery (14). Some of the MR studies of carotid arterial plaques include imaging and characterization of normal and pathologic arterial walls (14), quantification of plaque size (76), and detection of fibrous cap "integrity" (80).

As mentioned previously, most in vivo studies of MR imaging and characterization of plaque have been performed in a multicontrast approach (i.e., T1, proton density, and T2 weighting) with high-resolution black-blood spin-echo and fast spin-echo MR sequences. As the name implies, the signal from flowing blood is rendered black by the use of preparatory pulses (e.g., RF spatial saturation or inversion recovery pulses) for better visualization of the adjacent vessel wall. Hatsukami et al (80) introduced the use of bright-blood imaging (i.e., three-dimensional [3D] fast time-of-flight imaging) to visualize fibrous cap thickness and morphologic integrity. This sequence provides enhancement of the signal from flowing blood and a mixture of T1 and proton density contrast weighting, which highlights the fibrous cap. Multicontrast MRI of human carotid plaque had high sensitivity and specificity for identification of unstable fibrous caps and may enable prospective identification of high-risk carotid plaques (81). Additionally, MR direct thrombus imaging using a T1-weighted turbo field echo sequence, which improves detection of methemoglobin, enabled accurate identification of complicated carotid lesions with thrombus in symptomatic patients who underwent imaging and subsequent endarterectomy (82,83). Measurement of carotid wall volume and maximum area using contrast 3D-enhanced MR has also been performed (84,85).

MR angiography (MRA) and high-resolution black-blood imaging of the vessel wall can be combined. MRA demonstrates the severity of stenotic lesions and their spatial distribution, whereas the high-resolution black-blood wall characterization technique may show the composition of plaques and facilitate risk stratification and selection of treatment modality. Spatial resolution has been improved recently ($\leq$250 µm) with the design of new phased-array coils (85,86) tailored for carotid imaging (87) and new imaging sequences, such as long echo-train fast spin-echo imaging with "velocity selective" flow suppression and double inversion recovery preparatory pulses (black-blood imaging) (85,86). Luo et al (84) performed high-resolution black-blood MRI in vivo on 37 patients with carotid artery disease who then underwent carotid endarterectomy. Following surgery, the carotid plaque specimens were again imaged ex vivo with high-resolution MR and revealed good correlation between in vivo and ex vivo measurements of maximum wall area, minimum lumen area, and wall volume. High-resolution MRI also had good sensitivity and specificity for determining the type of carotid lesion based on the American Heart Association classification system (88–90). MR has been used to identify intraplaque hemorrhage (91) and differentiate intraplaque and juxtaluminal hemorrhage/thrombus in advanced human carotid atherosclerosis (92).

The use of gadolinium-based contrast agents has enabled improved characterization of carotid plaque by not only improving visualization of the arterial lumen but also by differential contrast enhancement of various plaque components. For example, Yuan et al (93) demonstrated an 80% enhancement of fibrous tissue while there was only a 29% enhancement of the necrotic core when comparing postcontrast-enhanced with noncontrast-enhanced high-resolution MRI.

MR has also been used to study differences in carotid plaque composition between different ethnic and racial groups (94).

IN VIVO MAGNETIC RESONANCE IMAGING STUDIES ON HUMAN AORTIC PLAQUE

In vivo black-blood MR characterization of atherosclerotic plaque in the human aorta has been reported (77,95). The principal challenges associated with MRI of the thoracic aorta include obtaining sufficient sensitivity for submillimeter imaging and excluding artifacts caused by respiratory motion and blood flow. Summers et al (95) used MRI to show that the wall thickness of the ascending aorta is increased in patients with homozygous familial hypercholesterolemia. Only conventional T1-weighted spin-echo images were obtained, and therefore, plaque composition was not analyzed (5). Fayad et al (77) assessed the composition of plaque in the thoracic aorta with T1-weighted, proton density-weighted, and T2-weighted images. Rapid high-resolution imaging was performed with a fast spin-echo sequence in conjunction with "velocity-selective" flow suppression preparatory pulses. The results of matched cross-sectional aortic imaging with MR and TEE correlated strongly for plaque composition and mean maximum plaque thickness. An example of MRI detection of human aortic plaque is demonstrated in Figure 24.1.

In asymptomatic subjects from the Framingham Heart Study (FHS), MR showed that the prevalence and burden (i.e., plaque volume/aortic volume) of aortic atherosclerosis increased significantly with age and was greater in the abdominal aorta compared with the thoracic aorta (96). It was also found that long-term measures of risk factors and the FHS coronary risk score are strongly associated with asymptomatic aortic atherosclerosis as detected by MR (97).

IN VIVO MAGNETIC RESONANCE IMAGING STUDIES OF CORONARY ARTERY PLAQUE

The ultimate goal is noninvasive imaging of plaque in the coronary arteries. Preliminary studies in a pig model showed that the difficulties encountered in imaging the coronary wall are caused by a combination of cardiac and respiratory motion artifacts in addition to the tortuous course, small size, and location of the coronary arteries (40,98). We applied the black-blood MR methods used in the human carotid artery and aorta to image the coronary arterial lumen and wall (79). The imaging method was validated in coronary lesions induced in Yorkshire albino swine with balloon angioplasty

(98). The intraobserver and interobserver assessment of variability by intraclass correlation for both MRI and histopathology showed good reproducibility, with the intraclass correlation coefficients ranging from 0.96 to 0.99. MRI was also able to visualize intralesional hematoma with a sensitivity of 82% and specificity of 84%.

After the animal experiments, high-resolution black-blood MRI of both normal and atherosclerotic human coronary arteries was performed. The difference in maximal wall thickness between normal subjects and patients (≥40% stenosis) was statistically significant. Fayad et al (79) investigated coronary plaque with MRI performed during breath-holding in order to minimize respiratory motion. To alleviate the need for breath-holding, Botnar et al (99) combined the black-blood fast-spin echo method with a real-time navigator for respiratory gating and real-time correction of slice position. High-resolution MR images of coronary artery vessel wall in healthy volunteers have also been obtained at 3T using a respiratory navigator and a real-time motion correction gradient echo sequence (100).

HUMAN IN VIVO MONITORING OF THERAPY WITH MAGNETIC RESONANCE IMAGING

MRI has become a powerful tool in quantifying the degree of plaque regression following administration of different pharmacotherapies when imaging animals or humans in vivo. We demonstrated that MR could be used in vivo to measure the effect of lipid-lowering therapy (statins) in asymptomatic untreated patients with hypercholesterolemia

and carotid and aortic atherosclerosis (101). Atherosclerotic plaques were visualized and measured with MR at different times after the initiation of lipid lowering therapy. Significant regression of atherosclerotic lesions was observed. Despite the early and expected hypolipidemic effect of the statins, a minimum of 12 months was needed to observe changes in the vessel wall. In fact, no changes were detected at 6 months. A decrease in the vessel wall area but no change in the luminal area was noted at 12 months, confirming the findings of previous experimental studies (71,72). After treating hyperlipidemic rabbits with aortic atherosclerosis with statins, selective peroxisomal proliferator-activated receptor-gamma (PPAR-gamma), or a combination, Corti et al (102) demonstrated that PPAR-gamma alone induced a significant regression in plaque but the largest regression was seen with PPAR-gamma and statin combination therapy. An illustration of plaque regression can be seen in Figure 24.4.

High-resolution MR of the popliteal artery and the response to balloon angioplasty was reported by Coulden et al (78). In all patients, the extent of the atherosclerotic plaque could be defined, such that even in segments of vessel that were angiographically "normal," atherosclerotic lesions with cross-sectional areas ranging from 49% to 76% of potential lumen area were identified. Following angioplasty, plaque fissuring and local dissection were easily identified, and serial changes in lumen diameter, blood flow, and lesion size were documented. This study showed that high-resolution MR can define the extent of atherosclerotic plaque in the peripheral vasculature and identify the changes of remodeling and restenosis following angioplasty.

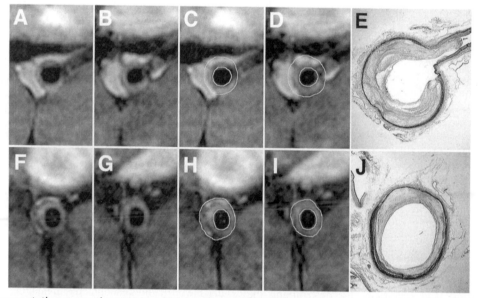

Figure 24.4. Representative magnetic resonance images of the abdominal aorta showing progression in the high cholesterol diet group (*upper panels*) and regression in the normal chow diet plus simvastatin plus peroxisomal proliferator-activated receptor-gamma agonist group (*lower panels*). The raw images at atherosclerosis (AT) baseline (**A,F**) and at the end of treatment (**B,G**), as well as the analyzed traced images at AT baseline (**C,H**) and at the end of treatment (**D,I**), are shown for the respective treatment groups. The right panels (**E,J**) show the matched histologic section at the end of treatment. (From Corti R, Osende JI, Fallon JT, et al. The selective peroxisomal proliferator-activated receptor-gamma agonist has an additive effect on plaque regression in combination with simvastatin in experimental atherosclerosis: in vivo study by high-resolution magnetic resonance imaging. *J Am Coll Cardiol* 2004;43:464–473, with permission.)

FUTURE APPLICATIONS

IMPROVEMENTS IN MAGNETIC RESONANCE TECHNIQUES FOR IMAGING PLAQUE

The spatial resolution of current MR techniques for imaging plaque is mainly limited by the available SNR. One way to increase the SNR directly is to improve the receiver coils.

New External Coils

We designed and tested a new cardiac coil for high-resolution MRI of human coronary plaques (86). Our new coil consists of an array (four-element phased-array coil: 2 square coils, each 7.3 cm × 7.3 cm, and 2 rectangular coils, each 6.4 cm × 9.7 cm) in which all of the coils are placed on the surface of the chest and MRI is performed on a 1.5T imager. We compared the SNRs in various regions of the heart with the new four-element anterior coil and with a general whole-heart coil (2 anterior and 2 posterior elements, each 20 cm × 12 cm). High-resolution imaging of the coronary wall and plaque was performed with two-dimensional spiral and black-blood fast spin-echo sequences in 15 normal subjects and 15 patients with proximal coronary disease. It is evident from the curves that the anterior array has an SNR advantage for depths to about 12 cm. High-resolution imaging of coronary plaque (≤0.5 mm in-plane resolution and 3–4 mm slice thickness) was achieved with our four-element anterior phased-array coil in all subjects. Proximally, our new coil produced images superior to those obtained with a general whole-heart coil. We believe this new approach can play an important role in applications such as high-resolution MR characterization of the wall in atherosclerotic proximal coronary arteries.

We have also developed coils that are optimized for carotid imaging at 1.5T (20). A new phased-array surface receiver coil consisting of a four-element bilateral array (5 cm × 5 cm in size, total of 8 channels) resonating at 63.64 MHz using distributed capacitors was developed. The individual 5-cm² coils of the array were etched on a flexible Kapton-clad material (DuPont, Wilmington, DE) and overlapped (to minimize mutual inductance) in a windowpane configuration. Actively switched PIN diodes were used for decoupling the coils during the transmit phase, as previously described by Fayad et al (85). Along the centerline, the overlapped coil elements were mounted on a 40 mm-wide flat piece of rigid plastic, while remaining sections were allowed to flex to accommodate various neck anatomies. Silicone foam was mounted over the coil assemblies, providing about an 8-mm distance between the coil traces and the subject's body. Figure 24.5 shows a version of the coil. With this coil, high-resolution black-blood carotid imaging (<0.5 cm in-plane resolution and slice thickness of 3 mm) was possible.

Targeted Magnetic Resonance Imaging of Molecular Components in Atherosclerotic Plaque

The ability to target specific molecules of plaques may greatly enhance detection and characterization of atheroscle-

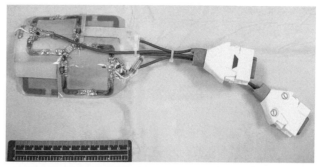

Figure 24.5. One side of eight-channel carotid phased-array coil showing four elements. Each array element is 5 cm², etched on a flexible Kapton-clad material, overlapped in a windowpane configuration, and resonated to 63.64 MHz using distributed capacitors. (From Itskovich VV, Mani V, Mizsei G, Aguinaldo JG, et al. Parallel and nonparallel simultaneous multislice black-blood double inversion recovery techniques for vessel wall imaging. *J Magn Reson Imaging* 2004;19:459–467, with permission.)

rotic and atherothrombotic lesions using MRI (103). Contrast agents linked to antibodies (104–107) or peptides (108,109) that target specific plaque components or molecules that localize to specific regions of atherosclerotic plaque (110–113) are examples of strategies that have been employed to image atherosclerosis with MR. The ability to target mononuclear cells such as monocytes, macrophages, and foam cells is an attractive means of identifying atherosclerosis since these cells have been shown to play a pivotal role in the progression of atherosclerosis to symptomatic disease (114,115). While current research is underway to target macrophages with gadolinium-based contrast agents that target the macrophage scavenger receptor, macrophages have only been imaged with iron oxide compounds (USPIOs, SPIOs) that are removed from the circulation by macrophages and other cells of the reticuloendothelial system (111–113). In a study by Kooi et al (112) on 11 symptomatic patients scheduled for carotid endarterectomy, 75% of ruptured or rupture-prone lesions demonstrated uptake of USPIOs compared with only 7% of stable lesions and a decrease in signal intensity of 24% on T2*.

Neovascularization has been shown to play an important role in atherosclerosis, and the integrin $\alpha_v\beta_3$ has been targeted to identify regions in the vessel wall undergoing neovascularization (105–107). Winter et al (107) recently demonstrated in a rabbit model of atherosclerosis that regions of neovascularization in plaque had a 47% increase in signal intensity following treatment with $\alpha_v\beta_3$-targeted nanoparticles.

Additional targets of interest for imaging of atherosclerotic plaque with molecular-specific MR contrast agents are oxidized low-density lipoprotein (oxLDL), tissue factor, endothelial integrins, matrix metalloproteinases, and extracellular matrix proteins such as tenascin-C. Choudhury et al (116) recently highlighted these targets (Fig. 24.6). While targeted nuclear imaging through the use of antibodies specific to oxLDL has demonstrated promises at detecting atherosclerosis (117), estimating plaque volume (118), and following progression/regression of atherosclerosis (119), we are unaware of any studies evaluating oxLDL as a target for molecular MRI of atherosclerosis. Additionally, molecules

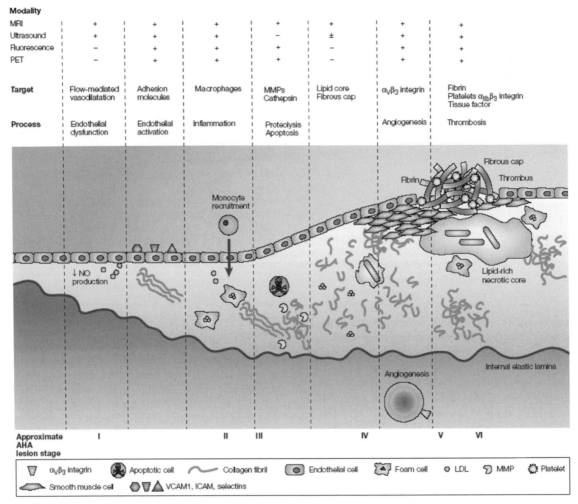

Modality								
MRI	+	+	+	+	+	+	+
Ultrasound	+	+	+	−	±	+	+
Fluorescence	−	+	+	−		+	+
PET	−	+	+	+	−	+	+

Target	Flow-mediated vasodilatation	Adhesion molecules	Macrophages	MMPs Cathepsin	Lipid core Fibrous cap	$\alpha_v\beta_3$ integrin	Fibrin Platelets $\alpha_{IIb}\beta_3$ integrin Tissue factor
Process	Endothelial dysfunction	Endothelial activation	Inflammation	Proteolysis Apoptosis		Angiogenesis	Thrombosis

Approximate AHA lesion stage: I II III IV V VI

Legend: ▽ $\alpha_v\beta_3$ integrin ☠ Apoptotic cell ⌇ Collagen fibril ⬭ Endothelial cell ▱ Foam cell ∘ LDL ⌇ MMP ✳ Platelet
◅ Smooth muscle cell ⬡▽▲ VCAM1, ICAM, selectins

Figure 24.6. Illustration of processes of atherogenesis ranging from prelesional endothelial dysfunction (*left*) through monocyte recruitment, to the development of complicated plaques complicated by thrombosis (*right*). The mechanisms are grossly simplified but focus on components (e.g., cell adhesion molecules, macrophages, connective tissue elements, lipid core, and fibrin) and processes (e.g., apoptosis, proteolysis, angiogenesis, and thrombosis) in plaque that have been imaged or that present useful potential imaging targets. Symbols indicate the feasibility (+ or −) of imaging using each of the modalities listed. (From Choudhury RP, Fuster V, Fayad ZA. Molecular, cellular and functional imaging of atherothrombosis. *Nat Rev Drug Discov* 2004;3(11):913–925, with permission.)

such as tissue factor (120) and endothelial integrins (120–122) such as E-selectin, P-selectin, intracellular adhesion molecule-1, or vascular cell adhesion molecule-1, have been targeted with antibodies linked to echogenic contrast agents. While these agents utilize echocardiography or nuclear imaging, the echogenic or nuclear contrast agent could easily be replaced by linking an MR contrast agent to the monoclonal antibody to target the molecule of interest. However, the identification of molecules found only in atherosclerotic plaque will ultimately enable improved detection of atherosclerotic plaque, assuming that the target is expressed in adequate quantity for detection by molecular MRI.

Gadofluorine M is a lipophilic, macrocyclic (1,528 Da), water-soluble, gadolinium chelate complex (Gd-DO3A-derivative) with a perfluorinated side chain. Sirol et al (110) and others (123) demonstrated that Gadofluorine M enhanced aortic wall imaging in Watanabe heritable hyperlipidemic rabbits but did not enhance the aorta of control rabbits.

Gadofluorine M increased signal intensity by 164% at 1-hour postcontrast and increased signal intensity 207% at 24-hours postcontrast (110). A strong correlation was found between the lipid-rich areas in histological sections and signal intensity in corresponding MR images (110) and suggests a high affinity of Gadofluorine M for lipid-rich plaques (Fig. 24.7).

Another recently developed imaging agent is a recombinant high-density lipoprotein (rHDL) molecule that incorporates gadolinium diethylenetriamine pentaacetic acid (Gd-DTPA) phospholipids (124). This imaging agent has a small diameter of 7 nm to 12 nm, is endogenous, does not trigger an immune reaction, and is easy to reconstitute (124). Tested in vivo in ApoE knockout mice, it demonstrated a 35% mean normalized enhancement ratio 24 hours following intravascular injection, and significant uptake of fluorescent rHDL was demonstrated by confocal microscopy (124). Figure 24.8 demonstrates the enhancement achievable with rHDL and provides an illustration of the contrast agent.

in advanced human carotid atherosclerotic lesions by in vivo magnetic resonance imaging. *Circulation* 2004;110:3239–3244.

95. Summers RM, Andrasko-Bourgeois J, Feuerstein IM, et al. Evaluation of the aortic root by MRI: insights from patients with homozygous familial hypercholesterolemia. *Circulation* 1998;98:509–518.

96. Jaffer FA, O'Donnell CJ, Kissinger KV, et al. MRI assessment of aortic atherosclerosis in an asymptomatic population: The Framingham Heart Study. *Circulation* 2000;102:II-458.

97. O'Donnell CJ, Larson MG, Jaffer FA, et al. Aortic atherosclerosis detected by MRI is associated with contemporaneous and longitudinal risk factors: The Framingham Heart Study (FHS). *Circulation* 2000;102:II-836.

98. Worthley SG, Helft G, Fuster V, et al. Noninvasive in vivo magnetic resonance imaging of experimental coronary artery lesions in a porcine model. *Circulation* 2000;101:2956–2961.

99. Botnar RM, Stuber M, Kissinger KV, et al. Noninvasive coronary vessel wall and plaque imaging with magnetic resonance imaging. *Circulation* 2000;102:2582–2587.

100. Botnar RM, Stuber M, Lamerichs R, et al. Initial experiences with in vivo right coronary artery human MR vessel wall imaging at 3 tesla. *J Cardiovasc Magn Reson* 2003;5:589–594.

101. Corti R, Fayad ZA, Fuster V, et al. Effects of lipid-lowering by simvastatin on human atherosclerotic lesions: a longitudinal study by high-resolution, noninvasive magnetic resonance imaging. *Circulation* 2001;104:249–252.

102. Corti R, Osende JI, Fallon JT, et al. The selective peroxisomal proliferator-activated receptor-gamma agonist has an additive effect on plaque regression in combination with simvastatin in experimental atherosclerosis: in vivo study by high-resolution magnetic resonance imaging. *J Am Coll Cardiol* 2004;43:464–473.

103. Lipinski MJ, Fuster V, Fisher EA, et al. Targeting of biological molecules for evaluation of high-risk atherosclerotic plaques with magnetic resonance imaging. *Nat Clin Pract Cardiovasc Med* 2004;1:48–55.

104. Kang HW, Josephson L, Petrovsky A, et al. Magnetic resonance imaging of inducible E-selectin expression in human endothelial cell culture. *Bioconjug Chem* 2002;13:122–127.

105. Kerwin W, Hooker A, Spilker M, et al. Quantitative magnetic resonance imaging analysis of neovasculature volume in carotid atherosclerotic plaque. *Circulation* 2003;107:851–856.

106. Anderson SA, Rader RK, Westlin WF, et al. Magnetic resonance contrast enhancement of neovasculature with alpha-(v)beta(3)-targeted nanoparticles. *Magn Reson Med* 2000;44:433–439.

107. Winter PM, Morawski AM, Caruthers SD, et al. Molecular imaging of angiogenesis in early-stage atherosclerosis with alpha(v)beta3-integrin-targeted nanoparticles. *Circulation* 2003;108:2270–2274.

108. Botnar RM, Perez AS, Witte S, et al. In vivo molecular imaging of acute and subacute thrombosis using a fibrin-binding magnetic resonance imaging contrast agent. *Circulation* 2004;109:2023–2029.

109. Johansson LO, Bjornerud A, Ahlstrom HK, et al. A targeted contrast agent for magnetic resonance imaging of thrombus: implications of spatial resolution. *J Magn Reson Imaging* 2001;13:615–618.

110. Sirol M, Itskovich VV, Mani V, et al. Lipid-rich atherosclerotic plaques detected by gadofluorine-enhanced in vivo magnetic resonance imaging. *Circulation* 2004;109:2890–2896.

111. Ruehm SG, Corot C, Vogt P, et al. Magnetic resonance imaging of atherosclerotic plaque with ultrasmall superparamagnetic particles of iron oxide in hyperlipidemic rabbits. *Circulation* 2001;103:415–422.

112. Kooi ME, Cappendijk VC, Cleutjens KB, et al. Accumulation of ultrasmall superparamagnetic particles of iron oxide in human atherosclerotic plaques can be detected by in vivo magnetic resonance imaging. *Circulation* 2003;107:2453–2458.

113. Trivedi RA, JM UK-I, Graves MJ, et al. In vivo detection of macrophages in human carotid atheroma: temporal dependence of ultrasmall superparamagnetic particles of iron oxide-enhanced MRI. *Stroke* 2004;35:1631–1635.

114. Falk E. Plaque rupture with severe pre-existing stenosis precipitating coronary thrombosis. Characteristics of coronary atherosclerotic plaques underlying fatal occlusive thrombi. *Br Heart J* 1983;50:127–134.

115. Ross R. Atherosclerosis—an inflammatory disease. *N Engl J Med* 1999;340:115–126.

116. Choudhury RP, Fuster V, Fayad ZA. Molecular, cellular and functional imaging of atherothrombosis. *Nat Rev Drug Discov* 2004;3:913–925.

117. Tsimikas S, Palinski W, Halpern SE, et al. Radiolabeled MDA2, an oxidation-specific, monoclonal antibody, identifies native atherosclerotic lesions in vivo. *J Nucl Cardiol* 1999;6:41–53.

118. Tsimikas S. Noninvasive imaging of oxidized low-density lipoprotein in atherosclerotic plaques with tagged oxidation-specific antibodies. *Am J Cardiol* 2002;90:22L–27L.

119. Tsimikas S, Shortal BP, Witztum JL, et al. In vivo uptake of radiolabeled MDA2, an oxidation-specific monoclonal antibody, provides an accurate measure of atherosclerotic lesions rich in oxidized LDL and is highly sensitive to their regression. *Arterioscler Thromb Vasc Biol* 2000;20:689–697.

120. Hamilton AJ, Huang SL, Warnick D, et al. Intravascular ultrasound molecular imaging of atheroma components in vivo. *J Am Coll Cardiol* 2004;43:453–460.

121. Villanueva FS, Jankowski RJ, Klibanov S, et al. Microbubbles targeted to intercellular adhesion molecule-1 bind to activated coronary artery endothelial cells. *Circulation* 1998;98:1–5.

122. Lindner JR, Song J, Christiansen J, et al. Ultrasound assessment of inflammation and renal tissue injury with microbubbles targeted to P-selectin. *Circulation* 2001;104:2107–2112.

123. Barkhausen J, Ebert W, Heyer C, et al. Detection of atherosclerotic plaque with Gadofluorine-enhanced magnetic resonance imaging. *Circulation* 2003;108:605–609.

124. Frias JC, Williams KJ, Fisher EA, et al. Recombinant HDL-like nanoparticles: a specific contrast agent for MRI of atherosclerotic plaques. *J Am Chem Soc* 2004;126:16316–16317.

125. Schmitz SA, Winterhalter S, Schiffler S, et al. USPIO-enhanced direct MR imaging of thrombus: preclinical evaluation in rabbits. *Radiology* 2001;221:237–243.

126. Johnstone MT, Botnar RM, Perez AS, et al. In vivo magnetic resonance imaging of experimental thrombosis in a rabbit model. *Arterioscler Thromb Vasc Biol* 2001;21:1556–1560.

127. Flacke S, Fischer S, Scott MJ, et al. Novel MRI contrast agent for molecular imaging of fibrin: implications for detecting vulnerable plaques. *Circulation* 2001;104:1280–1285.

128. Yu X, Song SK, Chen J, et al. High-resolution MRI characterization of human thrombus using a novel fibrin-targeted paramagnetic nanoparticle contrast agent. *Magn Reson Med* 2000;44:867–872.

129. Winter PM, Caruthers SD, Yu X, et al. Improved molecular imaging contrast agent for detection of human thrombus. *Magn Reson Med* 2003;50:411–416.

130. Sirol M, Aguinaldo JGS, Graham G, et al. Fibrin-targeted contrast agent for improvement of in vivo acute thrombus detection with magnetic resonance imaging. *Atherosclerosis* 2005. In press.

131. Luk-Pat GT, Gold GE, Olcott EW, et al. High-resolution three-dimensional in vivo imaging of atherosclerotic plaque. *Magn Reson Med* 1999;42:762–771.

132. Pachot-Clouard M, Vaufrey F, Darasse L, et al. Magnetization transfer characteristics in atherosclerotic plaque components assessed by adapted binomial preparation pulses. *MAGMA* 1998;7:9–15.

133. Steinman DA, Rutt BK. On the nature and reduction of plaque-mimicking flow artifacts in black blood MRI of the carotid bifurcation. *Magn Reson Med* 1998;39:635–641.

134. Berg A, Sailer J, Rand T, et al. Diffusivity- and T2 imaging at 3 Tesla for the detection of degenerative changes in human-excised tissue with high resolution: atherosclerotic arteries. *Invest Radiol* 2003;38:452–459.

25

Plaque Characterization— Computed Tomography

Christoph R. Becker

DEVELOPMENT OF CORONARY ATHEROSCLEROSIS

Coronary atherosclerosis begins as early as the first decade of life with endothelial dysfunction, proliferation of smooth muscle cells, and deposition of fatty streaks in the coronary artery wall (1). At the later stage of this still clinically silent disease, these lesions may further accumulate cholesterol within the intima and media coronary artery wall layer, with a fibrous cap separating the lipid pool from the coronary artery lumen (2). Inflammatory processes with invasion of macrophages and activation of matrix-metallo proteases may cause consecutive weakening of the fibrous cap (3).

Such vulnerable plaques can rupture when exposed to shear stress, and the thrombogenic lipid material may enter the bloodstream. In the most unfortunate event, thrombus progression turns the vulnerable plaques into culprit lesions that occlude the coronary vessels, leading to myocardial ischemia, ventricular fibrillation, and death (4). Alternatively, studies show that plaque erosions with consecutive thrombus formation constitute approximately 40% of cases of sudden coronary death (5). Plaque erosions are more commonly seen in young women and men 50 years of age, and are associated with smoking, especially in premenopausal women.

In the initial stadium of atherosclerosis, the coronary vessel widens at the location of the atherosclerotic plaques. The phenomenon is called "positive remodeling" and explains why such plaques may not be seen by cardiac catheter (6) (Fig. 25.1). Nonfatal plaque rupture or erosion at end stage may heal, organize, and subsequently calcify. Fibrocalcified lesions may reduce vessel lumen diameter (negative remodeling), with consecutive reduction of blood flow and myocardial ischemia.

ESTIMATION OF CARDIAC EVENT RISK

In many patients, unheralded myocardial infarction (MI) associated with a mortality of approximately 20% is the first sign of coronary artery disease (CAD). The risk of an event strongly depends on risk factors such as hypertension, hypercholesteremia, smoking habits, family history, age, and gender. Based of these risk factors, algorithms such as the Framingham (7), PROCAM (8), and SCORE (9) provide an estimation of the midterm (10-year) risk for an individual subject to experience a cardiac event. According to most of

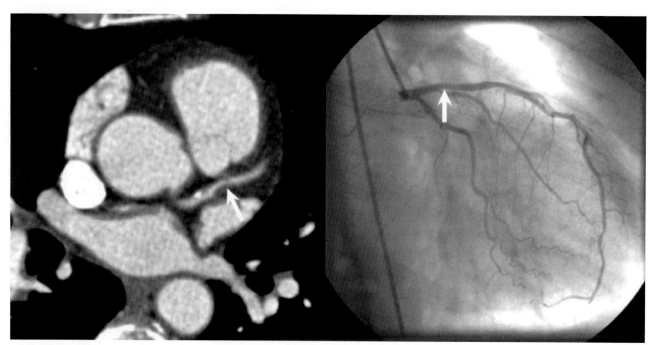

Figure 25.1. Noncalcified lesion (*left arrow*) in the proximal left anterior descending coronary artery. The lesion is difficult to assess in the coronary angiogram (*right arrow*) because of positive remodeling.

the international guidelines, patients with a midterm risk of less than 10% are considered to be at low risk and usually require advice for a healthy lifestyle but no specific therapy. Patients with a midterm risk of more than 20% are considered to be at high risk and, therefore, may be termed patients with a CAD equivalent. Similar to patients with established CAD, these asymptomatic patients may require intensive intervention for risk reduction, such as lifestyle changes and lifetime medial treatment.

Approximately 40% of the population is considered to have a moderate (10% to 20%) midterm risk of CAD. All of the currently available risk stratification schemes suffer from the lack of accuracy to correctly determine the risk, and uncertainty exists as to how to treat patients identified as intermediate risk. Providing information to reassure and/or treat intermediate-risk patients is a high priority. Currently, besides testing for myocardial ischemia (e.g., by treadmill testing), assessment of the atherosclerotic plaque burden provides valid information for further risk stratification in patient cohorts (10).

Tests for myocardial ischemia, such as electrocardiographic (ECG) stress testing, are better suited to diagnose patients with ischemic CAD than to assess clinically silent atherosclerosis in the coronary arteries. Determination of the intimal media thickness (IMT) and ankle bracelet index (ABI) by ultrasound and Doppler focus on the assessment of the atherosclerotic plaque burden in the carotid and peripheral arteries, respectively. However, only computed tomography (CT) and magnetic resonance imaging (MRI) have the ability to noninvasively assess the extent of the atherosclerotic plaque burden in the coronary arteries. MRI is superior to CT in terms of soft-tissue differentiation (11). However, CT is currently superior to MRI in terms of spatial and temporal resolution to image the small and constantly moving structures such as the coronary arteries. Therefore,

CT is the only reliable and practicable tool to investigate the entire coronary artery tree and to quantify the atherosclerotic plaque burden noninvasively (12).

COMPUTED TOMOGRAPHY TECHNIQUE

Initially, coronary CT was performed with electron beam CT (EBCT) since lack of any moving items allowed for exposure times as short as 100 ms. Scan acquisition in EBCT is triggered by the ECG signal to the mid-diastole phase of the cardiac cycle to further reduce cardiac motion artifacts (Table 25.1. The initial intent of EBCT was to measure myocardial perfusion (13). However, EBCT can also detect coronary calcifications as a surrogate marker for coronary atherosclerosis (14). Further attempts have also been made to use this scanner for CT angiography (CTA) and plaque imaging of the coronary arteries. However, low spatial resolution (3 mm) and high image noise of EBCT limits the investigation to the most proximal part of the coronary arteries (15).

Conventional mechanical CT scanners with an x-ray tube and detector ring rotating around the patient have also increased in speed within recent years. The scan mode dedicated to coronary multidetector-row (MD) CT is called retrospective ECG gating (16). In this technique, the spiral CT scan is acquired with a small pitch (table feed per gantry rotation), and image reconstruction is performed in the slow motion diastolic phase of the cardiac cycle. Coronary calcium quantities measured with the first clinical available MDCT scanner with four detector rows and temporal resolution of 250 ms are well comparable to EBCT (17,18).

TABLE 25-1	Acquisition Parameters for Computed Tomography			
	EBCT	4-MDCT	16-MDCT	64-MDCT
Spatial resolution	3 mm	3 mm	0.8 mm	0.4[a] mm
Temporal resolution	100 ms	250 ms	210–195[b] ms	165 ms
Scan time	20 sec	20 sec	20 sec	10 sec
Contrast for CTA	–	–	120 ml @ 4 ml/s	80 ml@ 5 ml/s
Radiation exposure[c]	CCS: 1 mSv	CCS: 2 mSv	CCS: 2 mSv	CCS: 2 mSv
	CTA: na	CTA: na	CTA: 10 mSv	CTA: 12 mSv

[a] With dual z-focus on x-ray tube.
[b] Depending on x-ray tube.
[c] May substantially be reduced in MDCT by applying ECG pulsing and a low-dose protocol.
EBCT, electron beam computed tomography; DCT, multidetector-row CT; CTA, CT angiography; CCS, coronary calcium scanning.

CORONARY CALCIUM SCREENING

A four detector-row CT with 500 ms gantry rotation time is the minimal requirement for a coronary calcium measurement. Coronary calcium screening can be performed by any MDCT without contrast media and with 3 mm slices. Overlapping slice reconstruction improves reproducibility of the coronary calcium quantification (19). Retrospective ECG gating is superior in acquiring the entire volume without any gaps and reconstructing the images with overlapping increment. An overlapping slice reconstruction may help to improve the reproducibility (19). Depending on the MDCT scanner, the scan time may range from 5 to 20 seconds, and the entire investigation is completed within 5 minutes. In total, 40 to 80 slices are generated with one investigation.

As a fundamental requirement for screening, the radiation exposure for coronary calcium scanning needs to be reduced to a minimum (1–2 mSv). In particular, when assessing coronary atherosclerosis in asymptomatic patients, redundant radiation should be avoided. On the base of the ECG signal, the x-ray tube current is switched to its nominal value during the diastolic phase and is reduced significantly during the systolic phase of the heartbeat. This technique is called prospective ECG tube current modulation or ECG pulsing, and is most effective in patients with low heart rates. If the heart rate is lower that 60 beats-per-minute, the radiation exposure will be reduced by approximately 50% (20).

Even the smallest calcifications will become visible by the reconstruction with a no-edge enhancing soft-tissue kernel. After the reconstruction, the image data are analyzed and postprocessed by a dedicated workstation. Upon identification of the specific lesions, the workstation automatically displays the quantities of coronary calcium as the Agatston score, volume equivalent, and absolute mass (Fig. 25.2). According to the method proposed by Agatston, any dense structure in the CT image greater than 130 HU in density is identified as calcification. The area of this calcification is multiplied by a factor that depends on the peak density of the lesion. A factor between 1 and 4 is used for a peak density of 130–199 HU, 200–299 HU, 300–399 HU, and greater than 400HU, respectively. The sum of all lesions in all four coronary vessels (left main, left anterior descending, circumflex, and right coronary artery) corresponds to the total Agatston score (14). This algorithm requires specific EBCT image quality and nonoverlapping slice thickness of 3 mm. Therefore, the Agatston quantification method is of limited value for MDCT.

Originally, the first investigations with the EBCT allowed for acquisition of half of the entire heart because no more than 20 slices could be acquired at once. With this approach, the limited reproducibility became obvious (21), and a number of authors have suggested algorithms to improve the reproducibility. To allow for a reproducible measurement of coronary calcium for follow-up investigations, it was necessary to introduce the calcium volume equivalent (22). With isotropic interpolation, overlapping slice acquisition can be simulated by a workstation, and the reproducibility of the quantification can be improved. However, real overlapping slice acquisition is always superior to isotropic interpolation (19) and should be used with MDCT. The volume score, as well as the Agatston score, is limited since the quantity of the calcium volume depends on the image quality and the values cannot easily be transferred from EBCT to MDCT.

In general, it is possible to quantify the absolute amount of coronary calcium by using a standard calibration phantom in CT (23). For this standardization, the calibration phantom must be scanned with those parameters that will be used later for patient investigation. As the mass of the calcium particles in the phantom are known, it is possible to measure the volume and density of the calcium from the CT image and then to calculate the calibration factor for absolute quantification.

In patient investigations, however, the accuracy of the measurement differs from patient to patient, depending on size. X-ray absorption is different in thin patients as compared to obese patients, where radiation exposure will lead to a beam hardening, resulting in a different density of the same amount of calcium. Therefore, the calibration phantom needs to be scanned with "fat rings" that simulate different patient sizes and deliver appropriate calibration factors (Fig. 25.3). As such, a topogram is used to determine the patient's chest diameter in order to select the appropriate calibration factor. In practice, the calibration phantom is measured without fat rings, with one fat ring, and with two fat rings. For

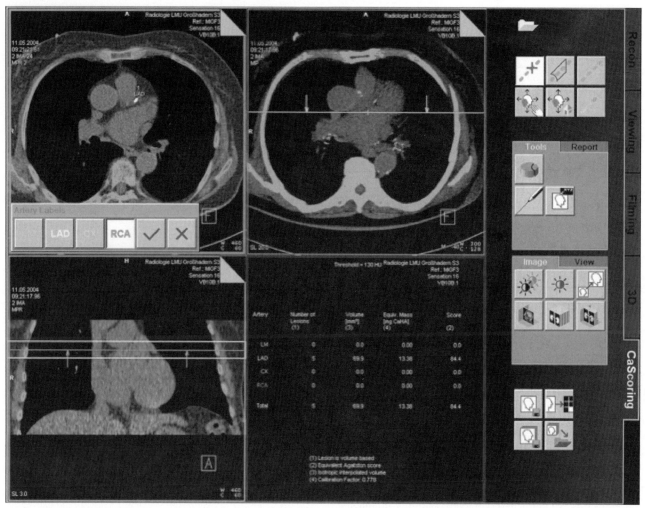

Figure 25.2. Coronary screening images are loaded into a dedicated workstation for quantification of coronary calcium. The software calculates the Agatston score, volume equivalent, and mass of coronary calcium in all of the four major coronary artery segments.

example, in patients with chest diameters measuring smaller than 30 cm, 30 to 38 cm, and larger than 38 cm, calibration factors with no fat ring, one fat ring, and two fat rings will be used, respectively, on each patient.

Recently, the International Consortium on Standardization in Cardiac CT tried to establish a standardized algorithm for coronary calcium measurements for all CT vendors. This consortium also tried to establish a database to collect data in a standardized fashion in order to provide reference values for the absolute mass of coronary calcium (24).

PLAQUE IMAGING BY COMPUTED TOMOGRAPHIC ANGIOGRAPHY

CTA for plaque imaging and detection of coronary artery stenoses requires the highest temporal and spatial resolution as provided by 16 detector-row and 64 detector-row CT. The 16 detector-row CT scanner overcame the limitation of long breath-hold time and allowed for imaging the entire coronary artery tree within 20 second. Recently, 64 detector-row CT scanners were introduced; they allow for scan times as short as 10 seconds and a temporal resolution of 165 ms with a gantry

rotation of 330 ms. The spatial resolution of each new CT scanner generation, with thinner collimation and rapidly moving z-focus on the x-ray tube, has improved from 1 to 0.4 mm (25). Currently, the spatial resolution of the 64 detector-row CT is only 50% below cardiac catheter (0.2 mm).

Homogenous and constant contrast in the coronary artery lumen is necessary to ensure reliable measurements of coronary artery plaque densities (26). Coronary artery enhancement depends mainly on contrast media density and injection rate (27). The use of a dual-head injector for the sequential injection of contrast media and saline is mandatory to keep the contrast bolus compact. In MDCT scanners with shorter scan times, a saline chaser bolus also results in a wash-out of contrast media from the right ventricle, helping to reduce artifacts caused by the influx of undiluted contrast media from the superior vena cava (28). The amount of contrast media necessary for a 16 detector-row and 64 detector-row CT angiography of the coronary arteries has dropped from 120 ml to 80 ml.

Even in 64 detector-row CT with 330 ms gantry rotation, an optimized partial scan view lasts approximately 165 ms. Reasonable good image quality for plaque imaging with this temporal resolution can only be achieved in patients with low heart rates, (e.g., <70 beats-per-minute) (29). To reduce

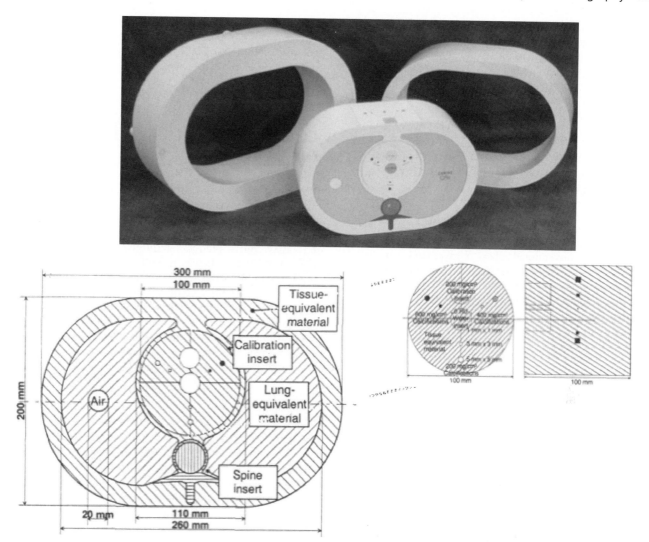

Figure 25.3. Calibration phantom and "fat rings" for calibrated measurement of coronary calcium. The calcium inlets contain known mass of calcium hydroxyapatite. Scanning with parameters used for patient investigation allows calculation of the calibration factor. The calibration factor needs to be adjusted to different body sizes to correct for beam hardening.

cardiac motion artifacts, the use of a beta-blocker may become necessary, aiming for a heart rate of 60 beats-per-minute or even less for patient preparation.

When considering beta-blocker administration, contraindications (bronchial asthma, AV block, severe congestive heart failure, aortic stenosis, etc.) (30) must be ruled out and informed consent must be obtained from the patient. When the patient's heart rate is significantly higher than 60 beats-per-minute, 50 to 200 mg of Metoprololtartrat can be administered orally 30 to 90 minutes prior to the investigation. Alternatively, 5 to 20 mg of Metoprololtartrat divided into four doses can be administered intravenously (30) immediately prior to scanning. Monitoring of vital functions, heart rate, and blood pressure is essential during this approach. The positive effects of beta-blockers on coronary CTA are fourfold: better patient compliance, less radiation exposure, less cardiac motion artifacts, and higher vascular enhancement.

Patients should be instructed not to press when taking deep breath in order to avoid the Valsalva maneuver. During the Valsalva maneuver, the intra-abdominal pressure in-

creases, with blood from the inferior vena cava entering the right atrium. With an increased pressure in the right atrium, blood mixed with contrast media from the superior vena cava is prevented from entering the right atrium. Furthermore, as a reflex, the increased blood volume in the right atrium leads to a decrease in heart rate. The Valsalva maneuver can last several seconds under breath-hold conditions. After release, high dense contrast media may enter the right atrium, and the heart rate recovers to its original or even slightly higher frequency (31). As a result, CTA may not be homogeneously enhanced and image quality may suffer from rapid changes of the heart rate.

After scan acquisition has been completed, reconstruction of the axial slices begins with a careful analysis of the ECG trace recorded with the helical scan. The image reconstruction interval is best seen placed between the T wave and the P wave of the ECG that corresponds to the mid-diastole interval, and the individual point-of-time adjustment for the reconstruction seems to improve image quality (29). The lower the heart rate, the easier it is to find the best interval for all three major branches of the coronary artery tree.

Paracardiac findings are frequently observed in CTA studies of the heart and should be reported. These findings include lymph node enlargement, pulmonary nodule esophageal hernias, or even tumors (32). These incidental findings should trigger an additional reconstruction with a larger field of view, or a more dedicated (CT) investigation might be recommended.

CLINICAL VALUE OF CORONARY CALCIUM

Coronary calcium is a specific marker for coronary atherosclerosis. Initially, such calcifications were detected by fluoroscopy or conventional chest x-ray. However, EBCT provides a more sensitive means to detect coronary calcifications than fluoroscopy. In a cohort of 584 patients, coronary calcium could be detected in 52% and 90% of patients by fluoroscopy and EBCT, respectively. However, only 109 patients within this entire cohort had proven CAD; therefore, detection of coronary calcium by EBCT is a poor method to discriminate between patients with and without CAD (14).

Arad et al were the first to report on the attempt to predict cardiac events with coronary calcium as detected by EBCT. In their cohort of 1,173 patients, they observed 26 soft events (percutaneous transluminal coronary angioplasty and bypass grafting) and hard events (myocardial infarction and death) in a period of 19 months. If the Agatston score was above 160, the odds ratio for an event was 20 to 35.4. Raggi et al (33) used age-specific and gender-specific percentiles derived from nearly 10,000 patients to identify those at increased risk for an event. Seventy percent of patients with an unheralded myocardial infarction (n = 172) were above the 75th percentile with their calcium score as compared to an asymptomatic cohort (n = 632) (33).

Current strategies provide two different values for the risk estimation—one by the conventional risk assessment and another by the amount of coronary calcium. It was recently hypothesized that the combined use of the Framingham risk assessment and the calcium measurement are superior to the use of the Framingham risk assessment alone (34). In the Framingham risk algorithm, higher age becomes the predominant factor above all others, an assumption that does not fit all patients. Therefore, Grundy has proposed an alternative method whereby the age score in Framingham is replaced by a scheme where the coronary calcium percentiles are taken into account. If the amount of coronary calcium falls between the 25th and 75th percentile, the Framingham risk score remains unchanged. If the amount of calcium is below the 25th or above the 75th percentile, the score is the same as for patients approximately 10 years younger or older, respectively (35).

The progression of coronary calcium in patients with hypercholesteremia may depend on the intensity of the statin therapy. In asymptomatic hypercholesteremic patients without therapy, statins, and more than 120 mg/dl cholesterol, the annual progression rate is 52 ± 36%, 25 ± 22%, and −7 ± 23%, respectively (36). However, a regression of coronary calcium appears very unlikely from the pathophysiological point of view. The reproducibility of the measurement of coronary calcium by CT is in the range of 10% and, therefore, a regression below this value may be very difficult to determine. Furthermore, it remains to be proved that the progression of coronary calcium results in an increased risk for a cardiac event.

COMPUTED TOMOGRAPHY PLAQUE ANALYSIS

The entire extent of coronary atherosclerosis with calcified and noncalcified plaques may become visible by the administration of contrast media. Plaques in heart specimens with low density plaques (40 HU) and high dense plaques (90 HU) may consist predominantly of lipid and fibrous tissue (37), respectively. It was recently reported that micro-CT with ultrahigh spatial resolution is able to distinguish between different plaque components such as lipid, fibrin, and calcium by the different Hounsfield units. In the early stages of atherosclerosis, the proliferation of smooth muscle cells initially increased the Hounsfield units of atherosclerotic plaques (38).

The current gold standard to detect coronary atherosclerosis *in vivo* is intravascular ultrasound (IVUS). Studies comparing IVUS with MDCT have shown a good correlation between the echogeneity and CT density of coronary atherosclerotic lesions (39). Schröder et al (40) were able to demonstrate that plaques with low, intermediate, and high echogeneity may correspond to plaques in MDCT with a density of 14 ± 26, 91 ± 21 HU, and 419 ± 194 HU, respectively, as compared to IVUS (Fig. 25.4). The sensitivity and specificity for CT to detect calcified and noncalcified coronary atheroscleroses are between 78% and 94%, respectively. However, the sensitivity to detect noncalcified plaques in a lesion-by-lesion comparison between CTA and IVUS is only 53% (41). Most likely, plaque erosions are more difficult to detect by MDCT than vulnerable plaque with a larger lipid core.

As mentioned previously, large lipid components are found predominantly in vulnerable plaques that are prone to rupture with consecutive thrombosis and occlusion of the coronary artery. Routine investigation of asymptomatic patients by coronary CTA is currently not indicated due to the high radiation burden and contrast media administration necessary for this investigation. Furthermore, the prospective value for the detection of noncalcified lesions has not been demonstrated to date and needs to be further investigated in clinical studies.

PLAQUE IMAGING IN SYMPTOMATIC PATIENTS

The assessment of atherosclerotic plaque burden in symptomatic patients may be of clinical interest. In a recently study, Leber et al (42) reported that noncalcified lesions were found predominantly in patients with acute MI, whereas calcified lesions were found more often in patients with chronic stable angina. In patients with acute coronary syn-

associated with isomerism of the bronchi, the two atria are not distinguishable.

VENOUS CONNECTIONS

SYSTEMIC VENOUS CONNECTIONS

MRI has demonstrated several anomalies of the systemic veins. The most common anomalous systemic venous connection is the persistent left-sided SVC, a remnant of the embryologic left anterior cardinal vein (6). By itself, a persistent left SVC is an incidental finding, although it can be seen in combination with other defects. Most commonly, the left SVC drains from the left brachiocephlic vein and joins the coronary sinus to drain into the right atrium. A right-sided SVC is usually present as well. The two SVCs may or may not be connected across the midline by a bridging vein. In the rare circumstance of atresia of the right SVC, the left SVC and coronary sinus are markedly dilated. Transverse MR images can depict the diameters of the venae cavae and of the coronary sinus. It is important to alert the surgeon to the presence of a left-sided SVC because it can affect cannulation of the heart during cardiac bypass and may divert flow away from the pulmonary circulation after certain types of surgical shunts (6).

Systemic vein anomalies can cause concern for a mediastinal mass on chest radiography. In this situation, MRI can be used for noninvasive diagnosis of the anomaly. As stated previously, the IVC insertion to the right atrium is nearly constant. However, there can be cases, especially with abnormal situs, where the IVC may drain into the left atrium, or in which some hepatic veins drain into one atrium and the rest drain into the other. These are usually associated with severe abnormalities of visceral situs as described previously (6). Interruption of the IVC with azygous continuation is readily demonstrated by MRI, which can be used to identify this anomaly when a dilated azygous vein suggests the possibility of IVC interruption.

PULMONARY VENOUS CONNECTIONS

Total anomalous pulmonary venous return

In the embryo, the pulmonary veins grow from the lung buds and come together to form a confluence, which normally incorporates into the posterior wall of the left atrium. However, if this confluence joins the circulatory system elsewhere, it creates the situation in which all of the pulmonary venous return is anomalous—total anomalous pulmonary venous return (TAPVC) (9). TAPVC is usually classified according to the location of the venous insertion. It may be supracardiac (type I), in which the pulmonary venous confluence usually drains into the SVC or into an anomalous left-sided vertical vein, which in turn drains into the left brachiocephalic vein. The left vertical vein is a derivative of the left anterior cardinal vein (9) (i.e., the same embryologic structure that in different patients may persist as a left-sided SVC). TAPVC at the cardiac level (type II) usually drains

into the right atrium or coronary sinus. In type III TAPVC, the pulmonary venous confluence drains below the diaphragm into the IVC or portal venous system. As the pulmonary veins pass below the diaphragm, there is often obstruction to flow, which results in pulmonary venous hypertension.

MRI has been shown to be highly accurate for the diagnosis of TAPVC (10), which can be diagnosed when MRI demonstrates that no pulmonary veins drain into the left atrium. MR tomograms and gadolinium-enhanced MRA can provide clues to the location of the anomalous connection by revealing enlargement of the SVC or coronary sinus, or the presence of a common pulmonary vein posterior to or above the left atrium.

Partial Anomalous Pulmonary Venous Connection

Partial anomalous pulmonary venous return (PAPVC) can be diagnosed when one, two, or three pulmonary veins drain anomalously into the systemic circulation. In PAPVC, the anomalous veins can drain into supracardiac (SVC, left vertical vein), cardiac (right atrium), or infracardiac (IVC) sites (9). In all cases of congenital heart disease, it is important to identify the connections of all four pulmonary veins, a function for which spin-echo MRI has been shown to be accurate (11) and which should improve with the use of gadolinium MRA (12) (Fig. 26.3).

PAPVC is a left-to-right shunt because oxygenated pulmonary venous blood is flowing into the right side of the heart. Therefore, ancillary findings of left-to-right shunting may be identified, including right atrial and possibly right ventricular enlargement depending on the magnitude of the shunt. The shunt can be quantified, as will be discussed.

PAPVC is associated with atrial septal defect (ASD) and occurs in almost all patients with sinus venosus ASD. Axial or coronal MR images can clearly depict the connections of

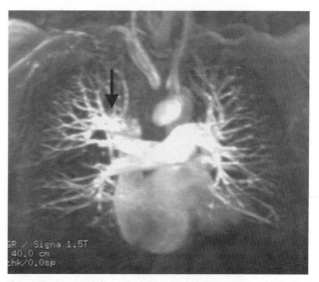

Figure 26.3. Partial anomalous pulmonary venous connection. Contrast-enhanced three-dimensional MRA shows anomalous connection of right upper pulmonary vein (*arrow*) to the superior vena cava. MRA, magnetic resonance angiography.

the pulmonary veins. These connections also can be demonstrated with gadolinium-enhanced MRA. MRI shows the right upper pulmonary vein entering the SVC above its junction, with the right atrium in the most frequent type of partial anomalous connection. Transverse MR images display the coronary sinus; a dilated sinus may be a sign of anomalous connection to this structure. MR images and gadolinium-enhanced MRA can depict the common right-sided pulmonary vein entering the IVC in patients with scimitar syndrome.

VENTRICLES AND ATRIOVENTRICULAR CONNECTIONS

Abnormalities of the AV connections consist primarily of discordant AV connections (such as congenitally corrected transposition of the great arteries) or of AV stenosis or atresia (such as tricuspid atresia, double-inlet ventricle, straddling AV valve) (2,3,13). The first step in analyzing AV connections is to identify the ventricles and determine their morphology.

Axial and coronal MR images through the ventricles can be used to identify these chambers as morphologically right or left. In early embryonic development, the heart is a straight tube with the two ventricles connected in series. The tube then folds over, placing the distal ventricle (the primitive right ventricle) beside and to the right of the primitive left ventricle (5,14, 15). Because the outflow of the primitive heart arises from the primitive right ventricle, the morphologic right ventricle has a muscular infundibulum. This muscular infundibulum and well-defined outflow region separate the right ventricular AV valve (the tricuspid valve) from the ventriculoarterial valve (5) (Fig. 26.4). These findings are identified readily on axial MRI, in which several axial slices usually separate the tricuspid valve and pulmonic valves. On the other hand, in the morphologic left ventricle, the AV valve and the outflow valve are in fibrous continuity (5) and will be seen on adjacent images in the axial plane. The AV valve of the morphologic right ventricle (the tricuspid valve) is slightly more apical in location than the AV valve of the morphologic left ventricle (the mitral valve). As a result, in the normal heart there is a small septum called the AV septum that divides the left ventricle from the right atrium (3,5).

The morphologic right ventricle has more trabeculations than the morphologic left ventricle. The ventricular septum at the apex is heavily trabeculated in the right ventricle but smooth in the left ventricle. A muscular band connecting

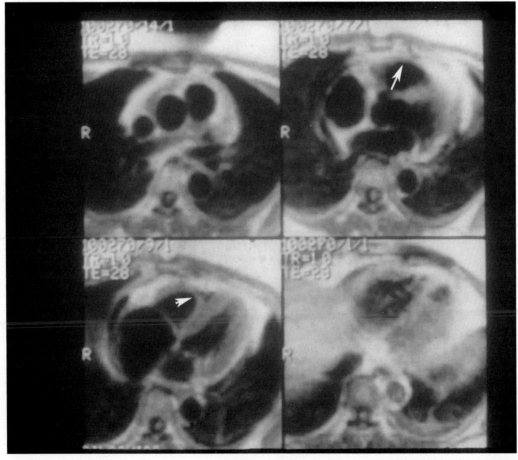

Figure 26.4. Ventricular characteristics. Spin-echo axial images arranged from cranial (*upper left*) to caudal (*lower right*) show a conus (complete tunnel of myocardium) (*arrow*) separating the pulmonary and tricuspid valves. This is a distinguishing feature of the right ventricle. The right ventricle also has a moderator band (*arrowhead*) and the tricuspid valve is positioned more ventral than the mitral valve.

the right ventricular free wall and septum is depicted on axial images (5) (Fig. 26.4).

ABNORMALITIES OF VENTRICULAR LOCATION/POSITION

The normal rightward bending of the primitive cardiac tube places the morphologic right ventricle on the right side of the heart. This rightward bending is called D-looping (the D for the Latin dextro, meaning right). If the primitive heart tube bends to the left, it is called L-looping (L for levo, meaning left) and the result is that the morphologic right ventricle is placed on the left side of the heart. The normal heart has a D ventricular loop. Any heart with the morphologic right ventricle on the left side of the heart may be said to have an L ventricular loop (13).

AV connections can be concordant or discordant. In normal concordant AV connections, the right atrium is connected to the right ventricle and the left atrium to the left ventricle. The AV valves remain with their respective ventricles, regardless of the type of ventricular loop. The mitral valve resides with the left ventricle, and the tricuspid valve is part of the right ventricle, except with double-inlet ventricle. Although the AV valves cannot be distinguished from each other by their morphology on MR images, the recognition of the ventricular morphology indicates the nature of the valve within the ventricle.

Right atrium-left ventricle and left atrium-right ventricle connections are discordant AV connections. Congenitally corrected transposition of the great arteries is an example of an anomaly with AV discordance.

Congenitally corrected transposition of the great arteries (Fig. 26.5) is the term used when the morphologic ventricles are on the wrong side of the heart (L loop) but the atria are in the appropriate location (normal atrial situs) and the great vessels come off the appropriate side of the heart (and, therefore, the inappropriate morphologic ventricles). Another common term used in classification systems is "AV and ventriculoarterial discordance" (1,3).

Corrected transposition can be understood as a ventricular inversion anomaly (i.e., the morphologic ventricles are transposed). The remaining structures (atria and great vessels) may be displaced to accommodate the abnormally located ventricles, but are otherwise normal. As a result, blood flows to the appropriate locations. On the right side, deoxygenated blood comes from the body into the right atrium, passes into a ventricle with fibrous continuity between its AV and ventriculararterial valves (i.e., a morphologic left ventricle), and ultimately into the pulmonary artery and the lungs. Oxygenated blood then returns to the left atrium, flows into a ventricle with a muscular outflow tract (i.e., a morphologic right ventricle), and eventually into the aorta and systemic circulation (16,17).

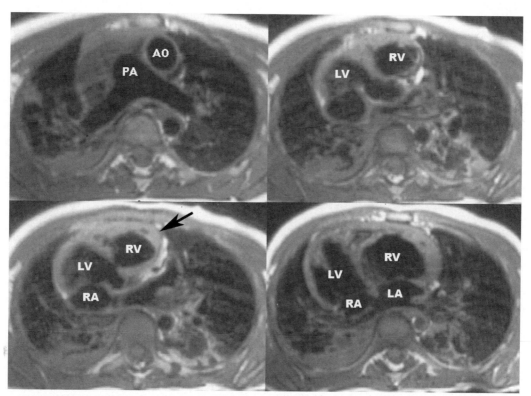

Figure 26.5. Situs solitus with corrected transposition and isolated dextrocardia. Spin-echo axial images arranged from cranial (*upper left*) to caudal (*lower right*). The right atrium (RA) is right-sided and left atrium (LA) is left-sided, indicating situs solitus. The right ventricle (RV) is positioned to left of the left ventricle (LV). Aorta (Ao) is anterior and leftward to the pulmonary artery (PA). Note the conus (*arrow*) and moderator band on the left-sided ventricle, indicating it is a morphologic right ventricle in an L-ventricular loop. Thus, this arrangement of connections is situs solitus, L-ventricular loop, l-transposition, which constitutes corrected TGA. The cardiac apex is right-sided, which indicated isolated dextrocardia. TGA, transposition of great arteries.

In almost all cases of AV discordance and ventriculoarterial discordance, the aorta is anterior to and to the left of the pulmonary artery, a spatial relationship known as "l-transposition." As a result, the position of the great vessels was often used to predict the position of the ventricles before the advent of cross-sectional imaging (17). However, the position of the great vessels is not always predictive of the ventricular morphology (17). Moreover, with MRI, ventricular morphology can be determined directly (18). Therefore, abnormalities of ventricular location should be defined by the position of the ventricles, and great vessel position should be described separately.

In corrected transposition, blood flows in the appropriate direction, and if there are no other abnormalities, patients are asymptomatic. However, the morphologic right ventricle is not designed to pump against systemic pressures for the long term, and patients may present with failure of the morphologic right ventricle (clinically left-sided heart failure) or arrhythmias when they reach their 40s or 50s (19). In more than 90% of patients with congenitally corrected transposition, other abnormalities may dominate the clinical picture. These patients are usually diagnosed in childhood. One associated anomaly is Ebstein's malformation (to be discussed) of the morphologic right ventricle. Ebstein's anomaly is an abnormality of the tricuspid valve, which is a part of the morphologic right ventricle. Therefore, Ebstein's anomaly with corrected transposition will cause obstruction of blood flow and/or regurgitation into the left atrium. Ventricular septal defect (VSD) and/or valvular or supravalvular pulmonic stenosis may also coexist (16,17).

INADEQUATE VENTRICULAR SIZE/ DECREASED FLOW THROUGH A VENTRICLE

In order for the cardiac chambers to grow to normal size and function, adequate blood must flow through them during embryonic life. If the AV or ventriculoarterial valves are stenotic, or if blood is preferentially shunted away from a ventricle, the ventricle fails to develop normally. Depending on the severity of the underlying problem, the lesser ventricle may be simply small or may be rudimentary with no visible lumen. Many clinicians and authors refer to this group of hearts as functionally "univentricular," a term that has created controversy among anatomists who have debated the strict definition of a ventricle (18). Nevertheless, "univentricular" is a helpful way to think about the surgical correction for this group of problems. In most cases, the surgeon's goal is to use the larger, more functional ventricle to pump blood to the systemic circulation. Most often, the smaller ventricle is bypassed by connecting the systemic venous return directly into the pulmonary arteries (20,21).

Tricuspid atresia

There is no direct communication between the right atrium and right ventricle in tricuspid atresia. The tricuspid valve may be imperforate, in which case a fibrous band will be seen. More commonly, the AV connection is absent, in which case fat from the AV groove is interposed between the atrium and ventricle (22,23) (Fig. 26.6).

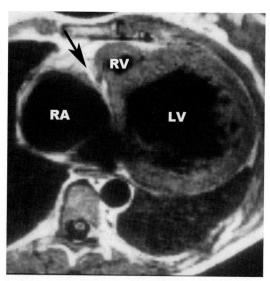

Figure 26.6. Tricuspid atresia. Spin-echo axial image shows a bar of fat and muscle (*arrow*) separating the right atrium (RA) from the hypoplastic right ventricle (RV). The left ventricle (LV) is enlarged.

If any blood is to reach the right ventricle, there must be an ASD to shunt blood from the right atrium to the left atrium, as well as a VSD to shunt blood from the left ventricle to the right ventricle. If both of these shunts are large and there is no pulmonic stenosis, the right ventricle may be close to normal size. On the other hand, if the ASD, VSD, and/or pulmonary outflow are small, the right ventricle may be small and rudimentary. Thus, in tricuspid atresia, the hemodynamics and, therefore, the chamber sizes are variable (24). A restrictive VSD is one in which the maximal diameter is less than the diameter of the pulmonary annulus in a person with normally related great arteries, or less than the diameter of the aortic annulus in a person with transposition of the great arteries. Differentiation of tricuspid atresia or with a large VSD from a single ventricle necessitates demonstration of the atretic valve. In tricuspid atresia, MRI depicts the size of the VSD in addition to hypoplasia or absence of the right ventricle inflow region. For accurate measurement of the defect, the imaging plane must be nearly perpendicular to the VSD.

The incidence of abnormalities of ventriculoarterial connection is high in tricuspid atresia. Twenty-five percent of patients with tricuspid atresia have "complete" transposition of the great vessels (to be discussed) in which the aorta arises from the diminutive right ventricle and the pulmonary artery arises from the larger, more functional, left ventricle (24). Most infants with tricuspid atresia undergo palliative correction, usually one or more of several types of systemic-to-pulmonary artery shunts. At 1 year of age, which many authors consider the minimal age for definitive correction (25), a Fontan procedure is performed. In this operation, all systemic venous blood is surgically rerouted to the pulmonary circulation, thus bypassing the right heart entirely. In its classic form, the Fontan procedure reroutes blood from the right atrium to the pulmonary artery; however, there are many adaptations, including extracardiac shunts that route blood directly from the IVC (26). Preoperatively, important selection criteria for the Fontan procedure include low mean pulmonary artery pressure and pulmonary vascular resistance

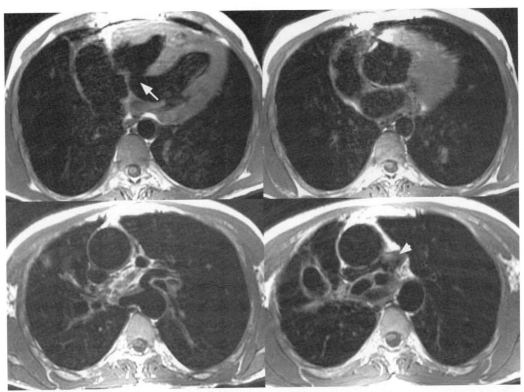

Figure 26.14. Pulmonary atresia with ventricular septal defect. Spin-echo axial images arranged from caudal (*upper left*) to cranial (*lower right*) demonstrate a single large artery (aorta) at the base of the heart, which overlies the ventricular septal defect (*arrow*). Right ventricular wall is hypertrophied. Note the central confluence (*arrowhead*) of the right and left pulmonary arteries distal to the atretic segment.

MRI. Assessment of blood supply to the lungs is achieved on both transverse and coronal images.

The pulmonary and bronchial arteries have bright signal on cine MRI and may be demonstrated better on this type of sequence than on spin-echo images. On transverse images at the level of the carina and immediately below, it is usually

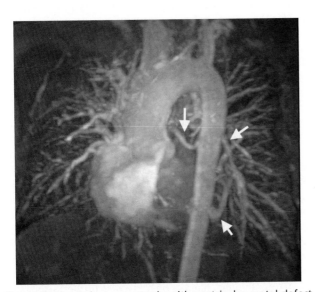

Figure 26.15. Pulmonary atresia with ventricular septal defect. Contrast-enhanced three-dimensional MRA in the coronal plane displays several large systemic-to-pulmonary artery collaterals (*arrows*) arising from the descending aorta. MRA, magnetic resonance angiography.

possible to distinguish between pulmonary and bronchial arteries. Pulmonary arteries are situated ventral to the bronchi, whereas bronchial arteries are located dorsal to the bronchi. Occasionally, a bronchial artery that arises from the subclavian arteries may be located ventral to the bronchi. The origin of bronchial arteries from the descending aorta can be observed on transverse and coronal images. Contrast-enhanced three-dimensional MRA in the coronal plane may be effective in demonstrating the blood supply to the lungs in pulmonary atresia with VSD (Fig. 26.15).

DOUBLE-OUTLET RIGHT VENTRICLE

The definition of double-outlet right ventricle (DORV) has been debated. Some authors include any situation in which both great vessels have more than 50% of their orifice over the right ventricle (Fig. 26.16). Other authors add the additional stipulation that the aortic valve and mitral valve lack their normal fibrous continuity (46). A VSD is almost always present in DORV (46). The location of the VSD, especially its relationship to the great arteries, is important for the determination of the type of surgical repair (47). On axial MRI, the location can be determined by identifying the great vessels and then inspecting the images immediately inferior in order to determine which great vessel outflow tract is confluent with the VSD. Normally, the infundibular portion of the septum separates one of the valves from the VSD (48). A VSD that is related to the aorta (subaortic) is the most common form of DORV, and in these cases, the surgical repair usually involves the creation of an intraventricular tunnel from the VSD to the aorta. If the VSD is on the pulmonic side of the infundibular

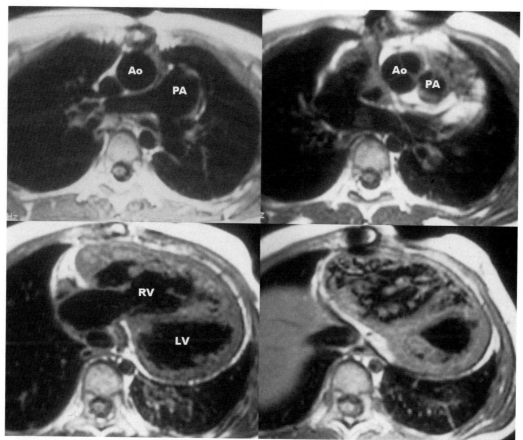

Figure 26.16. Double-outlet right ventricle. Spin-echo axial images arranged from cranial (*upper left*) to caudal (*lower right*). At the base of the heart, the aorta (Ao) and pulmonary artery (PA) lie side-by-side. Both great arteries are connected to the right ventricle (RV). There are coni beneath both great arteries, and trabeculation of the right ventricular side of the ventricular septum. LV, left ventricle.

septum (subpulmonic), the surgical options are more variable (47). DORV with a subpulmonic defect is often referred to as the Taussig-Bing heart (47). If the VSD is immediately inferior to both great vessels, it is called "doubly committed," and if distant from both is called "noncommitted." Both of these defects are less common.

Axial MRI can depict the relationship of the great arteries at the level of the ventriculoarterial valves. In DORV, the great arteries usually have a side-by-side relationship at the base of the heart, but in some cases, the aorta is anterior to the pulmonary artery and slightly to the left or right of the pulmonary artery. MR images can show the origins of the great vessels from the right ventricular outflow tract. The location of the VSD can also be seen on axial MR images. MRI shows that neither ventriculoarterial valve is in direct fibrous continuity with the mitral valve. A complete ring of myocardium is present between the two ventriculoarterial valves and the two AV valves.

Other important aspects of DORV include the presence of valvular and subvalvular obstruction and the presence of associated anomalies. A wide variety of associated anomalies have been reported. Of note, coarctation of the aorta is frequently found in patients with subpulmonic VSD.

TRUNCUS ARTERIOSUS

If the primitive truncus arteriosus does not divide, the aorta and pulmonary artery do not develop normally and a single

arterial trunk forms over both ventricles. A VSD is always present. Truncus arteriosus was initially classified by Collet and Edwards based on the origin of the pulmonary artery from the common arterial trunk (49). In type I, a septum divides the origin of the aorta and pulmonary trunk. In type II, the right and left pulmonary arteries are close to each other but arise separately from the pulmonary trunk. In type III, right and left pulmonary arteries arise further laterally. In type IV, no pulmonary vessels arise from the aorta but branches from the descending thoracic aorta supply the pulmonary vasculature. However, this latter classification has received criticism, primarily since type IV truncus is in fact pulmonary atresia with VSD.

Transverse, sagittal, and coronal images at the base of the heart can demonstrate a large truncus arising above the VSD and aligned over both the right and left ventricles (Fig. 26.17). In type I truncus, the origin of a main pulmonary artery from the truncus can be defined. Transverse scans can reveal the relative sizes of the two ventricles. A large single vessel arising from the base of the heart can also be observed on sagittal images in pulmonary atresia. Differentiation between truncus and pulmonary atresia is done by showing a small infundibular chamber on transverse images in the latter anomaly. Sagittal or coronal images are useful for depicting the truncus and demonstrating the origin of the pulmonary arteries from the truncus (Fig. 26.17). MR images, usually thin (3-mm) tomograms, are used to assess the size of the

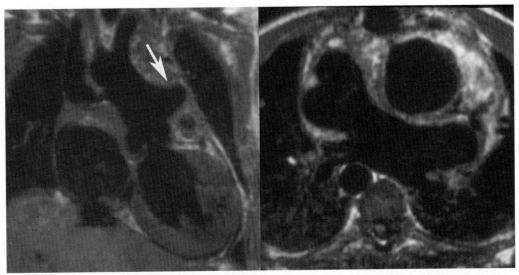

Figure 26.17. Truncus arteriosus, Type I. Spin-echo images in coronal (*left*) and axial (*right*) planes demonstrate a large single artery arising from the heart. The pulmonary artery (*arrow*) arises from the left side of the truncus and the aortic arch is right-sided.

right and left pulmonary arteries. MRI in transverse and sagittal planes is also used to evaluate the caliber of anastomosis after placement of a Rastelli conduit for the repair of the truncus. Demonstration of focal stenoses of the distal anastomoses or of the central pulmonary artery requires thin transverse tomograms. These can also be depicted by contrast-enhanced MRA.

INTRACARDIAC SHUNTS

VENTRICULAR SEPTAL DEFECT

Perimembranous Ventricular Septal Defect

VSDs are classified according to the affected part of the ventricular septum. The ventricular septum has a complex,

three-dimensional structure. Inferiorly, the ventricular septum runs parallel to the plane between the cardiac apex and base. Superiorly, the ventricular septum curves around the right ventricular outflow tract. The membranous part of the ventricular septum is a small area just inferior to the root of the aorta, nestled between the right coronary cusp and the noncoronary cusp (5). Most VSDs in this region extend beyond the anatomic membranous ventricular septum and are often called "perimembranous" (Fig. 26.18). The membranous ventricular septum has complex embryology, with contributions from several primitive structures, and is one of the last parts of the interventricular septum to form (15). It is, therefore, the most common location for a VSD.

Supracristal Ventricular Septal Defect

The crista supraventricularis is a muscular ridge that defines the outlet part of the right ventricle. It is often difficult to

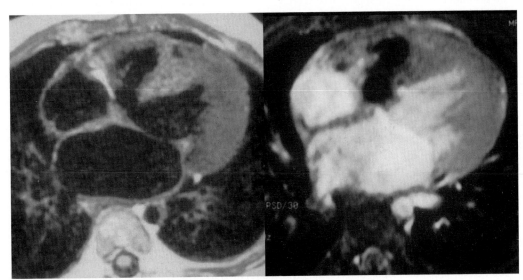

Figure 26.18. Ventricular septal defect. Spin-echo images (*left*) and gradient-echo (*right*) axial images show a defect in the perimembranous ventricular septum. A signal void at the defect is projected into the right ventricle.

see on axial images because it runs parallel to the scan plane. However, the supracristal part of the ventricular septum can be defined as the part of the ventricular septum inferior to the right and left coronary cusps (50). (Note that this is the infundibular part of the ventricular septum, and is anterior and superior to the membranous septum.) A supracristal VSD is located just below the pulmonary valve and the aortic valve and, therefore, is often called "subaortic" (Fig. 26.19). Prolapse of the right coronary cusp into the septal defect, resulting in aortic insufficiency, is a complication of supra-cristal VSD (51).

Muscular Ventricular Septal Defect

The thick part of the septum that is more apical in location than the membranous part is the muscular septum. VSDs can be multiple in this location. Due to the trabeculation on the right side of the heart, they are often difficult to visualize at surgery and must be clearly delineated by imaging.

ATRIAL SEPTAL DEFECT

Ostium Primum Septal Defect

The atrial septum is derived from several structures that to-gether divide the primitive atria into two chambers. During the course of this division, several septa and ostia form and involute in the process of making the final interatrial septum. ASD is usually named according to embryologic septal com-munications that fail to close normally. The first such ostium to form is called the "ostium primum," which is defined by the first interatrial septum, called the "septum primum." If the ostium primum persists, it causes a defect in the in-teratrial septum at the junction of the atrial and ventricular septa, appropriately called an "ostium primum septal de-fect." This defect is part of the spectrum of AV septal defects described previously (52) (Fig. 26.10).

Ostium Secundum Atrial Septal Defect

After the septum primum forms, a second primitive septum, the septum secundum, develops and eventually forms the

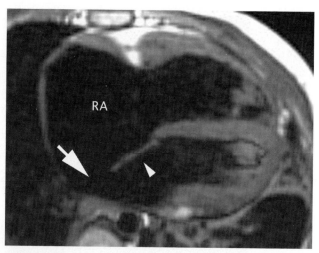

Figure 26.20.   Secundum atrial septal defect. ECG-gated trans-axial spin-echo image shows the defect (*arrow*) in the atrial sep-tum (*arrowhead*). ECG, electrocardiogram.

posterior and inferior part of the interatrial septum, including the foramen ovale. Deficiencies of this part of the septum are the most common type of ASD (Fig. 26.20). A patent foramen ovale is at the same site (52).

Sinus Venosus Atrial Septal Defect

The sinus venosus is the confluence of veins from the body that join the right atrium and form the smooth, posterior wall of the right atrium. Deficient incorporation of the sinus venosus creates an ASD near the junction of the right atrium with SVC (Fig. 26.21). This part of the interatrial septum also normally creates part of the separation of the superior right pulmonary vein from the left atrium so that when a sinus venosus ASD is present, the right superior pulmonary vein inserts into the bottom of the SVC at the site of connec-tion with the right atrium (52).

PATENT DUCTUS ARTERIOSUS

The connection between the aorta and pulmonary artery can be discerned on MR images. The ductus as an isolated anom-

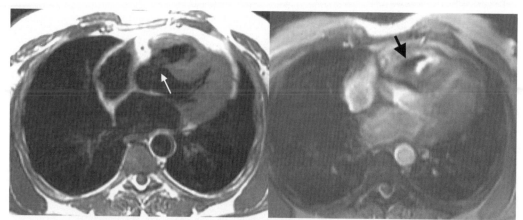

Figure 26.19.   Supracristal ventricular septal defect. Spin-echo images (*left*) and cine MR (*right*) images in axial plane demonstrate a defect (*white arrow*) in the outlet portion of the septum. A flow void (*black arrow*) projects into the upper region of the right ventricular outflow region.

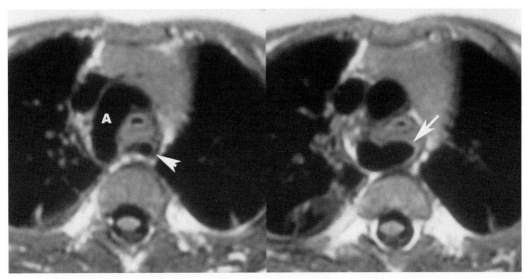

Figure 26.26. Right aortic arch with aberrant left subclavian artery. Spin-echo axial images (*left*) show the right arch **(A)** and aberrant left subclavian artery (*arrowhead*). Another axial image shows the diverticulum (*arrow*) of the descending arch, which is the site of origin of left subclavian artery.

forming a complete ring (Fig. 26.27). The right-sided arch is larger and higher in 80% of cases. Surgical ligation of the smaller arch is the treatment of choice. Axial and sagittal images can be used for preoperative measurement of the two arches.

FUNCTION

In addition to depiction of morphology, the use of MRI for reliable and in many cases unique measurements of function is due to technological improvements. The two main techniques for functional evaluation are gradient-echo cine and VEC-cine phase-contrast MR imaging.

GRADIENT-ECHO CINE

Gradient-echo sequences can be referenced to the ECG to produce multiple acquisitions through a cardiac cycle. By retrospective gating of these acquisitions over several cycles, a series of images corresponding to multiple phases of the cardiac cycle are created. These can be played in a cine loop to show cardiac motion, allowing qualitative and quantitative evaluation of wall motion, contractility, and wall thickening. Precise measurements of volumes and mass can be made without assumptions about geometry. This is especially helpful in cases with functionally univentricular hearts in which the ventricles may have unusual geometry, and in which the performance of both the larger more functional ventricle as well as that of the smaller rudimentary ventricle

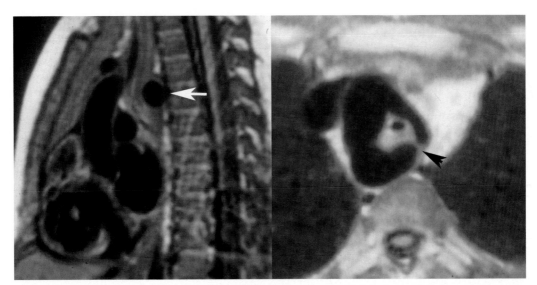

Figure 26.27. Double aortic arch. Spin-echo images in sagittal (*left*) and axial (*right*) planes display posterior compression of the trachea by a retroesophageal component (*arrow*) of a double arch. The axial plane shows that the right arch is the larger of the two as well as a short atretic posterior segment (*arrowhead*) of the left arch.

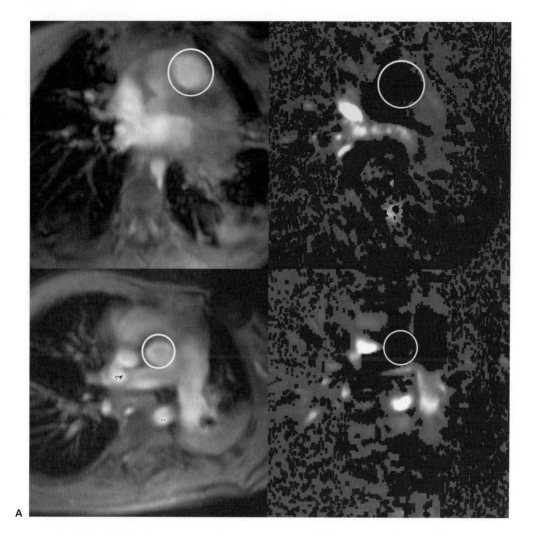

A

Qp/Qs

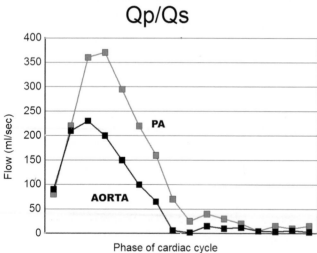

B

Figure 26.28. **(A)** Atrial septal defect. Magnitude (*left*) and phase (*right*) images from velocity-encoded cine MR in planes perpendicular to the long axis of the pulmonary artery (*above*) and proximal ascending aorta (*below*). Regions of interest surround the aorta and pulmonary artery. **(B)** Flow versus time curves for the aorta and pulmonary artery. Because of the left-to-right shunt, the area under the pulmonary artery curve is greater. The area under each curve provides a direct measurement of the pulmonary-to-systemic flow ratio (2.1/1.0).

is important for determining prognosis and for surgical planning (60).

Ventricular Volumes/Ejection Fraction

Cine images in the short-axis plane are used to quantify ventricular volumes, ejection fraction, and ventricular mass.

For each short-axis image, an end-diastolic image is selected and a region of interest (ROI) is created by tracing the inner (endocardial) border of the myocardium. The area of the ROI is multiplied by the slice thickness. Repeating this process for all the end-diastolic images and summing them yields the end-diastolic volume. The same process is performed for all of the end-systolic images to calculate end-systolic volume. This allows for the calculation of ejection fraction without any assumptions about the geometry of the ventricle and can be performed for either the left or right ventricle.

Ventricular Mass

For measurement of ventricular mass, an ROI is traced around the outer (epicardial) border of the myocardium to define an area that includes the myocardium and the ventricular cavity. A second ROI is drawn along the epicardial border of the myocardium. Subtraction of the latter area from the former yields the area of the myocardium on each image. The area of myocardium on each slice is multiplied by the slice thickness, and the areas obtained from all slices that encompass the heart are summed to obtain the ventricular volume. This volume is multiplied by the density of myocardium, 1.05 g/ml (25), to calculate the ventricular mass.

PHASE-CONTRAST VELOCITY/FLOW MEASUREMENTS

In phase-contrast imaging, the signal intensity encodes the velocity of blood at each pixel. ECG-gated phase-contrast images in which each image shows the velocity at a different time in the cardiac cycle can be produced. These are cine images, and are referred to as VEC MRI. A ROI drawn around a blood vessel will give the mean velocity within the vessel at that point in the cardiac cycle. The cross-sectional area of the vessel can be multiplied by the spatial mean velocity to obtain the flow in the blood vessel (27).

ASSESSMENT OF FUNCTIONAL SEVERITY OF COARCTATION OF THE AORTA AND MEASUREMENT OF COLLATERAL FLOW

The functional severity of a coarctation can be estimated with VEC MRI (57,61,62) (Fig. 26.25). VEC MRI sequences are ideally prescribed from an oblique sagittal image in the plane of the aortic arch. The VEC MRI acquisition should be performed in a plane orthogonal to the direction of blood flow. To quantify the collateral circulation, blood flow is estimated at two different locations, one at the proximal aorta just distal to the coarctation site and the other in the descending aorta at the level of the diaphragm (62). Flow is greater in the proximal aorta than in the distal aorta in normal persons. In coarctation, however, blood flow may be greater distally, indicating retrograde collateral flow into the aorta through the intercostal arteries and other branches of the thoracic aorta. To calculate the collateral blood flow, aortic flow distal to the coarctation site is subtracted from the flow at the level of the diaphragm. The degree of collateral flow may be an important factor in operative planning.

The pressure gradient across the coarctation is another important parameter in surgical planning. The peak flow velocity can be estimated by performing VEC MRI through the narrowest segment of the aorta (61), and the pressure gradient can be calculated with the modified Bernoulli equation $\Delta P = 4 v^2$, where ΔP is the pressure gradient in millimeters of mercury and v is the peak flow velocity in meters per second.

QUANTIFICATION OF SHUNTS

Studies have established the usefulness of VEC MRI for quantifying the pulmonary-to-systemic flow ratio (Qp/Qs), and the correlation with oximetry at cardiac catheterization is good (63,64). VEC MRI is also useful for monitoring changes in the volume of the shunt over time (64). Shunt quantification is based on the comparison of right ventricular and left ventricular stroke volumes. VEC MRI is used to ascertain the effective stroke volume (Fig. 26.28). VEC MRI flow measurements are obtained in both the ascending aorta and main pulmonary artery (64). In a normal subject, blood flow is equal in these two vessels. If a patient has a left-to-right shunt with an ASD, VSD, or partial anomalous pulmonary venous connection, flow in the pulmonary artery will

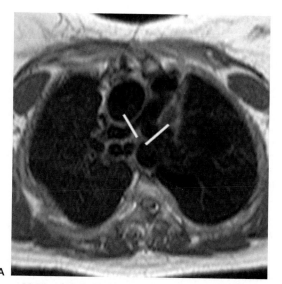

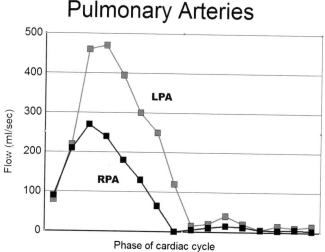

Figure 26.29. **(A)** Sites of acquisition of velocity encoded (phase-contrast) cine MR sequence for the right and left pulmonary arteries. **(B)** Flow versus time curve for right and left pulmonary arteries demonstrate drastically impaired flow in right pulmonary artery.

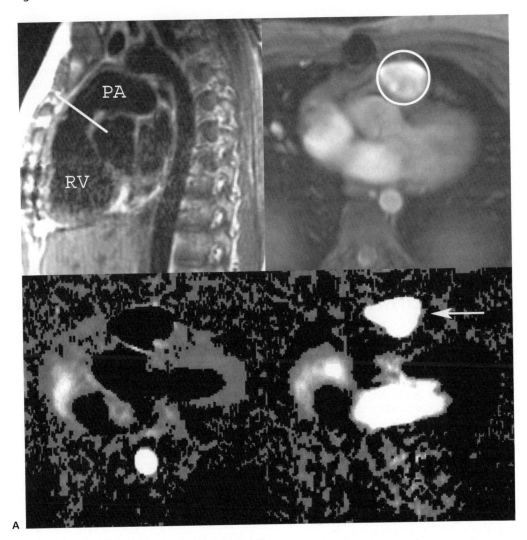

Pulmonary Regurgitation

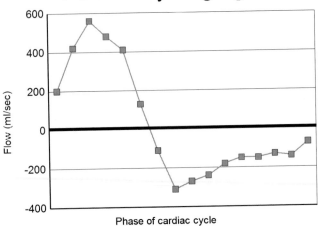

Figure 26.30. **(A)** Postoperative tetralogy of Fallot. Sagittal spin-echo image (*upper left*), axial magnitude image (*upper right*), and phase images in systole (*lower left*) and diastole (*lower right*). Phase-contrast images show forward flow in systole (dark voxels) and retrograde flow in diastole (bright voxels) (*arrow*). Region of interest for flow measurements is shown on the pulmonary artery. **(B)** Flow versus time curve displays the forward and retrograde flow in the pulmonary artery. Area under negative component of the curve yields a direct quantification of the volume of regurgitation.

be greater than aortic flow by the quantity of the shunt. On the other hand, with a patent ductus arteriosus, aortic flow is greater than pulmonary blood flow, and shunt volume is calculated by subtracting pulmonary flow from aortic flow. The opposite relationships are true in patients with right-to-left shunts.

MEASUREMENT OF PULMONARY FLOW

VEC MRI has the unique capability to measure differential blood flow in the right and left pulmonary arteries (65) (Fig. 26.29). VEC MRI can, therefore, provide important information about patients with a disparity of blood flow between

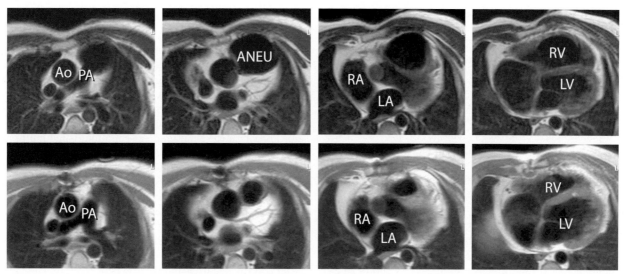

Figure 27.9. Same patient as in Figure 27.8. TOF with repair in the past. Black-blood spin-echo imaging before re-repair (*upper row*) and after re-repair with pulmonary homograft and reduction of the right ventricular outflow tract (RVOT) aneurysm (*lower row*). The RV end-diastolic volume (EDV) reduced from 500 mL preoperatively to 260 mL postoperatively. After the procedure, the effective RV ejection fraction (EF) remained moderate, although RV EF was significantly increased from 11% preoperatively to 36% postoperatively. RV, right ventricle; LV, left ventricle; RA, right atrium; LA, left atrium; ANEU, RVOT aneurysm; Ao, aorta; PA, pulmonary artery.

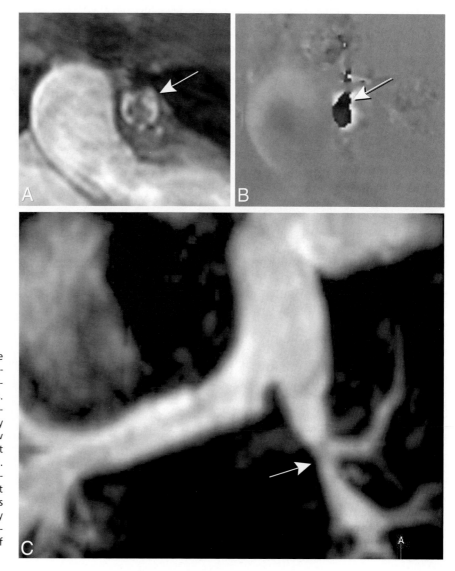

Figure 27.10. An 18-year-old female patient with a history of pulmonary atresia (extreme form of TOF) with pulmonary conduit repair at the age of 6 years. At follow-up, conduit stenosis was observed on flow mapping, represented by severe aliasing caused by increased flow velocity through the pulmonary conduit "valvular stenosis" (*arrows* in **A** and **B**). Also, a moderate pulmonary regurgitation (PR) of 30% was observed (not shown). In addition, there was stenosis of the proximal left pulmonary artery "supravalvular stenosis" on gadolinium-enhanced MRA with a vessel diameter of 7 mm at the stenosis **(C)**.

well (33,34). LV function may be hampered because of adverse RV-to-LV interaction, in which a pressure- or volume-overloaded RV causes dysfunction of the interventricular septum (30).

A recently recognized feature associated with TOF is dilatation of the aortic root and related aortic regurgitation (35). This phenomenon is probably caused by previous long-standing aortic volume overload, with increased aortic flow attributable to the right-to-left shunting before repair (36). In addition to hemodynamic factors, intrinsic wall abnormalities of the aortic wall (similar to patients with Marfan syndrome) have been observed in these patients as well (37). Both an aneurysmatic aortic root and aortic regurgitation may necessitate aortic root replacement (38) and can be assessed with black-blood images of the aortic root and flow mapping across the aortic valve. Figure 27.11 shows an example of dilatation of the ascending aorta associated with TOF.

Timely detection and monitoring of these morphologic and functional abnormalities requires an integrated imaging protocol, focused on assessment of biventricular function, depiction of the pulmonary vascular tree, and assessment of function of the pulmonary, aortic, and tricuspid valves. A complete overview of the imaging protocol in patients with TOF is shown as an example in Table 27.1.

Imaging Protocol

After scout images are obtained, an axial stack of black-blood turbo spin-echo images is acquired to outline cardiac and noncardiac anatomy. A double-oblique transverse stack of images along the aortic root can be used for measurement of aortic root diameters to exclude possible dilatation of the aortic root. Next, axial gradient-echo multislice multiphase imaging is performed to quantify LV and RV function, with special focus on RV function and the magnitude of RV hypertrophy and dilatation. Fifteen minutes after a contrast-enhanced MRA has been obtained to visualize the pulmonary vascular tree, delayed enhancement imaging can be performed to identify scarring of both ventricles, especially at the site of the RVOT. While one waits for the delayed enhancement sequence, flow mapping across the pulmonary artery, aorta, and tricuspid valve is performed for calculation of pulmonary and aortic regurgitant volumes and/or magnitude of stenosis, and RV diastolic function, respectively (Table 27.1).

TRANSPOSITION OF THE GREAT ARTERIES

Clinical Considerations

TGA is defined as atrial situs solitus, normal (concordant) connection between atria and ventricles, and abnormal (dis-

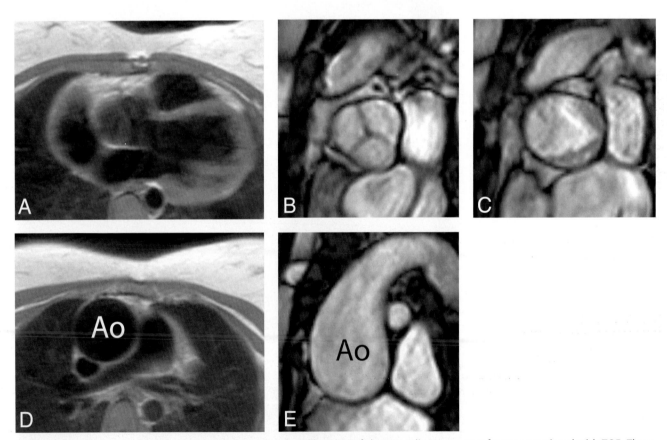

Figure 27.11. The same patient as in Figure 27.10, showing dilatation of the ascending aorta as a feature associated with TOF. There were no signs of aortic valve stenosis or regurgitation. Note the normal aortic root diameter on transverse black-blood spin-echo imaging **(A)** with a normal aspect of the closed and opened aortic valve on oblique sagittal fast gradient-echo imaging **(B,C)**. Dilatation of the ascending aorta (Ao) shown on transverse black-blood spin-echo imaging **(D)** and oblique sagittal fast gradient-echo imaging **(E)**.

TABLE 27-1	Imaging Protocol	
Sequence No.	**Sequence Type**	**Scan Duration (min)**
1.	Scout images	1
2.	Axial black-blood spin-echo	7
3.	Four-chamber multiphase gradient-echo	2
4.	Multislice multiphase gradient-echo	6
5.	Double-oblique transverse stack of images perpendicular to aortic root, black-blood spin-echo	6
6.	Timing MRA pulmonary artery	4
7.	MRA pulmonary artery	7
8.	Flow mapping pulmonary trunk	5
9.	Flow mapping tricuspid valve	5
10.	Flow mapping ascending aorta	5
11.	Look-Locker type sequence apply correct inversion recovery time to:	2
12.	Delayed-enhancement two-chamber orientation (3D-volume)	2
13.	Delayed-enhancement four-chamber orientation (3D-volume)	2
14.	Delayed-enhancement short-axis orientation (3D-volume)	2
Total scan duration time (min)		**56 min**

MRA, magnetic resonance angiography; 3D, three-dimensional.

cordant) ventriculo-arterial connections. The aorta arises from the RV, and the pulmonary artery arises from the left ventricle (LV). It accounts for 4.5% of all congenital cardiac malformations (39). Because the pulmonary circulation is isolated from the systemic circulation, TGA is a life-threatening CHD requiring palliative treatment after birth, followed by corrective surgery during the first year of life.

Before the introduction of the arterial switch operation in 1975 (40), TGA was corrected at the atrial level, redirecting systemic venous blood from the superior vena cava and inferior vena cava to the LV and pulmonary venous blood from the pulmonary veins to the RV (Fig. 27.12), using artificial or pericardial tissue (Mustard technique) or atrial tissue (Senning technique, Fig. 27.13). Although a "physiologic" correct circulation is created, normal anatomic relations are not restored, and the RV remains subjected to systemic loading conditions, followed by compensatory hypertrophy (Fig. 27.14). This results in late RV failure in up to 10% of patients with an atrial redirection operation (41). Other adverse effects like obstruction and leakage of the venous pathways and atrial arrhythmias frequently occur (42,43). Evaluation of biventricular function and depiction of the venous pathways in patients with an atrial redirection or after the arterial switch procedure can be performed best by gradient-echo MRI (Figs. 27.13 through 27.15).

Exercise-MRI can be used to detect subtle ventricular dysfunction, which may not be apparent at rest. The systemic ventricular SV increase in response to bicycle exercise is significantly smaller in patients with atrially corrected TGA compared with controls (14). A recent MRI study using the

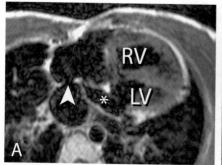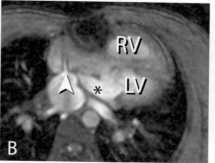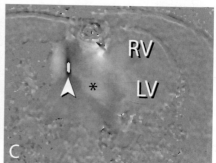

Figure 27.12. Spin-echo **(A)**, gradient-echo **(B)**, and phase-contrast **(C)** MRI in the transverse plane in a patient with a Mustard repair for TGA. A stenosis in the pulmonary venous conduit was observed (*arrowheads* in **A** and **B**) causing high flow velocities during systole (*arrowhead* in **C**). LV, left ventricle; RV, right ventricle. *Systemic venous conduit.

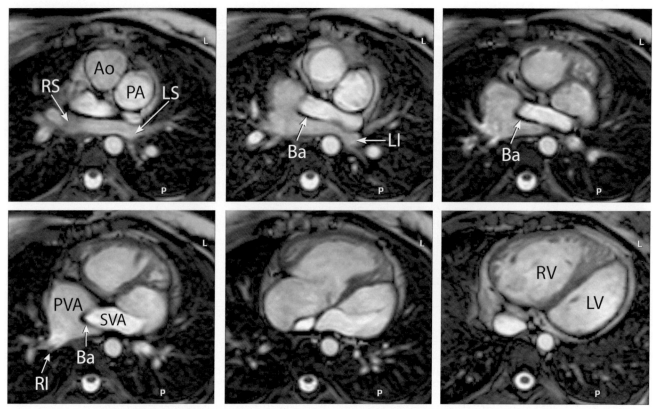

Figure 27.13. A 36-year-old female patient with TGA and Senning repair in the past. Fast gradient-echo images. The aorta arises from the RV. The RV is hypertrophied and sustains the systemic circulation. The pulmonary artery arises from the LV and sustains the pulmonary circulation. Pulmonary veins: LS, left superior; LI, left inferior; RS, right superior; RI, right inferior. Note how the pulmonary venous flow is directed to the RV and how the flow from the superior vena cava (SVC) and inferior vena cava (IVC) is directed to the LV by the intra-atrial baffle (Ba). PVA, pulmonary venous atrium; SVA, systemic venous atrium; Ao, aorta; PA, pulmonary artery.

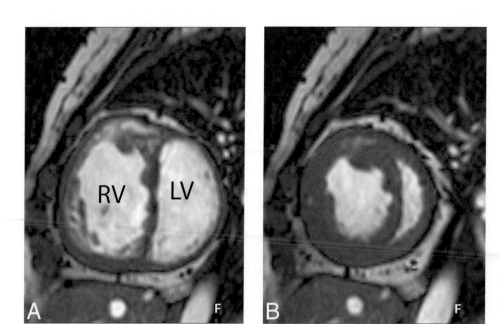

Figure 27.14. A 34-year-old female patient with TGA after Mustard repair in the past. Fast gradient-echo images in short axis, at end-diastolic **(A)** and end-systolic phases **(B)**. The RV sustains the systemic circulation and is hypertrophied and enlarged: RV EDV was 246 mL; LV EDV was 144 mL. RV function was moderately impaired with an EF of 45%. LV EF was 74%.

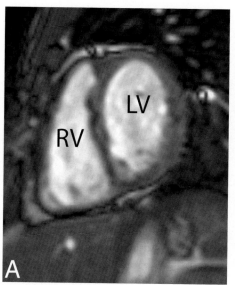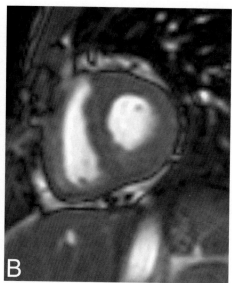

Figure 27.15. An 18-year-old male patient with TGA after arterial switch repair. Fast gradient-echo images in short axis, at end-diastolic **(A)** and end-systolic phases **(B)**. LV sustains the systemic circulation. RV appears slightly hypertrophied but not enlarged. LV EDV was 185 mL, and RV EDV was 163 mL. Good biventricular systolic function: LV EF was 60%, and RV EF was 65%. Note the differences compared with Figure 27.14.

same bicycle exercise protocol in patients with TGA showed distinct regional wall-motion disturbances of the anterior and free wall of the RV, with an increase of these RV wall-motion disturbances during exercise (44). This may be caused by regional perfusion abnormalities, as could be explained by the hypertrophy of the RV itself (the need for oxygen is not met by the supply) (45) or by preoperatively preexisting perfusion defects (46). Abnormal diastolic ventricular inflow patterns may suggest early manifestation of ventricular dysfunction, even in the absence of systolic dysfunction (14,42,47). At an early stage, diastolic dysfunction may precede the onset of systolic dysfunction (48).

Currently, the arterial switch procedure is the operation of choice with which normal anatomic relations are restored. Good mid-term (49,50) and long-term (51,52) results have been reported. With this procedure the great vessels are transected and switched, with reimplantation of the coronary arteries into the neo-aorta. The originally posterior branch pulmonary arteries are brought anterior to the aorta with the so-called Lecompte maneuver (Fig. 27.16).

Direct postoperative complications include myocardial perfusion defects, caused by problems in the transfer of coronary arteries (53). During the first year after surgery the incidence of coronary artery events ranges between 7.2% and 7.8% (50,53,54). A recent study using contrast-enhanced MRA of the coronaries and delayed enhancement suggested that coronary artery problems are not a long-term problem, showing no significant coronary stenoses and the absence of unexpected myocardial infarction areas (4) (Fig. 27.2). Evaluation of perfusion status was suggested to be restricted to patients with known complications after coronary reimplantation (4). Long-term complications after the arterial switch operation also include dilatation of the aortic root with subsequent aortic regurgitation (55–57). An echocardiography study showed an incidence of 35% of n c ortic regurgitation, which was progressive in 23% of the patients (57).

After the arterial switch operation, stenoses at the level of the pulmonary truncus and the peripheral pulmonary branches occur at a rate of 1% per year (58). Black-blood

imaging and gadolinium-enhanced MRA proved to be superior in the detection of stenoses in the great vessels when compared with transthoracic echocardiography, especially for stenoses in the peripheral pulmonary branches (Figs. 27.17 and 27.18) (2,58–61). An example of compensatory hypertrophy of the RV is shown in Figure 27.19. Information on specific hemodynamic changes in the great vessels after the arterial switch procedure can be obtained with gradient-echo multislice multiphase MRI (62). With this technique, narrowing of the (mainly right) pulmonary artery has been observed during systole, caused by expansion of the ascending aorta during systole (62). Velocity mapping can additionally be used to evaluate possible hemodynamic significance of these pulmonary artery stenoses (Fig. 27.18).

An abnormal diastolic RV inflow pattern may also be observed after the arterial switch procedure. An example is

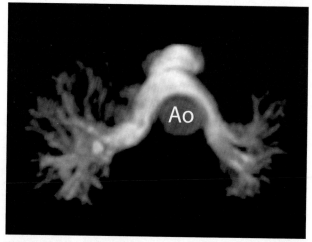

Figure 27.16. Same patient as in Figure 27.15 with TGA after arterial switch repair with Lecompte maneuver at early infancy. Gadolinium-enhanced MRA showing the typical arrangement of pulmonary arteries in relationship to the ascending aorta (Ao). The pulmonary arteries are well developed and show no stenoses.

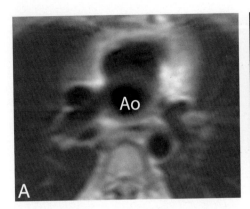

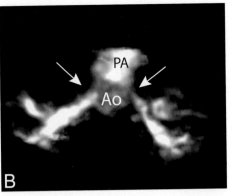

Figure 27.17. A 7-year-old female child with TGA after arterial switch repair. Axial black-blood spin-echo image **(A)** and corresponding gadolinium-enhanced maximum intensity projection MRA **(B)**. The arterial switch repair is complicated with severe pulmonary stenosis at the proximal left and right pulmonary arteries (left >right). See also Figures 27.18 and 27.19.

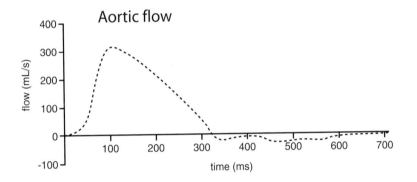

Figure 27.18. Same patient as in Figures 27.17 and 27.19. TGA after arterial switch repair. Flow mapping across the aorta and the main pulmonary artery. Note the broad and collapsed flow curve for pulmonary flow compared with the aortic flow curve, which is explained by the increased resistance to flow through the main pulmonary artery caused by the peripheral pulmonary stenosis at the proximal left and right pulmonary arteries.

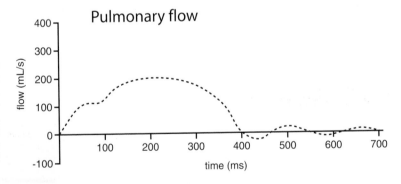

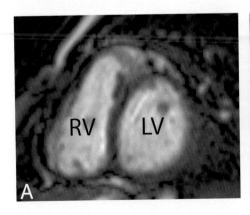

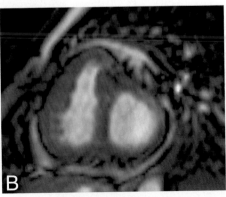

Figure 27.19. Same patient as in Figures 27.17 and 27.18. TGA after arterial switch repair. Fast gradient-echo images in short axis, at end-diastolic **(A)** and end-systolic phases **(B)**. The LV sustains the systemic circulation. Severe RV hypertrophy to compensate for the severe pulmonary stenosis as shown in Figure 27.17.

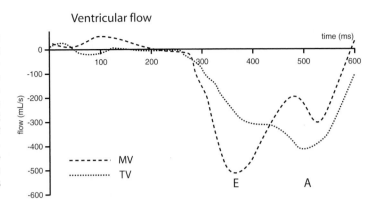

Figure 27.20. Same patient as in Figures 27.15 and 27.16: TGA after arterial switch repair. Flow mapping across the mitral valve (MV) and tricuspid valve (TV) for diastolic ventricular inflow patterns. Normally, a biphasic inflow pattern is recognized with two peaks representing early inflow **(E)** and late atrial kick **(A)**. At this age, the E/A ratio should be >1, that is, the first peak (E) larger than the last peak (A). This is the case for the left ventricular inflow across the MV, indicating normal relaxation of the LV. However, for the RV inflow, the E/A ratio was <1, indicating abnormal relaxation for the RV after arterial switch repair and slight RV hypertrophy. The pulmonary valve was normal, as were the pulmonary arteries.

shown in Figure 27.20, with slight hypertrophy of the RV, but without signs of pulmonary stenosis.

Imaging Protocol

After initial scout images and an axial stack of black-blood turbo spin-echo images, a double-oblique transverse stack of images along the aortic root is used for measurement of aortic root diameters, identical to the Fallot protocol. Axial or short-axis gradient-echo multislice multiphase imaging is performed to quantify biventricular function, with special attention to possible wall-motion abnormalities and the patency of the surgically created connections: both conduits after atrial repair and the site of anastomosis of the great vessels after the arterial switch. In patients undergoing arterial switch, a cine gradient-echo sequence is applied along the pulmonary trunk to identify the spatial relationship between the pulmonary branches and aorta. Temporary stenoses of pulmonary branches during systole can be detected when the aorta "swells" during the expulsion phase and compresses the adjacent pulmonary branches. Flow mapping across the pulmonary artery and the aorta are acquired for assessment of pulmonary or aortic regurgitation or stenosis. In addition, flow mapping across the mitral valve and tricuspid valve is obtained to evaluate ventricular inflow patterns and possible regurgitation. If indicated, an MRA of the pulmonary vascular tree and delayed enhancement imaging of both ventricles can finally be performed.

AORTIC COARCTATION

Clinical Considerations

Coarctation of the aorta accounts for 5% of all CHD and is defined as a congenital narrowing of the aorta, most commonly located in a juxtaductal position just distally to the origin of the left subclavian artery (63,64) (Fig. 27.1A,B). A wide spectrum of narrowing of the aorta can be observed, from a discrete narrowing to a hypoplastic aortic arch, whether it is associated or not associated with intracardiac defects like a VSD or aortic valve pathology. Classic symptoms are heart failure and an increased blood pressure proximal to the narrowing, as well as a low perfusion status of the body distally to the coarctation (63,64).

Treatment consists of surgical intervention with resection and end-to-end anastomosis or usage of a subclavian flap,

or balloon angioplasty. Serial follow-up of these patients is mandatory because of the considerable incidence of aneurysm formation and re-coarctation, which varies from 8% to 67%, depending on the procedure of choice, time of follow-up, and the age at which the intervention was performed (63,64). One third of all patients become or remain hypertensive, despite their lesion being corrected, with an increased risk of accelerated atherosclerosis and end-organ damage (65). Compensatory LV hypertrophy can be evaluated by gradient-echo multislice multiphase imaging. MRI proved to be the most cost-effective approach to diagnose complications at the site of repair, by comparison of sensitivity and specificity of various imaging modalities and their costs (63).

High numbers of bicuspid aortic valves have been reported in patients with coarctation, ranging between 25% and 85% (65–67). In addition to the clear association between bicuspid aortic valves and aortic valve pathology, the incidence of aortic valve pathology is higher in studies of patients with coarctation and a bicuspid aortic valve compared with those without coarctation, emphasizing the additional role of the coarctation in the development of aortic valve problems (65,68,69). Dilation of the ascending aorta during follow-up can be found in 28% to 44% of patients after repaired coarctation, without previous aortic valve intervention (65,69). Patients with coarctation and a bicuspid aortic valve are at risk for ascending aortic dissection, probably caused by dilatation of the ascending aorta and persistent hypertension (37). Close follow-up is necessary to time surgical intervention for aortic aneurysm.

Imaging Protocol

After initial scout images and an axial stack of black-blood turbo spin-echo images, a double-oblique transverse stack of images along the aortic root is used for depiction of aortic valve morphology and measurement of aortic root diameters. Next, axial gradient-echo multislice multiphase imaging is performed to assess biventricular function. A stack of thin consecutive black-blood slices in the oblique sagittal direction through the plane of the aortic arch allows detailed visualization of the ascending aorta, aortic arch, and descending aorta, which is sensitive for the detection and follow-up of recoarctation and aneurysms. Contrast-enhanced MRA of the thoracic aorta with 3D reconstruction can clearly demonstrate the spatial relationship between the stenosis, the other arch vessels, and possible collateral vessels. Flow mapping is performed across the aortic valve for detection of aortic valve stenosis or regurgitation. In the case of re-coarctation, velocity mapping across the aorta at the level of the ascending aorta, just distal to the level of the re-coarctation and at the level of the diaphragm, can be obtained for quantification of the pressure gradient across the re-coarctation and for calculation of the magnitude of possible collateral flow, by subtraction of the proximal aortic flow from the distal one (64). Flow mapping may be difficult to perform just distal to the coarctation site because of turbulent flow and increased flow velocity. In that case, shunt quantification may be performed by measuring just before the level of the coarctation or more distally. It should be noted, however, that collateral flow might be missed in the latter.

FONTAN CIRCULATION

Clinical Considerations

In 1971 Fontan described a surgical correction for the treatment of tricuspid atresia (70). This type of operation has become the treatment of choice in a heterogeneous group of congenital cardiac malformations characterized by the presence of a single (systemic) ventricle. The procedure establishes a circulation in which the systemic venous return directly enters the pulmonary arteries, bypassing the heart except for the atrioventricular variant (Figs. 27.21 and 27.22). Different types of connections can be implemented, including total cavopulmonary connection, atriopulmonary

connection, and atrioventricular connection. The introduction of a fenestration in the systemic venous tunnel wall improved the outcome of the procedure in high-risk cases by decreasing the incidence of early pericardial effusions after the procedure and maintaining LV output in times of hemodynamic stress (71).

The state of the systemic ventricle is important in the presurgical planning because ventricular hypertrophy and abnormal wall motion impair the surgical outcome (72). In the postoperative period ventricular function may deteriorate over time and should be followed carefully (72,73). EF may deteriorate 1 to 2 years after a Fontan operation compared with preoperative data (73). Gradient-echo multislice multiphase MRI is ideally suited to assess the complex morphology and function of the systemic ventricle before and after construction of the Fontan circulation (74,75). Both 3D-reconstructed MRA and spin-echo MRI can be used for detection of conduit obstruction (76). In adult patients, a diameter of the conduit measured with spin-echo MRI of less then 15 mm suggests that a significant pressure gradient within the conduit can be expected, whereas a diameter of more then 20 mm diameter is regarded as the optimal diameter (76).

The dimensions of the right and left pulmonary arteries, expressed as the McGoon ratio, are one of the most powerful risk factors for death or a dysfunctional Fontan circuit. This includes summation of the diameter of the distal but immediately pre-branching portion of the right and the left pulmonary artery, divided by the diameter of the descending aorta

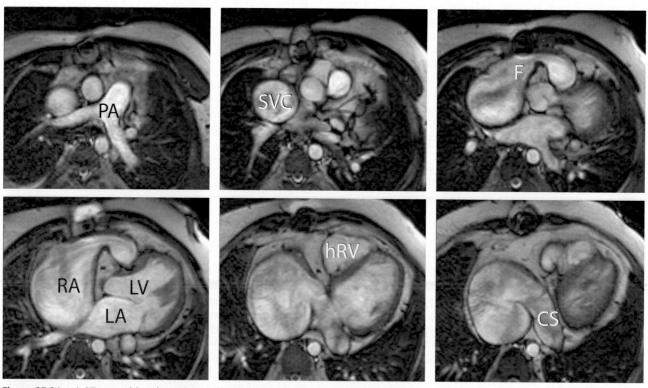

Figure 27.21. A 27-year-old male patient with tricuspid atresia and hypoplastic RV after correction by Fontan circulation. Axial fast-field gradient-echo images showing the Fontan circulation consisting of a patch connecting the dilated right atrium with the hypoplastic RV and main pulmonary artery. Note the dilated coronary sinus and superior vena cava, despite the open Fontan connection. Normal pulmonary arteries. LV, left ventricle; hRV, hypoplastic right ventricle; F, Fontan circulation; RA, right atrium; PA, pulmonary artery; CS, coronary sinus; SVC, superior vena cava.

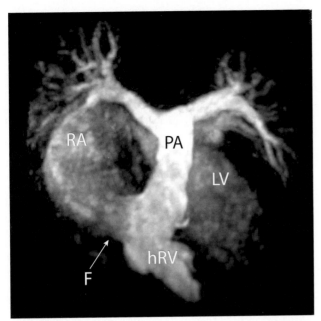

Figure 27.22. The same patient as in Figure 27.21. Gadolinium-enhanced MRA of the Fontan circulation, consisting of a patch (F) connecting the dilated right atrium with the hypoplastic RV and main pulmonary artery (after correction of infundibular pulmonary stenosis and correction of atrium septum defect and ventricular septum defect). Note the open Fontan connection between the right atrium and the hypoplastic RV and pulmonary artery. Normal pulmonary arteries. LV, left ventricle; RA, right atrium; hRV, hypoplastic right ventricle; PA, pulmonary artery.

measured just above the diaphragm (77). An increased risk for death or a dysfunctional Fontan circuit can be expected when the ratio is less than 1.8, because this is associated with flow obstruction through the pulmonary vascular tree. Unobstructed flow passage is of eminent importance considering the low propelling pressure of the vena cava system (77).

Flow mapping can be used to provide information on flow patterns within the different types of Fontan connections (78,79). In patients with an atriopulmonary connection, flow was biphasically pulsatile during the course of the cardiac cycle, but with a relatively small difference between the maximal and minimal velocities. After atrioventricular connection, a systolic arterial flow pattern can be found in the pulmonary arteries of half of the patients, indicating that the RV significantly sustains pulmonary blood flow (78).

Imaging Protocol

After initial scout images, axial and sagittal stacks of black-blood turbo spin-echo images are acquired for depiction of the often complex cardiac anatomy. Axial gradient-echo multislice multiphase imaging is performed to quantify systemic ventricular function and to assess the morphologic dynamics of the Fontan circulation (Fig. 27.21). Flow mapping across the aorta, the left and right pulmonary arteries, and the mitral valve is performed to evaluate flow patterns and to determine the magnitude of possible stenoses within the different types of Fontan connections, which are characterized by turbulent flow and increased flow velocity. The

session is finished with a contrast-enhanced MRA of the pulmonary vascular tree for optimal depiction of the spatial relationship of the Fontan connections (Fig. 27.22). Diameters of the right and left pulmonary arteries for the McGoon ratio can be obtained from axial imaging or the 3D-reconstructed MRA, and the diameter of the descending aorta can be obtained from axial spin-echo or gradient-echo imaging.

FUTURE PERSPECTIVE

Future applications of MRI in the setting of CHD will include new MRI sequences, subsequent improvement of clinical decision making in patients with corrected or palliated CHD, and the emerging field of interventional MRI.

New MRI techniques like SENSE provide improved assessment of cardiac function and morphology by offering better imaging quality. This may further help in the understanding of cardiac dysfunction in patients with CHD (80). New techniques will also provide faster MRI protocols, making it more attractive for widespread clinical usage, and will (partially) overcome the limitation of long breath holds that apply to the younger patient population (8). Furthermore, ultrafast or real-time MRI allows the assessment of dynamic processes such as the cardiac response to exercise (81) and changes in cardiac function during recovery from exercise (14). These new MRI techniques may help in the early detection of cardiac dysfunction and regional ischemia, which is important in the management of patients with CHD.

MRI may play an increasing role in clinical decision making in various patient groups with CHD, by serial assessment of cardiac parameters at fixed time points during follow-up. For example, the timing of PVR after total correction of TOF is a controversial issue, but it has been observed that PVR may lead to normalization of RV volume when performed before the RV reaches 150% of its normal size (2,29,82). These kinds of information derived from MRI studies may be helpful for improvement of patient-management strategies.

Cardiac catheterization procedures guided with MRI are an exciting new option, combining the unique advantages of MRI with catheter-driven interventions (see Chap. 37). Razavi et al recently showed that cardiac catheterization guided by MRI with radiographic support is feasible, moving a stage further toward complete MRI-guided cardiac catheterization (83). This will include advantages especially for the pediatric population, considering the essential role of cardiac catheterization in the diagnosis and treatment of CHD, and the concern for long-term complications associated with radiation burden.

REFERENCES

1. Jara H, Barish MA. Black-blood MR angiography. Techniques, and clinical applications. *Magn Reson Imaging Clin N Am* 1999;7(2):303–317.
2. Kondo C, Takada K, Yokoyama U, et al. Comparison of three-dimensional contrast-enhanced magnetic resonance angiography and axial radiographic angiography for diagnosing con-

genital stenoses in small pulmonary arteries. *Am J Cardiol* 2001;87(4):420–424.

3. Flamm SD, Muthupillai R. Coronary artery magnetic resonance angiography. *J Magn Reson Imaging* 2004;19(6): 686–709.

4. Taylor AM, Dymarkowski S, Hamaekers P, et al. MR coronary angiography and late-enhancement myocardial MR in children who underwent arterial switch surgery for transposition of great arteries. *Radiology* 2005;234(2):542–547.

5. Helbing WA, Bosch HG, Maliepaard C, et al. Comparison of echocardiographic methods with magnetic resonance imaging for assessment of right ventricular function in children. *Am J Cardiol* 1995;76(8):589–594.

6. Helbing WA, Rebergen SA, Maliepaard C, et al. Quantification of right ventricular function with magnetic resonance imaging in children with normal hearts and with congenital heart disease. *Am Heart J* 1995;130(4):828–837.

7. Niezen RA, Helbing WA, van der Wall EE, et al. Biventricular systolic function and mass studied with MR imaging in children with pulmonary regurgitation after repair for tetralogy of Fallot. *Radiology* 1996;201(1):135–140.

8. Tsao J, Boesiger P, Pruessmann KP. k-t BLAST and k-t SENSE: dynamic MRI with high frame rate exploiting spatiotemporal correlations. *Magn Reson Med* 2003;50(5):1031–1042.

9. Roest AA, Helbing WA, Kunz P, et al. Exercise MR imaging in the assessment of pulmonary regurgitation and biventricular function in patients after tetralogy of Fallot repair. *Radiology* 2002;223(1):204–211.

10. Rebergen SA, van der Wall EE, Helbing WA, et al. Quantification of pulmonary and systemic blood flow by magnetic resonance velocity mapping in the assessment of atrial-level shunts. *Int J Card Imaging* 1996;12(3):143–152.

11. Brenner LD, Caputo GR, Mostbeck G, et al. Quantification of left to right atrial shunts with velocity-encoded cine nuclear magnetic resonance imaging. *J Am Coll Cardiol* 1992;20(5): 1246–1250.

12. Beerbaum P, Korperich H, Gieseke J, et al. Rapid left-to-right shunt quantification in children by phase-contrast magnetic resonance imaging combined with sensitivity encoding (SENSE). *Circulation* 2003;108(11):1355–1361.

13. Oosterhof T, Mulder BJ, Vliegen HW, de Roos A. Cardiovascular magnetic resonance in the follow up of patients with corrected tetralogy of Fallot: a review. *Am J Cardiol* 2005 (in press).

14. Roest AA, Kunz P, Helbing WA, et al. Prolonged cardiac recovery from exercise in asymptomatic adults late after atrial correction of transposition of the great arteries: evaluation with magnetic resonance flow mapping. *Am J Cardiol* 2001;88(9): 1011–1017.

15. Roest AA, de Roos A, Lamb HJ, et al. Tetralogy of Fallot: postoperative delayed recovery of left ventricular stroke volume after physical exercise assessment with fast MR imaging. *Radiology* 2003;226(1):278–284.

16. de Roos A, Niezen RA, Lamb HJ, et al. MR of the heart under pharmacologic stress. *Cardiol Clin* 1998;16(2):247–265.

17. Hoffman JI, Kaplan S. The incidence of congenital heart disease. *J Am Coll Cardiol* 2002;39(12):1890–1900.

18. Anderson RH, Tynan M. Tetralogy of Fallot—a centennial review. *Int J Cardiol* 1988;21(3):219–232.

19. Lillehei CW, Cohen M, Warden HE, et al. Direct vision intracardiac surgical correction of the tetralogy of Fallot, pentalogy of Fallot, and pulmonary atresia defects; report of first ten cases. *Ann Surg* 1955;142(3):418–442.

20. Van Arsdell GS, Maharaj GS, Tom J, et al. What is the optimal age for repair of tetralogy of Fallot? *Circulation* 2000;102(19 Suppl 3):III123–III129.

21. Murphy JG, Gersh BJ, Mair DD, et al. Long-term outcome in patients undergoing surgical repair of tetralogy of Fallot. *N Engl J Med* 1993;329(9):593–599.

22. Gatzoulis MA, Balaji S, Webber SA, et al. Risk factors for arrhythmia and sudden cardiac death late after repair of tetralogy of Fallot: a multicentre study. *Lancet* 2000;356(9234): 975–981.

23. Waien SA, Liu PP, Ross BL, et al. Serial follow-up of adults with repaired tetralogy of Fallot. *J Am Coll Cardiol* 1992; 20(2):295–300.

24. Bove EL, Byrum CJ, Thomas FD, et al. The influence of pulmonary insufficiency on ventricular function following repair of tetralogy of Fallot. Evaluation using radionuclide ventriculography. *J Thorac Cardiovasc Surg* 1983;85(5):691–696.

25. Gatzoulis MA, Till JA, Somerville J, et al. Mechanoelectrical interaction in tetralogy of Fallot. QRS prolongation relates to right ventricular size and predicts malignant ventricular arrhythmias and sudden death. *Circulation* 1995;92(2):231–237.

26. Kondo C, Nakazawa M, Kusakabe K, et al. Left ventricular dysfunction on exercise long-term after total repair of tetralogy of Fallot. *Circulation* 1995;92(9 Suppl):II250–II255.

27. Therrien J, Siu SC, McLaughlin PR, et al. Pulmonary valve replacement in adults late after repair of tetralogy of Fallot: are we operating too late? *J Am Coll Cardiol* 2000;36(5): 1670–1675.

28. Vliegen HW, Van Straten A, de Roos A, et al. Magnetic resonance imaging to assess the hemodynamic effects of pulmonary valve replacement in adults late after repair of tetralogy of Fallot. *Circulation* 2002;106(13):1703–1707.

29. Therrien J, Provost Y, Merchant N, et al. Optimal timing for pulmonary valve replacement in adults after tetralogy of Fallot repair: a magnetic resonance imaging study. *Am J Cardiol* 2005;95:779–782.

30. Davlouros PA, Kilner PJ, Hornung TS, et al. Right ventricular function in adults with repaired tetralogy of Fallot assessed with cardiovascular magnetic resonance imaging: detrimental role of right ventricular outflow aneurysms or akinesia and adverse right-to-left ventricular interaction. *J Am Coll Cardiol* 2002;40(11):2044–2052.

31. Tulevski II, Hirsch A, Dodge-Khatami A, et al. Effect of pulmonary valve regurgitation on right ventricular function in patients with chronic right ventricular pressure overload. *Am J Cardiol* 2003;92(1):113–116.

32. Chaturvedi RR, Kilner PJ, White PA, et al. Increased airway pressure and simulated branch pulmonary artery stenosis increase pulmonary regurgitation after repair of tetralogy of Fallot. Real-time analysis with a conductance catheter technique. *Circulation* 1997;95(3):643–649.

33. Geva T, Sandweiss BM, Gauvreau K, et al. Factors associated with impaired clinical status in long-term survivors of tetralogy of Fallot repair evaluated by magnetic resonance imaging. *J Am Coll Cardiol* 2004;43(6):1068–1074.

34. Ghai A, Silversides C, Harris L, et al. Left ventricular dysfunction is a risk factor for sudden cardiac death in adults late after repair of tetralogy of Fallot. *J Am Coll Cardiol* 2002;40(9): 1675–1680.

35. Ishizaka T, Ichikawa H, Sawa Y, et al. Prevalence and optimal management strategy for aortic regurgitation in tetralogy of Fallot. *Eur J Cardiothorac Surg* 2004;26(6):1080–1086.

36. Niwa K, Siu SC, Webb GD, et al. Progressive aortic root dilatation in adults late after repair of tetralogy of Fallot. *Circulation* 2002;106(11):1374–1378.

37. Bonderman D, Gharehbaghi-Schnell E, Wollenek G, et al. Mechanisms underlying aortic dilatation in congenital aortic valve malformation. *Circulation* 1999;99(16):2138–2143.

38. Dodds GA, III, Warnes CA, Danielson GK. Aortic valve replacement after repair of pulmonary atresia and ventricular

septal defect or tetralogy of Fallot. *J Thorac Cardiovasc Surg* 1997;113(4):736–741.

39. Hoffman JI. Incidence of congenital heart disease: I. Postnatal incidence. *Pediatr Cardiol* 1995;16(3):103–113.

40. Jatene AD, Fontes VF, Paulista PP, et al. Successful anatomic correction of transposition of the great vessels. A preliminary report. *Arq Bras Cardiol* 1975;28(4):461–464.

41. Williams WG, Trusler GA, Kirklin JW, et al. Early and late results of a protocol for simple transposition leading to an atrial switch (Mustard) repair. *J Thorac Cardiovasc Surg* 1988; 95(4):717–726.

42. Roest AA, Lamb HJ, van der Wall EE, et al. Cardiovascular response to physical exercise in adult patients after atrial correction for transposition of the great arteries assessed with magnetic resonance imaging. *Heart* 2004;90(6):678–684.

43. Sampson C, Kilner PJ, Hirsch R, et al. Venoatrial pathways after the Mustard operation for transposition of the great arteries: anatomic and functional MR imaging. *Radiology* 1994; 193(1):211–217.

44. Tops LF, Roest AAW, Lamb HJ, et al. Exercise-MRI of regional systemic right ventricular function after intra-atrial repair for transposition of the great arteries. *Radiology* 2005 (in press).

45. Hornung TS, Kilner PJ, Davlouros PA, et al. Excessive right ventricular hypertrophic response in adults with the Mustard procedure for transposition of the great arteries. *Am J Cardiol* 2002;90(7):800–803.

46. Redington AN, Rigby ML, Oldershaw P, et al. Right ventricular function 10 years after the Mustard operation for transposition of the great arteries: analysis of size, shape, and wall motion. *Br Heart J* 1989;62(6):455–461.

47. Rebergen SA, Helbing WA, van der Wall EE, et al. MR velocity mapping of tricuspid flow in healthy children and in patients who have undergone Mustard or Senning repair. *Radiology* 1995;194(2):505–512.

48. Nishimura RA, Abel MD, Hatle LK, et al. Assessment of diastolic function of the heart: background and current applications of Doppler echocardiography. Part II. Clinical studies. *Mayo Clin Proc* 1989;64(2):181–204.

49. Kirklin JW, Blackstone EH, Tchervenkov CI, et al. Clinical outcomes after the arterial switch operation for transposition. Patient, support, procedural, and institutional risk factors. Congenital Heart Surgeons Society. *Circulation* 1992;86(5): 1501–1515.

50. Pretre R, Tamisier D, Bonhoeffer P, et al. Results of the arterial switch operation in neonates with transposed great arteries. *Lancet* 2001;357(9271):1826–1830.

51. Haas F, Wottke M, Poppert H, et al. Long-term survival and functional follow-up in patients after the arterial switch operation. *Ann Thorac Surg* 1999;68(5):1692–1697.

52. Losay J, Touchot A, Serraf A, et al. Late outcome after arterial switch operation for transposition of the great arteries. *Circulation* 2001;104(12 Suppl 1):I121–I126.

53. Tzifa A, Tulloh RM. Coronary arterial complications before and after the arterial switch operation: is the future clear? *Cardiol Young* 2002;12(2):164–171.

54. Legendre A, Losay J, Touchot-Kone A, et al. Coronary events after arterial switch operation for transposition of the great arteries. *Circulation* 2003;108(Suppl 1):II186–II190.

55. Hourihan M, Colan SD, Wernovsky G, et al. Growth of the aortic anastomosis, annulus, and root after the arterial switch procedure performed in infancy. *Circulation* 1993;88(2): 615–620.

56. Hutter PA, Thomeer BJ, Jansen P, et al. Fate of the aortic root after arterial switch operation. *Eur J Cardiothorac Surg* 2001; 20(1):82–88.

57. Formigari R, Toscano A, Giardini A, et al. Prevalence and predictors of neoaortic regurgitation after arterial switch opera-

tion for transposition of the great arteries. *J Thorac Cardiovasc Surg* 2003;126:1753–1759.

58. Williams WG, Quaegebeur JM, Kirklin JW, et al. Outflow obstruction after the arterial switch operation: a multiinstitutional study. Congenital Heart Surgeons Society. *J Thorac Cardiovasc Surg* 1997;114(6):975–987.

59. Beek FJ, Beekman RP, Dillon EH, et al. MRI of the pulmonary artery after arterial switch operation for transposition of the great arteries. *Pediatr Radiol* 1993;23(5):335–340.

60. Blakenberg F, Rhee J, Hardy C, et al. MRI vs echocardiography in the evaluation of the Jatene procedure. *J Comput Assist Tomogr* 1994;18(5):749–754.

61. Hardy CE, Helton GJ, Kondo C, et al. Usefulness of magnetic resonance imaging for evaluating great-vessel anatomy after arterial switch operation for D-transposition of the great arteries. *Am Heart J* 1994;128(2):326–332.

62. Gutberlet M, Boeckel T, Hosten N, et al. Arterial switch procedure for D-transposition of the great arteries: quantitative midterm evaluation of hemodynamic changes with cine MR imaging and phase-shift velocity mapping-initial experience. *Radiology* 2000;214(2):467–475.

63. Therrien J, Thorne SA, Wright A, et al. Repaired coarctation: a "cost-effective" approach to identify complications in adults. *J Am Coll Cardiol* 2000;35(4):997–1002.

64. Konen E, Merchant N, Provost Y, et al. Coarctation of the aorta before and after correction: the role of cardiovascular MRI. *AJR Am J Roentgenol* 2004;182(5):1333–1339.

65. Roos-Hesselink JW, Scholzel BE, Heijdra RJ, et al. Aortic valve and aortic arch pathology after coarctation repair. *Heart* 2003;89(9):1074–1077.

66. Presbitero P, Demarie D, Villani M, et al. Long term results (15–30 years) of surgical repair of aortic coarctation. *Br Heart J* 1987;57(5):462–467.

67. Stewart AB, Ahmed R, Travill CM, et al. Coarctation of the aorta life and health 20–44 years after surgical repair. *Br Heart J* 1993;69(1):65–70.

68. Ward C. Clinical significance of the bicuspid aortic valve. *Heart* 2000;83(1):81–85.

69. Nistri S, Sorbo MD, Marin M, et al. Aortic root dilatation in young men with normally functioning bicuspid aortic valves. *Heart* 1999;82(1):19–22.

70. Fontan F, Baudet E. Surgical repair of tricuspid atresia. *Thorax* 1971;26(3):240–248.

71. Bridges ND, Lock JE, Mayer JE Jr, et al. Cardiac catheterization and test occlusion of the interatrial communication after the fenestrated Fontan operation. *J Am Coll Cardiol* 1995; 25(7):1712–1717.

72. Chin AJ, Franklin WH, Andrews BA, et al. Changes in ventricular geometry early after Fontan operation. *Ann Thorac Surg* 1993;56(6):1359–1365.

73. Fogel MA, Weinberg PM, Chin AJ, et al. Late ventricular geometry and performance changes of functional single ventricle throughout staged Fontan reconstruction assessed by magnetic resonance imaging. *J Am Coll Cardiol* 1996;28(1): 212–221.

74. Fogel MA, Weinberg PM, Fellows KE, et al. Magnetic resonance imaging of constant total heart volume and center of mass in patients with functional single ventricle before and after staged Fontan procedure. *Am J Cardiol* 1993;72(18): 1435–1443.

75. Altmann K, Shen Z, Boxt LM, et al. Comparison of three-dimensional echocardiographic assessment of volume, mass, and function in children with functionally single left ventricles with two-dimensional echocardiography and magnetic resonance imaging. *Am J Cardiol* 1997;80(8):1060–1065.

76. Sampson C, Martinez J, Rees S, et al. Evaluation of Fontan's operation by magnetic resonance imaging. *Am J Cardiol* 1990; 65(11):819–821.

77. Fontan F, Fernandez G, Costa F, et al. The size of the pulmonary arteries and the results of the Fontan operation. *J Thorac Cardiovasc Surg* 1989;98(5 Pt 1):711–719.

78. Be'eri E, Maier SE, Landzberg MJ, et al. In vivo evaluation of Fontan pathway flow dynamics by multidimensional phase-velocity magnetic resonance imaging. *Circulation* 1998;98 (25):2873–2882.

79. Morgan VL, Graham TP Jr, Roselli RJ, et al. Alterations in pulmonary artery flow patterns and shear stress determined with three-dimensional phase-contrast magnetic resonance imaging in Fontan patients. *J Thorac Cardiovasc Surg* 1998; 116(2):294–304.

80. Fogel MA, Weinberg PM, Hubbard A, et al. Diastolic biomechanics in normal infants utilizing MRI tissue tagging. *Circulation* 2000;102(2):218–224.

81. Weiger M, Pruessmann KP, Leussler C, et al. Specific coil design for SENSE: a six-element cardiac array. *Magn Reson Med* 2001;45(3):495–504.

82. Hazekamp MG, Kurvers MM, Schoof PH, et al. Pulmonary valve insertion late after repair of Fallot's tetralogy. *Eur J Cardiothorac Surg* 2001;19(5):667–670.

83. Razavi R, Hill DL, Keevil SF, et al. Cardiac catheterisation guided by MRI in children and adults with congenital heart disease. *Lancet* 2003;362(9399):1877–1882.

28

Adult Congenital Heart Disease

Philip J. Kilner and Sonya V. Babu-Narayan

This chapter considers the uses of magnetic resonance imaging (MRI) and magnetic resonance angiography (MRA) in the assessment of adolescents and adults with congenital heart disease (CHD), an important group of patients whose numbers are increasing yearly, largely because of the success of surgical and catheter interventions. The effects of congenital disease, surgery, and acquired disease may combine to create varied and challenging pathology (1–3). Residual structural and functional abnormalities generally must be followed on a lifelong basis, preferably at a specialist referral center. Appropriate imaging facilities represent a key aspect of such a center. Cardiovascular MR can make outstanding contributions to the assessment of CHD in adults, in whom body size and the results of surgery tend to limit echocardiographic access. The costs of imaging should be weighed against the potential costs of inappropriate management, which can entail complicated repeated surgery and extended hospitalization.

Imaging specialists need not be deterred by the anatomic variability found in these patients, as discussion with the CHD specialist can clarify questions to be answered, and the comprehensive anatomic coverage offered by MRI almost always provides useful diagnostic information. Variations of anatomy and function do, however, mean that decisions on cine imaging planes and sequences generally must be made during acquisition. It is not only anatomic structures that vary—surgical techniques have also evolved and changed. Operations for conditions such as transposition of the great arteries (TGA) and single-ventricle heart have changed radically during the last few decades, and those investigating older patients need to be aware of both previous and current surgical practices. A number of reviews of MRI of CHD have been published (4–6), and information on the investigation and management of malformations has been put together by the Canadian Consensus Conference on Adult Congenital Heart Disease (7), conveniently accessible through the website of the Canadian Adult Congenital Heart Network (see www.cachnet.org for information on managing congenital heart defects).

The diagnostic contributions of MRI, such as the evaluation of extracardiac vessels, tend to complement those of transoesophageal echocardiography (8), though the latter can be more effective than MRI for imaging thin, mobile intracardiac structures such as the atrial septum, valve structures, and the vegetations of endocarditis. Diagnostic cardiac catheterization is now needed more rarely than in the past, and interventional catheterization may be expedited after MRI and transesophageal echocardiography. Further, information from MRI can direct cardiac catheterization and thus shorten radiation exposure. However, adequate assessments of coronary artery stenoses or pulmonary vascular resistance still rely on invasive investigations.

Novel work on MRI-guided catheterization has begun on humans (9), including attempted measurement of pulmonary vascular resistance by MRI flow combined with catheter pressure measurement (10).

Many adults with CHD have a complex clinical history with multiple complementary investigations, and our experience is that collaborative presentation and discussion can be important, allowing a comprehensive picture to be built up that can clarify questions of clinical management and further the process of learning. At such meetings, MRI studies should be shown interactively by a computer linked to a projector, with programs for the display and interrogation of multislice, cine, velocity, and three-dimensional (3D) MRA acquisitions. We use a program called *CMRTools* (Imperial College, London, United Kingdom) that is Digital Imaging and Communications in Medicine (DICOM)-compatible and runs on personal computers.

Cardiovascular MRI can provide functional as well as anatomic information, including the location and severity of stenoses (e.g., aortic coarctation or pulmonary artery stenosis), severity of regurgitation (e.g., pulmonary regurgitation), size and function of the heart chambers (the right and left ventricles), and measurements of shunt flow. In adults with CHD, the underlying cardiac anatomy is likely to have been assessed previously. Although it is important to understand the descriptions, they should not necessarily be assumed to be correct and should be reviewed in the light of new information gained at MRI study. The terminology used for malformed cardiovascular anatomy is described in Chapter 20.

TECHNIQUES

MULTISLICE IMAGING

In CHD, it is advisable to acquire coronal and sagittal as well as transaxial multislice images. Using either rapid acquisition by half-Fourier acquisition single-shot turbo spin-echo (HASTE), a dark-blood sequence, steady-state free precession (SSFP), or a bright-blood sequence, stacks of up to approximately 20 slices can be acquired, one slice per heart beat, in a single breath-hold. These acquisitions then serve as scout images for accurate location of subsequent breath-hold cine acquisitions.

CINE IMAGING

SSFP imaging, which gives good contrast between blood and myocardium, is used widely for cine acquisitions. These acquisitions are well suited for imaging and measuring ventricular function and mass and for visualizing valve leaflets. Where there is jet flow through a stenotic or regurgitant orifice, SSFP cine imaging can outline a coherent jet core, if present, because of the localized loss of signal from shear layers (Fig. 28.1). Rapid acquisition makes it possible to interrogate a jet area precisely and repeatedly. The approach of "cross-cutting"—locating an orthogonal slice though a partially visualized feature such as a valve orifice or jet—is an effective way of "homing in" on a particular feature of interest by MRI.

PHASE VELOCITY MAPPING

Phase-shift velocity mapping, if correctly implemented, can be an accurate and versatile way of measuring flow (11–13). Design of MRI systems with rapidly switching gradients for cardiovascular acquisition has, however, led to potential

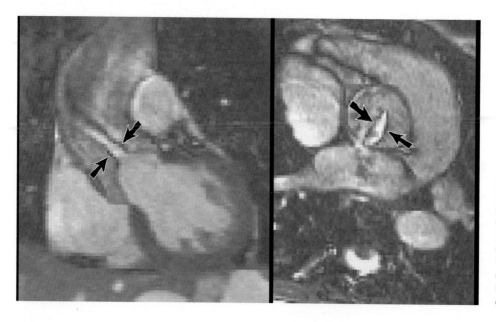

Figure 28.1. Systolic jet of moderate aortic stenosis shown by steady-state free precession (SSFP) cine imaging (echo time = 1.6 ms) in a coronal plane (*left*) and transecting the jet and aortic root (*right*). The arrows point to lines of signal loss caused by shear, outlining the relatively bright jet core.

inaccuracies in velocity mapping, particularly when used for measurement of regurgitant fraction or shunt flow. In these cases, slight shift of the background phase due to eddy currents and Maxwell gradients can introduce significant errors in flow calculation. Manufacturers have gradually become aware of these problems and have implemented modifications of hardware and software to avoid or counteract them in more recent systems. Unfortunately, however, it cannot be assumed that all systems in current clinical use are accurate in this respect.

Phase-shift velocity mapping is based on the frequency changes experienced by nuclei moving relative to applied magnetic gradients (11–13). The direction, steepness, and timing of the applied gradients can be chosen so that flows with a range of velocities, from low-velocity venous to high-velocity poststenotic flows, can be measured accurately. Clinical uses include measurements of cardiac output (14), shunt flow (15), collateral flow (16), regurgitant flow (17), and jet velocities through stenoses. However, for successful clinical application, the operator should have an understanding not only of the anatomy and pathophysiology of operated CHD, but also of the available technical choices for velocity mapping. It is necessary to select a plane, echo time, velocity-encoding direction, and velocity sensitivity appropriate for a particular investigation.

Velocity can be encoded in directions that lie either in or through an image plane. The mapping of velocities through a plane transecting a vessel (velocity encoded in the direction of the slice-selection gradient) allows the measurement of flow volume. The cross-sectional area of the lumen and the mean axially directed velocity within that area are measured for each phase through the heart cycle. From these data, a flow curve is plotted, and systolic forward flow and any diastolic reversed flow are computed by integration.

To calculate shunt flow, both aortic and pulmonary artery flows are measured. Two separate acquisitions are generally needed, except in cases of TGA, in which the aorta and pulmonary trunk usually run almost parallel to each other. For aortic flow measurement, a suitable plane transects the aortic root at the level of the sinotubular junction, and for pulmonary flow measurement, a suitable plane transects the pulmonary trunk proximal to its bifurcation. Pulmonary regurgitation is common after repair of tetralogy of Fallot, and in such cases, the repaired outflow tract and pulmonary trunk are tethered by scarring. However, if the mobility of the aortic and pulmonary valves is normal, especially in cases in which the root is dilated, the diastolic regurgitant flow can be significantly underestimated because of compliance and movement of the arterial root relative to the imaging plane. A potential solution to this problem will be movement of the acquisition plane to follow valve movement through the heart cycle, also know as "motion tracking."

Through-plane velocity mapping can be used to delineate an atrial septal defect (ASD) (18) and measure the velocities and cross-sectional areas of jets through stenotic orifices (19). It can be helpful in mapping velocities in a plane aligned with the direction of flow, with velocity encoded in the read gradient direction, which must also be aligned with the direction of jet flow. This allows depiction of the jet in relation to upstream and downstream regions. It is necessary, however, to locate the image plane correctly by cross cutting.

Jet-velocity mapping can be particularly valuable for assessing stenoses in which ultrasonic access is limited, such as in aortic coarctation (native or repaired) (20), ventriculo-pulmonary conduits, pulmonary artery branch stenoses, and obstructions at the atrial or atriopulmonary level following a Mustard, Senning, or Fontan operation.

THREE-DIMENSIONAL ANGIOGRAPHY AND CORONARY ANGIOGRAPHY

Although 3D MRA by time-of-flight or phase-contrast techniques do not require the injection of a contrast agent, gadolinium-enhanced angiography combines fast acquisition with very good resolution. The main roles of MRA in adults with CHD are depiction of anomalous pulmonary or systemc venous return, depiction of the geometry and dimensions of the aorta in the presence of coarctation with a view to balloon dilatation and stenting, and depiction of the size and distribution of aortopulmonary collaterals and surgical shunts in pulmonary atresia (Fig. 28.2).

Contrast-enhanced MRA is generally acquired in a breath-hold without cardiac gating, but this approach may not be suitable for coronary angiography due to the relative importance of cardiac motion. For angiographic visualization of anomalous origins of the coronary arteries, we use 3D SSFP acquisitions, either in a single breath-hold or with

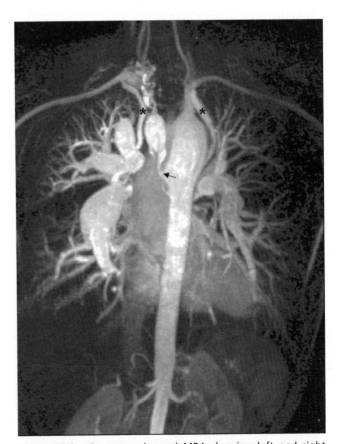

Figure 28.2. Contrast-enhanced MRA showing left and right Blalock-Taussig shunts (*) and an aortopulmonary collateral (*arrow*) supplying abnormal pulmonary artery branches in a patient with pulmonary atresia. MRA, magnetic resonance angiography.

diaphragm monitoring acquired during a limited part of respiratory cycles over a period of minutes. In the diagnosis and assessment of Kawasaki disease, contrast-enhanced MR angiography can be used to visualize coronary artery aneurysms or stenosis.

MEASUREMENT OF RIGHT VENTRICULAR FUNCTION AND MASS

Ventricular measurements have been described in greater detail elsewhere. In CHD, measurements of the right ventricle are at least as important as those of the left ventricle, but they pose particular challenges. The right ventricular cavity is crossed by coarse trabeculations, particularly near the apex. These become thickened and significant in summed volume when the right ventricle is hypertrophied. But even if clearly visualized, trabeculations are difficult to outline individually because of their complex structure. Furthermore, the base of the right ventricle tends to be more difficult to delineate that that of the left ventricle. After repair of tetralogy of Fallot, the right ventricular outflow tract (RVOT) can be dilated and dyskinetic, and may have no effective pulmonary valve. All these factors can make it difficult to decide on the limits of the right ventricle. In our center, we count a dilated or aneurysmal outflow tract as part of the right ventricle, not least as it lies beneath the pulmonary valve annulus and belongs to the right ventricle (17). Hence, the measurement of the ejection fraction is lower than measurements that attempt to exclude the non-contracting region. A particular center or research facility must establish a reproducible protocol for the acquisition and analysis right ventricular function, which despite difficulties is likely to prove more reliable than those obtained by any other imaging modality.

LATE GADOLINIUM ENHANCEMENT

Late gadolinium enhancement imaging makes use of the property of intravenously injected gadolinium chelate, a paramagnetic contrast agent, to linger in extracellular spaces in scarred myocardial tissue after its concentration has begun to fall in the bloodstream. Imaging at least 5 to 20 minutes after injection, depending on the dose of gadolinium given, allows infarcted tissue to be highlighted. An inversion recovery sequence is used, which with appropriate adjustment of parameters allows healthy myocardium to appear dark, contrasting with the bright signal of scarred myocardium (21).

Clinically, this can shed diagnostic light when there are unexpected areas of wall-motion abnormality. Specifically, late gadolinium enhancement MRI may provide assessment of anomalous coronary arteries, hypertrophic cardiomyopathy, and arrhythmogenic right ventricular cardiomyopathy (ARVC). In research, the techniques of late gadolinium enhancement imaging have been used for investigation of ventricular scarring in patients with CHD, particularly after surgery. Scarring has been found to be common in distinct locations. These are often directly attributable to the interventions performed (e.g., scarring of the wall of the partially resected infundibulum in patients after repair of tetralogy of Fallot) (22). Scarring of the systemic right ventricle in patients who previously underwent Mustard or Senning proce-

dures for transposition of the great arteries was found to relate to adverse ventricular function and incidence of arrhythmias (23). Longer-term follow-up will be needed to investigate the potential prognostic value of this finding.

APPLICATIONS OF MAGNETIC RESONANCE IMAGING/MAGNETIC RESONANCE ANGIOGRAPHY IN SPECIFIC DISEASES

LEFT VENTRICULAR OUTFLOW TRACT OBSTRUCTION AND AORTIC STENOSIS

In congenital valvar and subvalvar aortic stenosis, it is important to clarify the level(s) and severity of stenosis by appropriate acquisitions. In Shone syndrome, there may be both subaortic and aortic stenosis, sometimes combined with mitral valve stenosis, and all should be looked for and assessed. Our approach is to acquire cine images of the left ventricular outflow tract (LVOT) in several planes—a three-chamber LVOT view followed by a coronal LVOT view orthogonal to it, and an aortic valve view transecting the sinus of valsalva at the point of coaptation of the leaflets.

Velocity mapping can be performed with in-plane velocity encoding in the three-chamber LVOT view followed by through-plane velocity mapping at several levels, appropriately labeled for subsequent analysis through the subaortic, aortic valve, and immediate supra-aortic regions.

When there is significant subaortic stenosis, it can be dificcult or impossible to be sure whether aortic valve stenosis also exists. Even a mobile valve will not open fully where a narrow jet passes through it, but comparison of jet velocities at different levels beneath, at, and above the valve should allow determination of the level of the main stenosis.

THE OUTFLOW TRACTS AFTER THE ROSS OPERATION

The Ross operation is used for replacement of a diseased aortic valve with the patient's own pulmonary valve (a pulmonary autograft in aortic position). This in turn necessitates replacement of the pulmonary valve, usually with a pulmonary homograft. It is the homograft in pulmonary position that most often gives cause for concern after the Ross procedure. We found that the homograft has a tendency to shrink and become stenotic, with up to 10% of patients developing a peak velocity appproaching 3 m/s in the first year or two after Ross operation. This shrinkage is usually self-limiting. It can be at one or both suture lines, or along the length of the tube of the conduit (24). MRI with in-plane and through-plane velocity mapping is useful to determine the level and severity of stenosis. Cine imaging of the LVOT and neoaortic sinus is also required to look for any dysfunction of the autograft valve and possible dilatation of the autograft root in aortic position.

AORTIC COARCTATION, RECOARCTATION, AND ANEURYSM

Aortic coarctation consists of narrowing or occlusion of the proximal descending thoracic aorta, in most cases just distal to the left subclavian artery branch but occasionally proximal to it. The geometry of the aorta is highly variable in adults with aortic coarctation, especially after different types of repair. The risks associated with repaired aortic coarctation are related to systemic hypertension in the upper body, which may be exacerbated by any residual coarctation; rupture of an aneurysm or false aneurysm is also a risk. In this setting, a resting peak velocity of 3 m/s is significant, particularly if associated with a diastolic prolongation of forward flow (diastolic "tail"), which is a useful indicator of the obstructive significance of coarctation.

When aortic coarctation is investigated in an adult (unoperated, balloon-dilated, or operated), a number of questions must be considered:

- Is blood pressure high in one or both arms?
- To what extent is it caused by obstruction resulting from coarctation?
- If operated, what type of surgery?
- Is diastolic prolongation of forward flow present?
- Do blood pressure and "gradient" rise markedly with exercise?
- Is associated aortic valve disease present?
- Is the left ventricle hypertrophied?
- How extensive is the collateral flow?
- What is the location and severity of the coarctation?
- Of what type is it (e.g., membrane or narrow segment)?
- What is the geometry of the aorta and its branches in the vicinity of the coarctation?
- Is dissection, aneurysm, or false aneurysm present?

No single modality answers all questions, but MRI with cine imaging and velocity mapping can generally determine the nature and severity of coarctation (25,26) and identify any dissecting or false aneurysms (27). Where relevant, gadolinium-enhanced MRA can provide additional information if a narrow tortuous segment or collateral vessels must be visualized (Fig. 28.3), but it may not reliably assess severity if the obstruction is caused by a relatively thin membrane; appropriately located cine imaging and velocity mapping are better for this purpose.

Poststenotic dilation is common. It appears as fusiform dilation beyond a stenosed or previously stenosed region and is usually distinguishable by its location and smooth contours from more sinister aneurysmal dilation, which may require reoperation or protection with a covered stent. True or false aneurysms may complicate repairs, particularly those incorporating patches of noncompliant fabric, such as Dacron. We recommend that patients with such patches be followed regularly with MRI examinations. Leakage of blood through a false aneurysm can lead to hemoptysis. In such cases, para-aortic hematoma is generally well visualized by MRI, appearing bright, usually with diffuse edges, on spin-echo images. Postoperative hematoma is common, however, and sometimes leaves a region of signal adjacent to the aorta, which may be distinguished from a developing false aneurysm only if a comparison of images over time is possible. For this reason, it is worth acquiring baseline postoperative images in adults who have undergone repeated surgery for coarctation. Dissecting aneurysm can result from attempted balloon dilation (28).

PATENT DUCTUS ARTERIOSUS

Patent ductus arteriosus is identifiable by MRI, if sought. Flow through a patent ductus arteriosus, usually directed

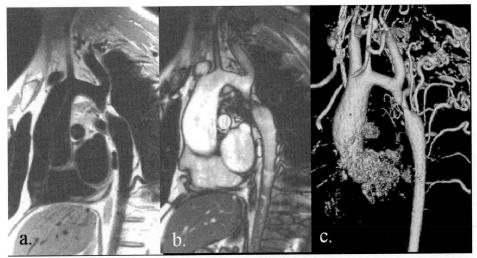

Figure 28.3. Unoperated aortic coarctation imaged by three different magnetic resonance techniques. The turbo spin-echo image **(A)** gives no blood signal and differentiated signal from other types of tissue. The SSFP cine image **(B)** gives bright blood with visualization of flow effects when viewed in cine mode. The 3D gadolinium contrast angiogram **(C)** shows the lumen of the aorta and collateral arteries. The 3D data set can be rotated and viewed from any angle. Although there was no visible orifice through the coarctation on 3D angiography, this patient was treated successfully by transcatheter balloon dilatation and stenting, the size and potential suitability of the stent having been determined from these images. SSFP, steady-state free precession; 3D, three-dimensional. (From Babu-Narayan SV, Kilner PJ. When to order cardiovascular magnetic resonance in adults with congenital heart disease. *Curr Cardiol Reports* 2003, 5:324–330, with permission.)

anteriorly in the top of the left pulmonary artery close to the pulmonary artery bifurcation, is detectable on cine images, especially if a relatively long time to echo (TE) of 14 ms is used to provide sensitivity to turbulence. Shunting can be assessed by measuring flow in the pulmonary trunk and aorta. Ascending aortic flow will be greater than pulmonary artery flow if duct flow is from the aorta to the pulmonary artery bifurcation. If true fast imaging with steady-state precession (true-FISP) is used for multislice assessment of the anatomy, pericardial fluid above the pulmonary artery bifurcation can cause a spot of bright signal that can be mistaken for a patent ductus arteriosus unless cine imaging is also used.

ATRIAL AND VENTRICULAR SEPTAL DEFECTS

Although ASDs and ventricular septal defects VSDs can often be assessed satisfactorily by echocardiography, MRI offers unrestricted access and makes it possible to determine shunt flow from the difference between measurements of flow in the pulmonary artery and aorta. In both VSD and ASD, a good way of searching for the defect is with a stack of multiple contiguous cine images. These can be acquired as a ventricular short-axis stack, working down the ventricles from base to apex, followed by an atrial short-axis stack, working back into the atria as far as the superior vena cava (SVC) from the basal slice. Each cine should be studied carefully for evidence of jet flow through a septal defect, with a further long-axis cine located to visualize any jet seen, followed by through-plane velocity mapping to measure the width and velocity of any transseptal jet.

PULMONARY HYPERTENSION

MRI cannot measure pulmonary vascular pressure or resistance directly, but it can give important indirect evidence of pulmonary arterial hypertension. For example, abnormal hypertrophy of the walls and trabeculations of the right ventricle and dilatation of the pulmonary trunk and proximal pulmonary arterial branches, with reduction of pulsatility, are typical appearances of pulmonary hypertension. With chronic pressure load, the hypertrophied and perhaps increasingly dilated right ventricle shows laborious and pro-

longed systolic contraction relative to the left ventricle, which leads to a paradoxical shift of the ventricular septum to the left at the onset of left ventricular diastole. In assessing and monitoring pulmonary hypertension, contrast-enhanced MR allows measurement of right ventricular mass and function and of cardiac output, which may be indexed to body surface area.

RIGHT VENTRICULAR OUTFLOW TRACT AND CONDUIT OBSTRUCTION

The RVOT and conduits from the right ventricle to the pulmonary artery are often inadequately visualized by ultrasonography; therefore, MRI can make important contributions in this region (24). For cine imaging and in-plane velocity mapping, an oblique sagittal slice located with respect to transaxial scouts is usually suitable. In some cases, it is also helpful to orient the plane with respect to coronal scouts. It is important to identify the level of stenosis. The level of the pulmonary valve can usually be identified on cine imaging by visualizing the valve cusps as they close at the onset of diastole (e.g., by the location of a regurgitant jet at the moment of valve closure). Obstruction may be subvalvar or supravalvar (e.g., at the distal suture line of a homograft conduit). An important variant is double-chambered right ventricle (Fig. 28.4),in which the right ventricle obstruction is subinfundibular, resulting from hypertrophied muscular ridges or bands beneath an infundibulum that is not hypertrophied and a pulmonary valve that is not stenosed. This can be corrected by surgical resection without the need for replacement of the pulmonary valve (29).

REPAIRED TETRALOGY OF FALLOT

Pulmonary regurgitation is common 20 to 30 years after repair of tetralogy of Fallot and is considered a risk factor for progressive right ventricular dysfunction, arrhythmia, and late sudden cardiac death. Implanted bioprosthetic valves have a finite lifespan, and the optimal timing of pulmonary valve replacement still causes debate. Information from MRI may be useful in the decision-making process, and MRI studies have shown evidence of functional improvements after pumonary valve replacement (30). Stenosis of the right or left pulmonary artery may occur, particularly

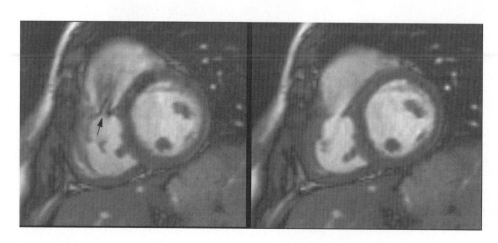

Figure 28.4. Double-chambered right ventricle. Stenosis in the cavity of the right ventricle is caused by hypertrophied myocardial ridges or bands. The arrow points to the jet through the narrowing in systole.

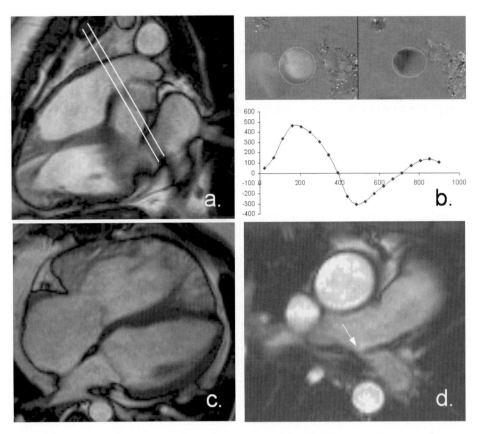

Figure 28.5. Pulmonary regurgitation measured by through-plane velocity mapping in a patient left with free pulmonary regurgitation after repair of tetralogy of Fallot. The oblique sagittal image **(A)** was used to locate the plane for velocity mapping in which cross-sectional area and mean flow velocity of the pulmonary artery (PA) lumen were measured in each phase of the cycle to give a plot of flow against time **(B)**. In this case, diastolic reversed flow was 40% of forward flow, and there was some forward flow in late diastole. This indicates free pulmonary regurgitation with "restrictive" right ventricular physiology. The four-chamber view at end diastole **(C)** shows function of the left ventricle and the muscular part of the right ventricle. An oblique transaxial slice **(D)** shows the pulmonary artery bifurcation with acute angulation and stenosis at the origin of the left pulmonary artery (*arrow*).

where a previous surgical shunt may have been closed, and pulmonary artery branch stenosis tends to worsen pulmonary regurgitation (31). Interestingly, in free pulmonary regurgitation without a functional pulmonary valve at all, the regurgitant fraction is only about 40% to 45% (diastolic reversed flow as a percentage of forward flow) (Fig. 28.5). The long-term follow-up of patients with a repaired tetralogy of Fallot should include measurement of the pulmonary regurgitant fraction by through-plane velocity mapping and measurement of the right ventricular function and volume, particularly the end-systolic volume increase, which is probably the best marker of right ventricular failure in response to volume overload. Measurement of right ventricular volume and function is not straightforward, however. In our experience, reproducible measurements require time and care. We have yet to find an automated method that works. The complex blood-myocardial borders of a volume-loaded and hypertrophied right ventricle, which for consistency we take to include any thin-walled, aneurysmal region of outflow tract up to the expected level of the pulmonary valve annulus, have to be painstakingly traced. A second observer is only likely to reproduce the measurements of a first observer if an agreed method of boundary recognition, including the right atrium-right ventricle and the right ventricle-pulmonary artery boundaries, is adhered to. Assessment should also include study of the pulmonary arteries and measurement of any aortic dilation.

EBSTEIN ANOMALY

Ebstein anomaly is a malformation of the tricuspid valve, with displacement of the septal and posterolateral leaflets toward the apex from their usual position at the atrioventricular junction (32). This is associated with atrialization of part of the right ventricle and varying degrees of tricuspid regurgitation. Depending on the severity of the malformation, the right atrium may become grossly enlarged. An ASD, VSD, tricuspid stenosis, or pulmonary stenosis may be present. In adults, MRI can be useful to assess the degree of right atrial dilation, the size and function of the right ventricle, and the severity of tricuspid regurgitation.

A simple, practical approach to imaging these patients is to acquire multiple transaxial cines, starting at the inferior border of the ventricles and working up to the level of the pulmonary arteries in 10 mm steps. This allows relatively comprehensive coverage to search for the jet or stream of tricuspid regurgitation, which may be surprisingly displaced through malposition of parts of the tricuspid valve. Once the regurgitant stream has been located and imaged in several slices, through-plane velocity mapping is valuable for determining the cross-sectional area of the regurgitant jet, which can be as broad as 1 cm or more in diameter. A transaxial stack of cines is also suitable for attempting to measure volumes of the functional part of the right ventricle in Ebstein patients, although the location of the tricuspid valve may not be easy to determine.

Cine imaging in a three-chamber LVOT view can show compression of the left ventricle by the distended right side of the heart, which may compromise left ventriclar filling in diastole. A four-chamber view should be acquired, aligned with the long axis of the left ventricle and tilted down anteriorly to pass through the abnormal tricuspid orifice. Cine imaging in additional planes through the tricuspid valve and RVOT may be helpful towards decision making regarding possible surgical repair of the tricuspid valve. Although echocardiography may better define the valve leaflets, MRI has the advantage of providing wide fields of view across the enlarged volume of the heart.

ARTERIAL SWITCH, MUSTARD, SENNING, AND RASTELLI OPERATIONS FOR TRANSPOSITION OF THE GREAT ARTERIES

In complete TGA, the atria and ventricles are normally related but the aorta and pulmonary artery are transposed with respect to the ventricles, resulting in ventriculoarterial discordance (Fig. 28.6). About two-thirds of such patients have no major additional malformations and are said to have "simple" transposition; the other one third have associated abnormalities, such as a VSD and pulmonary or subpulmonary stenosis. Since unoperated simple transposition is not compatible with long-term survival, patients seen as adults are likely to have undergone surgery. The current surgical approach to simple transposition is usually to switch the great arteries with respect to the ventricles in the first years of life, a technically difficult operation that requires reinsertion of the coronary arteries in the neoaorta root (formerly the pulmonary artery) (33–35). Such patients may be referred for MRI if there is concern regarding RVOT or branch pulmonary artery obstruction.

As the switch procedure has only come into widespread use in the last decade, most surviving adults will have had a Mustard or Senning procedure (Fig. 28.7), in which the flow paths are switched at the level of the atria, the ventriculo-

arterial connections having been left discordant (36). Blood is redirected at the atrial level with a baffle (Mustard operation) or with part of the in-turned atrial wall (Senning operation). A physiologic correction is achieved, although the right ventricle continues to support the systemic circulation. The imaging of patients after a Mustard or Senning operation requires an assessment of the pulmonary venous flow path, which passes from the pulmonary veins to the right of the curved baffle to the tricuspid valve. Both channels of the systemic venous flow paths must also be assessed. Channels from the superior and inferior venae cavae converge on the mitral valve, which lies to the left of the saddle-shaped baffle. It takes experience to assess the patency of all three atrial flow paths. Oblique planes for cine imaging and velocity mapping may be located with respect to sagittal scouts. Because it can be difficult to align a single plane with both the superior and inferior caval pathways, cross cuts may be needed to decide whether or not the pathways are stenosed. Obstruction can occur in one or more of the atrial flow paths, typically between the baffle and a ridge that may represent tissue where the native atrial septum was resected. Such obstruction at the atrial level does not generate jets with a very high velocity; a peak diastolic velocity between 1 and 2.5 ms may be found distal to a narrowing that is significantly obstructive. Gradual obstruction of one of the two caval flow paths is generally well tolerated as the azygous vein(s) dilates to divert flow to the other caval pathway. Because the hypertrophied right ventricle is delivering systemic pressure in these patients, it may be important to assess its function by volume measurements and assess any tricuspid regurgitation.

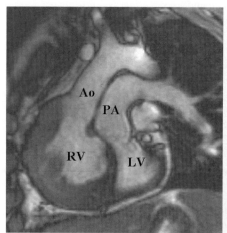
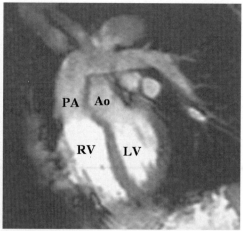
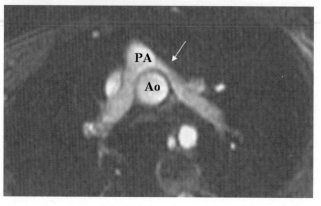

Figure 28.6. Transposed great arteries (*above left*) compared with the corrected ventriculoarterial connections in a different but comparable patient after arterial switch procedure for TGA (*above and below right*). The ascending aorta, which originally arose anteriorly from the right ventricle, has been switched with the pulmonary trunk. The left pulmonary artery (*arrow*) is now mildly compressed. Ao, aorta; LV, left ventricle; RV, right ventricle; PA, pulmonary artery; TGA, transposition of the great arteries.

29

Magnetic Resonance Imaging and Computed Tomography of the Thoracic Aorta

Rossella Fattori and Vincenzo Russo

In the past few years, considerable interest in aortic diseases has been shown in the medical literature. The prevalence of aortic disease seems to be increasing in the Western population, likely corresponding to aging of the population in addition to heightened clinical awareness. The continuous advances in our understanding of aortic pathology have been based on molecular and cellular studies elucidating the mechanisms of many pathologic conditions of the aorta and the complex interaction of this vessel with the cardiovascular system. However, increased clinical observation of aortic disease, demonstrated in epidemiologic studies, and a more appropriate definition of its pathologic substrate, reported in recent literature, may also reflect concurrent outstanding progress in imaging techniques. Among the imaging modalities, magnetic resonance (MR) and computed tomography (CT) offer the greatest versatility.

With its ability to delineate the intrinsic contrast between blood flow and vessel wall, and acquire images in multiple planes with a wide field of view, magnetic resonance imaging (MRI) provides a high degree of reliability in the diagnosis of aortic diseases, acute and chronic. MRI is totally noninvasive and can be repeated, so that the progression of the disease over time can be evaluated. Functional information can be obtained by gradient-echo sequences and phase mapping, which quantify blood-flow volume and velocity, so that our knowledge of aortic function can be expanded. The new magnetic resonance angiography (MRA) techniques have enhanced the noninvasive evaluation of vascular pathology, providing a high degree of spatial and contrast resolution and in many instances making invasive x-ray angiography an obsolete procedure for the detection of aortic diseases. In addition, the ability to differentiate tissue structures at a power of resolution in the order of micrometers provides an incomparable accuracy for the analysis of atherosclerotic plaque. At present, MRI microscopy, intravascular MRI, and spectroscopy are emerging techniques that will be used to understand atherosclerotic disease and its contributing pathogenic mechanisms more clearly.

Noninvasive vascular system imaging using computed tomography angiography (CTA) has become an important technique in the evaluation of vessels and has already been proven to yield high accuracy in the assessment of the thoracic-abdominal aorta and its major branches. Helical single-detector CT (SDCT), introduced to clinical routine imaging in the early 1990s, revolutionized body imaging through the use of slip-ring technology, demonstrating its superiority over conventional angiography in different applications (1–3). It created volume acquisition of image data using continuous patient translation during gantry rotation. The advantage of a three-dimensional (3D) data set allows for visual vessel assessment from any angle, and it rapidly became a standard diagnostic tool for large vessel investigation. However, the visualization of small aortic branches and extended vascular territories has been limited because of the restricted volume coverage (20–30 cm in one breath hold with moderate slice collimation). Another limitation of this technique was breathing and pulsation artifacts because of the long scan time (often >30 seconds) and the slow gantry rotation time (1 second), without any cardiac gating.

The development of multidetector-row CT (MDCT) in the late 1990s represented the most significant recent advancement in helical CT. Thinner collimations, faster gantry rotation times, large detector arrays, powered x-ray tubes, and increased table speed dramatically improved image quality and expanded the applications and indications of CT noninvasive vascular imaging. MDCT angiography provides a low-risk, efficient, and cost-effective evaluation of the arterial vascular system, allowing greater vessel length and smaller diameter to be visualized. In a single study, information of the vessel lumen and wall may be obtained together with extravascular information (4).

The latest development of MDCT scanners, in the early 2000s, with the use of 8, 16, 32, or even 64 detector-rows, now gives a submillimeter, isotropic 3D data acquisition of extended anatomic ranges, enabling high-quality vascular imaging with two-dimensional and 3D artifact-free reconstructions from virtually any angle and in any desirable plane (5–10).

ACQUIRED DISEASES OF THE THORACIC AORTA

AORTIC DISSECTION

Aortic dissection is characterized by a laceration of the aortic intima and inner layer of the aortic media that allows blood to course through a false lumen in the outer third of the media. Dissection can occur throughout the length of the aorta, and the two most common classifications are based on the anatomic location and extension of intimal flap. According to the DeBakey classification, in type I dissection the intimal tear originates in the ascending aorta and the intimal flap extends below the origin of the left subclavian artery; in type II dissection the intimal tear is confined to the ascending aorta; and in type III dissection the entry tear develops after the origin of the subclavian artery and extends distally. The Stanford classification simply classifies an aortic dissection irrespective of the site of the entry tear as type A if the ascending aorta is involved and as type B if the ascending aorta is spared. The Stanford classification is fundamentally based on prognostic factors: Type A dissection requires urgent surgical repair, whereas most of type B dissections can be successfully managed with medical therapy.

Acute aortic dissection is a life-threatening condition requiring prompt diagnosis and treatment (11). The 14-day period after onset has been designated as an acute phase because the rates of morbidity and mortality are highest during this period. The estimated mortality rate of untreated aortic dissection is 1% to 2% per hour in the first 24 hours after onset and 80% within 2 weeks. Early and accurate detection of the dissection and a delineation of its anatomic details are critical for successful management. However, because physical findings may be absent or misleading and symptoms may mimic those of other disorders, such as myocardial ischemia and stroke, the diagnosis of aortic dissection is often missed at initial evaluation (12,13). The anatomic characteristics of the dissection indicate the type of surgical technique and affect both the surgical success rate and long-term results. Thus, in dissection, the diagnostic goal is, regardless of the imaging modality used, not only a clear delineation of the intimal flap and its extension but also detection of the entry and reentry sites, presence and degree of aortic insufficiency, and flow in the aortic branches (14). Transcatheter endovascular reconstruction of type B aortic dissection is a new option for the treatment of both acute and chronic dissection (15,16). In endovascular techniques, the success of the procedure is strictly related to a detailed anatomic definition of the features of the dissected aorta. The identification of the entry and reentry sites, the relationship between true and false lumina and the visceral vessels, and any involvement of the iliac arteries are crucial in patient selection and stent-graft design (Fig. 29.1).

Magnetic Resonance Imaging Technique and Findings

In a suspected case of aortic dissection, the standard examination should begin with spin-echo sequences acquired with high-resolution parameters and preparatory pulses to nullify the blood signal and obtain a better definition of the aortic wall structures (Table 29.1). In the axial plane the intimal flap is detected as a straight linear image inside the aortic lumen. The true lumen can be differentiated from the false lumen by the anatomic features and flow pattern. The true lumen shows a signal void, whereas the false lumen has a higher signal intensity. In addition, the visualization of remnants of the dissected media as cobwebs adjacent to the outer wall of the lumen may help to identify the false lumen. The leakage of blood from the descending aorta into the periaortic space, which can appear with high signal intensity and result in a left-sided pleural effusion, is usually better visualized on axial images. A high signal intensity of a pericardial effusion indicates a bloody component and is considered a sign of impending rupture of the ascending aorta into the pericardial space. A detailed anatomic map of aortic dissection must indicate the type and extension of dissection and distinguish the origin and perfusion of branch vessels (arch branches, celiac, superior mesenteric, renal arteries, and coronary arteries) from the true or false channels. Therefore, a further spin-echo sequence on the sagittal plane should be performed to define the extension of the dissection in the thoracic and abdominal aorta and in the aortic arch branches (Fig. 29.2).

Adjunctive gradient-echo sequences or phase-contrast images can be instrumental in identifying aortic insufficiency and entry or reentry sites (Fig. 29.3), as well as in differentiating slow flow from thrombus in the false lumen (17,18). However, because the diagnosis of aortic dissection

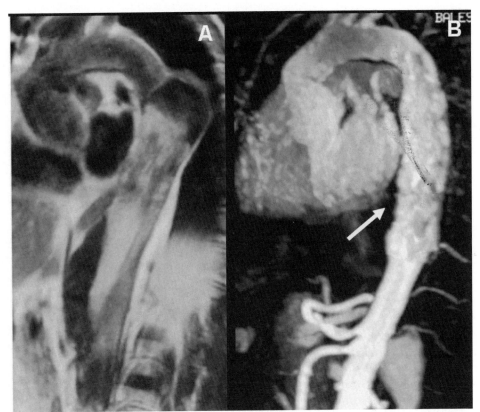

Figure 29.1. **(A)** Spin-echo sagittal image of type B dissection. Double aortic lumen is 4 cm below the left subclavian artery. False lumen (high signal intensity) is severely dilated. **(B)** Magnetic resonance angiography (MRA) of the same patient after stent graft treatment (*arrow*): aortic remodeling with complete thrombosis of the false lumen. The metallic structure of the stent graft produces minimal artifacts in the upper portion of the descending aorta.

TABLE 29-1	Magnetic Resonance Study Modality in Acute Aortic Syndromes	
Sequence/Plane	**Diagnostic Findings**	**Anatomic Details**
Aortic Dissection		
Spin-echo axial/sagittal	Intimal flap/true-false lumen	Periaortic hematoma Pericardial effusion
Gradient-echo axial/sagittal	Intimal flap/true-false lumen Aortic insufficiency	Thrombosis false lumen/entry and reentry sites
Magnetic resonance angiography	Intimal flap/true-false lumen	Origin/perfusion of supra aortic, coronary, abdominal vessels
Intramural Hematoma		
Spin-echo axial/sagittal T1 weighted	Abnormal wall thickness, crescentic shape High signal intensity (T1)	Periaortic hematoma Pericardial effusion
Spin-echo axial T2 weighted	High signal intensity (recent) Low signal intensity (old)	Pericardial, pleural, mediastinal effusion: increased signal intensity
Magnetic resonance angiography	No utility	
Penetrating Aortic Ulcer		
Spin-echo axial/sagittal	Crater-like outpouching/ circumscribed dissection/intramural hemorrhage	Periaortic hematoma/pleural effusion Diffuse aortic wall atherosclerosis
Gradient echo sagittal	No utility	
Magnetic resonance angiography	Crater-like outpouching/ saccular pseudoaneurysm	Relationship with aortic arch or abdominal vessels

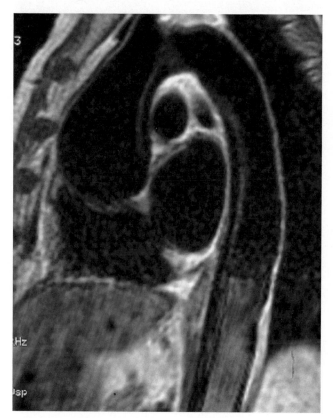

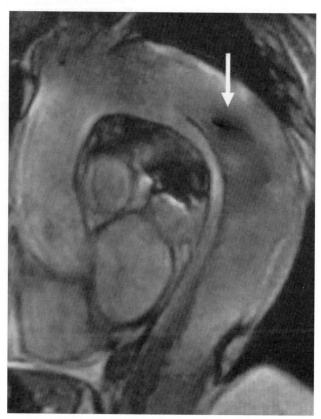

Figure 29.2.   Spin-echo sagittal image of type A dissection. The intimal flap is visible as subtle linear image in the ascending and descending aortas.

Figure 29.3.   Gradient-echo sagittal image of type B dissection. Flow turbulence (signal void, *arrow*) in the descending aorta indicates the entry site.

is not dependent on functional gradient-echo images, these sequences should be reserved for clinically stable patients.

The third step in the diagnosis of aortic dissection and the definition of its anatomic detail relies on the use of gadolinium-enhanced 3D MRA. Because 3D MRA is rapidly acquired without any need of electrocardiograph (ECG) triggering, this technique may be used even for severely ill patients. Because it is not nephrotoxic and causes no other adverse effects, gadolinium can be used in patients with renal failure or low cardiac output. With spin-echo sequences, artifacts caused by imperfect ECG gating, respiratory motion, or slow blood pool can result in intraluminal signal, simulating or obscuring an intimal flap. In gadolinium-enhanced 3D MRA, the intimal flap is easily detected and the relationship with aortic vessels is clearly depicted (Figs. 29.4 and 29.5). Entry and reentry sites appear as a segmental interruption of the linear intimal flap on axial or sagittal images (Fig. 29.6). The analysis of MRA images should not be limited to viewing maximum intensity projection (MIP) images or surface-shaded display; it should also include a complete evaluation of reformatted images in all three planes to confirm or improve spin-echo information and exclude artifacts. In MRA postprocessing displays, the appearance of the dissected aorta is similar to that on conventional catheter angiograms, but diagnostic information such as the intimal flap can be masked. Combining the spin-echo with MRA images completes the diagnosis and anatomic definition (19). However, two cases of intramural hematoma (IMH) missed by MRA (20) raise concern about using MRA as the sole modality for suspected aortic dissection.

At present, MRI is one of the most accurate tools in the detection of aortic dissection. A high degree of spatial resolution and contrast and the capability for multiplanar acquisition provide excellent sensitivity and specificity that approximate 100% in the published series (19,21–23). With modern scanners a comprehensive study of the entire aorta is completed in less than 10 minutes, and the patient's ECG, blood pressure, and oxygen saturation can be monitored, even during assisted ventilation. The implementation of open systems may soon allow a wider use of MRI even in acute pathology.

Aortography has long been considered the method of choice in suspected aortic dissection, despite the risk of catheter manipulation and injection of high-flow contrast in a dissected aorta. With the advent of noninvasive imaging modalities, its low accuracy has been demonstrated; the reported sensitivity is 77% to 90% and the specificity is 90% to 100%. The superiority of transesophageal echocardiography (TEE), CT, and MRI in comparison with angiography has been widely reported in the literature (12–14,21).

In general, TEE is a reliable method with excellent sensitivity, and a great advantage is that it can be performed at the bedside in patients too unstable for transportation. However, artifacts and "blind areas," such as the distal portion of the ascending aorta, can influence specificity in an operator-dependent manner. Because TEE information is limited to the thoracic aorta, sometimes with suboptimal display of the aortic arch, a second imaging modality encompassing the entire aorta is advisable in stable patients.

TABLE 29-3	General Strategy and Computed Tomography Study Findings of the Thoracic-Abdominal Aorta Diseases	

Disease	Type of Scan	Findings
Aortic Dissection	**Pre-contrast**	Displaced calcified intima
	Contrast Enhanced	Intimal flap
		True-false lumen flow
		False lumen filling defects (thromboses)
		Size of true and false lumen
		Visceral-epiaortic vessel's involvement
		Entry and re-entry sites
Intramural Hematoma (IMH)	**Pre-contrast**	Concentric area of high density around lumen
	Contrast Enhanced	Displaced calcified intima (subintimal location)
		Wall thickening
		+/− Aortic dilation
Aortic Ulcer	**Pre-contrast**	Dislodgment of the intimal calcifications
	Contrast Enhanced	+/− Wall enhancement
		"Collar button" contrast-filled ulceration
		Pseudoaneurysms, intimal flap
Aortic Aneurysms	**Pre-contrast**	Size (caliber, length, tortuosity)
	Contrast Enhanced	Extension/relationship with epiaortic/visceral vessels
		Necks
		Mural thromboses
		Calcifications
Aortic Trauma	**Pre-contrast**	Mediastinal hemorrhage
	Contrast Enhanced	Aortic contour abnormality (intima-media disruption)
		Focal caliber change or dissection flap
		Contrast media extravasation
Aortitis	**Pre-contrast**	Irregular calcified aortic wall
	Contrast Enhanced	Periaortic density (inflammation) and adjacent gas collection

ages, oxyhemoglobin shows intermediate signal intensity, whereas in the subacute phase (>8 days), methemoglobin shows high signal intensity. However, when the signal intensity is medium to low, it can be difficult to distinguish IMH from mural thrombus. T2-weighted spin-echo sequences may help in differentiating the two entities: Signal intensity is high in recent hemorrhage but low in chronic thrombosis. In a retrospective study of 22 cases, Murray et al (46) described three cases with recurrence of symptoms and unfavorable evolution in which MR signal intensity changes consistently with recurrent bleeding. The progression of IMH to overt dissection and rupture has been reported in 32% of cases, particularly with the involvement of ascending aorta (Fig. 29.11). Instability of the hematoma and recurrent bleeding, which can be detected by MRI, are important parameters in assessing the need for surgical repair.

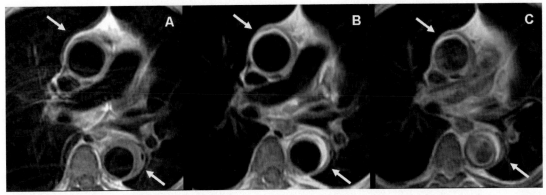

Figure 29.10. **(A,B)** T1-weighted spin-echo axial image of intramural hematoma (IMH) of the ascending and descending aortas; the abnormal wall thickening (*arrows*) presents intermediate signal intensity in **(A)** (oxyhemoglobin, acute phase) and high signal intensity in **(B)** (methemoglobin, subacute phase). **(C)** T2-weighted spin-echo image signal intensity is high in acute phase (recent hemorrhage).

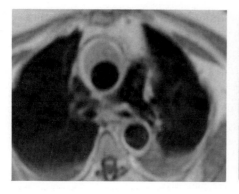 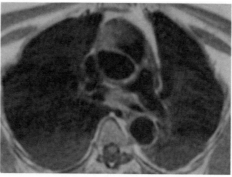

Figure 29.11. Spin-echo axial images of IMH evolved in classic dissection in the acute **(A)** and chronic **(B)** phases. **(A)** The high signal intensity of hematoma is visible in ascending and descending aortas. **(B)** Three months later the hematoma presents low signal intensity and partial area of reabsorption: An intimal flap is visible.

Computed Tomography Findings

Unenhanced CT imaging finding of IMH is a crescent-shaped area of hyperdensity in the aortic wall or circumferential wall thickening, corresponding to a hematoma in the medial layer that extends cephalic and caudal beneath a displaced calcified intima, with a constant relationship to the wall (subintimal location) (42,47–50) (Fig. 29.12). The hematoma may, or may not, compress the aortic lumen (51). It is important to perform unenhanced CT as the first imaging evaluation, because contrast agent within the vessel may obscure IMH. Unlike the false lumen in typical aortic dissection, the crescent-shaped area of IMH remains unenhanced after contrast material administration, and no intimal tear is seen on contrast-enhanced CT scan. Aortic dilatation could be present. One useful observation that may help differentiate IMH from a thrombosed false lumen of a classic intimal dissection is that the latter tends to longitudinally spiral around the aorta, whereas the former tends to maintain a constant circumferential relationship with aortic wall. Another finding that can be seen in the setting of IMH is intense enhancement and thickening of the aortic wall external to the hematoma, which may represent adventitial inflammation.

Several investigators have attempted to assess the usefulness of CT findings for predicting the progression of aortic IMH to overt dissection, but the relationship between them remains unclear. However, findings such as IMH type A, aortic diameter of more than 50 mm, thick hematoma with compression of the false lumen, and pericardial or pleural effusion are useful for predicting progression to aortic dissection (49,52–55).

Axial images alone will suffice for detection of IMH or penetrating ulcers in most cases, but 3D review is useful to discriminate both from irregular mural thrombus and to plan endovascular or surgical therapy and to map the full extent of IMH.

AORTIC ULCERS

In 1934 Shennan (56) was the first to describe penetrating atheromatous ulcers of the thoracic aorta. In elderly, hypertensive patients with severe atherosclerotic involvement of the aortic wall, usually in the descending aorta, a plaque may ulcerate into the media. Aortic ulcer is characterized by rupture of the atheromatous plaque disrupting the internal elastic lamina. Extension of the ulcerated atheroma into the media may result in an IMH or localized intramedial dissection, or the plaque may break through to the adventitia and form a saccular pseudoaneurysm. The adventitia may also rupture, in which case only the surrounding mediastinal tissues contain the hematoma. Aortic ulcers occur almost only in the descending aorta, but location in the aortic arch or ascending aorta has occasionally been reported. The clinical features of penetrating atherosclerotic ulcers may be similar to those of aortic dissection, but the ulcers should be considered a distinct entity with a different management and prognosis. Hypertension, advanced age, and systemic atherosclerosis are common predisposing factors. Persistent pain,

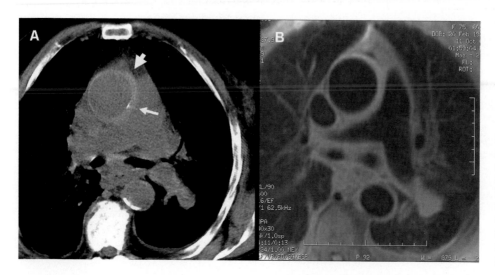

Figure 29.12. IMH. **(A)** Computed tomography (CT) image showing a crescent-shaped area of attenuation in the aortic wall (*arrowhead*) and a displaced calcified intima (*arrow*). **(B)** T1-weighted spin-echo image of the same patients presenting intermediate signal intensity (acute phase).

hemodynamic instability, and sign of expansion should trigger surgical treatment, whereas asymptomatic patients can be managed medically and monitored with imaging follow-up. Movsowitz et al (57) analyzed 45 cases of aortic ulcers reported in the medical literature and found an incidence of transmural rupture of 8%. A different prognostic profile was reported by Coady et al (42): Among 19 patients with a diagnosis of penetrating ulcer, 8 (42%) had ruptured ulcers before surgical treatment. Because penetrating ulcer is much less common than classic dissection and imaging findings may be subtle, careful awareness of its insidious behavior is particularly important for successful management.

Magnetic Resonance Imaging Findings

The MRI diagnosis of aortic ulcers is based on the visualization of a crater-like ulcer located in the aortic wall (Fig. 29.13). Mural thickening with high or intermediate signal intensity on spin-echo sequences may indicate extension of the ulcer into the media and the formation of an IMH. MRA is particularly suitable for depicting aortic ulcers (Fig. 29.14) along with the irregular aortic wall profile seen in diffuse

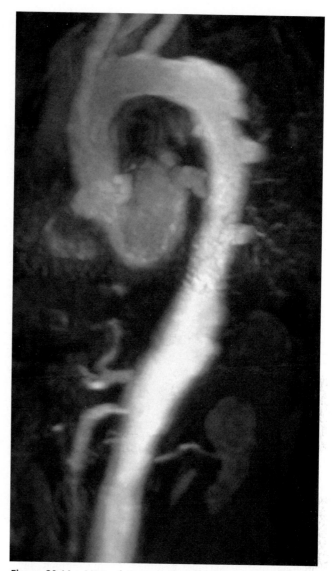

Figure 29.14. MRA of the same patient. The ulcers appear as contrast-filled outpouching protruding on the vessel profile.

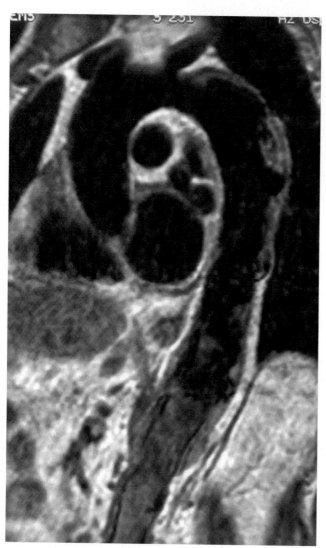

Figure 29.13. Spin-echo sagittal image of severe aortic atheromatous plaques and multiple penetrating ulcers of the descending aorta.

atherosclerotic involvement (58). The aortic ulcer is easily recognized as a contrast-filled outpouching of variable extent with jagged edges, which may result in a large pseudoaneurysm (59). The disadvantage of MRI with respect to CT is the failure to visualize dislodgment of the intimal calcifications, frequently observed in aortic ulcers.

Computed Tomography Findings

In PAUs the plaque rupture and disruption of the internal elastic lamina are manifest on unenhanced CT as extensive atherosclerosis and IMH of variable extent. Frequently the IMH is focal because of medial fibrosis caused by atherosclerosis (60). Displaced intimal calcifications are also often seen. On CTA, penetrating ulcer appears as a discrete "collar button" contrast-filled ulceration, similar to that of a peptic ulcer (Fig. 29.15) (42,47–50,61). Lesions can be single or multiple. It seems more eccentric than irregular mural thrombus and may be associated with wall thickening and enhancement, pseudoaneurysms, dissection, or rupture (48). Athero-

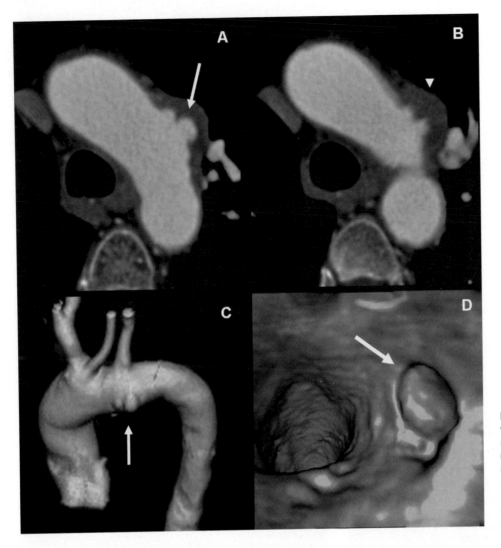

Figure 29.15. MDCT images illustrate penetrating atherosclerotic ulcer and IMH of the aortic arch. **(A,B)** Axial image of a double penetrating ulcer (*arrow*) with IMH (*arrowhead*). **(C,D)** Volume-rendering **(C)** and virtual endoscopy **(D)** images showing ulcers (*arrows*).

matous ulcers that are confined to the intimal layer sometimes have a radiologic appearance similar to that of penetrating ulcers. Therefore, particular attention should be taken in making diagnosis of a PAU if the lesions are discovered incidentally in an asymptomatic patient and if associated IMH is absent (58). CT has the advantage, as well as in IMH, to visualize dislodgment of the intimal calcifications that are very frequently observed in aortic ulcers. CTA, as well as MR, has permitted accurate, noninvasive follow-up of both PAU and IMH with reliability for detecting change that allows conservative management approaches to be explored and early intervention to be indicated.

MDCT can depict small, penetrating atherosclerotic ulcers and can demonstrate complex spatial relationships, mural abnormalities, and extraluminal pathologic conditions, which may offset this weakness (42).

POSTOPERATIVE EVALUATION OF AORTIC DISSECTION

The objective of surgical treatment of aortic dissection is to prevent aortic rupture in the proximal portion of the ascending aorta. Early and accurate detection by new imaging modalities and aggressive surgical approach have contributed

to a decrease in operative mortality from 40% to 50% in the 1970s to 5% to 7% in recent series (62–64). Nevertheless, survivors after initial repair still remain at considerable risk of future complications. A persistent distal false lumen has been reported in 75% to 100% of cases. Second entry tears in the descending aorta or aortic arch, which are common, are responsible for patency of the distal dissection, which is associated with an unfavorable prognosis. It is recognized that dilation and subsequent rupture of the distal aorta is the most common cause of death of patients after surgery for aortic dissection. Prosthetic graft degeneration or infection (Fig. 29.16), and malfunction of the prosthetic aortic valves are additional causes of postoperative complications. Therefore, after aortic dissection repair every patient must be carefully monitored with imaging according to a strict schedule, and the timing is crucial. Heinemann et al (65) suggested a first imaging session at discharge, so that a relatively normal baseline postoperative image of the new anatomic situation is available. Subsequent examinations are scheduled on the basis of absolute diameter (<5 cm once per year; >5 cm every 6 months) and the expansion rate on two subsequent follow-ups. Rupture is often preceded by a period of rapid aneurysm expansion, and detection of this phenomenon can identify patients at high risk of rupture, thereby decreasing the risk-to-benefit ratio of prophylactic surgical repair. The

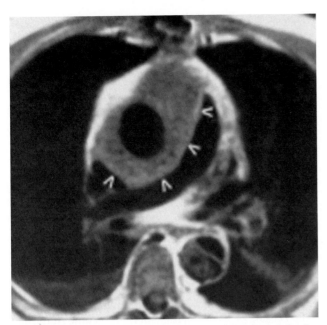

Figure 29.16. Spin-echo axial image of a periprosthetic infective collection (*arrowheads*) in a patient who underwent surgery for aortic dissection.

reported expansion rate for dissected segments ranges between 1.2 and 4.3 mm per year. However, a yearly expansion rate of 5.6 mm has been reported by Bonser et al (66) in aneurysms with a diameter of more than 60 mm. The presence of partial thrombosis of the false lumen seems to protect against dilation; an aortic growth rate of 3.4 mm per year in dissection with partial thrombosis of the false lumen versus an increase of 5.6 mm per year in dissection with no thrombosis of the false lumen has been reported (67). Therefore, in patients who have undergone surgery for aortic dissection, an appropriate follow-up should take into account an accurate measurement of the residual aorta to identify high-risk patients at an early time.

Magnetic Resonance Imaging

MRI is recognized as one of the imaging modalities of choice in postoperative evaluation (68–71). MRI measurements of parameters are highly reproducible, and reproducibility is an essential component of serial examinations, in which minimal change in dimension may represent a prognostic finding or indicate a need for preventive surgical strategies. Residual dissection is easily detected on spin-echo images, and gradient-echo sequences or phase-display images can be used to distinguish thrombosis of the false lumen from slow flow.

Slight thickening around the graft is a common finding caused by perigraft fibrosis (71,72). However, large or asymmetric thickening around the tube-graft may represent localized hematoma caused by an anastomotic leakage. Suture detachment with leakage has been reported in particular after composite graft replacement of the ascending aorta. Reoperation for bleeding at the site of repair has been reported after composite graft operation in 8% of patients after 30 days and in 4% of patients after 1 year. The higher incidence of bleeding has been reported at the site of reimplanted coronary arteries. Gadolinium-enhanced MRI with standard spin-

echo sequences can provide detailed information on suture detachment (73); the site of bleeding appears as high signal intensity within the hematoma. Moreover, gadolinium-enhanced MRA is particularly effective in depicting the complex postoperative anatomy and elucidating the prosthetic tube, distal and proximal anastomoses and residual distal dissection, and eventually dilated segments (Fig. 29.17). Reimplanted coronary arteries or reimplanted supraaortic vessels can be also visualized by MRA, and particular attention should be paid to evaluating these sites for possible postoperative weakness. Aneurysm of reimplanted coronary ostium has been reported after composite graft replacement of ascending aorta with the Bentall technique. In the Cabrol technique, intraoperative thrombosis or distortion of the prosthetic limb connecting the right coronary artery to the main prosthetic tube may cause myocardial infarction. Contrast-enhanced MRA can visualize the proximal segment of reimplanted coronary arteries and detect and monitor proximal coronary aneurysms (Fig. 29.18).

COMPUTED TOMOGRAPHY

The role of CTA as an appropriate imaging modality in postoperative evaluation of surgical or endovascular aortic repair is surely increased by the introduction of MDCT scanners.

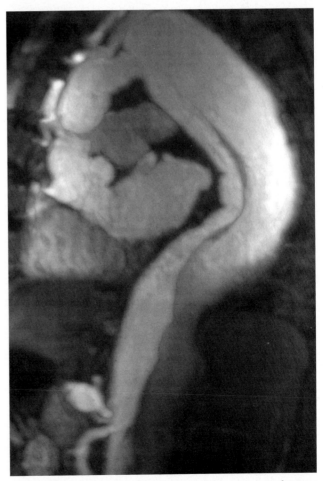

Figure 29.17. MRA of a patient who underwent surgery for type A dissection. The prosthetic tube is visible in the ascending aorta and aortic arch. Residual dissection is seen in the descending aorta, with dilation of the false lumen.

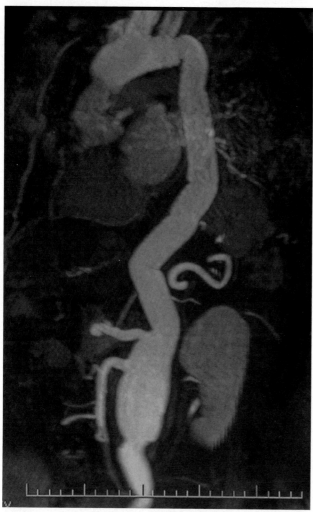

Figure 29.18. MRA of a patient who underwent multiple operations for type A dissection. In the ascending aorta, the origin of reimplanted coronary arteries is well depicted. Right coronary artery is visible up to its distal portion.

High anatomic details and images quality derived from thinner collimations, volumetric acquisition, and superior aortic enhancement are the hallmarks of this technique. Especially with MPR and 3D volume-rendering features, it is easy and clear to see the postoperative anatomy and the success or complication of any aortic repair modality, particularly during follow-up (Figs. 29.19 and 29.20) (3,74–78). Artifacts from metallic stents and surgical clips do not represent a problem with this new generation of scanners because of thinner collimations, fast gantry rotation time plus half rotation reconstruction algorithm (180 degrees), and kernel convolution filters (Fig. 29.21).

AORTIC ANEURYSMS

Aortic aneurysm is a localized or diffuse dilation involving all layers of the aortic wall, exceeding the expected aortic diameter by a factor of 1.5 or more. Aortic aneurysm is the thirteenth most common cause of death in United States. Because of the increasing age of population and environmental factors, it is expected that aortic aneurysm will occur more frequently in the near future.

Thoracic Aneurysm

Between 1951 and 1980, the incidence of thoracic aortic aneurysm was estimated to be 3.5 cases per 100,000 persons per year. Recently, a population-based study of thoracic and thoracoabdominal aortic aneurysm reported an incidence of 10.9 cases per 100,000 persons per year, revealing an increased rate of occurrence of the disorder (79). This phenomenon is not completely explained: The complex multifactorial mechanism, which leads to an alteration of the media and the formation of an aneurysm, is still under investigation. Most aneurysms are atherosclerotic in nature, usually fusiform and long. Saccular false aneurysms may also develop in patients with atherosclerosis as the result of a penetrating ulcer. The natural history is diverse, reflecting a broad spectrum of underlying causes. Although many studies have identified risk factors related to the formation and progression of aortic aneurysms, none has fully explained the cause of the disorder. Atherosclerosis is less commonly found in aneurysm of the ascending aorta than in those of the descending aorta. However, atherosclerosis should be considered a concomitant process and not a direct cause of aneurysm formation and growth. Aortic medial degeneration has been demonstrated in most aneurysms, regardless of their cause and location. The structural integrity of the adventitia is also lost as an aneurysm forms and expands. In the ascending aorta, gradual degenerative changes of the media can be related to congenital disorders of the extracellular matrix associated with an alteration of the elastic fibers, such as Marfan syndrome (Fig. 29.22). Moreover, a genetic predisposition to the development of thoracic and abdominal aneurysms in families, without evidence of collagen-vascular disease, has been documented.

The overall survival of patients with thoracic aortic aneurysms has improved significantly in the past few years. The estimated 5-year risk of rupture of a thoracic aneurysms with a diameter between 4 and 5.9 cm is 16%, but it increases to 31% for aneurysms 6 cm or more. Because the only well-documented risk factor for aortic rupture is increasing size of aneurysm, the major goal in the imaging evaluation of an aortic aneurysm is accurate measurement of its size (66).

Magnetic Resonance Imaging Findings

MRI is effective in identifying and characterizing thoracic and abdominal aortic aneurysms. Standard spin-echo sequences are helpful in evaluating alterations of the aortic wall and periaortic space (Fig. 29.23). Periaortic hematoma and areas of high signal intensity within the thrombus may indicate instability of the aneurysm and are well depicted on spin-echo images. Atherosclerotic lesions are visualized as areas of increased thickness with high signal intensity and irregular profiles. Use of the sagittal plane allows assessment of location and extent of the aneurysm and avoids partial volume effects. With the fat-suppression technique, the outer wall of the aneurysm can be easily distinguished on MR images by the periadventitial fat tissue, so that the aneurysm diameter can be accurately measured. The high level of reproducibility of MRI measurements ensures optimal reliability in monitoring the expansion rate (70). Gadolinium-enhanced T1-weighted MRI and MRA may play an important role in preoperative evaluation. Contrast-enhanced 3D MRA can provide precise topographic information about the

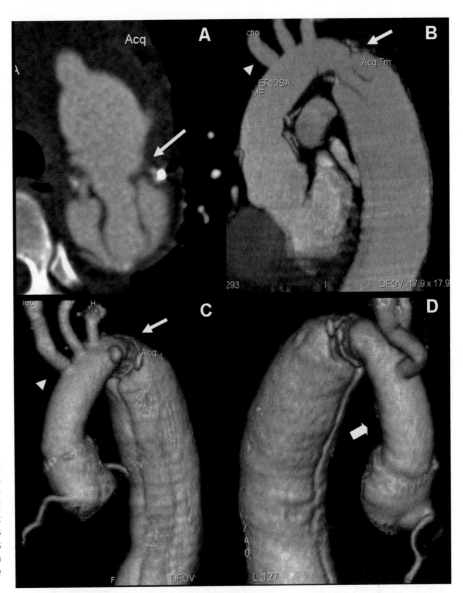

Figure 29.19. MDCT images showing a postoperative evaluation of a type A dissection treated with surgical prosthesis of ascending aorta (Bentall technique) and aortic arch (Elephant Trunk technique). Surgical anastomosis (*arrow*), supraaortic vessel reimplants (*arrowhead*), and prosthetic tube with coronary reimplants (*large arrow*) are well recognized by CT scan.

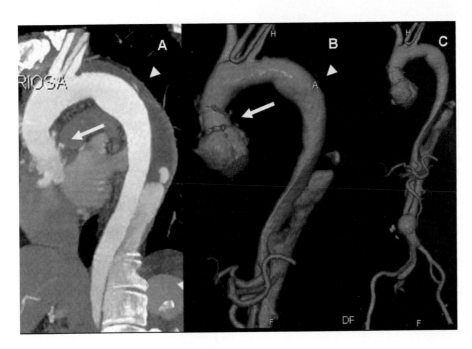

Figure 29.20. MDCT images of a patient who underwent surgery for type A aortic dissection. CT easily detects the prosthetic tube in ascending aorta (*arrows*) and the residual dissection in descending aorta, partially thrombosed (*arrowheads*).

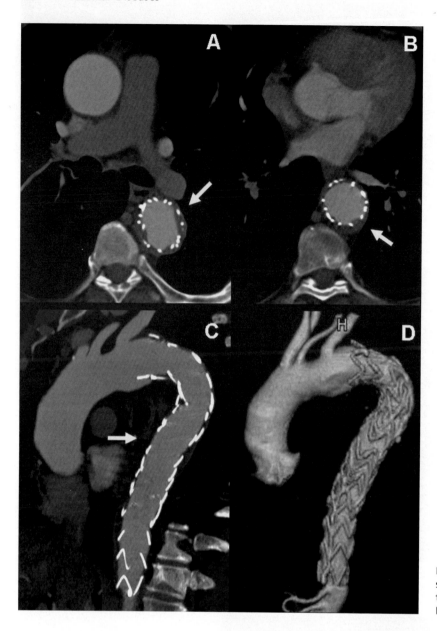

Figure 29.21. Postoperative evaluation after stent-graft apposition (*arrows*) in type B dissection; metallic artifacts are minimized with MDCT scanners.

extent of an aneurysm and its relationship to the aortic branches (Fig. 29.24) (20,80–82). The homogeneous enhancement of flowing blood within the lumen facilitates the delineation of thrombus. Stenosis of the aortic branch arteries can be detected with high rate of sensitivity, and x-ray angiography is not necessary (83,84).

Postoperative neurologic deficit secondary to spinal cord ischemia is a serious and unpredictable complication of surgery performed on the descending aorta. Because selective angiography of the spinal arteries is time consuming, difficult, and potentially hazardous, preoperative evaluation of the Adamkiewicz artery has been uncommon. The capability of contrast MRA to visualize the Adamkiewicz artery reported in the literature represents an important advance in planning the surgical repair of a thoracic aneurysm (85).

Computed Tomography Findings

Helical CT and, better, MDCT can easily detect aneurysms and facilitate surgical planning by delineating the extent of

the aneurysm and the involvement of aortic branches (Fig. 29.25). In 1996 Quint and colleagues (86) found that an analysis of transverse sections and multiplanar reformations was 94% accurate, with a positive predictive value of 95% and a negative predictive value of 93% for successfully predicting the need for hypothermic circulatory arrest. MDCT with enhanced resolution, image quality, and features could now be close to 100% accuracy.

Because of the tortuosity and curvature of the thoracic aorta, aneurysm sizing is performed most accurately when double-oblique tomograms are generated perpendicular to the aortic flow lumen. To date, information concerning the risk of aneurysm rupture and expansion rate is based on measurements made from transverse sections, where true diameters can be overestimated.

Until analysis tools are available to automatically identify the center of the flow channel, create true perpendicular tomograms, and compute accurate cross-sectional areas and mean diameters, the creation of true vessel cross sections is probably not practical for routine applications unless sizing

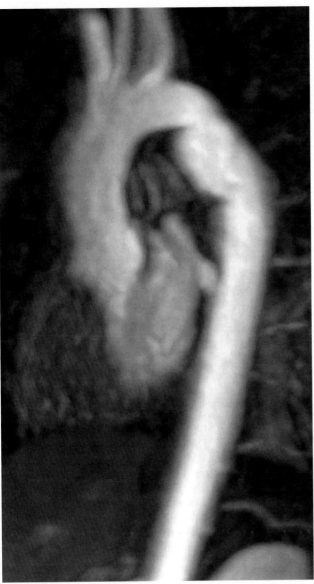

Figure 29.29. MRA of traumatic aortic lesion. The relationship with arch vessels is well depicted.

of pseudoaneurysm formation at the site of arterial puncture. Moreover, MRI can be useful in evaluating the response to medical treatment by depicting decreases in wall thickness of the involved arteries. In patients who undergo surgery for aortitis, recurrence of the inflammatory process is frequently reported that caused dehiscence of the sutures. A strict, lifelong follow-up is therefore mandatory in patients with aortitis, both before and after surgery.

Computed Tomography Findings

CT is an effective technique for depicting aortic infections and infected aneurysm, but an early diagnosis of infectious aortitis before luminal dilatation remains difficult because CT features overlap with retroperitoneal fibrosis, hemorrhage, and lymphadenopathy.

The CT appearance of abdominal aortic infection has been described by different authors in the past years (103–108). It consists of an irregular calcified aortic wall, periaortic density representing inflammation and/or hematoma, and adjacent gas collection, mostly in the presence of dilated aortic lumen. Aneurysms result from weakening or disruption of the aortic wall by an infectious process; therefore they represent pseudoaneurysm, usually saccular (109). Associated osteomyelitis, enlarged lymph nodes, and renal infarctions have also been reported (105–108). Early stages of aortic wall infection are rarely observed (106–108) as periaortic soft tissue densities with rim enhancement in predominant anterior and left lateral distributions, sparing the retroaortic region (inflammation). In some cases distributions could be circumferential and the rim could be hypodense and without contrast enhancement, located between the periaortic mass and aortic mural calcification (edema or necrosis) (110).

Subtle changes of the aortic wall during the early phase of aortitis can be detected on spiral CT with contrast enhancement of the inflamed segments. However, the high density of contrast medium inside the vessel lumen may cause artifacts in the adjacent aortic wall, so that these images may be unsuitable for detecting early mural changes. In conclusion, the CT finding of hazy periaortic density with gas adjacent to the aortic wall should suggest the presence of acute bacterial aortitis. This appearance may herald im-

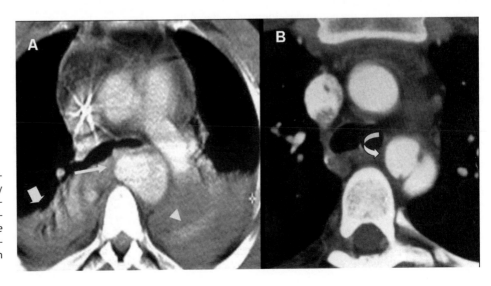

Figure 29.30. CT images of traumatic lesions. **(A)** Aortic injury (*arrow*) with periaortic hemorrhage (*arrowhead*), pleural effusion, and lung contusion (*large arrow*). **(B)** Posttraumatic pseudoaneurysm of the isthmic region (*curved arrow*).

TABLE 29-4	Presley Trauma Center Computed Tomography Grading System: Grades and Computed Tomography Findings	

Grade	Subgrade	CT Findings
Grade I Normal Aorta	**Ia**	Normal thoracic aorta No mediastinal hematoma
	Ib	Normal thoracic aorta Mediastinal hematoma (para-aortic)
Grade II Minimal Aortic Injury	IIa	Small (<1 cm) pseudoaneurysm Indeterminate <1 cm intimal flap or thrombus No mediastinal hematoma
	IIb	Small (usually <1 cm) pseudoaneurysm Indeterminate <1 cm intimal flap or thrombus Mediastinal hematoma (para-aortic)
Grade III Confined Thoracic Aortic Injury	IIIa	>1 cm regular, well-defined pseudoaneurysm Intimal flap or thrombus No ascending aorta, arch, or great vessel involvement Mediastinal hematoma
	IIIb	>1 cm regular, well-defined pseudoaneurysm Intimal flap or thrombus Ascending aorta, arch, or great vessel involvement Mediastinal hematoma
Grade IV Total Aortic Disruption	IV	Irregular, poorly defined pseudoaneurysm Intimal flap or thrombus Mediastinal hematoma

CT, computed tomography. (Modified from Gavant ML. Helical CT grading of traumatic aortic injuries. Impact on clinical guidelines for medical and surgical management. *Radiol Clin North Am* 1999;37(3):553–574, vi, with permission.)

pending rupture of the aorta, even in the absence of aneurysmal dilatation (110,111).

CONGENITAL AORTIC DISEASES

AORTIC ARCH ANOMALIES

During fetal life six pairs of aortic arches form to join the two dorsal aortae with the aortic sac that will become the ascending aorta. At the end of development, some of the arches disappear, and the third, fourth, and sixth aortic arches give rise to the adult vascular structures. Aortic arch anomalies result from either abnormal regression of an embryonic arch that normally remains patent or persistent patency of a structure that normally regresses (Table 29.5) (112).

Aberrant right subclavian artery, the most common type of vascular anomaly, affects 0.5% of the population. The reported prevalence ranges from 0.4% to 2%, with the condition occurring in approximately 1 in 200 births. The right subclavian artery arises from the left embryonic aortic arch. At the end development an aberrant right subclavian artery originates in the proximal portion of the descending aorta and passes posterior to the esophagus to form an incomplete vascular ring. The right subclavian artery may arise from an outpouching known as diverticulum of Kommerell, which represents persistence of the most distal portion of the embryonic right arch. Usually, an aberrant right subclavian ar-

tery does not cause any symptom and is an incidental finding on MRI or CT of the chest. Sometimes, with aging, the right subclavian artery becomes tortuous and ectatic and may cause an esophagus indentation or obstruction (113).

A right aortic arch passes to the right of the trachea and may descend either to the right or to the left of the thoracic

TABLE 29-5	Anomalies of the Aortic Arch Complex

Anomalies of Course or Composition of the Aorta

  A. Double aortic arch
  B. Aberrant right subclavian artery
  C. Aberrant innominate or left common carotid arteries with or without trachea compression
  D. Subclavian steal
  E. Ductus arteriosum sling
  F. Circumflex retroesophageal aortic arch
  G. Right aortic arch with or without retroesophageal component

Anomalies of Length, Size or Continuity of the Aorta

  A. Cervical aorta
  B. Pseudocoarctation of the aorta
  C. Hypoplasia of the aorta
  D. Complete interruption of the aortic arch

spine. It occurs in approximately 0.1% of adults. Two types of right aortic arch are described: right aortic arch with mirror image brachiocephalic branching and right aortic arch with aberrant left subclavian artery. The origin of the aberrant left subclavian artery may have a focal enlargement. Both types are frequently associated with other congenital cardiac anomalies. Usually, a right aortic arch with left subclavian artery does not in itself cause any symptoms. However, if the ligamentum arteriosum is on the left side, a vascular ring is formed by the right aortic arch, anterior left common carotid artery, ligamentum arteriosum, and retroesophageal left subclavian artery.

Double aortic arch is characterized by the presence of both a left and right aortic arch; these arise from a branching of the ascending aorta, pass on both sides of the trachea and esophagus, and join posteriorly to form the descending aorta, which may lie to the right or left of the vertebral column. The luminal size of the two arches in relation to each other varies considerably, and one of them, usually the left, may be partially or completely atretic. The double aortic arch is a vascular ring that can produce severe symptoms if it compresses the trachea and esophagus.

Cervical arch is a rare anomaly in which the aortic arch extends into the soft tissues of the neck before turning down on itself, forming the descending aorta. The anomalous high position of the aortic arch may sometimes produce symptoms related to tracheal compression, such as stridor or dyspnea. The presence of pulsatile neck mass is the most characteristic finding.

Magnetic Resonance Imaging Findings

MRI is particularly valuable in detecting aortic arch anomalies because of its ability to image multiple projections with a large field of view. When an aortic arch anomaly is suspected, a systematic approach should be used to examine the anatomic structures in each subsequent slice. Spin-echo images in the axial plane can detect the abnormal vessel and its relationship with the esophagus and trachea (Fig. 29.31). Additional information can be derived from the coronal and sagittal planes and thin-slice thickness to demonstrate the origin of the aberrant vessels. Kersting-Sommerhoff et al (114) demonstrated the ability of spin-echo MRI to detect aortic arch anomalies in 16 patients. At present, contrast-enhanced MRA is the method of choice to assess aortic arch anomalies because it can provide an accurate overview of the aortic arch and associated vascular malformation noninvasively in a 3D format (Fig. 29.32) (115,116). Postprocessing by MIP and surface rendering provides a 3D impression that can be useful in understanding the abnormal mediastinal anatomy, which is particularly helpful in planning an optimal surgical approach. The combination of MRA and spin-echo MRI is more effective than catheter angiography in preoperative evaluation because MRI can display the abnormal aortic arch and arch vessels along with any compression of the mediastinal structures.

AORTIC COARCTATION

Coarctation is a common congenital anomaly in which an abnormal plication of the tunica media of the posterior aortic

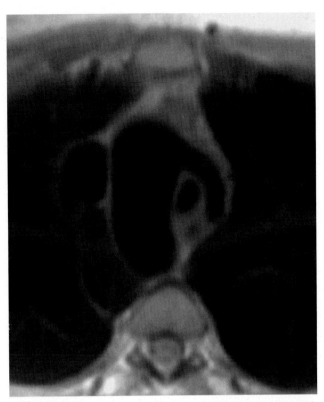

Figure 29.31. Spin-echo axial image of right aortic arch with aberrant left subclavian artery joining the trachea and esophagus.

wall proximal to the ligamentum arteriosum causes a fibrous ridge to form that protrudes into the aorta and causes an obstructive lesion. The stenotic segment can be focal (aortic coarctation), diffuse (hypoplastic aortic isthmus), or complete (aortic arch interruption).

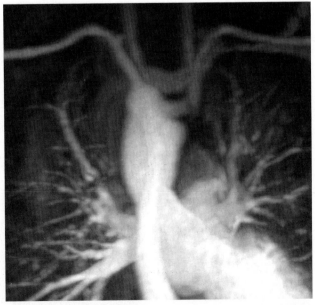

Figure 29.32. MRA of right aortic arch: The aberrant left subclavian artery arises from the right arch.

Magnetic Resonance Imaging Findings

Spin-echo sagittal images show the morphologic features of the coarctation. An anatomic display of the extent and severity of the stenotic segment is the first important step in the diagnosis and quantification of the disease. Aortic coarctation is easier to identify on the sagittal plane; on axial images, partial volume effects may lead to an underestimation of the severity of coarctation. The aortic arch and arch vessels are also well depicted on the sagittal plane. By the measurement of aortic diameter at the isthmus and above the diaphragm, morphologic indexes of the coarctation can be determined. The severity of the stenosis is expressed as the ratio of diameter or cross-sectional area at the isthmus to the same parameters measured in the abdominal aorta. However, although the detection of anatomic narrowing of the aorta establishes the diagnosis of coarctation, an assessment of its clinical significance depends on determining its hemodynamic effects. Cine MRI has been applied to evaluate flow turbulence across the coarctation; the severity of coarctation is quantified on the basis of the length of flow void. Further functional information can be provided by MR flow mapping, which can define the severity of the stenosis by measuring velocity jets at the level of coarctation. Moreover, flow mapping is able to quantify the flow pattern and volume of collateral flow in the descending aorta (117). The volume of collateral flow is another important parameter of the severity of coarctation, and this information may be crucial in the choice of surgical strategy. 3D MRA can display the extent and severity of the coarctation without partial volume errors and spin dephasing artifacts (Fig. 29.33). Collateral vessels, which indicate the severity of hemodynamic effects of the anatomic coarctation, are also displayed, and this information is also important in planning surgical repair.

Postoperative Findings

Several therapeutic strategies are available for the treatment of aortic coarctation, depending on the morphology of the

aortic arch and coarctation, and the age and clinical condition of the patient. Surgery for aortic coarctation is recommended at an early age because long-term results seem to be better. Recently, interventional procedures and balloon angioplasty have come into wide use and provide good results especially in mild or moderate cases. An accurate selection of favorable anatomy by high-resolution imaging modalities is particularly important in interventional procedure to ensure a low rate of complications and restenosis (118).

Residual coarctation and aortic arch hypoplasia may be responsible for postoperative hypertension, more frequently associated with surgical techniques such as coarctation resection with end-to-end anastomosis. An increased risk for aneurysm formation at the site of repair has been reported after both synthetic patch aortoplasty and subclavian-flap arterioplasty. Moreover, restenosis, aortic dissection, and pseudoaneurysms have been reported after balloon angioplasty. Therefore, careful follow-up is recommended for patients who have undergone repair of an aortic coarctation, independent of surgical technique used and timing of the repair (119). Echocardiography is widely applied in the postoperative evaluation of aortic coarctation repair. With color Doppler, it can provide useful data on the gradient across the coarctation, which identifies restenosis. However, evaluation of aortic arch anatomy can often be made difficult by limited acoustic windows, especially in adults. MRI has long been used in the follow-up of repaired aortic coarctation; it provides an optimal depiction of the thoracic aorta with multiplanar standard spin-echo sequences. Additional diagnostic information can be obtained with contrast-enhanced MRA. MRA better visualizes the aortic arch and proximal portion of the descending aorta, which may have a tortuous or kinked course. Postoperative complications, such as recoarctation, Dacron patch aneurysm (Fig. 29.34), and anastomotic pseudoaneurysm are well displayed by postprocessing methods (120). Because postoperative complications may not produce any symptoms, MRA of aortic coarctation after surgical repair should be recommended routinely.

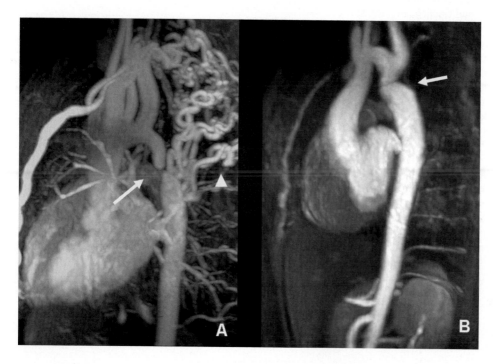

Figure 29.33. MRA of aortic coarctation: focal stenotic segment at the isthmic zone below a large left subclavian artery **(A,B).** Where the stenosis is more severe **(A)**, it is possible to see many collateral vessels (*arrowhead*).

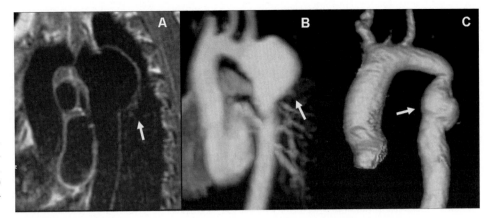

Figure 29.34. Patients underwent surgery for aortic coarctation. Spin-echo sagittal image **(A)**, MRA MIP **(B)**, and 3D MRA **(C)** showing a large Dacron patch aneurysm.

AORTIC PSEUDOCOARCTATION

Pseudocoarctation is a rare anomaly of the thoracic aorta that occurs when the third to seventh embryonic dorsal segments fail to fuse properly to form the aortic arch. It results in elongation of the aortic arch and the first portion of the descending aorta, fixed by the ligamentum arteriosum, so that an abnormal kinking develops. Despite the abnormal tortuosity and morphologic aspects, similar to those of aortic coarctation, no significant gradient develops through the kinking. It is usually asymptomatic, but hypertension may occasionally be present. With aging, turbulent flow can cause progressive dilation of the pseudocoarctation, and aortic dissection is frequently reported.

MRI is able to identify pseudocoarctation and is particularly useful in differentiating it from true coarctation. On spin-echo images, the abnormal kinking may be visualized in the axial and sagittal plane. The morphology of the aortic tortuosity is similar to that of coarctation, but no fibrous ridge is present. The elongated and high position of the aortic arch, the absence of collateral vessels on MRA, and the absence of significant stenosis on reformatted images in the axial and sagittal planes are characteristic features diagnostic of pseudocoarctation.

ANEURYSM OF THE VALSALVA SINUS

Aneurysm of the Valsalva sinus is a rare congenital anomaly of the structural layers of the aortic wall characterized by the absence of the medial layer. This abnormality is usually limited to one of the Valsalva sinuses, most frequently the right coronary Valsalva sinus. Because of the absence of the elastic components of the medial layer, the Valsalva sinus is asymmetrically dilated even in the neonatal age. Aneurysm of the Valsalva sinus does not produce any symptoms, and a high incidence of aortic rupture has been reported in young patients in whom the disease was not suspected. In a neonate with severely dilated Valsalva sinuses, the differential diagnosis should include the neonatal variant of Marfan syndrome. The aortic abnormality is visible on spin-echo MR images and MR angiograms (121). The abnormal dilation of the aortic sinuses is typically asymmetric, whereas in Marfan syndrome the dilation involves the aortic root uniformly. Rupture of sinus aneurysm is usually into the right atrium; it creates a left-to-right shunt, which can be visualized by gradient-echo sequences. Criteria for surgical timing in unruptured aneurysms have not been developed. Regardless of the absolute size of an aneurysm, progressive enlargement on serial studies may constitute indication for surgical repair.

COMPUTED TOMOGRAPHY STUDY OF CONGENITAL AORTIC DISEASE

Before the advent of faster scanners, CT study of congenital aortic disease was unfeasible because of low image quality and scanning planes (thick collimations and just transaxial plane), radiation dose, and iodinated contrast material. With helical CT or MDCT, it is possible to avoid image quality and scanning plane problems, to use a lower quantity of contrast agent, and to use technical improvements or tricks to reduce radiation dose.

CT scan is not as frequently used in pediatric patients as in adults because of the good reliability of echocardiography and MRI techniques in pediatric patients, but with the great anatomic detail of MDCT two-dimensional and 3D reconstruction, CT studies are improving.

In the literature, CT angiographic evaluations were performed in cases of aortic arch anomalies and coarctation, pulmonary artery anomalies, venous anomalies, and complex heart disease with success (122,123). CT has the advantages of easy availability and very short scanning times. It is also possible to set the lowest diagnostic tube current according to the patient's weight and age; in addition, doubling the pitch reduces radiation dose by half (123). Sedation times are significantly shorter than those required for MRI (2–10 minutes vs. 30–45 minutes), and it is possible to use nonionic contrast material with medium iodine concentration (200–300 mgI/mL) administered at a dose of 2 mL/kg, which is better with the bolus tracking technique for contrast peak optimization (122). The decision to image with CT versus MRI should be based on the availability (equipment and scheduling), patient's ability to cooperate (children), and clinical goal.

REFERENCES

1. Van Hoe LS, Baert AL, Gryspeerdt S, et al. Supra and juxta-renal aneurysms of the abdominal aorta: preoperative assess-

ment with thin-section spiral CT. *Radiology* 1996;198(2): 443–448.

2. Kaatee R, Van Leeuwen MS, De Lange EE, et al. Spiral CT angiography of the renal arteries: should a scan delay based on a test bolus injection or a fixed scan delay be used to obtain maximum enhancement of the vessels? *J Comput Assist Tomogr* 1998;22(4):541–547.

3. Armerding MD, Rubin GD, Beaulieu CF, et al. Aortic aneurysmal disease: assessment of stent-graft treatment-CT versus conventional angiography. *Radiology* 2000;215(1):138–146.

4. Katz DS, Jorgensen MJ, Rubin GD. Detection and follow-up of important extra-arterial lesions with helical CT angiography. *Clin Radiol* 1999;54(5):294–300.

5. Rubin GD, Shiau MC, Leung AN, et al. Aorta and iliac arteries: single versus multiple detector-row helical CT angiography. *Radiology* 2000;215(3):670–676.

6. Rubin GD. MDCT imaging of the aorta and peripheral vessels. *Eur J Radiol* 2003;45(Suppl 1):S42–S49.

7. Lawler LP, Fishman EK. Multi-detector row CT of thoracic disease with emphasis on 3D volume rendering and CT angiography. *Radiographics* 2001;21(5):1257–1273.

8. Lawler LP, Fishman EK. Multidetector row computed tomography of the aorta and peripheral arteries. *Cardiol Clin* 2003; 21(4):607–629.

9. Wintersperger BJ, Nikolaou K, Becker CR. Multidetector-row CT angiography of the aorta and visceral arteries. *Semin Ultrasound CT MR* 2004;25(1):25–40.

10. Wintersperger BJ, Herzog P, Jakobs T, et al. Initial experience with the clinical use of a 16 detector row CT system. *Crit Rev Comput Tomogr* 2002;43(4):283–316.

11. Coady MA, Rizzo JA, Goldstein LJ, et al. Natural history, pathogenesis and etiology of thoracic aneurysms and dissection. *Card Clin North Am* 1999;17(4):615–633.

12. Bansal RC, Krishnaswamy C, Ayala K, et al. Frequency and explanation of false negative diagnosis of aortic dissection by aortography and transesophageal echocardiography. *J Am Coll Cardiol* 1995;25:1393–1401.

13. Spittel PC, Spittel JA, Joyce W, et al. Clinical features and differential diagnosis of aortic dissection: experience with 236 cases (1980 trough 1990). *Mayo Clin Proc* 1993;68: 642–651.

14. Cigarroa JE, Isselbacher EM, De Sanctis RW, et al. Diagnostic imaging in the evaluation of suspected aortic dissection. Old standard and new direction. *N Engl J Med* 1993;328: 35–43.

15. Nienaber CA, Fattori R, Lund G, et al. Nonsurgical reconstruction of thoracic aortic dissection by stent-graft placement. *New Engl J Med* 1999;140:1338–1345.

16. Dake MD, Kato N, Mitchell RS, et al. Endovascular stent-graft placement for the treatment of acute aortic dissection. *N Engl J Med* 1999;140:1546–1552.

17. Nitatori T, Yokoyama K, Hachiya J, et al. Fast dynamic MRI of aortic dissection: flow assessment by subsecondal imaging. *Radiat Med* 1999;17(1):9–14.

18. Chang JM, Friese K, Caputo GR, et al. MR measurement of blood flow in the true and false channel in chronic aortic dissection. *J Comput Assist Tomogr* 1991;15:418–423.

19. Bogaert J, Meyns B, Rademakers FE, et al. Follow-up of aortic dissection: contribution of MR angiography for evaluation of the abdominal aorta and its branches. *Eur Radiol* 1997; 7:695–702.

20. Krinsky G, Rofsky N, De Corato DR, et al. Thoracic aorta: comparison of Gadolinium-enhanced three dimensional MR angiography with conventional MR imaging. *Radiology* 1997;202:183–193.

21. Nienaber CA, von Kodolitsch Y, Nikolas V, et al. The diagnosis of thoracic aortic dissection by noninvasive imaging procedures. *N Engl J Med* 1993;328:1–9.

22. Sommer T, Fehske W, Holzknecht, et al. Aortic dissection: a comparative study of diagnosis with spiral CT, multiplanar transesophageal echocardiography and MR imaging. *Radiology* 1996;199:347–352.

23. Fisher U, Vossherich R, Kopka L, et al. Dissection of the thoracic aorta: pre- and postoperative findings of turbo-FLASH MR images in the plane of the aortic arch. *AJR Am J Roentgenol* 1994;163:1069–1072.

24. Moore AG, Eagle KA, Bruckman D, et al. Choice of computed tomography, transesophageal echocardiography, magnetic resonance imaging, and aortography in acute aortic dissection: International Registry of Acute Aortic Dissection (IRAD). *Am J Cardiol* 2002;89(10):1235–1238.

25. Erbel R, Engberding R, Daniel W, et al. Echocardiography in diagnosis of aortic dissection. *Lancet* 1989;1(8636):457–461.

26. Clague J, Magee P, Mills P. Diagnostic techniques in suspected thoracic aortic dissection. *Br Heart J* 1992;67(6): 428–429.

27. Barbant SD, Eisenberg MJ, Schiller NB. The diagnostic value of imaging techniques for aortic dissection. *Am Heart J* 1992; 124(2):541–543.

28. Small JH, Dixon AK, Coulden RA, et al. Fast CT for aortic dissection *Br J Radiol* 1996;69(826):900–905.

29. Chung JW, Park JH, Im JG, et al. Spiral CT angiography of the thoracic aorta radiographics. *Radiographics* 1996;16(4): 811–824.

30. Sebastia C, Pallisa E, Quiroga S, et al. Aortic dissection: diagnosis and follow-up with helical CT. *Radiographics* 1999;19(1):45–60.

31. Fisher RG, Chasen MH, Lamki N. Diagnosis of injuries of the aorta and brachiocephalic arteries caused by blunt chest trauma: CT vs aortography. *AJR Am J Roentgenol* 1994; 162(5):1047–1052.

32. Lee DY, Williams DM, Abrams GD. The dissected aorta: part II. Differentiation of the true from the false lumen with intravascular US. *Radiology* 1997;203(1):32–36.

33. Williams MP, Farrow R. Atypical patterns in the CT diagnosis of aortic dissection. *Clin Radiol* 1994;49(10):686–689.

34. LePage MA, Quint LE, Sonnad SS, et al. Aortic dissection: CT features that distinguish true lumen from false lumen. *AJR Am J Roentgenol* 2001;177(1):207–11.

35. Nelsen KM, Spizarny DL, Kastan DJ. Intimointimal intussusception in aortic dissection: CT diagnosis. *AJR Am J Roentgenol* 1994;162(4):813–814.

36. Karabulut N, Goodman LR, Olinger GN. CT diagnosis of an unusual aortic dissection with intimointimal intussusception: the wind sock sign. *Comput Assist Tomogr* 1998;22(5): 692–693.

37. Rubin GD. Helical CT angiography of the thoracic aorta. *J Thorac Imaging* 1997;12(2):128–149.

38. Batra P, Bigoni B, Manning J, et al. Pitfalls in the diagnosis of thoracic aortic dissection at CT angiography. *Radiographics* 2000;20(2):309–320.

39. Krukemberg E. Beiträge zur Frage des Aneurysma dissecans. *Beitr Pathol Anat Allg Pathol* 1920;67:329–351.

40. Fattori R, Bertaccini P, Celletti F, et al. Intramural posttraumatic hematoma of the ascending aorta in a patient with a double aortic arch. *Eur Radiol* 1997;7:51–53.

41. Nienaber CA, von Kodolitsch Y, Petersen B, et al. Intramural hemorrhage of the thoracic aorta. Diagnostic and therapeutic implication. *Circulation* 1995;92:1465–1472.

42. Coady MA, Rizzo JA, Elefteriades JA. Pathologic variants of thoracic aortic dissections. Penetrating atherosclerotic ul-

cers and intramural hematomas. *Cardiol Clin* 1999;17(4): 637–657.

43. Yamada T, Takamiya M, Naito H, et al. Diagnosis of aortic dissection without intimal rupture by X-ray computed tomography. *Nippon Igaku Hoshasen Gakkai Zasshi* 1985;45(5): 699–710.

44. Keren A, Kim CB, Hu BS, et al. Accuracy of multiplane transesophageal echocardiography in diagnosis of typical acute aortic dissection and intramural hematoma. *J Am Coll Cardiol* 1996;28:627–636.

45. Moore A, Oh J, Bruckman D, et al. Transesophageal echocardiography in the diagnosis and management of aortic dissection. An analysis of data from the International Registry of Aortic Dissection (IRAD). *J Am Coll Cardiol* 1999;33–2(A): 470A.

46. Murray JG, Manisali M, Flamm SD, et al. Intramural hematoma of the thoracic aorta: MR imaging findings and their prognostic implications. *Radiology* 1997:204:349–355.

47. Quint LE, Williams DM, Francis IR, et al. Ulcerlike lesions of the aorta: imaging features and natural history. *Radiology* 2001;218(3):719–23.

48. Kazerooni EA, Bree RL, Williams DM. Penetrating atherosclerotic ulcers of the descending thoracic aorta: evaluation with CT and distinction from aortic dissection. *Radiology* 1992;183(3):759–765.

49. Sueyoshi E, Matsuoka Y, Imada T, et al. New development of an ulcerlike projection in aortic intramural hematoma: CT evaluation. *Radiology* 2002;224(2):536–541.

50. Castaner E, Andreu M, Gallardo X, et al. CT in nontraumatic acute thoracic aortic disease: typical and atypical features and complications. *Radiographics* 2003;23 Spec No:S93–110.

51. Ledbetter S, Stuk JL, Kaufman JA. Helical (spiral) CT in the evaluation of emergent thoracic aortic syndromes. Traumatic aortic rupture, aortic aneurysm, aortic dissection, intramural hematoma, and penetrating atherosclerotic ulcer. *Radiol Clin North Am* 1999;37(3):575–589.

52. Ide K, Uchida H, Otsuji H, et al. Acute aortic dissection with intramural hematoma: possibility of transition to classic dissection or aneurysm. *J Thorac Imaging* 1996;11(1):46–52.

53. Kaji S, Nishigami K, Akasaka T, et al. Prediction of progression or regression of type A aortic intramural hematoma by computed tomography. *Circulation* 1999;100(19 Suppl): II281–286.

54. Choi SH, Choi SJ, Kim JH, et al. Useful CT findings for predicting the progression of aortic intramural hematoma to overt aortic dissection. *J Comput Assist Tomogr* 2001;25(2): 295–299.

55. Sueyoshi E, Matsuoka Y, Sakamoto I, et al. Fate of intramural hematoma of the aorta: CT evaluation. *J Comput Assist Tomogr* 1997;21(6):931–938.

56. Shennan T. Dissecting aneurisms. Medical Research Council Special Report series no. 193:1934.

57. Movsowitz HD, Lampert C, Jacobs LE, et al. Penetrating atherosclerotic aortic ulcers. *Am Heart J* 1994;128:1210–1217.

58. Hayashi H, Matsuoka Y, Sakamoto I, et al. Penetrating atherosclerotic ulcer of the aorta: imaging features and disease concept. *Radiographics* 2000;20(4):995–1005.

59. Yucel EK, Steinberg FL, Egglin TK, et al. Penetrating atherosclerotic ulcers: diagnosis with MR imaging. *Radiology* 1990; 177:779–781.

60. Welch TJ, Stanson AW, Sheedy PF 2nd, et al. Radiologic evaluation of penetrating aortic atherosclerotic ulcer. *Radiographics* 1990;10(4):675–685.

61. Sawhney NS, DeMaria AN, Blanchard DG. Aortic intramural hematoma: an increasingly recognized and potentially fatal entity. *Chest* 2001;120(4):1340–1346.

62. Chung JW, Park JH, Im JG, et al. Spiral CT angiography of the thoracic aorta. *Radiographics* 1996;16(4):811–824.

63. Fann JI, Smith JA, Miller CD, et al. Surgical management of aortic dissection during a 30 years period. *Circulation* 1995; 92(suppl II):110–121.

64. Svensson LG, Crawford SE. Statistical analyses of operative results. In: *Cardiovascular and vascular disease of the aorta.* Philadelphia: W.B. Saunders Company; 1997:432–455.

65. Heinemann M, Laas J, Karck M, et al. Thoracic aortic aneurysms after acute type A aortic dissection: necessity for follow-up. *Ann Thorac Surg* 1990;49:580–584.

66. Bonser RS, Pagano D, Lewis ME, et al. Clinical and pathoanatomical factors affecting expansion of thoracic aortic aneurysms. *Heart* 2000;84(3):277–283.

67. Fattori R, Bacchi Reggiani ML, Bertaccini P, et al. Evolution of aortic dissection after surgical repair. *Am J Cardiol* 2000; 86(8):868–872.

68. Moore NR, Parry AJ, Trottman-Dickenson B, et al. Fate of the native aorta after repair of acute type A dissection: a magnetic resonance imaging study. *Heart* 1996;75:62–66.

69. Mesana TG, Caus T, Gaubert J, et al. Late complications after prosthetic replacement of the ascending aorta: what did we learn from routine magnetic resonance imaging follow-up? *Eur J Cardiothorac Surg* 2000;18(3):313–320.

70. Kawamoto S, Bluemke DA, Traill TA, et al. Thoracoabdominal aorta in Marfan syndrome: MR imaging findings of progression of vasculopathy after surgical repair. *Radiology* 1997;203:727–732.

71. Gaubert J, Moulin G, Mesana T, et al. Type A dissection of the thoracic aorta. Use of MR imaging for long term follow-up. *Radiology* 1995:363–369.

72. Loubeyre P, Delignette A, Boneloy L, et al. MRI evaluation of the ascending aorta after graft-inclusion surgery: comparison between an ultra-fast contrast-enhanced MR sequence and conventional cine-MRI. *J Magn Reson Imaging* 1996;6: 478–483.

73. Fattori R, Descovich B, Bertaccini P, et al. Composite graft replacement of the ascending aorta: leakage detection with gadolinium-enhanced MR imaging. *Radiology* 1999;212: 573–577.

74. Quint LE, Francis IR, Williams DM, et al. Synthetic interposition grafts of the thoracic aorta: postoperative appearance on serial CT studies. *Radiology* 1999;211(2):317–324.

75. Rydberg J, Kopecky KK, Lalka SG, et al. Stent grafting of abdominal aortic aneurysms: pre-and postoperative evaluation with multislice helical CT. *J Comput Assist Tomogr* 2001;25(4):580–586.

76. Mita T, Arita T, Matsunaga N, et al. Complications of endovascular repair for thoracic and abdominal aortic aneurysm: an imaging spectrum. *Radiographics* 2000;20(5):1263–1278.

77. Sakai T, Dake MD, Semba CP, et al. Descending thoracic aortic aneurysm: thoracic CT findings after endovascular stent-graft placement. *Radiology* 1999;212(1):169–174.

78. Riley P, Rooney S, Bonser R, et al. Imaging the post-operative thoracic aorta: normal anatomy and pitfalls. *Br J Radiol* 2001; 74(888):1150–1158.

79. Clouse WD, Hallett JW, Shaff HV, et al. Improved prognosis of thoracic aortic aneurysm: a population based study. *JAMA* 1998;9:280:1926–1929.

80. Debatin JF, Hany TF. MR-based assessment of vascular morphology and function. *Eur Radiol* 1998;8:528–539.

81. Neimatallah MA, Ho VB, Dong Q, et al. Gadolinium-enhanced 3D magnetic resonance angiography of the thoracic vessels. *J Magn Reson Imaging* 1999;10:758–770.

82. Prince MR, Narasimham DL, Jacoby WT, et al. Three dimensional gadolinium-enhanced MR angiography of the thoracic aorta. *AJR Am J Roentgenol* 1996;166:1387–1397.

83. Weishaupt D, Ruhm SG, Binkert Ca, et al. Equilibrium-phase MR angiography of the aortoiliac and renal arteries using a blood pool contrast agent. *Am J Roentgenol* 2000;175(1): 189–195.

84. Holland AE, Barentsz JO, Skotnicki S, et al. Preoperative MRA assessment of the coronary arteries in an ascending aortic aneurysm. *J Magn Reson Imaging* 2000;11:324–326.

85. Yamada N, Okita Y, Minatoya K, et al. Preoperative demonstration of the Adamkiewicz artery by magnetic resonance angiography in patients with descending or thoracoabdominal aortic aneurysms. *Eur J Cardiothorac Surg* 2000;18(1): 104–111.

86. Quint LE, Francis IR, Williams DM, et al. Evaluation of thoracic aortic disease with the use of helical CT and multiplanar reconstructions: comparison with surgical findings. *Radiology* 1996;201(1):37–41.

87. Bortone AS, De Cillis E, D'Agostino D, et al. Endovascular treatment of thoracic aortic disease: four years of experience. *Circulation* 2004;110(11 Suppl 1):II262–267.

88. Pate JW, Fabian TC, Walker W. Traumatic rupture of the aortic isthmus: an emergency? *World J Surg* 1995;19: 119–126.

89. Mirvis SE, Shanmuganathan K. MR imaging of thoracic trauma. *Magn Reson Imaging Clin N Am* 2000;8(1):91–104.

90. Fattori R, Celletti F, Bertaccini, et al. Delayed surgery of traumatic aortic rupture: role of magnetic resonance imaging. *Circulation* 1996;94:2865–2870.

91. Fattori R, Celletti F, Descovich B, et al. Evolution of post traumatic aneurysm in the subacute phase: magnetic resonance imaging follow-up as a support of the surgical timing. *Eur J Cardiothorac Surg* 1998;13:582–587.

92. Mirvis SE, Kostrubiak I, Whitley NO, et al. Role of CT in excluding major arterial injury after blunt thoracic trauma. *AJR Am J Roentgenol* 1987;149(3):601–605.

93. Mirvis SE, Shanmuganathan K, Miller BH, et al. Traumatic aortic injury: diagnosis with contrast-enhanced thoracic CT—five-year experience at a major trauma center. *Radiology* 1996;200(2):413–422.

94. Scaglione M, Pinto A, Pinto F, et al. Role of contrast-enhanced helical CT in the evaluation of acute thoracic aortic injuries after blunt chest trauma. *Eur Radiol* 2001;11(12): 2444–2448. Epub 2001 Feb 23.

95. Creasy JD, Chiles C, Routh WD, et al. Overview of traumatic injury of the thoracic aorta. *Radiographics* 1997;17(1): 27–45.

96. Marotta R, Franchetto AA. The CT appearance of aortic transection. *AJR Am J Roentgenol* 1996;166(3):647–651.

97. Kuhlman JE, Pozniak MA, Collins J, et al. Radiographic and CT findings of blunt chest trauma: aortic injuries and looking beyond them. *Radiographics* 1998;18(5):1085–1106; discussion 1107–1108.

98. Gavant ML, Menke PG, Fabian T, et al. Blunt traumatic aortic rupture: detection with helical CT of the chest. *Radiology* 1995;197(1):125–133.

99. Gavant ML. Helical CT grading of traumatic aortic injuries. Impact on clinical guidelines for medical and surgical management. *Radiol Clin North Am* 1999;37(3):553–574, vi.

100. Dyer DS, Moore EE, Mestek MF, et al. Can chest CT be used to exclude aortic injury? *Radiology* 1999;213(1):195–202.

101. Choe YH, Kim DK, Koh EM, et al. Takayasu arteritis: diagnosis with MR imaging and MR angiography in acute and chronic active stages. *J Magn Reson Imaging* 1999;10(5): 751–757.

102. Berkmen T. MR Angiography of aneurysms in Beçhet disease: a report of four cases. *J Comput Assist Tomogr* 1998; 22:202–206.

103. Pripstein S, Cavoto FV, Gerritsen RW. Spontaneous mycotic aneurysm of the abdominal aorta. *J Comput Assist Tomogr* 1979;3(5):681–683.

104. Atlas SW, Vogelzang RL, Bressler EL, et al. CT diagnosis of a mycotic aneurysm of the thoracoabdominal aorta. *J Comput Assist Tomogr* 1984;8(6):1211–1212.

105. Vogelzang RL, Sohaey R. Infected aortic aneurysms: CT appearance. *J Comput Assist Tomogr* 1988;12(1):109–112.

106. Gonda RL Jr, Gutierrez OH, Azodo MV. Mycotic aneurysms of the aorta: radiologic features. *Radiology* 1988;168(2): 343–346.

107. Blair RH, Resnik MD, Polga JP. CT appearance of mycotic abdominal aortic aneurysms. *J Comput Assist Tomogr* 1989; 13(1):101–104.

108. Gomes MN, Choyke PL. Infected aortic aneurysms: CT diagnosis. *J Cardiovasc Surg (Torino)* 1992;33(6):684–689.

109. Chan P, Lan CK, Wan YL. Salmonella choleraesuis bacteremia and mycotic aneurysm of abdominal aorta—report of five cases. *Changgeng Yi Xue Za Zhi* 1989;12(2):115–120.

110. Rozenblit A, Marin ML, Veith FJ, et al. Endovascular repair of abdominal aortic aneurysm: value of postoperative follow-up with helical CT. *AJR Am J Roentgenol* 1995;165(6): 1473–1479.

111. Mantello MT, Panaccione JL, Moriarty PE, et al. Impending rupture of nonaneurysmal bacterial aortitis: CT diagnosis. *J Comput Assist Tomogr* 1990;14(6):950–953.

112. Thiene G, Frescura C. Etiology and pathology of aortic arch malformations. In: Nienaber CA, Fattori R, eds. *Diagnosis and treatment of aortic diseases.* Norwell, MA: Kluwer Academic Publisher; 1999:225–269.

113. Bakker DA, Berger RM, Witsenburg M, et al. Vascular rings: a rare cause of common respiratory symptoms. *Acta Paediatr* 1999;88(9):947–952.

114. Kersting-Sommerhoff BA, Sechtem UP, Fisher MR, et al. MR imaging of congenital anomalies of the aortic arch. *AJR Am J Roentgenol* 1987;149(1):9–13.

115. Delabrousse E, Kastler B, Bernard Y, et al. MR diagnosis of a congenital abnormality of the thoracic aorta with an aneurysm of the right subclavian artery presenting as a Horner's syndrome in an adult. *Eur Radiol* 2000;10(4):650–652.

116. Carpenter JP, Holland GA, Golden MA, et al. Magnetic resonance angiography of the aortic arch. *J Vasc Surg* 1997;25: 145–151.

117. Julsrud PR, Breen JF, Felmlee JP, et al. Coarctation of the aorta: collateral flow assessment with phase-contrast MR angiography. *AJR Am J Roentgenol* 1997;169:1735–1742

118. Paddon AJ, Nicholson AA, Ettles DF, et al. Long-term follow-up of percutaneous balloon angioplasty in adult aortic coarctation. *Cardiovasc Intervent Radiol* 2000;23(5): 364–367.

119. Therrien J, Thorne SA, Wright A, et al. Repaired coarctation: a "cost-effective" approach to identify complications in adults. *J Am Coll Cardiol* 2000;15;35(4):997–1002.

120. Bogaert J, Kuzo R, DymorKovski S, et al. Follow-up of patients with previous treatment for coarctation of the thoracic aorta: comparison between contrast enhanced MR angiography and fast spin-echo MR imaging. *Eur Radiol* 2000;10: 1047–1054

121. Baur LH, Vliegen HW, van der Wall EE, et al. Imaging of an aneurysm of the sinus of Valsalva with transesophageal echocardiography, contrast angiography and MRI. *Int J Card Imaging* 2000;16(1):35–41.

122. Gilkeson RC, Ciancibello L, Zahka K. Pictorial essay. Multidetector CT evaluation of congenital heart disease in pediatric and adult patients. *AJR Am J Roentgenol* 2003;180(4): 973–980.

123. Haramati LB, Glickstein JS, Issenberg HJ, et al. MR imaging and CT of vascular anomalies and connections in patients with congenital heart disease: significance in surgical planning. *Radiographics* 2002;22(2):337–347; discussion 348–349.

30

Magnetic Resonance Angiography of Abdominal Aorta and Renal and Mesenteric Vessels

Frank J. Thornton and Thomas M. Grist

Acquired pathology of the abdominal aorta and its visceral branches is ubiquitous and requires accurate evaluation for optimal and appropriate management. The current trend, which favors noninvasive imaging of vascular pathology over the gold standard of conventional angiography, requires a robust and reproducible alternative approach. Magnetic resonance angiography (MRA) represents such a technique, with the abolition of invasive catheterization, nephrotoxic contrast material, and ionizing radiation as real intrinsic advantages. Circumventing the use of iodine-based contrast materials is especially desirable in patients with atherosclerotic disease of the abdominal aorta, as these patients are also likely to have compromised renal function.

Abdominal MRA without and with gadolinium contrast medium has been applied successfully to the assessment of native renal (1–3), transplant renal (4), hepatic, mesenteric (5), and pancreatic vessels as well as portal venous hypertension (6,7) and follow-up of aneurysm size (8) and vasculitides. Contrast-enhanced (CE) MRA is ideal for monitoring the postoperative aorta, particularly for perigraft infection and pseudoaneurysm formation at the anastomoses. Current challenges include its application to endovascular stent follow-up for endoleak detection and follow-up of native aneurysm sac size (9).

Noncontrast MRA techniques, including black-blood, spin-echo, and bright-blood gradient-recalled echo (GRE) sequences have less utility in the abdomen compared to other vascular territories, although phase-contrast flow analysis still has widespread use in assessing the hemodynamic significance of vascular pathology.

An optimal breath-hold is a prerequisite to diagnostic image quality. Where vascular pathology is accompanied by cardiac decompensation, seen most frequently in the pediatric and elderly patient population, breath-holding presents a significant limitation to data acquisition, often resulting in degradation of the image data set from motion artifact. The evolution of magnetic resonance imaging (MRI) hardware and gradient technology, increasingly efficient imaging strategies, and the development of new contrast agents is surmounting this problem and continues to propel abdominal MRA towards new horizons.

This chapter presents practical and current MRA imaging protocols and discusses the most prevalent disease processes in the abdominal aorta, renal arteries, and mesenteric vessels. Frequently encountered problems and pitfalls of interpretation will be considered, and finally, current and prospective advances in abdominal MRA will be addressed.

ABDOMINAL MAGNETIC RESONANCE ANGIOGRAPHY TECHNIQUES

PRESCAN SETUP

Currently, a 1.5 Tesla (T) magnet is used most frequently for diagnostic abdominal MRA. "Open" low-field magnets should be reserved for obese patients unable to fit the regular magnet or for claustrophobic patients. For the latter group, sedation may allow imaging in a high-field magnet, although this must be balanced against the requirement for breath-hold performance.

Patients are imaged supine, with their arms placed above their head or folded across their chest to prevent wrap artifact into the imaged field-of-view (FOV). Oxygen may be administered to optimize breath-hold capacity or the patient can be hyperventilated prior to image acquisition. Coaching

the patient and performing a test breath-hold prior to placing the patient in the scanner can pay dividends, facilitating better patient compliance and tailoring of the sequences to the patient's maximum breath-hold (10).

A surface phased-array coil is employed to maximize signal-to-noise ratio (SNR) and is positioned to cover the required region of interest, usually from the suprarenal abdominal aorta to the external iliac arteries. In obese or tall individuals, the body coil may be used to ensure coverage, although this will compromise SNR. Based upon the patient's weight and the specific indications for the study, a power injector is loaded with double-dose or triple-dose (0.2–0.3 mmol/kg) gadolinium contrast medium and connected to the patient via an antecubital venous cannula (20 or 22 G).

PRECONTRAST IMAGING

Coronal and sagittal localizers are acquired during inspiration using an ungated two-dimensional (2D) true steady-state free precession (SSFP) sequence (Fast Imaging Employing Steady-State Acquisition [FIESTA], GE Healthcare Systems; True Fast Imaging with Steady State Precession [TrueFISP], Siemens Medical Systems, or Balanced Fast-Field Echo [FFE], Philips Medical Systems), which provides intrinsic tissue contrast and bright-blood images that allow easy prescription of the imaged FOV. Alternatively, rapid black-blood localizers can be performed, including single-shot fast-spin echo techniques (SSFSE, HASTE) (Fig. 30.1).

An axial fat-saturated, fast-turbo spin-echo T2 sequence is performed from diaphragm to the iliac crest to help characterize incidentally seen mass lesions and to document renal cysts.

CONTRAST-ENHANCED MAGNETIC RESONANCE ANGIOGRAPHY

All abdominal MRA protocols should include a CE three-dimensional (3D) spoiled GRE MRA sequence. The volume acquisition allows multiplanar reconstructions (MPR) and full or sub-volume maximum intensity projection (MIP) reconstructions in any desired plane. The acquisition of data for aorta and renal vessel imaging is acquired conventionally in the coronal plane and in the sagittal plane for mesenteric vessels. The imaging volume is prescribed from the localizers to include the abdominal aorta from above the celiac artery origin (juxtadiaphragmatic) to the common femoral vessels. Careful attention to the localizer images will help avoid anatomy exclusion artifacts. These can occur where there is vascular tortuosity in the presence of chronic hypertension or advanced atheromatous disease, as well as in the

Figure 30.1. Routine sequences. A collage of source images from a basic contrast-enhanced renal MRA study is shown. **(A)** Coronal localizer using nongated 2D steady-state free procession (SSFP) technique. This provides T2*/T1 weighting, which can be useful in characterizing some of the incidentally noted abdominal findings. **(B)** Axial T2 fast-recovery, fast-spin echo also used to characterize incidentally noted lesions within the abdominal viscera, such as renal cysts and liver nodules. **(C)** Coronal precontrast 3D spoiled gradient-echo acquisition followed by **(D)** an arterial phase, source image depicting the renal artery ostia and the origin of the celiac axis and superior mesenteric artery. The precontrast sequence allows evaluation of signal-to-noise ratio and coverage prior to injection

(continues)

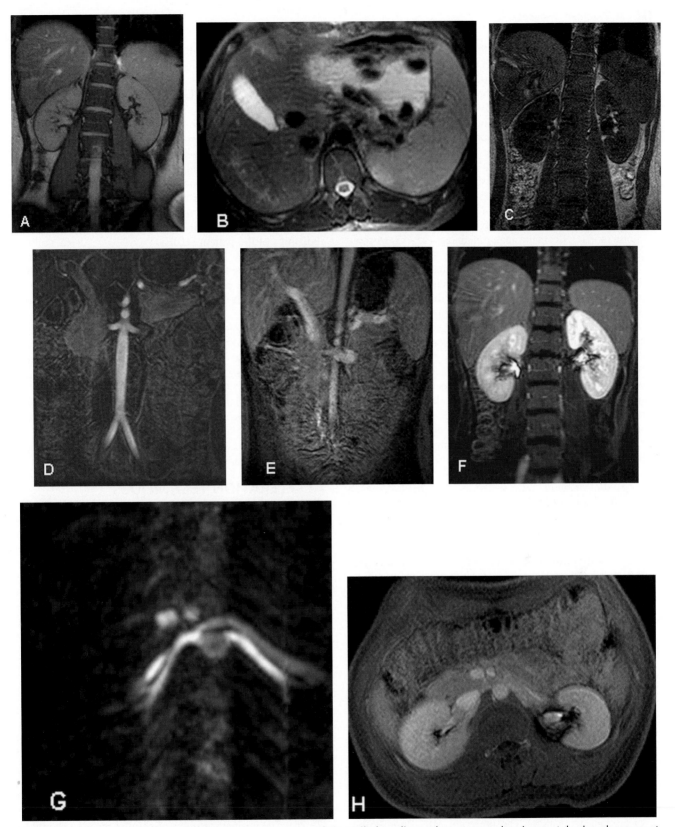

Figure 30.1. *(continued)* of contrast. **(E)**. Venous phase coronal 3D spoiled gradient-echo sequence showing portal vein enhancement and left renal vein enhancement. This acquisition is necessary to depict normal venous drainage from the kidneys and normal enhancement of the inferior vena cava. It can also be useful in the context of intimal dissection to describe the relative enhancement of the true and false lumen. **(F)** Postcontrast 3D volume acquisition designed to maximize signal-to-noise ratio, which allows calculation of renal volumes and is useful in surveying the other abdominal contents. **(G)** Axial postcontrast 3D phase-contrast image. This sequence is useful in evaluating for hemodynamic significance of lesions seen on the contrast-enhanced component of the study. Local dephasing from a hemodynamically significant narrowing will cause signal dropout within the stenosis. **(H)** Represents an axial postcontrast fast-spoiled gradient-echo sequence that allows a survey of the abdominal viscera and other abdominal and pelvic contents for other findings. The parameters used in each of these sequences are described in Table 30.1.

event of accessory renal vessels that may arise as low as the iliac vessels. The presence of extra-anatomic bypass conduits (axillary-femoral or femoral-femoral grafts) may be visible on localizer images but should be known to the technologist prior to imaging. Such complex neoanatomy should have direct radiologist supervision where possible.

An initial precontrast 3D acquisition is performed to assess for coverage, SNR, and the presence of artifact (Fig. 30.1). This also serves as a "mask" for subtraction purposes. Arterial CE MRA requires acquisition of image data during peak arterial phase of contrast passage. This requires close correlation of injection rate and volume with acquisition speed. The injection rate is designed to optimize contrast-to-noise ratio (CNR) in the acquired images (11–13). A fixed injection rate of 2.0–4.0 ml/s is generally used, followed by a flush of 20 ml normal saline to ensure that the full contrast dose is delivered. The low-spatial frequency data acquired during central k-space filling determines the image contrast. Therefore, peak gadolinium concentration within the vessel of interest should coincide with filling of central k-space. In centric or elliptic-centric acquisitions, where central k-space is filled early in the acquisition, a more rapid injection is required. Although less susceptible to artifact from poor breath holding, these sequences require more accurate injection timing. For the same reason, with shorter acquisition strategies and with more sophisticated pulse sequences, substantially lower contrast doses ("single dose," i.e., 20 cc) may be used. When parallel imaging is employed, the injection rate can be increased proportional to the acceleration factor, which helps offset some of the SNR loss experienced with parallel imaging. With sequential k-space strategies, a slower injection is permitted, as central k-space is acquired over a longer time. This is a more forgiving technique when accurate timing is not possible or where a power injector is not available. If image acquisition is begun too early, where T1 shortening is still in rapid flux, severe ringing artifact will be present. In the presence of large abdominal aneurysms or dissections with slow flow, where there is considerable delay in the homogeneous mixing of gadolinium contrast, the elliptic-centric and even centric k-space filling techniques may be detrimental, causing suboptimal evaluation of the lumen and even misdiagnosis in the case of dissection. For this reason, a venous phase-delayed MRA sequence is acquired. This also serves to evaluate venous anatomy and can help characterize incidental findings such as liver hemangiomas.

Timing of contrast injection has evolved from a hand-injection technique with imaging at a fixed or "inspired" delay time to use of a test injection, an automated bolus detection algorithm (SmartPrep, GE Healthcare, Waukesha, WI), or real-time visualization of contrast passage (MR Fluorotrigger, GE Healthcare Systems; CareBolus, Siemens Medical Systems; and Bolus-Track, Philips Medical Systems) that allows more accurate and optimal timing of central k-space data acquisition. The preferred MRI fluoroscopic technique allows the operator to choose when image acquisition should begin by viewing real-time images of the vessel of interest during contrast medium injection (14). When optimal contrast is seen on the rapidly acquired 2D images, the operator triggers ("fluorotriggering") the 3D MRA acquisition. This technique can be compromised by interoperator variability but in general is a dependable method for accurate timing. The operator has discretion over the start of image

acquisition and can vary this depending on the k-space filling strategy being utilized.

ADDITIONAL SEQUENCES

Three-dimensional phase contrast (Tab. 30.1) has clinical application for characterizing renal artery stenosis (RAS) (1,15). This method relies on the velocity-induced signal loss associated with highly turbulent flow near a hemodynamically significant stenosis. For optimal sensitivity to the dephasing effect of turbulence at the stenosis, the echo time should be increased to 8 ms and the velocity encoded value (VENC) should be 25–50 cm/s based on the expected hemodynamics of the patient (10).

A postcontrast fat-suppressed 3D-spoiled gradient-echo sequence is designed to increase SNR and to allow evaluation of the renal parenchyma and calculation of renal volume. Renal masses, cysts, and infarcts are well seen on this sequence.

Cine 2D phase-contrast sequences (Tab. 30.1), cardiac-gated breath-hold sequences, may also be used to determine further functional information used to predict intervention outcome and triage patients to intervention versus medical treatment (10).

As MRI continues to develop, the renal MRA examination will likely expand to include extensive functional information about creatinine clearance, baseline flow, and response to pharmacologic agents, as well as spectroscopy, diffusion, perfusion, and other techniques (16–19)

ACCELERATION TECHNIQUES

Much of the current efforts to optimize MRA strategy relate to improving acquisition speed. When further acceleration is required, as in pediatric patients or respiratory compromised adults, a number of options are available (20–23).

Using a minimum repetition time (TR) (~4 ms) and echo time (TE) (~1 ms) is recommended. Accurate volume prescription with minimum slice number to cover the region of interest may allow some time gain. Simply increasing the bandwidth will reduce scanning time but will decrease SNR. Flip angle is generally set at 20° to 45°. Rectangular FOV is employed to take advantage of the decreased anterior-to-posterior dimensions relative to inferior-to-superior FOV dimensions. Typical sequence parameters are as follows: TR/TE/Flip/BW = 3.8/1.0/30°/62.5. More recently, parallel imaging, with eponyms such as SENSE (Sensitivity Encoding, Philips Medical Systems), iPAT (Integrated Parallel Acquisition Techniques, Siemens Medical Systems), and ASSET (Array Spatial Sensitivity Encoding Technique, GE Medical Systems) (24) has been applied to abdominal MRA. These ultrafast MRI techniques use the unique geometry of phased-array coils to spatially encode the image faster (25,26). The intrinsic artifacts of parallel imaging should be familiar to the radiologist (26). Simultaneous data is acquired in multiple detectors in the form of arrays of radiofrequency coils. As SNR increases with the square root of imaging time, any attempt to increase acquisition speed will adversely influence SNR (Fig. 30.2) (27). The several-fold increase in imaging speed facilitates more rapid injection of contrast medium, which allows recovery of both SNR and higher contrast resolution (28,29). As mentioned previously, aneurysm is an important preoperative diagnosis, as it may cause adhesions between the bowel, particularly duodenum and the aorta as well as encasement of the ureters (Fig. 30.4). These findings can precipitate aortic-enteric fistula formation and urinary tract obstruction and make aneurysm surgery more complicated, with increased morbidity and mortality. MRI is an ideal modality to follow interval change in disease if a nonsurgical approach is employed (43,44).

Takayasu arteritis, a large vessel arteritis, most commonly affects young women.

A new classification of angiographic findings in patients with Takayasu arteritis was proposed at the International Conference on Takayasu Arteritis (Table 30.2) (45). Type V is the most common, and type IV is observed in India and Thailand but is very rare in the United States and Japan.

Inflammation of the aorta from any cause can result in aortic dilation. Also, it can cause fibrous thickening and ostial stenosis of major branches, which in the abdomen can cause mesenteric ischemia (46) or central hypertension due to RAS. Immune disorders known to affect the aorta include serum sickness, cryoglobulinemia, systemic lupus erythema-

TABLE 30-2	Classification of Takayasu Arteritis

Type I involves great vessels.

Type IIa involves the ascending aorta, aortic arch, and its branches.

Type IIb involves the type IIa region plus the thoracic descending aorta.

Type III involves the thoracic descending aorta, abdominal aorta, and/or renal arteries.

Type IV involves only the abdominal aorta and/or renal arteries.

Type V involves the whole aorta and its branches.

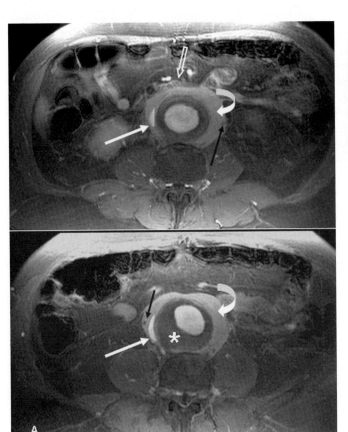
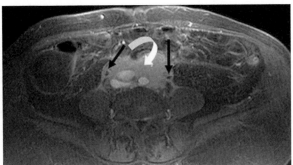
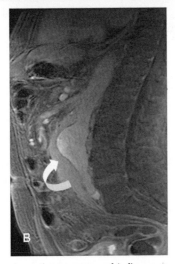

Figure 30.4. Inflammatory aneurysm. Images from two different patient studies show the presence of inflammatory aneurysms in the abdominal aorta. **(A)** Axial postcontrast (fat-suppressed T1 images) at two levels in the infrarenal abdominal aorta show an enhancing rind of inflammatory soft tissue surrounding the aneurysm sac (*curved arrow*). **(B)** Axial postcontrast (fat-suppressed T1 images) image from below the level of the bifurcation (*above*) and a sagittal delayed postcontrast image that outlines the craniocaudal extent of the inflammatory process (*below*). The inflammatory tissue encases both the ureters (**A,B,** *black arrows*) and the inferior vena cava (**A,** *white arrow*). The third part of the duodenum is adherent and incorporated in the inflammatory process (**A,** *open white arrow*). Also demonstrated is a circumferential layer of mural thrombus (**A,** *asterisk*) within the aneurysm sac. These images highlight the importance of an axial postcontrast survey of the abdomen and pelvis to provide these additional points of information to the surgeon. Prior knowledge of this inflammatory process that involves the inferior vena cava, duodenum, and ureters may help to minimize the postoperative morbidity associated with open repair of these aneurysms.

tosus (SLE), rheumatoid arthritis, Henoch-Schönlein purpura, and postinfectious or drug-induced immune complex disease. Also, antineutrophil cytoplasmic autoantibody (ANCA) can affect the large vessels, as in Wegener's granulomatosis, polyangiitis, and Churg-Strauss syndrome. Other antibodies such as antiglomerular basement membrane (i.e., Goodpasture syndrome) and antiendothelial (i.e., Kawasaki disease) also can be culprits.

Within the abdomen, vasculitides primarily involving large vessels include giant cell arteritis and Takayasu arteritis (47). Polyarteritis nodosa and Kawasaki disease involve medium-sized vessels; Wegener granulomatosis, Churg-Strauss syndrome, microscopic polyangiitis, Henoch-Schonlein syndrome, systemic lupus erythematosus, rheumatoid vasculitis, and Behcet syndrome involve small vessels. Radiologic findings often overlap, thus making a specific diagnosis impossible by imaging. Transplant rejection, inflammatory bowel diseases, and paraneoplastic vasculitis can also afflict the large vessels. The advantage of MRA in evaluating the abdominal vessels for these conditions lies in the panoramic vascular assessment provided and the better characterization of wall thickening and enhancement compared with all other modalities. To produce a useful differential diagnosis, the imaging specialist must be able to recognize the type of stenosis and the configuration of collateral circulatory pathways. MRA provides a high resolution detail of vessel wall thickness and lumen configuration (44). It allows the measurement of wall enhancement as a reflection of edema and inflammation (Fig. 30.5). By reduction of enhancement on follow-up, MRA also serves as a surrogate marker for disease activity and can be combined with other modalities, such as positron emission tomography (PET) imaging, to follow activity (43).

PREOPERATIVE MAGNETIC RESONANCE ANGIOGRAPHY OF THE AORTA

The two primary approaches to abdominal aortic aneurysm repair are open laparatomy with transperitoneal or retroperitoneal placement of a synthetic tubular graft or the increasingly more frequent endovascular deployment of a stent graft (EVAR, endovascular aneurysm repair) to exclude the native aneurysm sac (48). Evaluation of the aneurysm sac for open repair requires less precision; however, assessment of the renal and mesenteric vessels is paramount as these may require endarterectomy or reimplantation. Defining the extent of the aneurysm to the bifurcation or into the iliac vessels is also critical in determining whether a bifurcating graft or tubular graft is used. Iliac artery involvement by aneurysmal dilatation has increased risk of morbidity (49).

More recently, the exclusion criteria for EVAR have become less rigid due to improvements in stent design. Preoperative precise definition of the required stent dimensions remains a prerequisite for successful outcome. Using the contrast-enhanced volume acquisition that allows comprehensive MPR and MIP postprocessing, much of the detail extracted from CTA studies, can be obtained equally from MRA imaging. A recent and evolving technique, EVAR requires accurate depiction of the aneurysm anatomy on an individual case basis in order to select a stent graft with

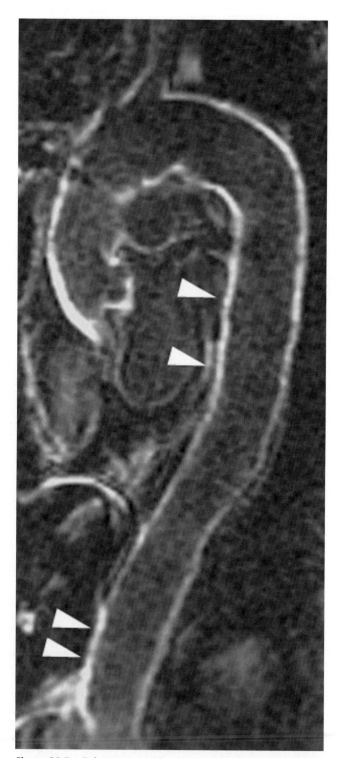

Figure 30.5. Takayasu arteritis: vessel wall enhancement. There is a nonuniform but marked enhancement of the aortic wall (*arrowheads*), both thoracic and abdominal, presumed to reflect active arteritis. A cardiac-gated, inversion-recovery gradient-echo sequence was used with an inversion time (TI) chosen at 120 ms to null blood signal. Imaging was performed 15 minutes after infusion of 0.2 mmol/kg of gadolinium contrast agent. Blood suppression maximizes contrast between vessel wall and background blood and soft tissues. (From Grist TM, Thornton FJ. Magnetic resonance angiography in children: technique, indications, and imaging findings. *Pediatr Radiol* 2005;35:26–39, with permission.)

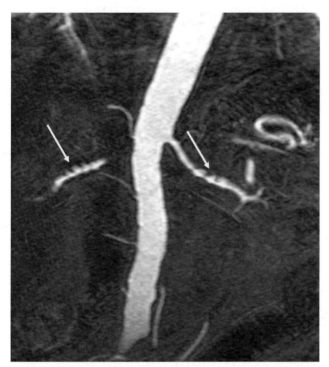

Figure 30.12. Fibromuscular dysplasia. Arterial phase, sub-volume coronal MIP image from a renal MRA study demonstrating luminal irregularity bilaterally in the distal renal arteries (*white arrows*). This "string-of-pearls" appearance is pathognomonic for fibromuscular dysplasia in the renal arteries.

lesions with intervening aneurysmal outpouching, usually seen in the medial form of FMD, whereas a smooth focal stenosis is usually seen in the intimal form of FMD. Micro-aneurysms and dissections are intrinsic complications of FMD and are independent of histological type. The "string-

of-pearls" appearance is typically seen in the middle to distal portion of the artery (Fig. 30.13).

Renovascular disease affects women more than men, with patients typically between 15 and 50 years of age. Overall, FMD accounts for less than 10% of cases of renal vascular hypertension and can be difficult to diagnosis by MRA. This is most true when the pathology involves the distal renal and segmental branches, where motion artifact that simulates FMD is frequently encountered, even in the presence of normal vessels. If there is a strong clinical suspicion for FMD, it may be appropriate to evaluate initially with conventional angiography. Although evaluation of postprocessed MIP and curved linear reformat images is useful, use of source images is essential to evaluate optimally. In patients with poor ability to breath-hold, the use of parallel imaging with an increased injection rate may help to minimize motion artifact.

GRADING OF RENAL ARTERY STENOSIS

Standardized descriptions of RAS include a description of the location in the renal artery. Ostial stenoses lie within 5 mm of the vessel origin (Fig. 30.14), while nonostial lesions have a leading edge more than 5 mm from the vessel origin. Branch stenoses lie within the subdivisions of the main renal artery (70).

Stenosis determination is made by measuring the ratio between the diameter of the narrowest segment of the imaged renal artery and the diameter of a normal or reference segment of the artery proximal to the stenosis or distal to any poststenotic dilation (71). A combined morphologic and functional MR examination significantly reduces interobserver variability, an acknowledged "Achilles heel" of 3D contrast-enhanced renal MRA when evaluated alone (Fig. 30.15). Combined interpretation offers more reliable and reproducible grading of RAS based on both stenosis morphology and hemodynamic effect (Table 30.4) (1,72).

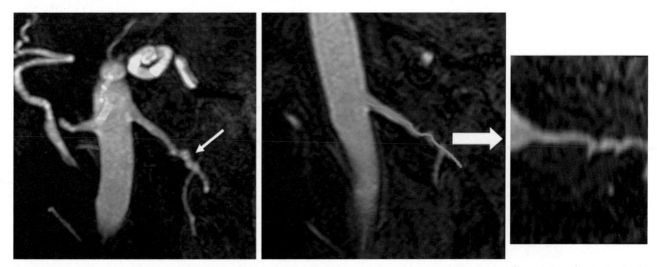

Figure 30.13. Fibromuscular dysplasia. Coronal sub-volume MIP demonstrating a characteristic "string-of-pearls" configuration in the distal left renal artery (*white arrow*). The appearances are consistent with fibromuscular dysplasia. Using a curved reformat technique, a tortuous vessel can be laid out in a linear format, which helps confirm the diagnosis. The product image on the right confirms the nonuniform luminal diameter of the distal left renal artery.

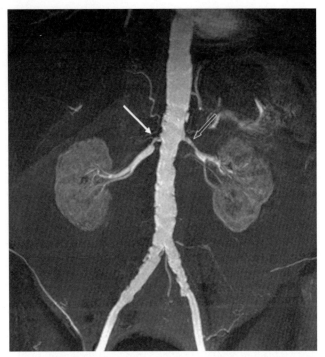

Figure 30.14. Renal artery stenosis. Coronal sub-volume MIP from a renal contrast-enhanced MRA study demonstrating a 1 cm long high-grade ostial stenosis in the origin of the right renal artery (*white arrow*). This was associated with significant signal dropout on 3D phase-contrast imaging (not shown). There is also diffuse moderate narrowing in the proximal left renal artery (*open arrow*), which was also hemodynamically significant. There is moderate luminal irregularity within the abdominal aorta and bilateral common iliac arteries, consistent with severe atheromatous disease.

PREOPERATIVE ASSESSMENT OF LIVING RENAL TRANSPLANT DONORS

Both MRI and CT offer useful preoperative assessment of renal transplant donor candidates, allowing a holistic approach with imaging of renal parenchyma, arterial, and venous structures as well as the ureters. Preprocedure discovery of underlying clinically occult renal pathology or renal vascular anomalies is critical for candidate selection.

A standard MRA protocol is generally utilized, with review of both source images, MPR, MIP, and volume-rendered postprocessed imaging for the presence of accessory renal vessels or early branching renal arteries (73). The number of renal veins is also evaluated, and the presence of retroaortic or circumaortic left renal venous anatomy is noted (74). The postcontrast axial fat-saturated T1 survey of the abdomen performed for all MRA studies can evaluate for renal masses or cysts, and in combination with T2-weighted imaging helps characterize these lesions.

Preoperative evaluation of transplant recipients is requested frequently to evaluate for underlying vascular pathology in the iliac arteries, the usual attachment site for the transplant renal artery. Stenosis of the iliac segment proximal to the transplant renal artery is an uncommon cause of graft dysfunction and hypertension, with physiological effects similar to a true transplant RAS (75). A standard MRA protocol centered upon the pelvic vessels is performed. An intrinsic limitation of MRI for this purpose is its poor sensitivity to calcifications in the vessel wall.

TRANSPLANT KIDNEY MAGNETIC RESONANCE ANGIOGRAPHY

Renal transplant artery stenosis is a common and potentially treatable cause of post-transplant hypertension and graft dysfunction (Fig. 30.16). Transplant renal artery occlusion is often suspected clinically prior to imaging and occurs most often in the early post-transplant period (Fig. 30.17). Transplant recipients with predisposition to peripheral vascular disease (PVD) may develop iliac artery lesions that simulate transplant RAS (75). Iliac artery stenosis may also develop at the site of an iatrogenic clamp injury. MRA provides a comprehensive evaluation of the renal transplant, including arterial and venous patency, parenchymal enhancement, and detection of peritransplant urinoma, hematoma and lymphocele and post-transplant lymphoproliferative disorder. Three-dimensional phase-contrast MRA is useful in characterizing suspected stenotic lesions seen on the contrast-enhanced MRA. Currently, pancreatic transplant is often performed with renal transplantation. The pancreatic trans-

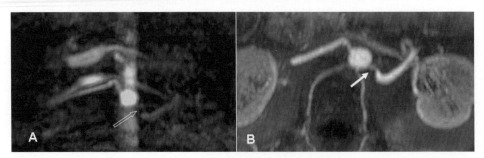

Figure 30.15. Renal artery stenosis. Axial three-dimensional phase-contrast image **(A)** and axial MIP reconstruction from a contrast-enhanced renal MRA **(B)** demonstrating a high-grade stenosis at the ostium of the left renal artery (*white arrow*). Signal dropout within the region of stenosis is seen on phase-contrast imaging (*open arrow*). This results from the nonlaminar or turbulent flow that causes local dephasing of protons and subsequent signal dropout.

TABLE 30-4	Grading of Renal Artery Stenosis Based on 3D Contrast-Enhanced MRA and 3D Phase-Contrast MRA	

Grade	3D CE MRA	3D PC MRA
Normal (0%–24%)	Normal	Normal
Mild (25%–49%)	Mild stenosis	Normal
Moderate (50%–75%)	Moderate stenosis	Stenosis +/−dephasing
Severe (75%–99%)	Stenosis >75%	Severe dephasing
Occlusion	Optimal image quality but cannot find renal artery	Optimal image quality but cannot find renal artery

3D, three-dimensional; MRA, magnetic resonance angiography; CE, contrast-enhanced; PC, phase contrast.
(From Dong Q, Chabra SG, Prince MR. MRA of abdominal aorta and renal and mesenteric arteries. In: Higgins CB, de Roos A, eds. MRI and CT of the Cardiovascular System, 1st ed. Philadelphia: Lippincott Williams & Wilkins, 2003:393–414, with permission.)

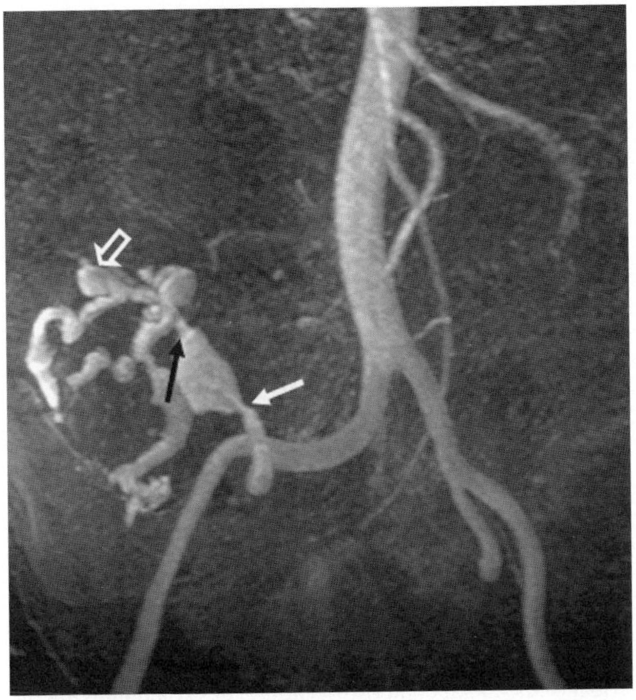

plant vascular anatomy, including occlusion of the artery, is well delineated by MRA (Figs. 30.17 and 30.18).

MESENTERIC MAGNETIC RESONANCE ANGIOGRAPHY

Mesenteric artery stenosis with associated mesenteric ischemia has a high incidence in the elderly population, and often is associated with weight loss and renal artery disease (Fig. 30.19) (76). MRA is a sensitive diagnostic tool for investigating chronic mesenteric ischemia, and CTA remains the modality of choice when acute mesenteric ischemia presents as an acute abdomen. Other conditions of the mesenteric vasculature that are well delineated with current MRA techniques include hepatic arterial variants, particularly in liver transplant donors and recipients (77–79), "nutcracker" syndrome (80), portosystemic venous thrombosis (81–83), and collateral networks, including Budd-Chiari Syndrome (84). Combined MRI and MRA techniques can be used to evaluate the vascular supply and vascular encasement or invasion by hepatic, biliary, and pancreatic neoplasms (85–87). Potential future applications include localization of bleeding sources in patients with gastrointestinal hemorrhage, which may be an ideal use for new blood-pool agents (88).

Coronal imaging allows evaluation of the aorta, hepatic vessels, and portal-venous system; however, if the clinical question relates to mesenteric artery stenosis, a sagittal acquisition is recommended. Imaging in the sagittal plane is less prone to aliasing, and using a smaller rectangular FOV with higher resolution is possible. Axial imaging is recommended if the primary question relates to hepatic arterial anatomy, parenchyma, or portal vein. To avoid aliasing in the slice direction, which is common with 3D MRA, use of a surface coil whose superior-inferior dimension is only slightly larger than the dimensions of the imaging volume is recommended (10).

Figure 30.16. Renal transplant rejection. Coronal MIP image from a three-dimensional contrast-enhanced MRA shows enhancement of the arterial vessels of a right lower quadrant renal transplant. The right internal iliac artery was previously anastomosed to the donor transplant artery. There is now a high-grade, hemodynamically significant stenosis at this site (*white arrow*). A large aneurysm of the main renal artery is present. There is extensive luminal irregularity within the segmental branches, consisting of alternating aneurysmal dilatations (*open arrow*) and stenoses (*black arrow*). The findings were consistent with the patient's diagnosis of chronic transplant rejection.

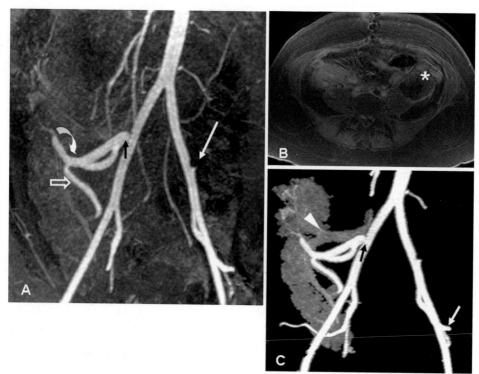

Figure 30.17. Occluded renal transplant artery. Images from a contrast-enhanced MRA study of the abdomen and pelvis in a patient postrenal and pancreas transplantation are shown. There is occlusion of the left-sided renal transplant artery at its origin from the distal left common iliac artery (*white arrow*). The axial postcontrast T1 survey of the abdomen and pelvis shows the nonenhancing parenchyma in the left kidney (*asterisk*). The pancreatic transplant arterial and venous anatomy is well depicted using sub-volume MIP **(A)** and automatic object detect postprocessing techniques **(B)**. The donor common iliac artery is attached to the recipient common iliac artery (*black arrow*). There is a minimal stenosis seen at this takeoff. The donor external iliac artery is anastomosed to the SMA, harvested with the pancreatic transplant (*curved arrow*). The donor internal iliac artery is anastomosed to the splenic artery also harvested with the pancreatic transplant organ (*open arrow*). On this examination it is difficult to localize the anastomotic site but there is no evidence of stenosis identified and no evidence of pseudoaneurysm formation or dissection. The confluence of the donor splenic and superior mesenteric veins (*arrowhead*) as well as the portal vein that drains into the inferior vena cava are also shown.

Pseudostenosis of the celiac artery caused by extrinsic compression from the median arcuate ligament where it joins the right and left diaphragmatic crus is a frequent artifact specific to the mesenteric artery evaluation (Fig. 30.20). This appearance is variable, since it relates to the degree of inspiration or expiration, but it has a characteristic asymmetry, with the visible impression on the superior wall of the vessel.

"Nutcracker" phenomenon refers to compression of the left renal vein between the aorta and the superior mesenteric artery, which results in renal venous hypertension and its clinical symptoms. This phenomenon is an unusual but well-accepted cause of hematuria (89,90).

Anatomic variants, most comprehensively described by Michels in 1955 (91), are common in the hepatic arterial anatomy (92). Most common is a replaced (17%) or accessory (8%) right hepatic artery that usually arises from the superior mesenteric artery. Less common variants include accessory left hepatic artery from the left gastric common hepatic artery (Fig. 30.21), that arises from the superior mesenteric artery, and a common celiac and superior mesenteric trunk. Knowledge of these variants is a prerequisite for successful liver resection or uneventful chemotherapy pump placement (87,92).

ARTIFACTS IN ABDOMINAL MAGNETIC RESONANCE ANGIOGRAPHY

SUSCEPTIBILITY ARTIFACT FROM STENT PLACEMENT

Susceptibility artifact presents as a signal void and occurs at the interface between materials of different magnetic susceptibility (93–95). MR artifacts associated with endovascular stents are related to both stent geometry (96) and the underlying metal composition of the stent (97–101). The effect of the metal composition dominates when imaging the stainless steel Palmaz stent or the cobalt-based alloy Easy Wallstent. Both of these prostheses cause large signal voids on 3D MRA images, making assessment of the stent lumen and patency impossible. The covered Corvita Stent is constructed from the same cobalt-based alloy as the Wallstent, although it contains a tantalum core that reduces the associated artifact. Although shortening the TE makes the associated artifact less pronounced, it is still too extensive to exclude the presence of even a significant stenosis. Conversely, stents made from nitinol, a nickel-titanium alloy (Crag Stent,

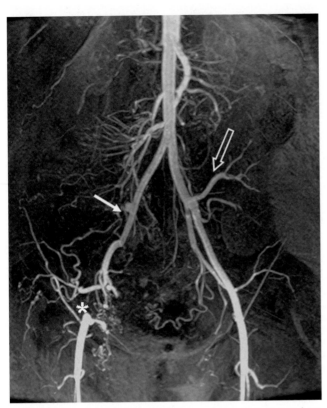

Figure 30.18. Occluded pancreatic transplant artery. Coronal, arterial-phase MIP image shows a widely patent transplant renal artery originating from the distal left common iliac artery (*open arrow*). There is occlusion of a right-sided pancreatic transplant artery arising from the right common iliac artery (*white arrow*). There is also extensive collateralization in the right pelvis resulting from occlusion of the right external iliac artery (*asterisk*).

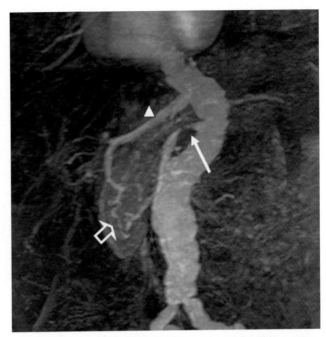

Figure 30.19. Superior mesenteric artery stenosis. Oblique coronal MIP image of a three-dimensional contrast-enhanced MRA data set demonstrating the celiac artery (*arrowhead*) and a high-grade stenosis of the superior mesenteric artery (*white arrow*). Collateral flow has been established through the gastroduodenal arcade and the peripancreatic arterial vessels (*open arrow*). These reconstitute flow to the superior mesenteric artery from the celiac artery beyond the level of the stenosis. Note the fusiform infrarenal abdominal aortic aneurysm.

Crag EndoPro system-1 Stent, Passenger Stent) or elgiloy, a nickel-chromium-cobalt alloy, cause only minor artifacts. The stent lumen can be assessed sufficiently to exclude the presence of a hemodynamically significant (>50% lumen narrowing) stenosis. Signal loss due to radiofrequency shielding inside nitinol stents (Faraday cage effect) imaged by CE MRA can be reduced by applying high flip angles in the order of 70° (99). Vanguard aortic aneurysm stents are also relatively immune to artifact. It would appear that the luminal patency of selected commercially available plain and covered stents can indeed be assessed with 3D contrast MRA. Shortening the TE (minimum) and increasing the flip angle to overcome the radiofrequency shielding tendency will help achieve this end. The importance of obtaining an accurate history regarding past endovascular stenting should be stressed, in addition to the type of stent deployed.

Gradient-echo sequences are particularly susceptible to metallic artifact, which is ironic as these sequences are ubiquitously employed for CE MRA. The spin-echo sequence employs a refocusing 180° pulse that negates the dephasing of stationary protons caused by ferromagnetic objects. When using GRE sequences, artifact can be minimized by using shorter TE values, which decreases the time for dephasing. Increasing the receiver bandwidth, using asymmetric echo acquisitions, increasing the FOV, reducing matrix size, or increasing the slice thickness may reduce the TE. The last

three choices, however, also increase voxel size, which may increase intravoxel dephasing.

POSTPROCESSING ARTIFACT

Source images may be summated for interpretation using several techniques, most commonly MIP reconstruction, volume-rendered techniques, and virtual endoluminal techniques (Figs. 30.22, 30.23, and 30.24). MIP processing reduces a 3D data set to a 2D projection image in any plane. This is achieved by projecting along parallel rays through the volume data and recording the maximum pixel intensity encountered along each ray. These can be full-volume or sub-volume MIP images. The latter can help avoid artifacts by removing irrelevant data from the 3D volume data set prior to processing. These images provide an aesthetic overview of the vascular territory being imaged but should only be interpreted in correlation with source images. A frequent artifact caused by MIP reconstruction is apparent stenosis (pseudostenosis) of a vessel or accentuation of a real stenotic lesion (10). MIP images can also conceal significant intraluminal lesions such as thrombus or dissection, making it essential to review these images with source images and sub-volume MIP images of the region of concern (Fig. 30.25). Virtual endoluminal postprocessing can provide additional information in a limited number of clinical situations.

Zerofill interpolation processing (ZIP) is a widely used postprocessing technique that improves the apparent resolution by interpolating images between the scanned images.

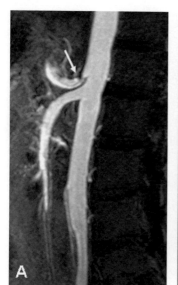
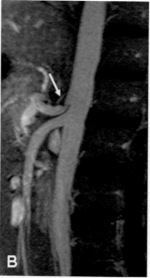
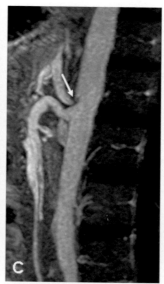
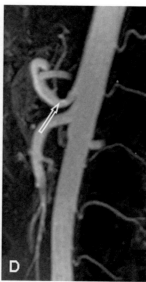

Figure 30.20. Extrinsic compression of the celiac axis by the median arcuate ligament. A selection of sagittal MIP images from contrast-enhanced MRA studies of the mesenteric vessels is demonstrated in a 51-year-old female patient. The patient presented with symptoms of vague upper abdominal pain. **(A)** From the arterial phase, this image demonstrates a high-grade stenosis at the origin of the celiac artery (*white arrow*). The narrowing is asymmetric and primarily affects the superior wall of the vessel. In the venous phase, inspiration **(B)** and expiration **(C)** acquisitions were performed, showing that on expiration the impingement on the celiac artery origin was accentuated (*white arrow*). The patient underwent laparoscopic release of the medial arcuate ligament and had a subsequent MRA study performed **(D)**. This shows a patent celiac artery significantly improved from the preoperative imaging studies. A tiny focus of signal "pileup" is seen from an adjacent surgical staple (*open* arrow). MIP, maximum intensity projection; MRA, magnetic resonance angiography.

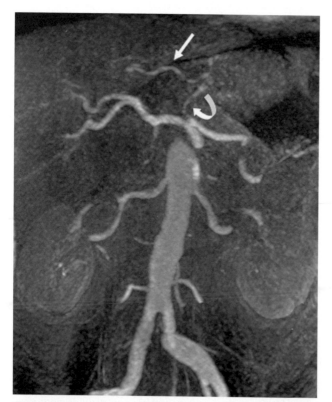

Figure 30.21. Hepatic arterial variant. Coronal arterial phase sub-volume MIP reconstruction demonstrating an accessory left hepatic artery (*white arrow*) arising from the left gastric artery (*curved arrow*). A comprehensive review of the source images is necessary to fully evaluate for hepatic arterial anomalies.

It allows reduction in scan time without loss of resolution. By converting a 256×256 matrix to a 512×512 matrix, the "stair-step" artifact can be eliminated from postprocessed images (102).

ANATOMY EXCLUSION AND WRAP ARTIFACT

When prescribing the 3D imaging volume from localizer images, it is important to include the entire vessel of interest within the volume. This can be particularly difficult when the image localizer is noisy, as is often the case in obese patients. Specific to the abdomen, it is important to be aware of prior extra-anatomic bypass surgery, usually axillary-femoral, so that the FOV can be prescribed adequately. This is also important when depiction of portosystemic collateral flow is required. A frequent artifact seen in imaging of renal transplant and renal failure patients is "wrapping" of the forearm dialysis graft into the FOV (Fig. 30.26). This occurs in the phase-encoding direction and is seen as spatial mismapping or wrapping around of the excluded body segment onto the opposite side of the acquired image. This artifact can also occur in 3D volume imaging from "front-to-back" if the body volume extends beyond the FOV in the slab-select dimension. This problem can be avoided by increasing the FOV to include the entire anatomy. This, however, will decrease the spatial resolution unless the number of phase-encoding steps is increased appropriately. Increasing the number of phase-encoding steps will increase the time of the scan, which in turn increases the risk of movement artifact, particularly in breath-hold situations. The role of the radiologist in these situations is paramount in deciding which parameters will allow the best study for a particular clinical situation.

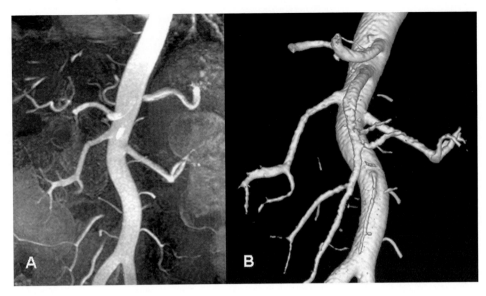

Figure 30.22. Postprocessing techniques. **(A)** Sub-volume MIP and **(B)** volume-rendered postprocessing represent two techniques frequently used for contrast-enhanced MRA evaluation. The images show widely patent renal arteries throughout their length and a smooth luminal contour to the abdominal aorta and proximal iliac vessels. Both of these postprocessing techniques can hide focal vascular lesions or can accentuate stenotic lesions and should always be reviewed in combination with the source images.

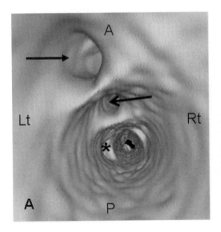

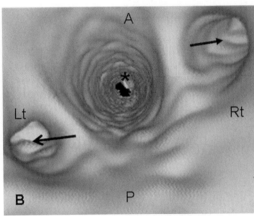

Figure 30.23. Postprocessing techniques. Virtual endoluminal surface-shaded reconstructions that depict the mesenteric arterial vessel (*black arrows*) ostia **(A)** and the renal artery (*black arrows*) ostia **(B)**. These images are oriented with the viewer looking down the aorta from above at the bifurcation (*asterisk*). A cine loop can be prepared to allow rapid evaluation of the lumen, intimal dissections, complex plaque formation, or other vascular abnormalities that are not optimally evaluated by routine MIP or volume-rendered postprocessing techniques.

Figure 30.24. Postprocessing techniques. **(A)** Coronal MIP image demonstrating a large posterior wall mural plaque in the infrarenal abdominal aorta. A further postprocessing technique **(B)**, virtual endoluminal rendering, often provides additional information regarding the character of mural plaque or its location relative to branch ostia. This technique requires some dexterity to perform and in general is only required in select cases.

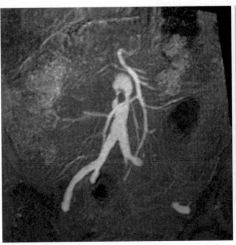

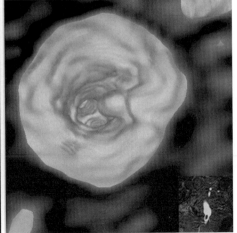

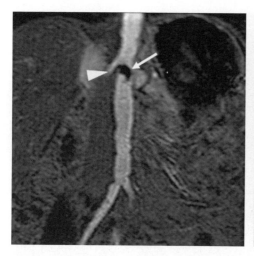
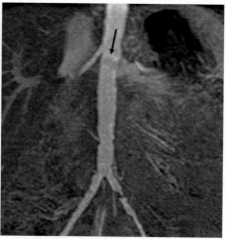

Figure 30.25. MIP pitfall. **(A)** A source image from a coronal three-dimensional contrast-enhanced acquisition during the arterial phase demonstrates a large plaque within the posterior wall of the juxtarenal abdominal aorta (*white arrow*). The plaque projects into the ostium of the right renal artery (*white arrowhead*). On a postprocessed MIP image **(B)**, the plaque is almost invisible (*black arrow*). This figure emphasizes the importance of reviewing source images rather than relying solely on MIP images for interpretation.

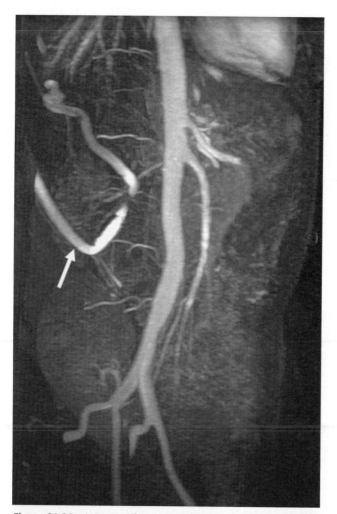

Figure 30.26. Wrap artifact. Arterial phase MIP image demonstrating wrap-around artifact. An enhancing dialysis graft from the opposite arm has wrapped into the image (*white arrow*). Wrap-around artifact results from use of a small field-of-view. Items outside of the field-of-view in the phase encoding direction will wrap into the opposite side of the image as shown.

CONTRAST-TIME ARTIFACT

Contrast-time artifacts represent one of the most common artifacts encountered in daily practice (13,103,104). They occur when data acquisition is not synchronized properly with arrival and passage of the contrast material in the vessels of interest. Three different scenarios may present.

Contrast material concentration may vary dramatically at time of imaging, causing rapid alteration in T1 of blood as k-space is being acquired. The latter presents as one or several dark and/or bright lines along the lumen of the vessel or adjacent to the vessel. This artifact is frequently referred to as "ringing" or Maki artifact due to the parallel nature of the lines inside and outside the vessel (Fig. 30.27) (105). Ringing artifact is encountered more frequently when centric or elliptical-centric 3D sequences are employed (105). Too rapid an injection rate can result in similar artifact. The underlying etiology relates to image acquisition while the gadolinium concentration and thus T1 relaxation is still in a state of rapid flux. This artifact may simulate the presence of a dissection when seen in the aorta and its major branches (10). Correlation of the image acquired during passage of contrast agent with an image acquired during recirculation, when the T1 relaxation of the blood has normalized, should confirm the presence or absence of a dissection. This artifact can also be readily differentiated from an aortic dissection, as it does not take a spiral course like a true intimal flap. Use of the fluorotriggering technique helps avoid ringing artifacts, particularly in patients with underlying cardiac failure where timing of contrast material is less predictable. It also avoids the problem of renal collecting system opacification seen with the "bolus-timing" technique when imaging the renal arteries.

MOTION ARTIFACT

Motion artifacts can be subdivided into those caused by respiratory motion, cardiac motion, or motion of body parts. Consistent breath-holding technique is essential for achieving diagnostic image quality in 3D MRA of the abdomen

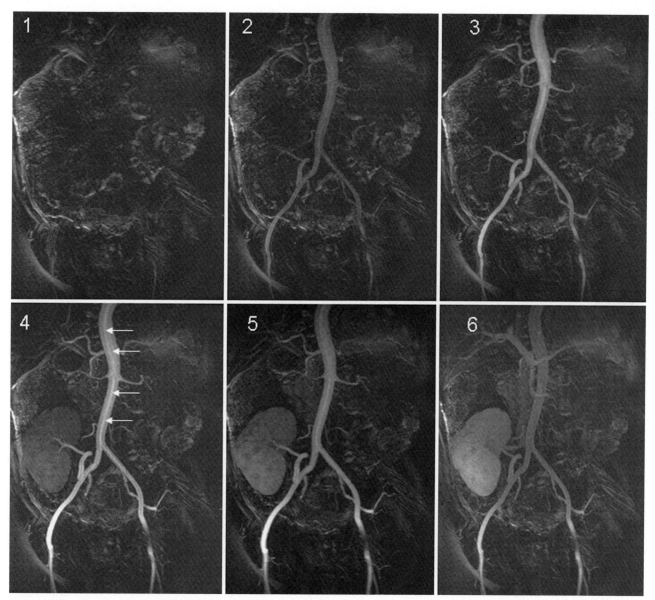

Figure 30.27. Ringing artifact. Six time frames from a time-resolved transplant renal contrast-enhanced MRA study. The study was requested to evaluate for arteriovenous fistula formation from a recent biopsy. The patient had persistent hematuria. The images show no evidence of parenchyma blush in the early arterial phase and no early venous filling. The addition of a time-resolved sequence for evaluation of such clinical questions allows for increased sensitivity. Note the bright line extending through the center of the aorta throughout its length and seen on almost all sequences (*arrow*). This is a characteristic ringing artifact, which must be distinguished from an intimal dissection flap. Usually, the artifact is gone by the late arterial phase, but somewhat unusual persisted in this case. MRA, magnetic resonance angiography.

(106). Artifact resulting from respiratory motion is most evident in vessels perpendicular to the direction of diaphragmatic motion. Imaging of the renal arteries may be nondiagnostic due to the degree of motion artifact, particularly in the distal vessel where respiratory motion has maximum influence (107). Tailoring the scan parameters to minimize imaging time can avoid this artifact. Parallel imaging techniques can play a pivotal role in achieving this end. Motion experienced in imaging the thoracic vessels may be resolved by cardiac gating, although this significantly extends scan time (108,109).

FUTURE PERSPECTIVE

ABDOMINAL MAGNETIC RESONANCE IMAGING WITH 3.0 TELSA

Presently, experience with abdominal MRA with 3.0 T capabilities is limited but has shown positive early results in evaluation of the abdominal vessels (110). This technology has been shown to hold great potential and is further compli-

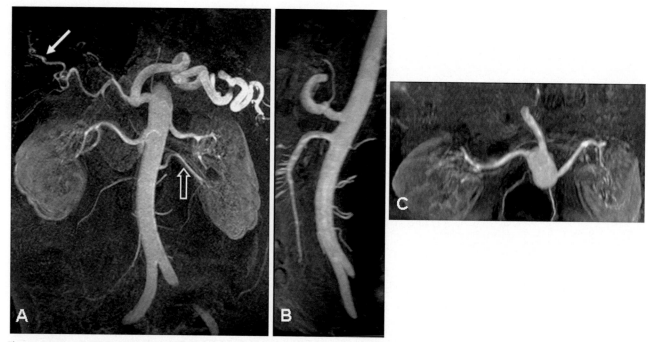

Figure 30.28. 3.0 Tesla (T) MRA. Coronal **(A)**, sagittal **(B)**, and axial **(C)** sub-volume MIP images from a contrast-enhanced renal MRA performed on a 3.0 T clinical magnet. The increased spatial resolution and signal-to-noise ratio allow depiction of the smaller hepatic arterial vessels (*arrow*), which are not always routinely appreciated on 1.5 T clinical scanners. Incidental note is made of an accessory left renal artery (*open arrow*).

mented by the concurrent advancement in phased-array surface-coil technology. The increased spin polarization intrinsic to higher magnetic fields provides a linear increase in SNR with magnetic field strength (Fig. 30.28). This can be employed in MRA to decrease scan time in order to utilize parallel imaging techniques without the current 1.5 T concerns over SNR loss (111). These benefits will allow shorter

breath-hold, less motion artifact, and potentially less contrast medium requirements.

The increased T1 values of tissue with 3.0 T and the relative stability of blood and gadolinium T1 values with field strength changes contribute to a further advantage of disproportionately increasing vessel—background tissue contrast-to-noise ratio. Challenges associated with increases

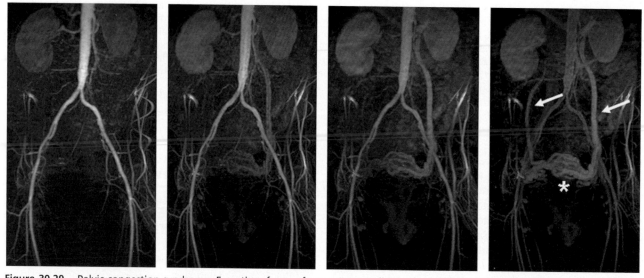

Figure 30.29. Pelvic congestion syndrome. Four time frames from a temporally resolved MRA sequence (EC-TRICKS, GE Healthcare, Waukesha, WI) showed dilatation of the gonadal vessels (*white arrows*), left greater than right, and extensive venous dilatation within the pelvis (*asterisk*). Correlation with the patient's symptoms and history confirmed diagnosis of pelvic congestion syndrome.

CONTRAST ADMINISTRATION

Intravascular contrast material administration is essential in CTA (5). Both technical factors and patient-related factors affect the process of contrast enhancement. It is important to achieve homogeneous intravascular enhancement during imaging. Arterial enhancement depends on iodine concentration of the contrast medium used and the injection protocol (8). More enhancement is achieved with higher iodine concentration. Faster injection rates also provide more enhancement, because a higher concentration of iodine is injected over time (8).

Several contrast injection protocols have been used for CTA. Uniphasic injection protocols with fixed scan delay, injection volume, and injection rate usually result in sufficient aortic enhancement (9). An interactive protocol, in which the injection of contrast medium is stopped manually, can be used to reduce the volume of contrast medium administered (10). Uniform, plateau-like arterial enhancement can only be achieved using a biphasic injection protocol (11). A biphasic injection protocol starts with a small bolus with a high flow rate, followed by a larger bolus with a lower flow rate (11). A saline flush is recommended to flush the veins and push the contrast column into the circulation to reduce the amount of contrast agent (5). Contrast injection for abdominal imaging is preferably administered in a cubital vein.

Major patient-related factors determining contrast enhancement are body habitus and cardiac status. In case of an abdominal aortic aneurysm (AAA), enhancement can be inhomogeneous because of turbulent flow (Fig. 31.1). Be-

cause of these and other differences in circulation dynamics between patients, scanning with a fixed delay is not recommended (11). Solutions to optimize scan delay for determination of the optimal enhancement phase in a single patient are bolus triggering and the use of a test bolus. With the first technique, a region of interest is placed in the distal descending aorta for abdominal CTA. During contrast injection, low-dose nonincremental scans are obtained in a dynamic fashion. The attenuation is monitored in the region of interest and when a predefined enhancement threshold is reached, for example, 150 Hounsfield Units, the CT scan starts automatically with a delay of a few seconds, depending on the type of CT scanner (5). The second technique uses a test bolus to determine patients' contrast transit time. A region of interest is placed in the distal descending aorta for abdominal CTA and during injection of 15 to 20 mL contrast medium, the test bolus, a series of low-dose nonincremental CT scans are obtained. An enhancement curve is then automatically calculated, and the time to maximum enhancement equals the mean contrast transit time. The time to maximum enhancement is set as the scan delay. However, scanning should be started after an extra delay of approximately 10 seconds, because with a large contrast bolus maximum enhancement is achieved later compared with a test bolus because of the accumulation of the contrast agent in the blood vessels (5).

With shorter acquisition times, the amount of contrast agent to be injected can be reduced, but higher injection rates are required for optimal enhancement. When parenchyma imaging is also required (e.g., in liver imaging), the volume of contrast medium cannot be reduced, because enhancement of the parenchyma depends on the total iodine dose (8).

Oral contrast administration is not advisable for vascular imaging; superposition of bowel loops filled with contrast medium can hamper the evaluation of the contrast-enhanced blood vessels, especially when reconstructions are obtained. However, when oral contrast administration is required for imaging, negative contrast medium (water) can be used, which will not disturb evaluation of the contrast-enhanced blood vessels.

SCANNING TECHNIQUE

Vascular imaging of the abdominal aorta and its side branches requires a high-resolution protocol to produce a near isotropic data set of thin overlapping cross-sectional images. Two-dimensional (2D) and 3D reconstructions of high quality can be produced from this data set. With 4- or 16-row MDCT, section thickness of 1 to 1.25 mm and 1 mm, respectively, can be obtained for high-resolution scanning. With thinner section thickness, scanning is not fast enough for covering the entire body volume of interest, whereas with 64-row MDCT, section thickness of 0.5 mm can be obtained routinely.

Our standard scan protocol for the Aquilion 16 (Toshiba Medical Systems, Toshiba cooperation, Tokyo, Japan) for the abdominal aorta and mesenteric vessels is performed in the supine position, with the arms elevated. Scanning is performed during inspiration and breath hold. Section thickness is 1 mm, helical pitch is 23, and reconstruction index and interval are 1 mm and 0.8 mm, respectively. The selected

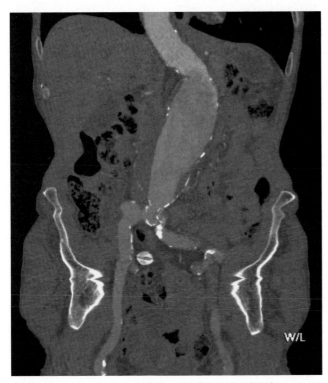

Figure 31.1. Coronal curved planar reformation (CPR) presentation in the abdominal aorta and right iliac artery in a patient with an abdominal aortic aneurysm (AAA). Inhomogeneous enhancement in the abdominal aorta and iliac arteries because of turbulent flow.

kV is 120, the mA varies between 250 and 300, and the rotation time is 400 ms. Arterial imaging is performed with an injection of 100 mL contrast agent (300 mg iodine/mL) at 4 mL/s, or 75 mL contrast agent (400 mg iodine/mL) at 3 mL/s, both followed by 40 mL of saline flush at the same injection rate with at least 18-gauge venous access, injected with a power injector (Medrad, Medrad Inc., Indianola, PA). Delay is determined by bolus triggering, and scanning starts with a delay of 10 seconds when an enhancement increase of 100 Hounsfield Units is reached.

For the renal arteries slice thickness is 0.5 mm, helical pitch is 23, and reconstruction index and interval are 0.5 mm and 0.4 mm, respectively. The selected mA is 300 kV (120), and rotation time (400 ms) is unchanged. Parameters can be changed individually depending on the patient's weight.

Standard vascular protocols for the Aquilion 64 (Toshiba Medical Systems) routinely use a slice thickness of 0.5 mm. Helical pitch is 53, and reconstruction index and interval are 0.4 mm and 0.3 mm, respectively.

POSTPROCESSING

A great challenge of MDCT is in dealing with a large data load (13), especially if an isotropic or near isotropic acquisition is performed (3). For example, routine 16-slice CTA of the abdominal aorta with a scan range of 30 cm performed with 1-mm collimation and a reconstruction index of 1 mm and reconstruction interval of 0.8 mm produces 375 images. With 64-slice CT, 1000 images are generated for the same scan volume with a reconstruction index and interval of 0.4 mm and 0.3 mm, respectively. Imaging the peripheral arteries generates even more images, because the scan volume is much larger. Workstation-based review is necessary not only to evaluate the axial images, which still remains the primary mode for evaluating the abdominal aorta (14), but also to generate reconstructed and 3D images (13). Several reconstruction techniques can be used, which allows better evaluation of the entire vasculature. The main visualization techniques are multiplanar reformation (MPR), maximum intensity projection (MIP), shaded surface display (SSD), and volume rendering (VR) (15).

An MPR is a 2D reconstruction in any coronal, sagittal, or oblique plane. MPR presentation is easy to use, but restricted to a single 2D plane. Therefore it is of limited value for vascular imaging, especially in tortuous arteries (Fig. 31.2). A more sophisticated technique is curved planar reformation (CPR). With CPR reformation, the display planes curve along an anatomic structure through the entire data set (16), for example, the abdominal aorta and a single iliac artery (Fig. 31.3), projected in a 2D image. This technique is a valuable tool for vascular imaging. We use a Vitrea workstation (Vital Images Incorporated, Plymouth, MN), which can generate CPRs semiautomatically. At the same time, additional perpendicular images are displayed, allowing better evaluation of diameters, stenosis, and thrombus composition, thereby improving visualization of eccentric lesions.

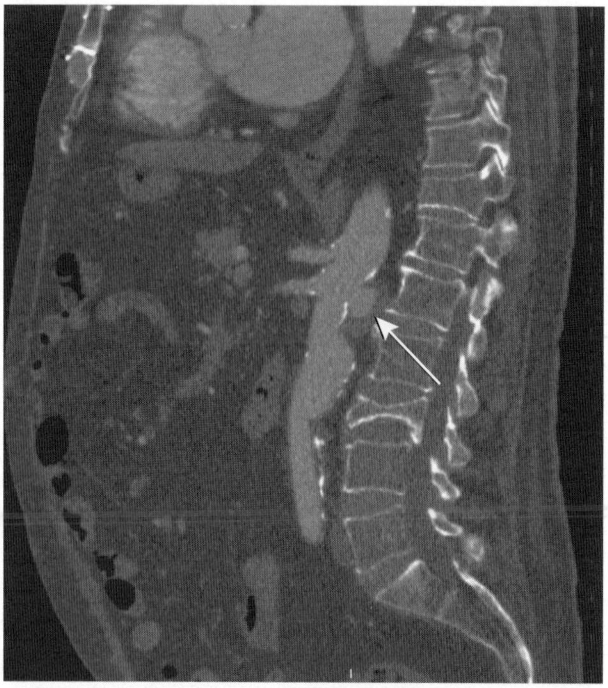

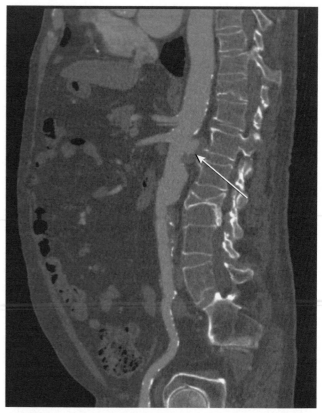

Figure 31.2. Multiplanar reformation (MPR) presentation in the mid-sagittal plane. Patient with an AAA and small penetrating ulcer posteriorly (*arrow*). The focus of interest (penetrating ulcer) is clearly depicted with this MPR technique, although the larger part of the aorta is not visualized in this plane. Note the osteoporotic collapse of the third lumbar vertebra.

Figure 31.3. Same patient as in Figure 31.2. CPR presentation in the sagittal plane through the aorta and right iliac artery. CPR presentation allows better evaluation of the vascular system through the entire data set, especially with tortuous atherosclerotic arteries. Penetrating ulcer (*arrow*).

MIP presentation visualizes only the brightest structures in a selected plane (e.g., anteroposterior) and provides an angio-like image presentation (Fig. 31.4) (14). Thick- or thin-slab MIP images can be obtained. Thin-slab images allow better visualization of complicated anatomic structures. A limitation of the MIP technique, because it is a projection technique, is that more attenuated structures like bones obscure the contrast-enhanced blood vessels (13). Editing to remove overlying structures from the MIP images is usually time-consuming. Another limitation of MIP presentation is the absence of the appreciation of depth relationships, especially in regions with a complex anatomy (13). MIP presentations are sometimes inadequate for visualizing small vascular structures, for example, accessory renal arteries in living-related kidney donors. Variants of MIP are minimum intensity projections and curved-slab MIP. The latter can include multiple vessels in a single image with improvement of the interpretation efficiency (12).

VR is the most complex technique (Fig. 31.5). With VR, every voxel value is assigned an opacity level, ranging from opacity to transparency. The opacification function can be applied to a selected region in the histogram of voxel opacity values, thereby visualizing the selected tissue of interest, for example, blood vessels (13). Colors can be applied to the attenuation histogram, to differentiate voxel values and, for

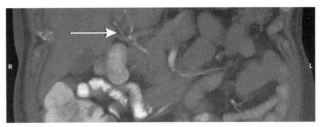

Figure 31.5. Coronal volume rendering (VR) presentation of the hepatic artery showing a separate artery for segment IV (*arrow*), where this artery usually arises from the left hepatic artery. This variant anatomy is a contraindication for living-related liver donation.

instance, to distinguish a calcified plaque from enhancing arterial lumen.

SSD presentations provide 3D images often without prior editing (Fig. 31.6) (13). SSD images are aesthetically pleasant looking, but have some important limitations in their diagnostic value. When displayed in CTA setting, calcifications and enhanced blood vessels are within the same threshold range. Calcified stenosis can therefore appear as local dilations in vascular imaging, resulting in underestimation of the stenosis (13). Also, in aneurysms with mural thrombus, the thrombotic parts are not displayed. This may result in displaying an apparently normal vessel even when a large

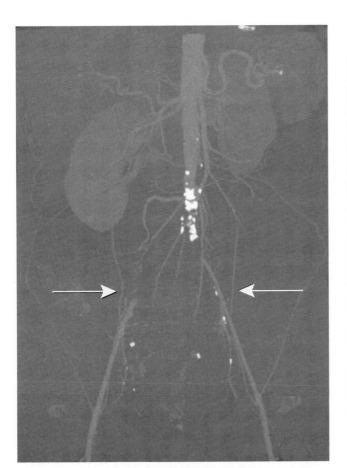

Figure 31.4. Maximum intensity projection (MIP) presentation in the anteroposterior plane in a patient with occlusion of the distal aorta and common iliac arteries. MIP presentation shows an angio-like image. Note the collateral vessels from the splanchnic circulation supplying the external iliac arteries (*arrows*).

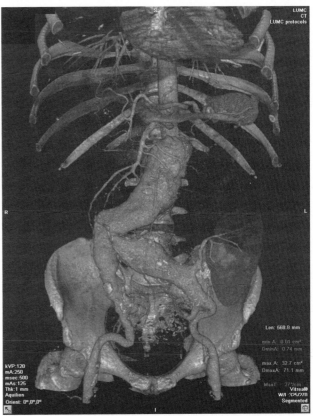

Figure 31.6. Three-dimensional (3D) shaded surface display (SSD) presentation in a patient with an AAA with extension in both iliac arteries. Note the transplant kidney in the left iliac fossa. The renal artery of the transplant kidney arises from the aneurysmatic left iliac artery.

aneurysm is present. VR and SSD presentations can be used for virtual endoscopy to evaluate the internal surface of tubular structures (13,17).

Additional visualization techniques like MIP and VR presentations are most often used in vascular imaging. The interpretation of an examination of the abdominal aorta takes approximately 20 minutes, using a dedicated workstation. Evaluating only 3D images is not an option because of the limitations that have been discussed. It is always important to review the cross-sectional images to obtain additional information (5).

CLINICAL APPLICATIONS

ABDOMINAL AORTA

Abdominal Aortic Aneurysm

Patients with AAA often remain without any symptoms until rupture occurs, with a high mortality rate. AAA occurs most often in middle-aged and elderly patients, and in more men than women with a ratio of 4:1. The pathogenesis of an AAA is complex. Risk factors for atherosclerosis and AAA are overlapping (18).

Aneurysms can be classified according to their cause (19). Most aneurysms are degenerative atherosclerotic aneurysms (Fig. 31.6). Atherosclerotic penetrating ulcers can cause small aneurysms (Figs. 31.2 and 31.3), with a high rupture rate up to 40% (20). Other types of aneurysms are infectious, inflammatory, traumatic, congenital, and postoperative anastomotic aneurysms. It is important to differentiate between these causes, because therapy strategies differ with the cause of the aneurysm. Aneurysms can also be classified according to their anatomic form (saccular, fusiform, true or false aneurysms) or their anatomic location (19). The latter allows classification of AAAs into thoracoabdominal aneurysms, suprarenal aneurysms (involvement of the aorta above the renal arteries), juxtarenal aneurysms (involvement of the aorta at the level of the lowest renal artery or within 5 mm distance from the lowest main renal artery), and infrarenal aneurysms (with a neck of normal aorta between the renal arteries and the beginning of the aneurysm).

The most important issue in evaluation of AAA is accurate diameter measurement, because the maximum diameter of the aneurysm is an important predictor for rupture. Aneurysms exceeding 5 cm in diameter have a higher rupture rate (21,22). Expansion rates of aneurysms are variable. Follow-up examinations are important for monitoring the expansion rate (22). Diameter measurements are usually larger with CT than with ultrasound (US) (23). With standardized measurements on CT or US in routine follow-up, changes in diameter can be detected easily. However, reliable information for optimal planning of endovascular intervention or surgery cannot be obtained by US alone.

It has been demonstrated that the maximum diameter of the aneurysm is not enough for estimation of rupture risk, because small aneurysms may also rupture (24,25). Peak wall stress distribution, which can be measured from the CT data in combination with patient-related factors such as blood pressure, seems to be superior for predicting rupture

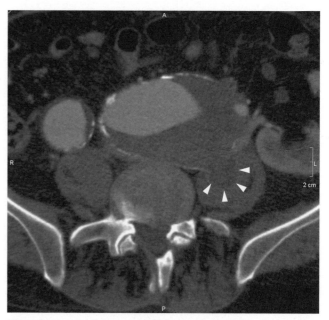

Figure 31.7. Axial computed tomography (CT) image in the same patient as in Figure 31.6, at the level of the common iliac arteries. Contained rupture of the left iliac aneurysm (*arrowheads*) with extension in the left psoas muscle.

risk compared with maximal aneurysm diameter measurements (26). Measuring peak wall stress might affect therapy strategy for small aneurysms with high wall stress and large aneurysms with low wall stress in patients at high risk for surgery (27). Further evaluation is needed to establish the value of peak wall stress distribution for use in the routine clinical practice.

Contained rupture may be observed in patients presenting with an acute symptomatic AAA if their condition allows CT imaging (Fig. 31.7). CT imaging may show a large retroperitoneal hematoma, and sometimes the location of rupture (Fig. 31.8).

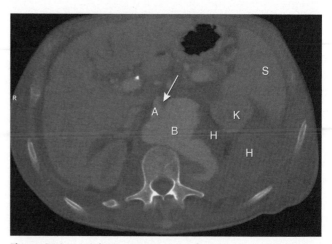

Figure 31.8. Axial VR presentation of an acute ruptured AAA. The site of aortic rupture is posterolateral left (*arrow*) with active bleeding (B) and a large retroperitoneal hematoma (H), displacing the left kidney (K) and spleen (S) anteriorly. Active bleeding causes compression and displacement of the aorta (A).

Exact evaluation of large aneurysms (>5 cm in diameter) is important for clinical decision making and planning therapy, and should provide all anatomic information necessary for planning surgery or endovascular aneurysm repair (EVAR) (28). In the past a combination of aortofemoral angiography and conventional cross-sectional single-slice CT has routinely been used for evaluation of AAA before EVAR. Calibrated angiography, performed with a marked catheter, was necessary for measurements of length and diameters because of the limitations of conventional CT to measure length along the vessel axis (29). But angiography has some disadvantages. It is an invasive method, and diameter measurements are inadequate because only the aortic lumen is visualized and mural thrombus cannot be detected (30). Therefore the assessment of the neck of the aneurysm and possible presence of aneurysmatic iliac arteries may be difficult. Accurate length measurements are more reliable with MDCT compared with x-ray angiography (30). The use of MDCT with 3D reconstructions allows all the information needed, thus eliminating x-ray angiography as a preoperative examination method (29,31,32). Intraobserver and interobserver correlations of aortoiliac length measurement are even better with CTA compared with x-ray angiography (30). When CPR presentations are made with images perpendicular to each other, the true vessel diameter is displayed and reliable measurements are easy to perform (Fig. 31.9) (33).

Evaluation of aneurysms should include the location, length, and diameter of the aneurysm, the extension proximal and distal, the status of the neck of the aneurysm, and the diameter and length of the iliac arteries, and iliac aneurysms, when present (33). Abnormalities of renal, visceral, iliac, and femoral arteries, the number and size of the accessory renal arteries and anatomic variants, and vessel configuration

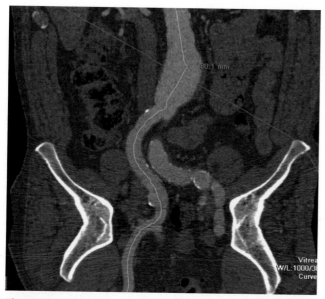

Figure 31.9. CPR presentation through the aorta and right iliac artery in a patient with an AAA. The line is perpendicular to the aortic lumen. The distance displayed (80.1 mm) represents the distance between the level of the lowest renal artery (*small line at the top*) and the largest aneurysm diameter. Diameter and length measurements for stent grafts are easy to perform with CPR presentations.

must also be evaluated (18,33). Furthermore, the cause of the aneurysm should be sought (19). Unenhanced CT in the evaluation of AAA before EVAR allows evaluation of calcifications. Contrast-enhanced CTA is required for evaluating anatomic information and performing measurements, necessary for stent-graft selection.

Endovascular Aortic Aneurysm Repair and Endoleak

Since it was first used in the early 1990s (34), EVAR has become increasingly accepted for treatment of infrarenal AAA. The stent graft, composed of a wired metal frame and prosthetic graft material, is inserted through the femoral arteries and excludes the aneurysm from the circulation, thereby preventing aneurysm rupture (33).

Recently published articles compared conventional and endovascular repair of AAA in randomized trials and concluded that on the basis of operative mortality and complications (the first 30 days after a procedure), endovascular repair of AAA is preferred over open repair (35,36). However, long-term follow-up is necessary to evaluate the benefits of EVAR over prolonged periods of time compared with surgery (35–37).

Successful EVAR relies on accurate preoperative AAA imaging for patient selection (31). Detailed measurements must be obtained, because endovascular stent-graft types and sizes are selected per patient and based on these measurements. A small error in stent-graft size can lead to major problems such as endoleak, stent migration, or other complications resulting in stent failure, the need for conversion to open repair, or even aneurysm rupture (29).

Most limitations for endovascular treatment of abdominal aneurysms are related to proximal neck anatomy of the aneurysm (38–40). Evaluation of the neck requires measurement of the neck length, tapering, degree of angulation, and evaluation of presence of mural thrombus. The length of the neck is the distance between the most caudal renal artery and the beginning of the aneurysm. When the neck length is shorter than 15 mm, sealing problems are likely to occur (41). Fenestrated stent grafts or stent grafts with suprarenal fixation can be used to solve this problem (42). Proximal fixation problems of the stent graft can occur when more than a 2-mm reverse taper is present in the neck of the aneurysm within the first centimeter below the renal arteries (38). Angulation of the neck is defined as the angle between the longitudinal axis of the proximal aortic neck and the longitudinal axis of the aneurysm (Fig. 31.10). Increased risk for complications occurs with moderate (40–59 degrees) or severe (>59 degrees) angulation of the neck, compared with mild (<40 degrees) angulation, even if the neck length is more than 2 cm (43). Reported complications are stent-graft migration, kinking, and insufficient sealing causing endoleak (41,43). Mural thrombus in the neck of the aneurysm may be another important and possible contraindication for EVAR, because this can cause insufficient sealing resulting in endoleak or embolism (44). Furthermore, nonsignificant aortic stenosis in the region of the aneurysm neck may hamper expansion of the stent graft and cause endoleak (Fig. 31.11). A careful search for accessory renal arteries is required. Accessory renal arteries originating from the aneurysm can cause endoleak after EVAR or lead to renal dys-

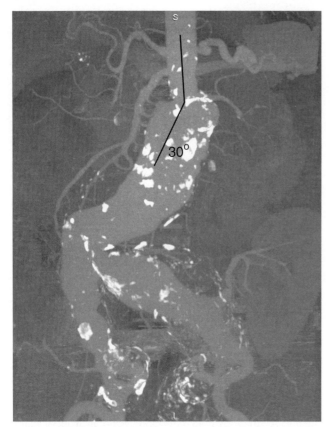

Figure 31.10. Coronal MIP presentation (same patient as in Figs. 31.6 and 31.7). Mild angulation of the aortic neck (30 degrees).

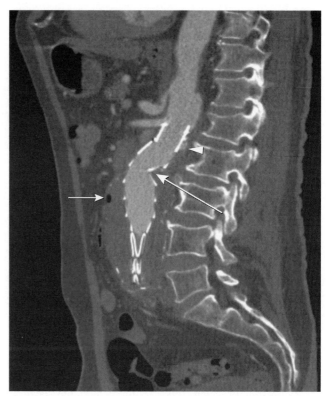

Figure 31.11. Mid-sagittal MPR presentation. Patient with an AAA 2 days after stent-graft placement. Calcified stenosis at the proximal end of the aneurysm, causing insufficient expansion of the stent graft (*large arrow*). Endoleak type 1a (*arrowhead*) resulting from insufficient proximal sealing, probably caused by the insufficient expansion of the stent graft, which was treated with a Palmaz stent (not shown). Note the small air collection anterior in the aneurysm sac (*small arrow*).

function when excluded from the circulation by the stent graft. When small, these arteries may be embolized before EVAR (Fig. 31.12). Other potential contraindications for EVAR are bilateral common iliac aneurysms that would require stenting with exclusion of both internal iliac arteries (41). Also, small vascular femoral access arteries may hinder the use of EVAR. This problem occurs more commonly in women than in men (41).

Complications, especially late complications, are far more frequent after EVAR compared with conventional abdominal aneurysm surgery (37). Routine follow-up is therefore required, and CT is used most often (45). We perform a triple-phase CT (unenhanced, arterial phase, and delayed phase) for follow-up. The first follow-up CT is performed before discharge from the hospital, 2 to 4 days after stent-graft placement; the second CT is performed after 6 months and then annually. Knowledge of normal morphologic changes and problems related to specific types of stent grafts is important (46–49). The complications most frequently reported are endoleak, stent migration, stent-graft kinking (Fig. 31.13), stent-graft thrombosis (Fig. 31.14), enlargement of the aneurysm, and infection (Fig. 31.15) that may cause pseudo-aneurysm formation (33,45). Signs of infection are soft tissue mass, stranding, fluid, and gas bubbles around the aorta (50). The proximal neck of the aneurysm dilates after EVAR in up to 30% of the patients (Fig. 31.16). When this dilation is severe, stent migration can occur, resulting in endoleak (51). Other less frequent complications are mostly directly related to the procedure, such as perfora-

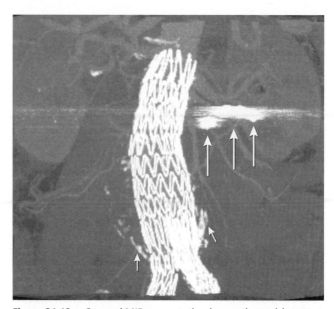

Figure 31.12. Coronal MIP presentation in a patient with a stent graft for an infrarenal aortic aneurysm. Metallic artifacts next to the stent graft (*large arrows*), caused by previous coiling of an accessory renal artery arising from the aneurysm. Note the calcifications in the excluded aortic aneurysm (*small arrows*).

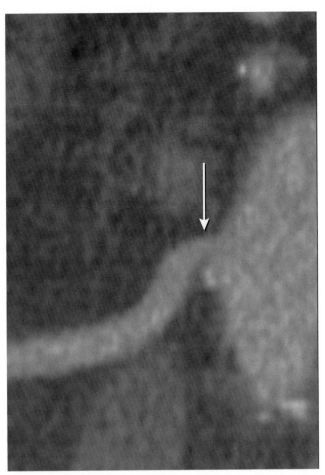

Figure 31.24. CPR presentation through the proximal right renal artery. Significant stenosis at the origin (*arrow*).

decreased size of the ipsilateral kidney, and delayed enhancement can also be noticed, and sustain the diagnosis of probably significant renal artery stenosis (68).

MDCT is well suited for evaluation of renal artery stenosis. However, we usually prefer MRI and MRA for evaluating patients with suspected renal artery stenosis. This is because impaired renal function is often present in these patients, which is a relative contraindication for administering iodinated contrast agent.

Other Applications

The most common primary tumor of the kidney is renal cell carcinoma (69). CT imaging for renal tumors has a dual role. First, CT can be used for diagnosis and characterizing renal masses suspect for malignancy. Second, CT allows evaluation of the relationship between the tumor and the major vessels and collecting system, and comprises the anatomic information necessary to decide whether a patient is suited for nephron-sparing surgery (69). Patients with a single kidney (e.g., after prior nephrectomy for tumor surgery) obtain great benefit when partial nephrectomy is performed, because dialysis may be avoided (70).

Evaluation of renal masses requires multiphase CT, combining an unenhanced phase, a corticomedullary phase, a nephrogenic phase, and an excretory phase (71). Vascular

analysis should reveal the arterial and venous anatomy and variants, and possible extension of tumor-thrombus into the renal veins. The vascular protocol is the same as that used for living renal donors described earlier. The surgical approach depends on the radiologic findings. An alternative that is increasingly used, when surgery is not preferable, is radiofrequency ablation or cryoablation (72).

VASCULAR LIVER IMAGING

Treatment of liver malignancies, either primary or secondary, is increasingly performed. Surgery, radiofrequency ablation, intra-arterial chemotherapy, and isolated liver perfusion are techniques applied. Therapeutic strategies depend on radiologic findings. For example, isolated liver perfusion is frequently performed in our hospital, but this cannot be performed when a right replaced hepatic artery is present. Dedicated vascular CT protocols are necessary for adequate visualization of the liver vasculature before surgical intervention. This is especially true for preoperative assessment for liver transplantation (73,74).

Living-donor liver transplantation was first developed to overcome organ shortage in the pediatric population, but it is also increasingly used in adults, mainly for the same reason (75). The goal of CT for potential liver donors is to evaluate the liver parenchyma and the hepatic and mesenteric anatomy (75–77).

Characterization of focal liver lesions requires multiphase imaging, combining different phases. Unenhanced phase, early arterial phase, late arterial phase, portal venous phase, and delayed phase can be used, depending on the type of lesion suspected (73,74). The early arterial phase allows good evaluation of the hepatic arteries and mesenteric circulation (73). The portal venous phase is used for the portal venous anatomy (78). Liver volumes should be measured before partial liver resection to estimate postoperative success in case of a living donor for transplantation, or for patients in whom partial liver resection for malignancies is planned. Liver insufficiency can occur postoperatively if the remaining liver volume is not enough (78). Assessment of the hepatic arterial anatomy is of utmost importance for living-donor liver transplantation. Anatomic hepatic artery variants are difficult to transplant because these arteries often are very small and may cause anastomotic problems. This problem does not occur during partial liver resection for malignancy.

Classic vascular anatomy of the celiac trunk and mesenteric vessels is present only in approximately 50% of the population (Fig. 31.25) (75–77). The most common variants are a right replaced hepatic artery, arising from the superior mesenteric artery (Fig. 31.26), and a left replaced hepatic artery, arising from the left gastric artery (73). An important variant in potential living liver donors is the arterial supply of segment IV, which normally arises from the left hepatic artery (Fig. 31.5). When this artery arises from the right hepatic artery, left liver lobe donation cannot be performed because adequate surgical anastomosis cannot be obtained. When there are doubts about the arterial anatomy, if one or more hepatic arteries are not visualized by MDCT, or when stenosis in the hepatic artery or their supplying arteries is suspected, x-ray angiography should be performed (77). Variants may be present in the venous system as well. The

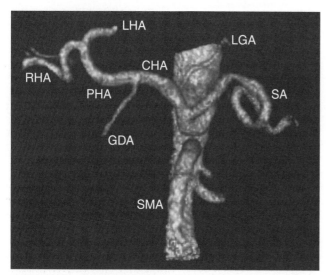

Figure 31.25. 3D SSD presentation of the normal hepatic anatomy. The left gastric artery (LGA), common hepatic artery (CHA), and splenic artery (SA) arise from the celiac trunk. The common hepatic artery divides into gastroduodenal artery (GDA) and proper hepatic artery (PHA). The latter divides into left hepatic artery (LHA) and right hepatic artery (RHA). SMA, superior mesenteric artery.

most frequently reported venous variant is an accessory right inferior hepatic vein (75). The biliary anatomy should be assessed as well (75).

MESENTERIC ISCHEMIA

CT examination of patients with suspected mesenteric ischemia involves evaluation of both the mesenteric vessels

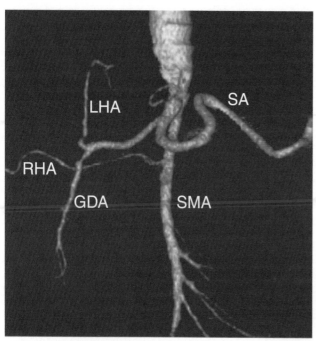

Figure 31.26. 3D SSD presentation image of a patient with a replaced RHA, arising from the superior mesenteric artery (SMA). See text of Figure 31.25 for abbreviations.

and the bowel walls (79,80). Mesenteric ischemia can be classified as acute, subacute, or chronic. CT signs of acute mesenteric ischemia are bowel wall thickening and edema, changes in enhancement, submucosal hemorrhage, mesenteric stranding, mesenteric fluid, and pneumatosis intestinalis (79–81). Acute mesenteric ischemia is caused by severe stenosis or occlusion of the superior mesenteric artery or vein, usually by an acute embolus or thrombosis. The severity, size, and site of the bowel affected depends on the cause of ischemia, the location and extent of the stenosis or occlusion, the duration of the process, and the presence of collateral vessels (80). Mesenteric venous thrombosis may present with subacute symptomatology over 1 to 4 weeks (80,81).

Chronic mesenteric ischemia is known as abdominal angina and usually caused by atherosclerosis (79). Symptoms of abdominal epigastric pain typically occur postprandial, when increased blood flow is required in the splanchnic arteries (celiac trunk, superior mesenteric artery, and inferior mesenteric artery). Chronic mesenteric ischemia generally occurs only when two or all three arteries are significantly stenosed, because of the presence of extensive collateral vessels between the splanchnic arteries (Fig. 31.4) (79). The diagnosis is made after exclusion of other abnormalities.

CT allows excellent visualization of the bowel walls, arterial anatomy with its collateral vessels, vascular variants, and anomalies (82–84). Arterial phase imaging allows optimal visualization of the splanchnic arteries. CPR is very useful for evaluating the degree of stenosis, because perpendicular CPR images centered on the central lumen line drawn through the stenosis are displayed simultaneously (Figs. 31.27 and 31.28). Most atherosclerotic stenoses are located proximally in the affected artery (79). Stenosis can be graded as nonsignificant or significant. Secondary signs of stenosis such as poststenotic dilation are generally recognized well. An acute embolus can be diagnosed as a filling defect in an enhanced artery.

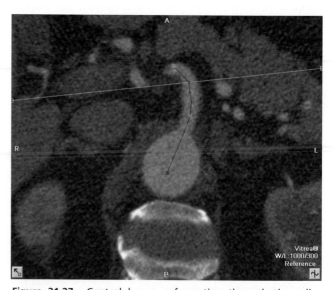

Figure 31.27. Central lumen reformation through the celiac trunk. This line is drawn manually when scrolling through the axial images. The resulting sagittal CPR presentation is shown in Figure 31.28.

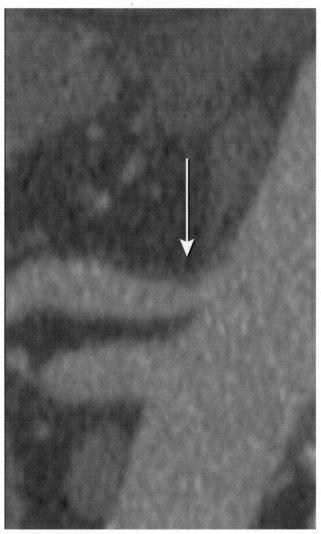

Figure 31.28. Sagittal CPR presentation shows 50% stenosis at the origin of the celiac trunk.

SUMMARY

CTA has rapidly gained wide acceptance for imaging of the aorta and its abdominal side branches because of its fast imaging with high spatial resolution. The introduction of 16-row and 64-row MDCT has especially advanced the technology and provides an alternative to x-ray angiography and MRA for several indications. Further studies should evaluate the cost-effectiveness of MDCT for specific abdominal indications, as has been performed for peripheral vascular imaging (85). Optimized injection protocols and specific contrast medium concentrations are required for further optimization.

REFERENCES

1. Rydberg J, Buckwalter KA, Caldemeyer KS, et al. Multisection CT: scanning techniques and clinical applications. *Radiographics* 2000;20:(6):1787–1806.

2. Hu H, He HD, Foley WD, et al. Four multidetector-row helical CT: image quality and volume coverage speed. *Radiology* 2000;215:(1):55–62.

3. Prokop M. General principles of MDCT. *Eur J Radiol* 2003; 45:S4–S10.

4. Saini S. Multi-detector row CT: principles and practice for abdominal applications. *Radiology* 2004;233:(2):323–327.

5. Napoli A, Fleischmann D, Chan FP, et al. Computed tomography angiography: state-of-the-art imaging using multidetector-row technology. *J Comput Assist Tomogr* 2004;28(Suppl 1): S32–S45.

6. Rubin GD. MDCT imaging of the aorta and peripheral vessels. *Eur J Radiol* 2003;45(Suppl)1:S42–S49.

7. Rubin GD, Shiau MC, Leung AN, et al. Aorta and iliac arteries: single versus multiple detector-row helical CT angiography. *Radiology* 2000;215:(3):670–676.

8. Fleischmann D. Use of high concentration contrast media: principles and rationale-vascular district. *Eur J Radiol* 2003; 45(Suppl 1):S88–S93.

9. Macari M, Israel GM, Berman P, et al. Infrarenal abdominal aortic aneurysms at multi-detector row CT angiography: intravascular enhancement without a timing acquisition. *Radiology* 2001;220:(2):519–523.

10. Ho LM, Nelson RC, Thomas J, et al. Abdominal aortic aneurysms at multi-detector row helical CT: optimization with interactive determination of scanning delay and contrast medium dose. *Radiology* 2004;232:(3):854–859.

11. Fleischmann D, Rubin GD, Bankier AA, et al. Improved uniformity of aortic enhancement with customized contrast medium injection protocols at CT angiography. *Radiology* 2000; 214:(2):363–371.

12. Raman R, Napel S, Rubin GD. Curved-slab maximum intensity projection: method and evaluation. *Radiology* 2003;229:(1): 255–260.

13. Rubin GD. 3-D imaging with MDCT. *Eur J Radiol* 2003; 45(Suppl 1):S37–S41.

14. Prokop M. Multislice CT angiography. *Eur J Radiol* 2000;36: (2):86–96.

15. Cody DD. AAPM/RSNA physics tutorial for residents: topics in CT. Image processing in CT. *Radiographics* 2002;22:(5): 1255–1268.

16. Nino-Murcia M, Jeffrey RB Jr., Beaulieu CF, et al. Multidetector CT of the pancreas and bile duct system: value of curved planar reformations. *AJR Am J Roentgenol* 2001;176:(3): 689–693.

17. Sun Z, Gallagher E. Multislice CT virtual intravascular endoscopy for abdominal aortic aneurysm stent grafts. *J Vasc Interv Radiol* 2004;15:(9):961–970.

18. Singh K, Bonaa KH, Jacobsen BK, et al. Prevalence of and risk factors for abdominal aortic aneurysms in a population-based study: The Tromso Study. *Am J Epidemiol* 2001;154: (3):236–244.

19. Chaikof EL, Blankensteijn JD, Harris PL, et al. Reporting standards for endovascular aortic aneurysm repair. *J Vasc Surg* 2002;35:(5):1048–1060.

20. Eggebrecht H, Baumgart D, Schmermund A, et al. Penetrating atherosclerotic ulcer of the aorta: treatment by endovascular stent-graft placement. *Curr Opin Cardiol* 2003;18:(6):431–435.

21. Nevitt MP, Ballard DJ, Hallett JW Jr. Prognosis of abdominal aortic aneurysms. A population-based study. *N Engl J Med* 1989;321:(15):1009–1014.

22. Glimaker H, Holmberg L, Elvin A, et al. Natural history of patients with abdominal aortic aneurysm. *Eur J Vasc Surg* 1991;5:(2):125–130.

23. Sprouse LR, Meier GH III, Lesar CJ, et al. Comparison of abdominal aortic aneurysm diameter measurements obtained

with ultrasound and computed tomography: is there a difference? *J Vasc Surg* 2003;38:(3):466–471.

24. Fillinger MF, Racusin J, Baker RK, et al. Anatomic characteristics of ruptured abdominal aortic aneurysm on conventional CT scans: implications for rupture risk. *J Vasc Surg* 2004;39:(6):1243–1252.

25. Nicholls SC, Gardner JB, Meissner MH, et al. Rupture in small abdominal aortic aneurysms. *J Vasc Surg* 1998;28:(5):884–888.

26. Fillinger MF, Marra SP, Raghavan ML, et al. Prediction of rupture risk in abdominal aortic aneurysm during observation: wall stress versus diameter. *J Vasc Surg* 2003;37:(4):724–732.

27. Fillinger MF, Raghavan ML, Marra SP, et al. In vivo analysis of mechanical wall stress and abdominal aortic aneurysm rupture risk. *J Vasc Surg* 2002;36:(3):589–597.

28. Qanadli SD, Mesurolle B, Coggia M, et al. Abdominal aortic aneurysm: pretherapy assessment with dual-slice helical CT angiography. *AJR Am J Roentgenol* 2000;174:(1):181–187.

29. Wyers MC, Fillinger MF, Schermerhorn ML, et al. Endovascular repair of abdominal aortic aneurysm without preoperative arteriography. *J Vasc Surg* 2003;38:(4):730–738.

30. Diehm N, Herrmann P, Dinkel HP. Multidetector CT angiography versus digital subtraction angiography for aortoiliac length measurements prior to endovascular AAA repair. *J Endovasc Ther* 2004;11:(5):527–534.

31. Blum U, Voshage G, Lammer J, et al. Endoluminal stent-grafts for infrarenal abdominal aortic aneurysms. *N Engl J Med* 1997;336:(1):13–20.

32. Willmann JK, Wildermuth S, Pfammatter T, et al. Aortoiliac and renal arteries: prospective intraindividual comparison of contrast-enhanced three-dimensional MR angiography and multi-detector row CT angiography. *Radiology* 2003;226:(3):798–811.

33. Rydberg J, Kopecky KK, Lalka SG, et al. Stent grafting of abdominal aortic aneurysms: pre-and postoperative evaluation with multislice helical CT. *J Comput Assist Tomogr* 2001;25:(4):580–586.

34. Parodi JC, Palmaz JC, Barone HD. Transfemoral intraluminal graft implantation for abdominal aortic aneurysms. *Ann Vasc Surg* 1991;5:(6):491–499.

35. Prinssen M, Verhoeven EL, Buth J, et al. A randomized trial comparing conventional and endovascular repair of abdominal aortic aneurysms. *N Engl J Med* 2004;351:(16):1607–1618.

36. Greenhalgh RM, Brown LC, Kwong GP, et al. Comparison of endovascular aneurysm repair with open repair in patients with abdominal aortic aneurysm (EVAR trial 1), 30-day operative mortality results: randomised controlled trial. *Lancet* 2004;364:(9437):843–848.

37. Lederle FA. Abdominal aortic aneurysm—open versus endovascular repair. *N Engl J Med* 2004;351:(16):1677–1679.

38. Dillavou ED, Muluk SC, Rhee RY, et al. Does hostile neck anatomy preclude successful endovascular aortic aneurysm repair? *J Vasc Surg* 2003;38:(4):657–663.

39. Mohan IV, Laheij RJ, Harris PL. Risk factors for endoleak and the evidence for stent-graft oversizing in patients undergoing endovascular aneurysm repair. *Eur J Vasc Endovasc Surg* 2001;21:(4):344–349.

40. Stanley BM, Semmens JB, Mai Q, et al. Evaluation of patient selection guidelines for endoluminal AAA repair with the Zenith Stent-Graft: the Australasian experience. *J Endovasc Ther* 2001;8:(5):457–464.

41. Carpenter JP, Baum RA, Barker CF, et al. Impact of exclusion criteria on patient selection for endovascular abdominal aortic aneurysm repair. *J Vasc Surg* 2001;34:(6):1050–1054.

42. Verhoeven EL, Prins TR, Tielliu IF, et al. Treatment of short-necked infrarenal aortic aneurysms with fenestrated stent-grafts: short-term results. *Eur J Vasc Endovasc Surg* 2004;27:(5):477–483.

43. Sternbergh WC III, Carter G, York JW, et al. Aortic neck angulation predicts adverse outcome with endovascular abdominal aortic aneurysm repair. *J Vasc Surg* 2002;35:(3):482–486.

44. Gitlitz DB, Ramaswami G, Kaplan D, et al. Endovascular stent grafting in the presence of aortic neck filling defects: early clinical experience. *J Vasc Surg* 2001;33:(2):340–344.

45. Armerding MD, Rubin GD, Beaulieu CF, et al. Aortic aneurysmal disease: assessment of stent-graft treatment-CT versus conventional angiography. *Radiology* 2000;215:(1):138–146.

46. Tillich M, Hausegger KA, Tiesenhausen K, et al. Helical CT angiography of stent-grafts in abdominal aortic aneurysms: morphologic changes and complications. *Radiographics* 1999;19:(6):1573–1583.

47. Mita T, Arita T, Matsunaga N, et al. Complications of endovascular repair for thoracic and abdominal aortic aneurysm: an imaging spectrum. *Radiographics* 2000;20:(5):1263–1278.

48. Dattilo JB, Brewster DC, Fan CM, et al. Clinical failures of endovascular abdominal aortic aneurysm repair: incidence, causes, and management. *J Vasc Surg* 2002;35:(6):1137–1144.

49. Haulon S, Devos P, Willoteaux S, et al. Risk factors of early and late complications in patients undergoing endovascular aneurysm repair. *Eur J Vasc Endovasc Surg* 2003;25:(2):118–124.

50. Macedo TA, Stanson AW, Oderich GS, et al. Infected aortic aneurysms: imaging findings. *Radiology* 2004;231:(1):250–257.

51. Napoli V, Sardella SG, Bargellini I, et al. Evaluation of the proximal aortic neck enlargement following endovascular repair of abdominal aortic aneurysm: 3-years experience. *Eur Radiol* 2003;13:(8):1962–1971.

52. Sawhney R, Kerlan RK, Wall SD, et al. Analysis of initial CT findings after endovascular repair of abdominal aortic aneurysm. *Radiology* 2001;220:(1):157–160.

53. Farner MC, Carpenter JP, Baum RA, et al. Early changes in abdominal aortic aneurysm diameter after endovascular repair. *J Vasc Interv Radiol* 2003;14:(2 Pt 1):205–210.

54. Kritpracha B, Beebe HG, Comerota AJ. Aortic diameter is an insensitive measurement of early aneurysm expansion after endografting. *J Endovasc Ther* 2004;11:(2):184–190.

55. Veith FJ, Baum RA, Ohki T, et al. Nature and significance of endoleaks and endotension: summary of opinions expressed at an international conference. *J Vasc Surg* 2002;35:(5):1029–1035.

56. Elkouri S, Panneton JM, Andrews JC, et al. Computed tomography and ultrasound in follow-up of patients after endovascular repair of abdominal aortic aneurysm. *Ann Vasc Surg* 2004;18:(3):271–279.

57. Pollock JG, Travis SJ, Whitaker SC, et al. Endovascular AAA repair: classification of aneurysm sac volumetric change using spiral computed tomographic angiography. *J Endovasc Ther* 2002;9:(2):185–193.

58. Stavropoulos SW, Baum RA. Imaging modalities for the detection and management of endoleaks. *Semin Vasc Surg* 2004;17:(2):154–160.

59. Rozenblit AM, Patlas M, Rosenbaum AT, et al. Detection of endoleaks after endovascular repair of abdominal aortic aneurysm: value of unenhanced and delayed helical CT acquisitions. *Radiology* 2003;227:(2):426–433.

60. Napoli V, Bargellini I, Sardella SG, et al. Abdominal aortic aneurysm: contrast-enhanced US for missed endoleaks after endoluminal repair. *Radiology* 2004;233:(1):217–225.

61. Gorich J, Rilinger N, Sokiranski R, et al. Endoleaks after endovascular repair of aortic aneurysm: are they predictable?-initial results. *Radiology* 2001;218:(2):477–480.

62. Kawamoto S, Montgomery RA, Lawler LP, et al. Multi-detector row CT evaluation of living renal donors prior to laparoscopic nephrectomy. *Radiographics* 2004;24:(2):453–466.

63. Rankin SC, Jan W, Koffman CG. Noninvasive imaging of living related kidney donors: evaluation with CT angiography and gadolinium-enhanced MR angiography. *AJR Am J Roentgenol* 2001;177:(2):349–355.

64. Rydberg J, Kopecky KK, Tann M, et al. Evaluation of prospective living renal donors for laparoscopic nephrectomy with multisection CT: the marriage of minimally invasive imaging with minimally invasive surgery. *Radiographics* 2001;21 Spec No:S223–S236.

65. Kawamoto S, Montgomery RA, Lawler LP, et al. Multidetector CT angiography for preoperative evaluation of living laparoscopic kidney donors. *AJR Am J Roentgenol* 2003;180:(6): 1633–1638.

66. Halpern EJ, Mitchell DG, Wechsler RJ, et al. Preoperative evaluation of living renal donors: comparison of CT angiography and MR angiography. *Radiology* 2000;216:(2):434–439.

67. Safian RD, Textor SC. Renal-artery stenosis. *N Engl J Med* 2001;344:(6):431–442.

68. Fleischmann D. Multiple detector-row CT angiography of the renal and mesenteric vessels. *Eur J Radiol* 2003;45(Suppl 1): S79–S87.

69. Sheth S, Scatarige JC, Horton KM, et al. Current concepts in the diagnosis and management of renal cell carcinoma: role of multidetector CT and three-dimensional CT. *Radiographics* 2001;21 Spec No:S237–S254.

70. Catalano C, Fraioli F, Laghi A, et al. High-resolution multidetector CT in the preoperative evaluation of patients with renal cell carcinoma. *AJR Am J Roentgenol* 2003;180:(5): 1271–1277.

71. Foley WD. Renal MDCT. *Eur J Radiol* 2003;45(Suppl 1): S73–S78.

72. Gervais DA, McGovern FJ, Arellano RS, et al. Renal cell carcinoma: clinical experience and technical success with radiofrequency ablation of 42 tumors. *Radiology* 2003;226:(2): 417–424.

73. Foley WD, Mallisee TA, Hohenwalter MD, et al. Multiphase hepatic CT with a multirow detector CT scanner. *AJR Am J Roentgenol* 2000;175:(3):679–685.

74. Foley WD. Special focus session: multidetector CT: abdominal visceral imaging. *Radiographics* 2002;22:(3):701–719.

75. Erbay N, Raptopoulos V, Pomfret EA, et al. Living donor liver transplantation in adults: vascular variants important in surgical planning for donors and recipients. *AJR Am J Roentgenol* 2003;181:(1):109–114.

76. Lee SS, Kim TK, Byun JH, et al. Hepatic arteries in potential donors for living related liver transplantation: evaluation with multi-detector row CT angiography. *Radiology* 2003;227:(2): 391–399.

77. Byun JH, Kim TK, Lee SS, et al. Evaluation of the hepatic artery in potential donors for living donor liver transplantation by computed tomography angiography using multidetector-row computed tomography: comparison of volume rendering and maximum intensity projection techniques. *J Comput Assist Tomogr* 2003;27:(2):125–131.

78. Onodera Y, Omatsu T, Nakayama J, et al. Peripheral anatomic evaluation using 3D CT hepatic venography in donors: significance of peripheral venous visualization in living-donor liver transplantation. *AJR Am J Roentgenol* 2004;183:(4): 1065–1070.

79. Cademartiri F, Raaijmakers RH, Kuiper JW, et al. Multi-detector row CT angiography in patients with abdominal angina. *Radiographics* 2004;24:(4):969–984.

80. Horton KM, Fishman EK. Multi-detector row CT of mesenteric ischemia: can it be done? *Radiographics* 2001;21:(6): 1463–1473.

81. Bradbury MS, Kavanagh PV, Bechtold RE, et al. Mesenteric venous thrombosis: diagnosis and noninvasive imaging. *Radiographics* 2002;22:(3):527–541.

82. Laghi A, Iannaccone R, Catalano C, et al. Multislice spiral computed tomography angiography of mesenteric arteries. *Lancet* 2001;358:(9282):638–639.

83. Lawler LP, Fishman EK. Celiomesenteric anomaly demonstration by multidetector CT and volume rendering. *J Comput Assist Tomogr* 2001;25:(5):802–804.

84. Horton KM, Fishman EK. 3D CT angiography of the celiac and superior mesenteric arteries with multidetector CT data sets: preliminary observations. *Abdom Imaging* 2000;25:(5): 523–525.

85. Visser K, Kock MC, Kuntz KM, et al. Cost-effectiveness targets for multi-detector row CT angiography in the work-up of patients with intermittent claudication. *Radiology* 2003;227: (3):647–656.

32

Magnetic Resonance and Computed Tomography Angiography of Peripheral Arteries

Martin N. Wasser and Albert de Roos

With the increasing average age of the population in the industrialized world, atherosclerotic disease of the peripheral vessels is gaining importance. Although atherosclerotic lesions occur in all vascular territories, the lower limbs are affected in 90% of cases. Presently, atherosclerosis in the lower limbs accounts for 50,000 to 60,000 percutaneous angioplasties, implantation of 110,000 vascular prostheses, and 100,000 amputations annually in the United States (1).

Before the planning of therapeutic actions, detailed information on localization, extent, and severity of the disease is essential. Conventional angiography has long served as the imaging modality of choice in this respect. However, x-ray angiography has definite risks and limitations, including the possibility of a severe contrast medium reaction, even when nonionic agents are used (2). Also, because approximately 70% of patients with severe occlusive peripheral disease have evidence of impairment of renal function (3), contrast-induced renal insufficiency is a matter of concern. Therefore, noninvasive alternatives, such as duplex ultrasound and magnetic resonance (MR) angiography, are increasingly used in the diagnostic workup of patients with peripheral arterial disease.

Contrast-enhanced magnetic resonance angiography (CE-MRA) has rapidly emerged as an attractive alternative to conventional angiography. The reason for this rapid acceptance in the "vascular community" is the close resemblance of CE-MRA images to conventional angiography. The contrast agent gadolinium diethylenetriamine pentaacetic acid (DTPA) in the dosages used for MRA is nonnephrotoxic (4). This means that also patients with impaired renal function can be examined with CE-MRA.

Recently, with the advent of multidetector row or multi-slice computed tomography (CT), a new modality has emerged for the noninvasive evaluation of the peripheral vasculature. Although this technique involves the use of radiation and iodinated contrast agents, the spatial resolution that can be obtained with multislice CT angiography (CTA) is superior to that of MR angiography. CTA has therefore rapidly become a serious competitor for MRA in evaluation of peripheral vascular disease in patients with nonimpaired renal function.

This chapter will provide an overview of the techniques and indications for CE-MRA and CE-CTA of the peripheral arteries of the lower limbs. Although atherosclerosis is the major cause of peripheral arterial disease, other abnormalities will also be addressed.

MAGNETIC RESONANCE ANGIOGRAPHY OF PERIPHERAL ARTERIES

GENERAL

As opposed to the older MRA techniques [phase contrast MRA (PCA) and time-of-flight (TOF) MRA], CE-MRA does not suffer from artifacts caused by turbulence and in-plane saturation. This makes CE-MRA easier to interpret than PCA or TOF-MRA. Also, the lack of in-plane saturation has enabled imaging in the coronal plane, allowing for coverage of much larger anatomic regions. In general, the most important advantage of CE-MRA, as opposed to conventional MRA, is the enormous reduction in examination time.

According to a meta-analysis published in 2000 (5), the sensitivity for detection of hemodynamically significant stenosis (>50% luminal reduction) ranged from 64% to 100% for two-dimensional (2D) TOF and 92% to 100% for three-dimensional (3D) CE-MRA. Specificity ranged from 68% to 96% for 2D TOF and 91% to 99% for 3D CE-MRA. This indicates that 3D CE-MRA is superior to 2D TOF for the detection of peripheral arterial disease. Especially for imaging of the proximal vessels in the legs, 2D TOF appears to be less reliable (sensitivity, 83% to 100%; specificity, 23% to 98%). In tortuous, elongated iliac arteries, 2D TOF may show false-positive results because of in-plane saturation or saturation of arterial signal by the venous presaturation slab. Short segments of signal void may be caused by either a short occlusion or a severe stenosis. Also, retrograde flow may not be recognized because of the venous presaturation slab.

Also in the femoropopliteal and infrapopliteal regions, CE-MRA appears to perform better than 2D TOF. Sensitivity ranges between 88% and 92% and between 94% and 100% for 2D TOF and CE-MRA, respectively, in evaluating the femoropopliteal region (specificity, 82% to 98% versus 97% to 99%). With respect to the infrapopliteal vessels, sensitivity/specificity are 89% to 98%/91% to 95% versus 91% to 94%/100% for 2D TOF and CE-MRA, respectively. Contrast-enhanced MRA is therefore the best MRA technique to evaluate arterial disease in the lower limbs, in terms of time-effectiveness and accuracy.

TECHNIQUES FOR PERIPHERAL CONTRAST-ENHANCED MAGNETIC RESONANCE ANGIOGRAPHY

Basics

The basic principle behind CE-MRA is imaging the arterial first pass of paramagnetic contrast agent in the vessels after intravenous injection (6). The injected contrast agent produces a strong shortening of the T1-relaxation time of blood. This results in high signal intensity of the arteries on T1-weighted, spoiled gradient-echo images. The delay between arterial and venous enhancement provides a time window for pure arterial imaging. This time window depends on the rate of contrast agent injection, but also on the anatomic region being imaged. In the upper limbs, venous return is much faster than in the lower limbs, requiring a much shorter measurement time. Because the technique depends on imaging of the first pass of contrast agent, timing the start of image acquisition after injection is essential. Various techniques have been developed to calculate this so-called scan delay, as will be explained later.

The quality of the MRA images with regard to selective arterial visualization, resolution, and volume of interest depends on both sequence parameters used and the contrast medium bolus geometry. Arterial enhancement depends on individual physiologic parameters, such as cardiac output and blood volume, but also on contrast agent application parameters, which can be manipulated (flow rate, dose, and saline flush volume). The T1-shortening of blood depends on the intravascular concentration of the contrast agent, which, in turn, depends on the rate of injection. In general, the higher the injection rate, the higher the concentration will be, although rates exceeding 5 mL per second do not result in further increase in signal intensity. In fact, intravascular signal may become lower at rates higher than 6 mL per second (7). On the other hand, a higher infusion rate results in faster venous return and a shorter bolus length, requiring a shorter measurement time. Always a compromise between imaging time, resolution and arterial/venous time window must be sought. Because for examination of the lower limbs the entire vascular tree from renal arteries to the ankles has to be imaged with high resolution (especially in the lower legs), a long arteriovenous time interval is necessary. Therefore, in the lower extremities injection rates of 0.5 to 1.5 mL per second are used. After injection of contrast agent, the venous system should be flushed with saline to push the contrast medium column from the arm veins into the circulation.

A heavily T1-weighted, spoiled gradient-echo sequence [short repetition time/echo time (TR/TE); flip angle, 25° to 50°] is used in which the achievable field of view, matrix size, scan volume, and number of partitions are determined by the arterial/venous time interval. Subtraction of pre- and postcontrast images is performed to visualize only the arteries for greater ease of image interpretation and to reduce artifacts (Fig. 32.1) (8). The obtained volumetric data set containing high intensity voxels corresponding to arteries can be postprocessed using the maximum-intensity-projection (MIP) algorithm. For improved diagnostic performance, review of the individual source images or reformatting images in the transverse plane is required.

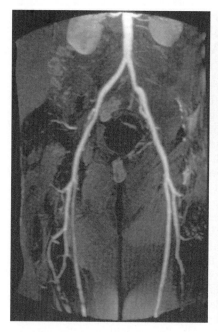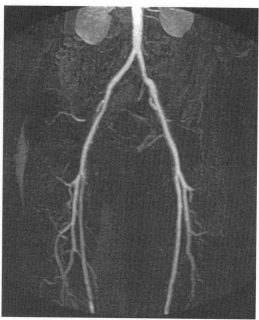

Figure 32.1. Nonsubtracted **(A)** and subtracted **(B)** CE-MRA images of the aortoiliac region. The subtracted image shows higher contrast/background ratio. More vessels can be seen on the subtracted image.

Timing of Image Acquisition

In CE-MRA, adequate timing of the start of data acquisition, with arrival of the contrast agent in the vessels of interest, is essential. Arterial enhancement must coincide with acquisition of central k-lines, and for improved arterial/venous differentiation, the central k-lines have to be sampled before venous return. Essentially, three methods have been developed to ensure proper timing.

Test Bolus

Adequate timing can be performed by measuring the circulation time after intravenous injection of a small test bolus (1 to 2 mL) of contrast agent, using a rapid dynamic imaging sequence. With this dynamic series, the arrival time of the test bolus after injection in the region of interest (ROI) can be imaged and, therefore, the scan delay can be calculated. To avoid pooling of the test bolus in veins, the tubing has to be flushed with saline. Both the test bolus and the final infusion should be injected at the same rate. This timing method is fairly robust and easy to perform. A disadvantage is that the method requires additional administration of contrast agent. It lengthens the total procedure time with 2 to 3 minutes. Also, in case of irregular heart action, the circulation time calculated from the test bolus may sometimes differ from that during injection of the final bolus.

Fluoroscopic Triggering

Fast imaging sequences can be used to visualize the influx of contrast into the region of interest. MRA data acquisition is then started automatically or manually [MR Smart-Prep (9), bolus track (10)]. A disadvantage of this method is the delay of 2 to 4 seconds that occurs between visualizing the arrival of the contrast bolus and actual start of acquisition. Also, time for breathing instructions, if required, may be too short.

Time-resolved Imaging

With ongoing improvements in hardware and gradient technology, the time required to image a large volume of interest with high resolution has greatly reduced. With a 2D slab, the entire anteroposterior diameter of the legs can be covered in 2 to 3 seconds (11). Therefore, by performing a dynamic volumetric series after intravenous injection of the contrast agent, the arterial phase will always be included in one of the data sets, thus obviating the need for bolus timing.

Imaging Strategies

For imaging of the leg vessels, a large anatomic region (approximately 100 cm) has to be covered. Because the longitudinal field of view of MR systems is limited to 45 to 50 cm, complete imaging of the lower extremity requires imaging of several regions (or "stations"). This means repositioning of the patient to the isocenter of the magnet. Two methods for imaging of the entire legs have been developed: so-called multistation/multi-injection imaging and the bolus chase method. In both techniques one has to ensure sufficient overlap between the separate stations. No studies have been performed comparing the two methods directly; however, because of its short examination time and more efficient use of contrast agent, the bolus chase technique is the current standard of practice.

Multistation/Multi-injection Imaging or Step-by-step Technique

With this technique, the three regions of the legs (aortoiliac, femoropopliteal, and infrapopliteal vessels) are imaged sequentially with two or three separate bolus injections of contrast medium (12). Imaging of each station involves acquisition of a mask data set, which is subtracted from the subsequent images obtained after contrast injection. Contrast agent can be injected at moderately high rates of 1 to 1.5

mL per second, ensuring high signal intensity in the vessels. The advantage of this technique is that it can be applied on any clinical scanner without use of special hardware, and imaging parameters can be tailored to every single station. The multistation/multi-injection technique, however, is not very time efficient (30 to 45 minutes per patient); a total contrast agent dose of 0.2 to 0.3 mmol/kg/patient is required, and the contrast-to-noise ratio of the subtracted images becomes less at the second and third stations as a result of circulating gadolinium (Fig. 32.2) (13). Using larger dosages in the subsequent stages can partly circumvent this decrease in signal intensity. Surface coils can be used for imaging of the different stations. Huber et al (14) achieved 100% sensitivity and 94% specificity for identifying 80 hemodynamically significant stenoses and 39 occlusions in 24 patients.

Bolus Chase or Moving-table Technique

In this technique, mask images of all three stations of the legs are made first (10,15–17). Then, during slow constant infusion of contrast agent, the flow of contrast through the legs is chased using a floating table. This technique requires application of special hardware to move the table to predefined positions. This can be done using homemade table-stopping devices or special MR-table hardware. The advantage of the moving-table technique is that it is very rapid (coverage of the entire legs in less than 4 minutes), requiring a relatively low dose of contrast agent (approximately 30 cc).

Formerly, a disadvantage of the stepping-table technique was that the three stations were imaged sequentially while the scan preparation had been optimized for only a single station. Recently, the method has become more flexible (10), and even dedicated surface coils can be used (18,19).

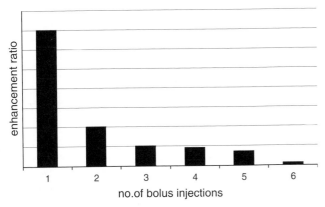

Figure 32.2. Enhancement ratios of subtracted images after repeated injection of gadolinium-DTPA in a flowing phantom model. Repeated injection results in substantially reduced contrast-to-noise ratios. In vivo, however, extravasation of contrast agent also occurs. The effect of intravascular accumulation of contrast will therefore be lower in vivo. (From Westenberg JJ, Wasser MN, van der Geest RJ, et al. Scan optimization of gadolinium-enhanced three-dimensional MRA of peripheral arteries with multiple bolus injections and in vitro validation of stenosis quantification. *Magn Reson Imaging* 1999;17:47–57, with permission.)

Although with the bolus-chase technique, imaging times of the various segments are short, early venous enhancement may sometimes cause difficulties in evaluation of the arteries of the lower leg. This venous overlay may be especially prominent in patients with diabetes, venous ulcers, or cellulitis. Enhancement of the veins in the third station, the lower legs, can be minimized by using an optimized imaging protocol: use of a biphasic injection protocol (e.g., 1 mL per second during 10 seconds and the rest with 0.5 mL per second), use of "centric" k-space acquisition, in which the contrast-determining k-lines are acquired first, and the use of parallel imaging. With simultaneous acquisition of spatial harmonics (SMASH) (20) or sensitivity encoding (SENSE) (21) techniques, combinations of coils can be used to compensate for omitted gradient steps. The increase in imaging speed can be used to reduce acquisition times or to increase resolution of the scan (22). Binkert et al (23) used a dual-bolus technique, in which they started with a dedicated calf MRA and—after a 15-minute interval—proceeded with the moving-table MRA. This led to better visualization of the infrapopliteal arteries with less venous overlay and therefore a significantly increased diagnostic accuracy, compared to moving-table MRA alone. Also, venous compression by means of a tourniquet, either at the midfemoral (24) or at infragenual level (25,26), can be used to slow down the flow in the vessels of the legs.

Image Presentation

To encourage acceptance of the technique by referring clinicians, one has to provide them with images to which they are accustomed and which appear similar to conventional angiography. The number of images should be limited as a practical concern for vascular surgeons. The images should be large to be viewed from a distance, displaying standard angiographic views. Also, bony landmarks should be provided for better orientation, similar to images of conventional angiography (Fig. 32.3).

PITFALLS

Although signal loss owing to turbulence and in-plane saturation is usually not present in CE-MRA, overestimation of the length of a stenosis can still occur, especially at high velocity rates at the stenotic area and a low concentration of contrast material (27).

If the contrast agent arrives in the vessel of interest *after* sampling of the central k-lines as a result of improper timing, a central dark line in the vessel can be seen, the so-called pseudodissection (28).

Care has to be taken to include all vessels of interest in the imaging volume. Inappropriate image coverage may mimic occlusion of tortuous arteries, such as the external iliac arteries (29). Therefore, it is recommended to present also sagittal or transverse views to demonstrate the entire imaging volume (Fig. 32.4).

Sometimes a ghost or phase artifact can be seen parallel to vessels with very high signal intensity (28) (Fig. 32.5). Also, subtraction misregistration artifact may occur. Clips

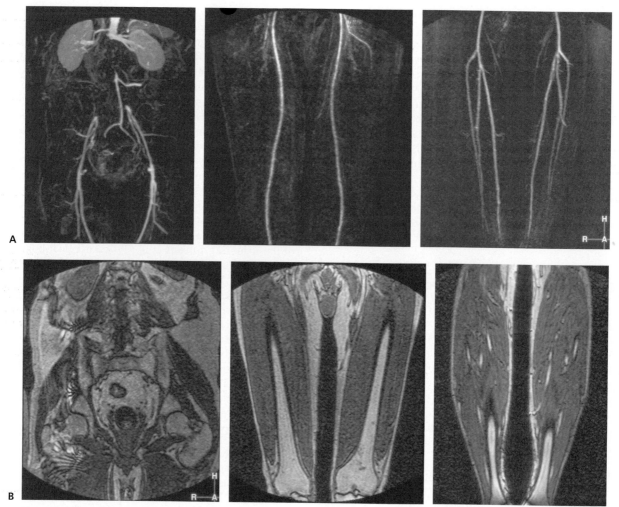

Figure 32.3. Peripheral MRA of the lower limbs in a patient with occlusion of the distal aorta and proximal common iliac arteries **(A)**. The nonsubtracted source images provide the bony land marks, especially of the joints **(B)**.

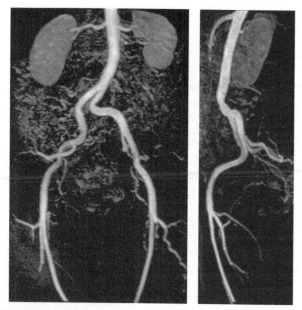

Figure 32.4. Coronal (*left*) and sagittal (*right*) CE-MRA MIP images of the aortoiliac region. Especially the sagittal view shows the elongated external iliac arteries in this patient.

and metallic stents may cause signal voids as a result of susceptibility artifacts (Fig. 32.6).

COMPUTED TOMOGRAPHY ANGIOGRAPHY OF PERIPHERAL ARTERIES

GENERAL

The introduction of multidetector row or multislice CT (MSCT) represented a revolutionary advance in CT technology. Compared with single-slice helical CT, multislice CT offers faster rotation times and simultaneous acquisition of multiple helices per rotation, resulting in shorter acquisition times, increased longitudinal volume coverage, lower dose contrast medium, and improved spatial resolution for assessing smaller arterial branches. With every new generation of multislice scanners, these advantages become more apparent, enabling increased table feed (and therefore shorter examination times) and increased spatial resolution. The developments take place so rapidly that, although there are already 64-slice scanners on the market, at the time of writing only

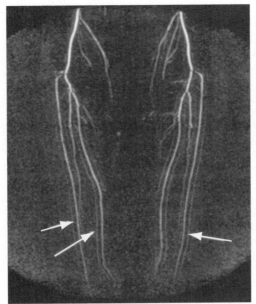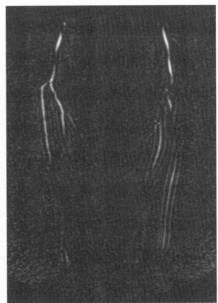

Figure 32.5. Example of ghost artifacts in images of the lower limbs (*arrows*): MIP (*left*) and source image (*right*).

studies with 4-slice scanners have been published (30–36). Overall figures for sensitivity and specificity for detection of hemodynamically significant stenoses are high (>90%), but agreement between digital cardiac angiography (DSA) and CTA is better for the inflow vessels than for the runoff vessels (33,36). The reason for this is probably because with 4-slice scanners within the available arteriovenous time window of 30 to 40 seconds, the longitudinal resolution (slice thickness) is limited to 3 mm. With 8-, 16-, or more slice scanners, spatial resolution can be much higher because of thin collimation and close section spacing. Adriaensen et al (37) assessed the therapeutic confidence of 4-slice CTA and found that physicians had less confidence in CTA than in DSA and requested more often further imaging tests after CTA (35%) than after DSA (14%). Such a study has not been done for 16-slice CTA (and also not for MRA). Only preliminary reports have been published on the use of 16-slice scanners. Balzer et al (38) reported agreement between

CTA and DSA for detecting >70%, 50% to 70%, and <50% stenosis to be 98%, 95%, and 91%, respectively.

Radiation dose is an issue in MSCT, but in the age group of patients with intermittent claudication, it is probably not very important. Moreover, the radiation dose in conventional angiography is approximately four times as high as in MSCT (30).

TECHNIQUE FOR PERIPHERAL COMPUTED TOMOGRAPHY ANGIOGRAPHY

As in CE-MRA, the principle behind peripheral multislice CTA is imaging the arterial phase of contrast enhancement before substantial interstitial or venous enhancement occurs. The advent of multislice scanning has enabled chasing of the contrast bolus while maintaining high spatial resolution. High spatial resolution is especially required for imaging of

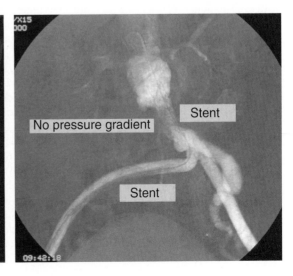

Figure 32.6. Patient with aorto-iliac bifurcation prosthesis and implantation of stents in the distal aorta and right iliac leg of the prosthesis. At MRA (*left*) susceptibility artifacts falsely suggest significant stenoses in the stents; no pressure gradient was found on angiography (*right*).

the infrapopliteal vessels. Using a 16-slice scanner in our department, we therefore choose to obtain 1-mm slices in the aortoiliac and femoral segments (to go for speed) and 0.5-mm slices in the infrapopliteal segments (to go for spatial resolution). Total acquisition time for imaging from the suprarenal aorta down to the toes is 30 to 35 seconds. With modern 16-slice scanners (with gantry rotation of 0.5 or 0.4 seconds), to run ahead of the bolus is even possible! The table feed should therefore not exceed 50 mm per second (39).

As in CE-MRA, the delay time between contrast injection and start of the scan may be determined by a test bolus (20 cc). A region of interest is drawn in the distal aorta, and, after injection of the test bolus, low dose scans of the ROI are obtained in a dynamic (nonincremental) fashion. The time to peak enhancement is then chosen as scan-delay time. Most often, automated bolus timing is performed, in which scanning is started after the enhancement in the region of interest has exceeded a predefined enhancement level (e.g., 100 HU). After this threshold is reached, scanning is started following a delay of 4 to 12 seconds. This delay is required to allow the scanner to move from the ROI-measurement level to the level at which scanning is to begin.

Because CT is less sensitive than MR for contrast enhancement, a larger volume of contrast agent (120 to 160 mL) has to be injected in CTA, compared to MRA at a higher rate (3 to 4 mL per second). The level of enhancement of the arteries depends on the infusion rate and the type of contrast agent used. If a contrast agent with an iodine concentration of 370 to 400 mg per cc is used, the injection rate can be lower than if a contrast medium with 300 mg iodine per cc is used. The total amount of contrast agent needed depends on the scan duration. Total duration of injection can be 5 to 10 seconds shorter than the actual scanning time (40). After injection of contrast agent, the venous system should be flushed with saline. Saline flushing prolongs arterial enhancement.

VISUALIZATION TECHNIQUES

In CTA, similar to MRA, postprocessing of the data and 3D reconstruction is primarily done using maximum intensity projection. Because it is a projection technique, structures with high attenuation, such as bones, are superimposed over the enhancing vessels. Therefore, before applying the MIP algorithm, segmentation of bony structures is necessary to visualize the vessels in their entirety (Fig. 32.7). An important disadvantage of MIP reformation is that calcified plaques and stents can obscure visualization of the lumen, especially when the calcium has a significant circumferential extent (Fig. 32.8). For a better overview of these difficult areas with calcifications and stents, a curved multiplanar reconstruction or central luminal line can be made (Fig. 32.9A). Large calcifications in the MIP can be removed by segmentation using the algorithm for bone removal (Figs. 32.9B, 32.10, and 32.11). This segmentation method, however, is too crude to be used in segments with small calcifications, i.e., in the lower legs (Figs. 32.12 and 32.13). Another disadvantage of the MIP algorithm is that vessel edges and stenoses may not be accurately mapped because of decreased attenuation or signal secondary to partial volume effects.

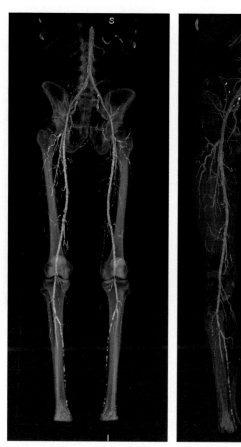

Figure 32.7. Volume rendering (*left*) and MIP projection (*right*) of a CTA study in a 62-year-old patient with diabetes mellitus (see also Fig. 32.13). To visualize the entire arterial tree in the MIP image, skeletal structures were removed by segmentation.

With improvements in computer technology, volume rendering is therefore increasingly used for 3D reconstruction of the data. In volume rendering, no data are discarded. Opacification of a voxel, ranging from transparency to total opacity, is assigned based on the attenuation coefficient. Because the image is inclusive off all voxels acquired, there are no surfaces. Because both opacification and lighting effects are coded in gray scale, color is often added to clarify the image features. Color is assigned on the basis of the attenuation coefficient of a voxel (Fig. 32.8).

CLINICAL APPLICATIONS OF PERIPHERAL MAGNETIC RESONANCE ANGIOGRAPHY AND COMPUTED TOMOGRAPHY ANGIOGRAPHY

ATHEROSCLEROSIS

Atherosclerosis is a systemic process that may cause stenosis, occlusion, or aneurysmal dilatation of the affected arteries.

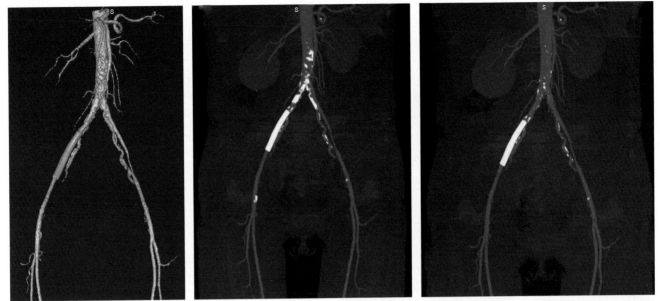

Figure 32.8. Volume rendering (*left*) and MIP image (*middle*) of a CTA examination in a 56-year-old man with atherosclerosis after stent placement in the right external iliac artery. Large calcified atherosclerotic lesions were present in the distal aorta and both common iliac arteries. The calcified plaques could be removed by segmentation, and evaluation of patency of the stent was not possible.

Steno-occlusive Disease

In patients with acute limb threatening ischemia, angiographic imaging is performed as soon as possible, followed by thrombolytic therapy in the same session. MRA or CTA has no role in the management of this condition.

In patients with chronic ischemia, however, MRA has emerged as a valuable alternative pretreatment procedure to catheter angiography. In analyzing MRA images of the lower limbs of patients with intermittent claudication, one has to understand what the treating physician wants to know. In other words, one has to "think as a vascular radiologist," and one has to be familiar with the clinical issues and the potential treatment options (41). Analyzing the proximal inflow to a lesion, the distal outflow from the lesion, and the lesion itself is important. If the inflow is impaired, a distal arterial reconstruction may be endangered. On the other hand, if the outflow is limited, a proximal reconstruction may be compromised. A general rule in vascular surgery is to first treat the most proximal lesions, because they usually have the greatest impact on flow to the limbs.

Regarding the lesion itself, it is important to report the localization, severity, and length of the stenosis. In general, hemodynamically significant stenoses, usually taken as >50% luminal narrowing, require treatment. In case of borderline stenosis (40% to 60%), it may be difficult to determine the hemodynamic significance of the lesion. This, however, also holds for conventional angiography, and, in these cases, intravascular pressure measurements are performed to assess the hemodynamic implications of a lesion (42). In almost all studies evaluating the value of MRA, conventional DSA is taken as the standard of reference. This standard, however, may not be as "gold" as one is inclined to believe. Eccentric plaques in the large proximal vessels may go undetected with DSA because of the limited number of projec-

tions (Fig. 32.14). In the renal arteries we found a sensitivity of only 70% for DSA in detecting hemodynamically significant stenoses when compared with intravascular pressure measurements (43). In the iliac arteries, Wikström et al (44) found sensitivities/specificities of 86%/88% for DSA, 81%/75% for MRA, and 72%/88% for duplex, in detection of significant stenoses using an aortofemoral pressure gradient of 20 mm Hg indicating hemodynamic significance. Probably, conventional angiography is also not an adequate standard of reference in analyzing runoff vessels, because CE-MRA demonstrated more patent vessels than did conventional angiography (Fig. 32.15) (45,46).

Duplex Doppler ultrasonography (US) is an accurate method to detect stenoses in the carotid arteries. Also in the lower limbs, duplex ultrasound has been shown to be a reliable noninvasive diagnostic modality (47,48). Duplex US, however, is operator-dependent, laborious, and it does not provide a complete road map for treatment planning.

Recently, a meta-analysis was done based on 9 papers on CE-MRA (216 patients) and 18 on color-guided duplex US (1,059 patients) (49). In all of these papers, conventional angiography was used as the gold standard. The pooled sensitivity of CE-MRA for assessing arterial disease (i.e., >50% luminal reduction) in these studies was 97% (95% CI: 95.7% to 99.3%) and for duplex US, 87.6% (95% CI: 84.4% to 90.8%). The pooled specificities were similar (96.2% for CE-MRA and 94.7% for duplex US). These figures for CE-MRA correspond to the ones reported in the meta-analysis mentioned earlier, comparing 2D TOF with CE-MRA.

In almost all duplex US studies, results for the different stations were reported, but this was done in only five of nine CE-MRA studies. Stratification per anatomic site was therefore not possible. In general, the interval between CE-MRA and conventional angiography was shorter (mean: 5

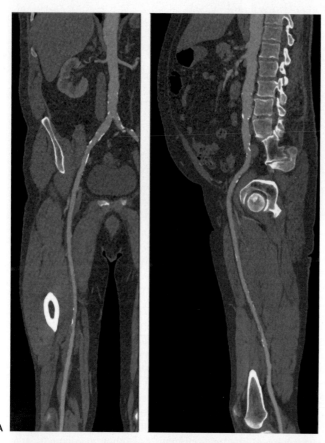

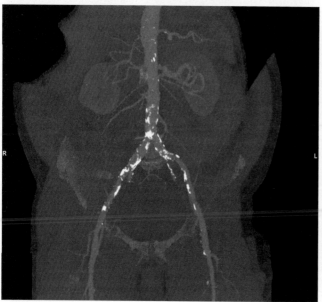

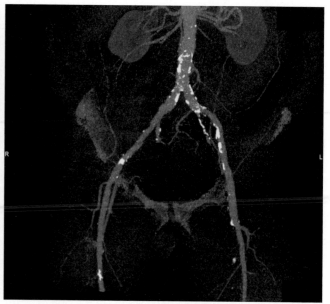

Figure 32.9. CTA images of a 56-year-old man with multiple atherosclerotic lesions in the distal aorta and iliac arteries. Curved multiplanar reformatted image or center luminal line reconstruction (**A**) shows patent right iliac arteries, despite extensive calcified plaques as visualized on the MIP reconstruction (**B**, *left*). After segmentation of the disfications, patency of the right iliac arteries is also visible on MIP (**B**, *right*).

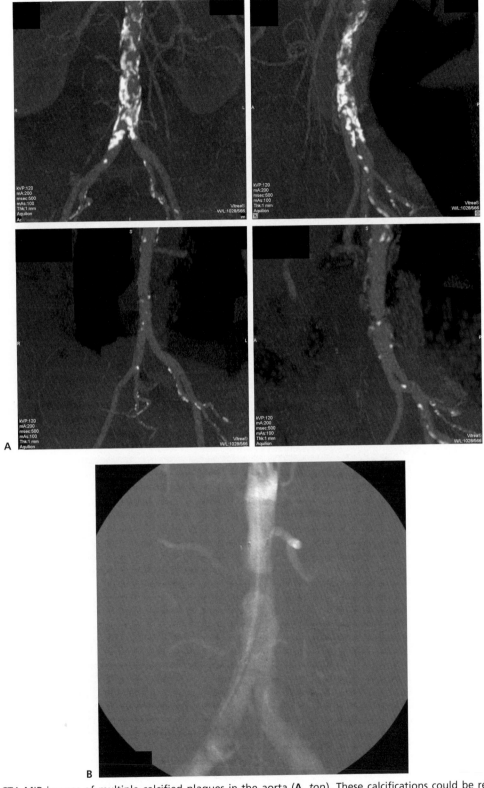

Figure 32.10. CTA-MIP images of multiple calcified plaques in the aorta (**A**, *top*). These calcifications could be removed from the images by segmentation (**A**, *bottom*). On the segmented images, a stenosis was appreciated in the distal aorta. This stenosis was also visible on DSA **(B)**.

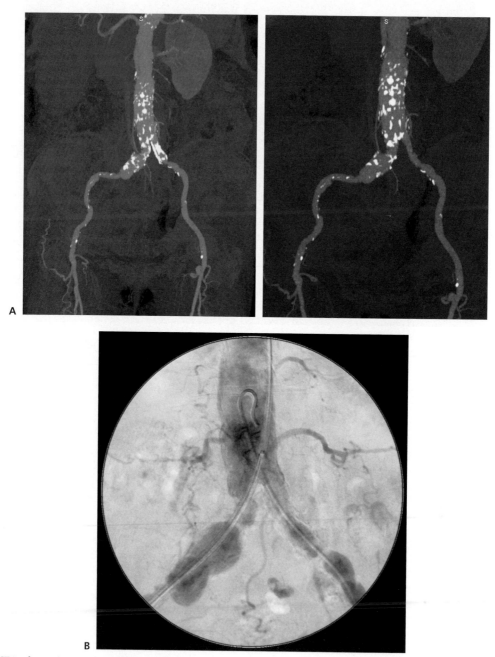

Figure 32.11. CTA of a patient with multiple calcifications in the distal aorta and iliac arteries **(A)**. An aneurysm of the right common iliac artery is seen, also visible on DSA **(B)**. Because of a large calcified plaque, patency of the left common iliac artery cannot be assessed **(A**, *left)*. After segmentation, the left common iliac artery appears patent **(B**, *right)*, which was confirmed at DSA **(B)**.

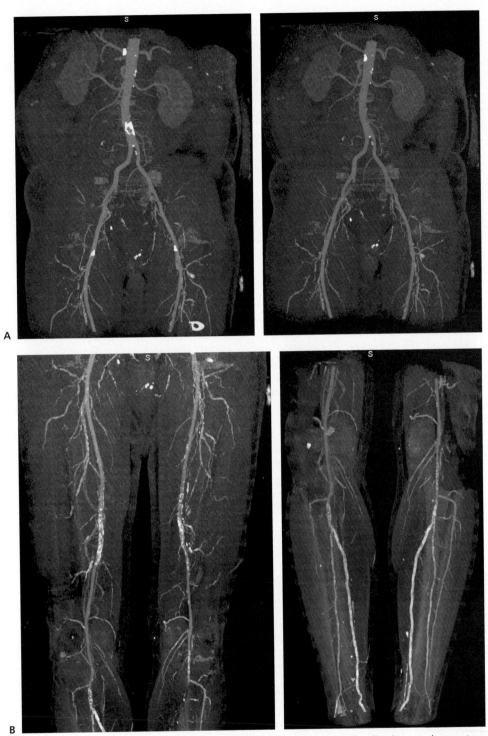

Figure 32.12. CTA of a 52-year-old patient with diabetes. A large calcified plaque in the distal aorta does not result in stenosis of the aorta **(A)**, before (*left*) and after (*right*) segmentation of the calcification. Smaller calcifications in the femoral and infrapopliteal arteries could not be removed **(B)**.

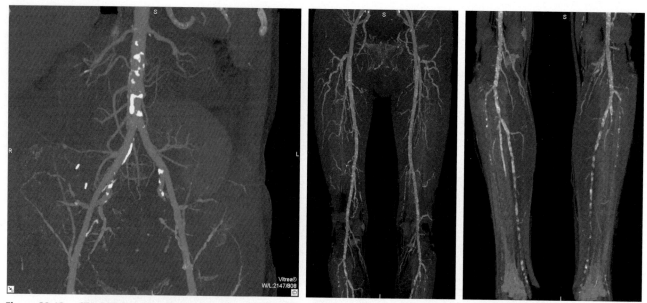

Figure 32.13. CTA-MIP images of a 53-year-old woman with diabetes. Extensive calcifications, especially in the infrapopliteal vessels, were not removable by segmentation.

days) than between duplex US and angiography (mean: 17 days). One might expect that as the interval between the studied examination and the reference examination increases, the discriminatory power of the studied examination decreases. This was indeed found for duplex US. The lower sensitivity of duplex US in the reported studies may therefore be partly attributed to the longer interval between duplex and angiography.

It appears that, because of its high sensitivity and specificity, CE-MRA may replace conventional angiography in the workup of patients with intermittent claudication (Figs. 32.15 to 32.18). Color-guided duplex US can then be reserved to determine the hemodynamic significance of stenoses found on CE-MRA.

As mentioned previously, mainly CTA studies using 4-slice scanners have been published with acceptable results (sensitivity for detection of significant stenoses >90%). Results with newer generation scanners will be better.

Intermittent claudication is commonly caused by stenosis or occlusion of vessels in the legs. Sometimes, however, the symptoms may be caused by severe stenosis or occlusion of the aorta (Leriche syndrome). Also, this entity can be visualized with CE-MRA (50) (Figs. 32.3 and 32.19).

ANEURYSMS

CE-MRA has been found to be adequate in demonstrating the extent of aortoiliac aneurysmal disease (51). Aneurysms

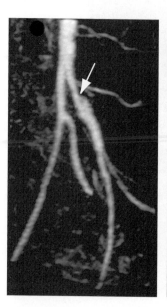
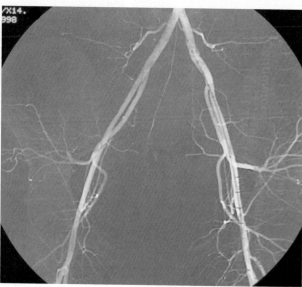

Figure 32.14. Patient with atherosclerotic lesion in the left common iliac artery, as visualized on MRA (*left*). The stenosis, located on the dorsal wall of the vessel, was not appreciated at angiography (*right*), although a pressure gradient of 25 mm Hg was measured.

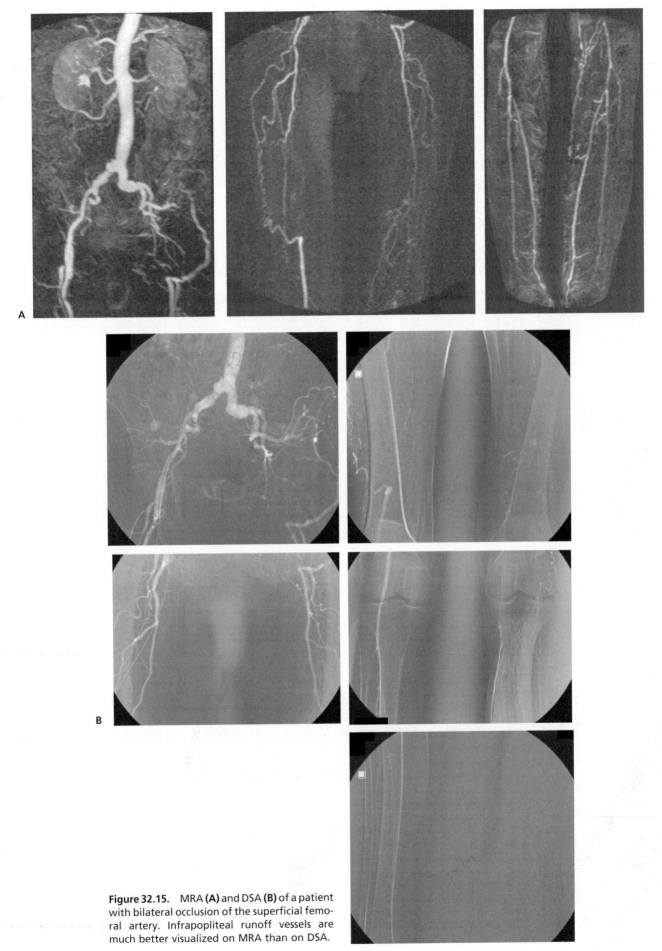

Figure 32.15. MRA **(A)** and DSA **(B)** of a patient with bilateral occlusion of the superficial femoral artery. Infrapopliteal runoff vessels are much better visualized on MRA than on DSA.

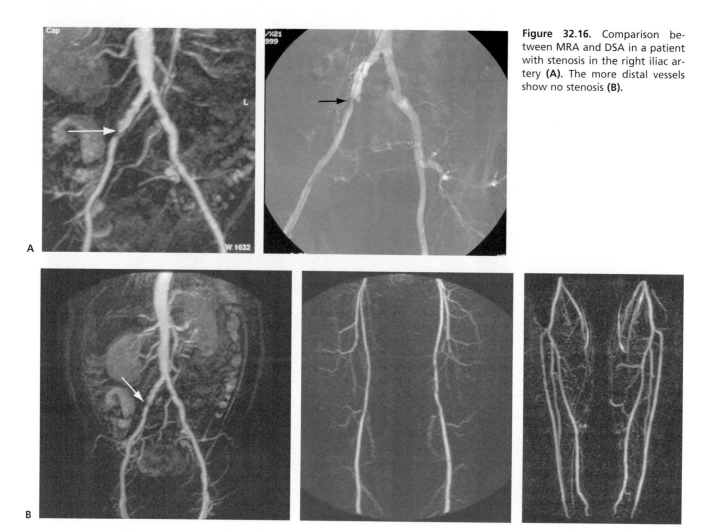

Figure 32.16. Comparison between MRA and DSA in a patient with stenosis in the right iliac artery **(A)**. The more distal vessels show no stenosis **(B)**.

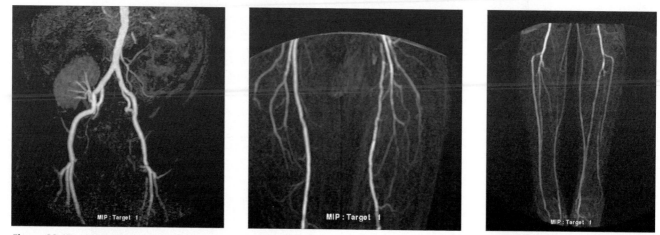

Figure 32.17. MRA-MIP images of a patient with a kidney transplant in the right iliac fossa and a short occlusion proximally in the left superficial femoral artery.

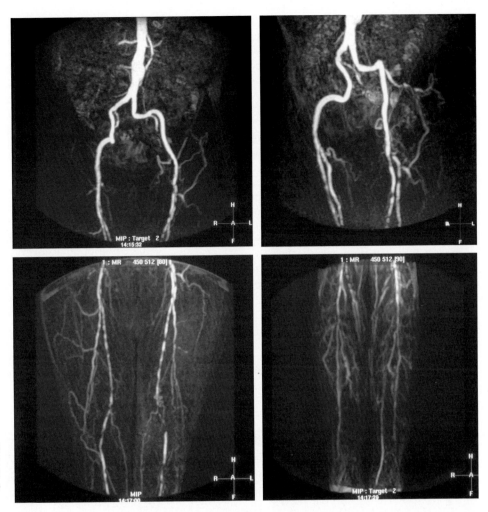

Figure 32.18. MRA of a patient with multiple bilateral stenoses in both femoral and infrapopliteal arteries and short occlusion in the left femoral artery.

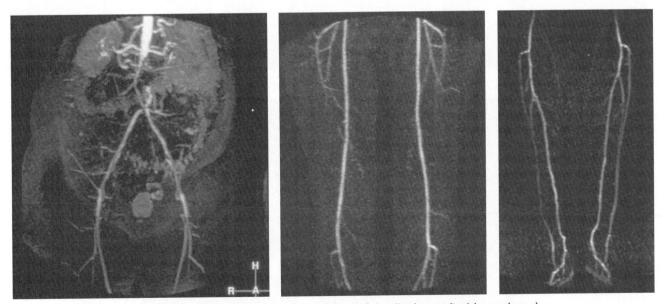

Figure 32.19. MRA of a patient with occlusion of the distal aorta (Leriche syndrome).

may also occur in the femoral and popliteal arteries. Popliteal aneurysm is an important entity, because up to one-third of patients have either distal embolization or severe acute limb ischemia from an unrecognized and nonpalpable popliteal aneurysm (52). Femoral aneurysms are less important and they may be followed conservatively (53,54). In a study in 313 patients with abdominal aortic aneurysms (AAA) who all underwent ultrasound examination of the femoropopliteal region, Diwan et al (55) encountered femoral and popliteal aneurysms in 12% of patients (36 patients with 51 peripheral aneurysms, of which 31 were popliteal aneurysms). The peripheral aneurysms occurred only in men with AAA (incidence 14%), no aneurysms were found in the 62 women with AAA. The reason for this sex difference is not known. In 14 (39%) of the 36 men with peripheral aneurysms, peripheral occlusive disease was present as opposed to 20 (9%) of the 215 men without peripheral aneurysm.

Also, popliteal aneurysms can be detected on CE-MRA. (Important: view individual coronal images, Fig. 32.20, or CTA.)

DIABETES

Diabetes-related angiopathy is an important cause of nontraumatic lower extremity amputations in the industrialized world. Diabetic patients often suffer from long segments of arterial occlusions, especially of the infrapopliteal vessels (Fig. 32.21). Surgical reconstitution of blood flow remains the most important therapeutic option for limb salvage in these patients. Improvements in bypass graft technology have enabled the use of the pedal arteries as target sites. For planning of distal revascularizations, information on distal vessels in the foot (including the pedal arch) is necessary. Some studies have indicated that even 2D TOF MRA can demonstrate patent distal vessels, not visible on conventional angiography (44,56). Kreitner et al (57) evaluated the value of CE-MRA in 24 diabetic patients, using the head coil for signal reception. All patients underwent angiography for comparison within 5 days. Seven vascular segments were evaluated in each extremity: distal anterior tibial artery, distal posterior tibial artery, distal peroneal artery, dorsal pedal artery, lateral plantar artery, medial plantar artery, and plantar arch. Of possible 168 segments, 74 were seen to be patent on DSA and 104 on CE-MRA. Thirty vessel segments that were suitable for distal grafting in 9 (38%) patients were seen exclusively on MRA. In seven of the nine patients this resulted in a change of treatment plans. Therefore, this study shows that in diabetic patients with severe peripheral occlusive disease, CE-MRA should be used for pedal bypass planning, instead of DSA.

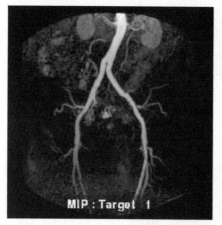
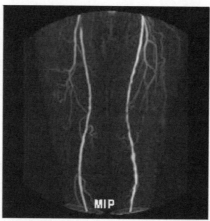
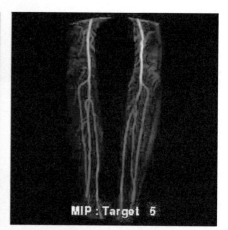

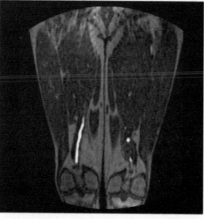
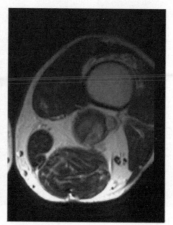

Figure 32.20. MRA of a patient with aneurysm of the left popliteal artery, not clearly visible on the MIP images but well recognizable on the unsubtracted images and transverse T2 transverse, sagital, coronal (TSE) images.

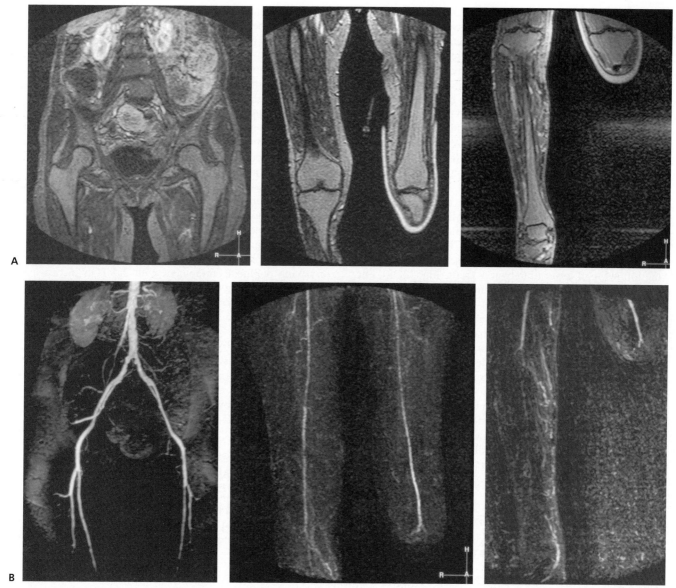

Figure 32.21. MRA of a patient with diabetes, after amputation of the left lower leg **(A)**. Persistent ulceration and ischemia of the right lower leg as a result of occlusion of the infrapopliteal arteries **(B)**.

SURVEILLANCE OF PERIPHERAL BYPASS GRAFTS

CE-MRA may also be used in the postoperative follow-up of arterial bypass grafts. Peripheral bypass grafts may consist of autologous saphenous vein, expanded polytetrafluoroethylene (PTFE) or Dacron. Autologous venous grafts have a superior patency rate compared to the other grafts, but still a 12% incidence of bypass graft stenosis in the first postoperative year. Eighty percent of stenosis occurs during the first postoperative year, and almost all occur in the first 18 months (58). In 60% of cases of stenosis this occurs with no initial clinical symptoms (58). Therefore, these bypasses are carefully monitored to detect stenosis in time to enable reconstitution of flow (secondary patency). Surveillance criteria, such as the ankle-brachial index, have been successfully tested. Also, duplex US is routinely performed for surveillance. Midgraft peak systolic velocity (PSV), PSV ratio

before and after stenosis can be calculated, or the entire graft can be visualized. Conventional angiography is performed when an abnormality at duplex US is found and when a vascular intervention is needed.

Duplex US is adequate in assessing graft patency, and it can detect stenoses adequately. However, duplex US is limited in detecting collateral flow, and also proximal lesions that may endanger future patency of the graft may be missed at duplex US.

Three studies evaluated the use of CE-MRA in surveillance of lower limb grafts. Bertschinger et al (59) evaluated 30 patients with 31 grafts who underwent both IA-DSA and CE-MRA. All abnormalities (10 stenoses, 9 occlusions, and 8 aneurysms or ectasias) could be visualized by CE-MRA (sensitivity, 100%). Because 6 segments could not be evaluated, specificity was 90.3%. Bendib et al (60) selected 23 patients with 40 vascular grafts with either clinical symptoms or abnormal duplex findings. All patients also underwent x-ray angiography. MRA depicted 38 grafts (95%) with 28 abnormalities. Two stenoses were overestimated. Some grafts had more than one abnormality. Sensitivity and specificity for detection of stenoses and occlusions of CE-MRA were 91% and 95%, respectively. In five cases, CE-MRA showed extra complications: four nonthrombotic ectasias not seen on ultrasound and one thrombotic ectasia, overlooked at conventional angiography. Meissner et al (61) performed MRA in 24 patients with 26 femorotibial or femoropedal grafts. The degree of stenosis at MRA was compared to findings at duplex US, and, in case of discrepancy, to DSA findings. In 109 of 117 evaluated segments (93%), MRA and duplex US showed concordant findings. In eight discordant segments in seven patients, duplex US overlooked four high-grade stenoses, correctly identified at MRA and confirmed by DSA. In no case did MRA miss an area of stenosis of sufficient severity to require treatment. These data strongly suggest that MRA is well suited as a screening method in the follow-up of lower limb bypass grafts (Fig. 32.22). Further study to analyze the cost-benefit ratio is required to assess whether CE-MRA can be used as the single follow-up examination and road map for additional reconstruction.

Using a 4-slice scanner, Willmann et al (62) found no statistically significant difference in sensitivity or specificity between CTA and duplex US for detection of hemodynamically significant bypass stenosis or occlusion, aneurismal changes, or arteriovenous fistulas.

CE-MRA also appears useful in the surveillance of extra-anatomic bypass grafts. These grafts are made of PTFE or Dacron; veins cannot be used. Possible reconstructions in the lower limbs are axillofemoral grafts, femorofemoral crossover bypasses (Fig. 32.23), and thoracic aortofemoral artery bypass grafts (63).

POPLITEAL ENTRAPMENT SYNDROME

Intermittent claudication in younger patients, without signs of atherosclerotic disease, may be caused by the so-called *popliteal entrapment syndrome*. The incidence of the syndrome in the general population is 0.16% to 3.5% (64). Popliteal entrapment is caused by an anomalous relationship between the gastrocnemic muscle and the popliteal artery (65). It can be the result of an anomalous course of the popliteal artery, medial to the medial head of the gastrocnemic muscle. An abnormal insertion of the medial head of the gastrocnemic muscle may also result in compression of the popliteal artery during exercise. Finally, also "functional entrapment" is reported, in which the popliteal artery is compressed by a hypertrophic gastrocnemic muscle with a normal anatomic relationship between the two structures (66). Potential treatment options are transsection of the anomalous medial gastrocnemic head or stent implantation in the popliteal artery. Thus far, conventional angiography in rest and during active plantar flexion against resistance is the method of choice to demonstrate popliteal artery compression during stress. DSA, however, does not show the cause of the entrapment syndrome.

Cross-sectional imaging may show the cause of entrapment. Di Cesare et al (67) examined six patients suspected of having popliteal entrapment with 2D TOF in rest and during active plantar flexion of the foot against resistance. In the transverse images, during stress the compressed popliteal artery could be visualized as well as anomalous anatomic relationships.

The diagnosis of popliteal entrapment can also be made with CE-MRA in rest and during stress. By using reconstructions of the nonsubtracted 3D data set, the anomalous anatomy can be visualized. Figure 32.24 shows compression of the popliteal artery by the gastrocnemic muscle during stress, as visualized by CE-MRA.

COMPARISON BETWEEN PERIPHERAL MAGNETIC RESONANCE ANGIOGRAPHY AND COMPUTED TOMOGRAPHY ANGIOGRAPHY

Thus far, no studies have been published comparing multi-slice CTA and MRA in assessment of patency of the peripheral vessel directly. Willman et al (68) compared the performance of CTA and MRA in evaluation of stenoses in the

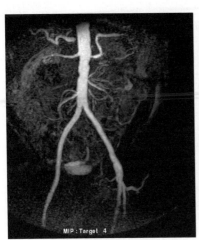
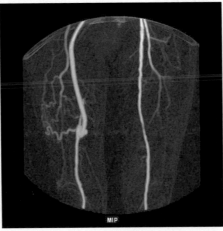
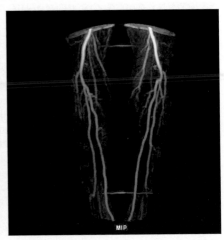

Figure 32.22. MRA-MIP images of a patient with an aortic bifurcation prosthesis. Distal anastomosis is shown on the external iliac artery (*left*) and on the superficial femoral artery (*right*).

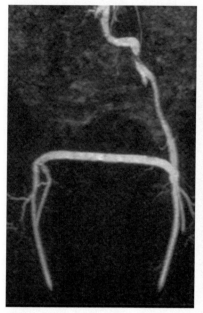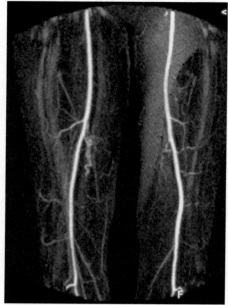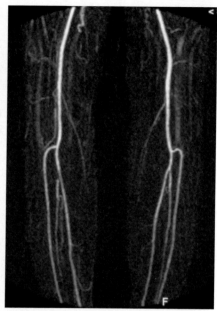

Figure 32.23. MRA-MIP images of a patient with a patent femorofemoral crossover bypass. The right iliac arteries are occluded.

renal and aortoiliac arteries and found no significant differences in detecting hemodynamically significant stenoses: sensitivity and specificity figures (two observers) were 92%/93% and 100%/99% for MRA and 91%/92% and 99%/99% for CTA, respectively. However, a significant difference in examination time occurred: on average, 24 minutes for CTA and 35 minutes for MRA. On the other hand, times required for 3D reconstruction and image interpretation were much longer for CTA (20 to 45 minutes) than for MRA (5 to 9 minutes). The most time-consuming procedure in CTA is segmentation of surrounding nonvascular structures.

They also examined patient acceptance of the various examination procedures. Patients found MS-CTA the least uncomfortable procedure and DSA the most uncomfortable procedure. Surprisingly, no statistically significant difference occurred in patient acceptance between DSA and MRA. The most disturbing factors in MRA are noise, having to keep still, and the lengthy procedure and arterial puncture and postprocedural application of pressure in DSA.

NEW DEVELOPMENTS

MAGNETIC RESONANCE ANGIOGRAPHY TECHNIQUE

Ongoing hardware and gradient improvements result in shorter scan times, enabling time-resolved imaging with high resolution. Time-resolved imaging will continue to improve with higher resolution, real-time reconstruction, and viewing capabilities (69). Besides obviating the need for contrast bolus timing, time-resolved imaging also adds an extra dimension to imaging of the peripheral arteries. Because of the dynamic nature of the series, visualizing differences in influx of contrast agent in the two limbs is possible, similar to conventional angiography. Also, the use of mag-

nets with higher field strengths (3 T) will result in improved visualization of small infrapopliteal vessels and better delineation of stenoses (70).

In addition, dedicated coils for peripheral vascular imaging will probably be more commonly used. These dedicated coils will not only result in images with higher resolution and signal-to-noise ratios, but—in case of phased array coils—also may aid in reducing imaging times by allowing acquisition of data in parallel.

MAGNETIC RESONANCE CONTRAST AGENTS

In MR arteriography of the lower limbs, when extracellular contrast agents, such as gadolinium-DTPA, are administered at a low infusion rate, venous enhancement occurs relatively late as a result of diffusion into the interstitium. The disadvantage of using low infusion rates is the dilution of contrast agent in the bloodstream, with resulting relatively moderate enhancement. Using higher infusion rates results in higher local concentration of the contrast agent in the vessels of interest, but at the cost of faster venous return and a shorter arterial/venous time window for imaging. A possible solution to this problem may be the use of higher concentration formulations, such as gadobutrol 1.0 molar (Gadovist, Schering, Berlin, Germany) (71,72). With these extracellular contrast agents, however, extravasation into the interstitium results in reduced contrast-to-background ratios.

Therefore, new contrast agents have been developed that stay within the blood compartment with no, or little, interstitial diffusion, the so-called *blood pool agents.* This does not necessarily imply prolonged residence of these agents in the body. In fact, for safety reasons, it is desirable that blood pool agents are excreted rapidly at almost "extracellular" speed, or even faster. The first generation of blood pool agents showed little interstitial diffusion, but

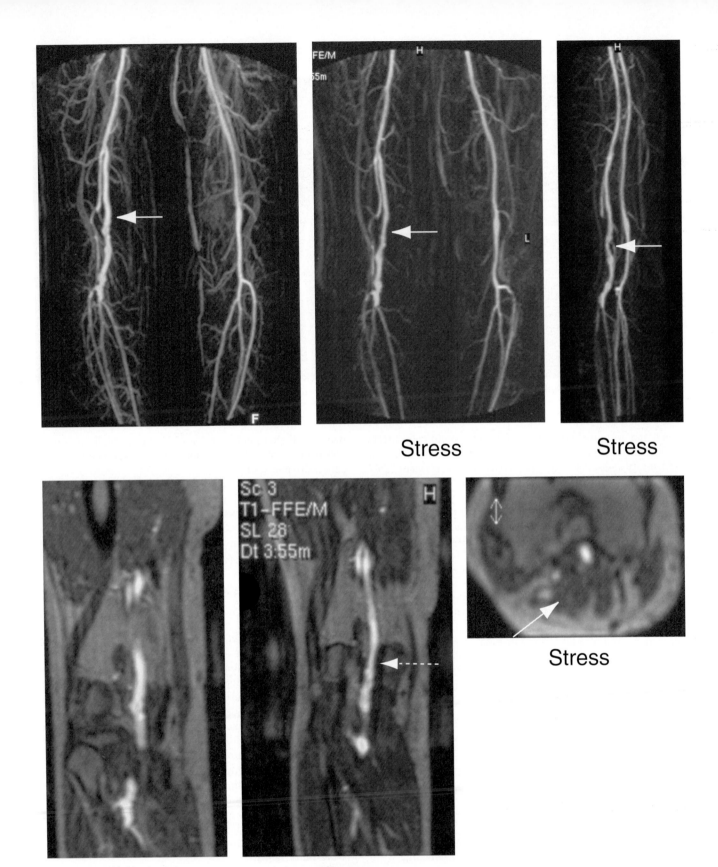

Stress

Stress

Stress

Stress

Figure 32.24. MRA images of a 27-year-old male long distance runner with recurrence of claudication. He previously underwent femoropopliteal bypass grafting for severe stenosis of the right popliteal artery. At rest, no stenosis is present. **(A)** During plantar flexion of the foot with extended knee joint, compression of the bypass by the gastrocnemic muscle can be seen on MRA: coronal (*middle*) and sagittal MIP projection (*right*). **(B)** Coronal unsubtracted source image and transverse reconstructed image of the MRA study show the compression of the bypass between the medial and lateral head of the gastrocnemic muscle and the medial femoral condyle.

long blood residence times, and never reached clinical testing. They consisted of paramagnetic chelates covalently bound to macromolecules, such as polylysine, albumin, polysaccharides, or lipids. The newer paramagnetic (Gd-based) blood pool agents have much faster clearing rates but show no, or little, interstitial diffusion. This has been accomplished by producing agents that bind reversibly to macromolecules, such as albumin, for instance, MS-325 (EPIX).

A separate paramagnetic contrast agent, MultiHance (Bracco), that binds weakly to albumin has been tested in clinical trials (73,74). Through the weak protein binding, interstitial diffusion is diminished but not absent. Multi-Hance, therefore, is not a blood pool agent *in sensu strictu*.

Comprising another class of blood pool agents are the superparamagnetic particles containing iron oxide, such as PEG-Ferron (Nycomed Amersham), AngioMark (EPIX), and Combidex (Advanced Magnetics).

The major advantage of both the paramagnetic and super-paramagnetic intravascular agents, and also of MultiHance, is the higher relaxivity as compared to the extracellular agents. This property can be used to obtain higher signal in the vessels or to lower the dose and injection volume requirement.

The major disadvantage of blood pool agents is the early venous enhancement leaving a small time window for arterial imaging. This early venous enhancement will not cause a problem in imaging of the larger vessels, such as the iliac and femoral arteries because of the possibilities of selective projection reconstructions. In the lower legs, however, this venous overlap will seriously deteriorate imaging of the arteries.

Considering the good results that have been obtained with extracellular agents, the problem of venous overlap has to be solved before blood pool agents can ever be successfully applied in peripheral MRA. Potential solutions to this problem can be found in the development of special postprocessing techniques, such as venous subtraction algorithms (75). Or, possibly, algorithms may be developed that incorporate phase information into the image and provide it as an overlay indicating the direction of flow, thus enabling arterial and venous differentiation, as in color Doppler (76).

COMPUTED TOMOGRAPHY ANGIOGRAPHY TECHNIQUE

Multidetector CT technology will continue to develop, enabling faster scanning with higher resolution. Possibly, the calcification problem will be solved, e.g., by performing a low-dose mask scan, followed by the regular CTA examination. Calcifications can then be removed by subtracting the scans. Also, postprocessing of CTA data will be made less cumbersome by introduction of automatic segmentation software.

SUMMARY

In 2003, Visser et al (77) concluded that CTA, compared to MRA, will be cost-effective if the costs are $300 or less, if

sensitivity for detection of significant stenoses is higher than 94%, and if 20% or fewer patients require additional workup. With using a 4-slice CT, it has been found that after CTA 35% of patients needed additional imaging before adequate treatment planning (37). CTA on 4-slice scanners is therefore not a cost-effective alternative to MRA. Considering the rapid progress in multidetector technology, however, CTA using newer generation CT scanners will probably prove cost-effective.

Which of the two modalities—CTA or MRA—will eventually prevail for imaging of the peripheral vessels is difficult to say. Considering the disadvantages of CTA (use of iodinated contrast agents and difficulties in assessment of patency of vessels, in case of calcified plaques), an indication for MRA will remain in patients with diabetes and impaired renal function. In other patients, it will depend on local facilities, infrastructure, and local experience to determine which of the two modalities will be used for noninvasive imaging of the peripheral arteries.

REFERENCES

1. Martin EC. Transcatheter therapies in peripheral and nonvascular disease. *Circulation* 1991;83:1–5.
2. Waugh JR, Sacharias N. Arteriographic complications in the DSA era. *Radiology* 1992;138:237–281.
3. Goldman K, Salvesen S, Hegedus V. Acute renal failure after contrast medium injection. *Invest Radiol* 1984;S19:S125.
4. Niendorf HP, Haustein J, Louton T, et al. Safety and tolerance after intravenous administration of 0.3 mmol/kg Gd-DTPA: results of a randomized, controlled clinical trial. *Invest Radiol* 1991;26(Suppl 1):221S–225S.
5. Nelemans PJ, Leiner T, de Vet HCW, et al. Peripheral arterial disease: meta-analysis of the diagnostic performance of MR angiography. *Radiology* 2000;217;105–114.
6. Prince MR, Yucel EK, Kaufman JA, et al. Dynamic gadolinium-enhanced three-dimensional abdominal MR arteriography. *J Magn Reson Imaging* 1993;3:677–881.
7. Kopka L, Vosshenrich R, Rodenwaldt J, et al. Differences in injecting rates on contrast-enhanced breath-hold three-dimensional MR angiography. *AJR* 1998;170:345–348.
8. Ho KY, de Haan MW, Kessels AG, et al. Peripheral vascular tree stenosis: detection with subtracted and nonsubtracted MR angiography. *Radiology* 1998;206:673–681.
9. Foo TKF, Saranathan M, Prince MR, et al. Automated detection of bolus arrival and initiation of data acquisition in fast, three-dimensional MR angiography image quality. *Radiology* 1997;203:275–280.
10. Leiner T, Ho KY, Nelemans PJ, et al. Three-dimensional contrast-enhanced moving-bed infusion-tracking (MoBi-track) peripheral MR angiography with flexible choice of imaging parameters for each field of view. *J Magn Reson Imaging* 2000; 11:368–377.
11. Frayne R, Grist TM, Swan JS, et al. 3D MR DSA: effects of injection protocol and image masking. *J Magn Reson Imaging* 2000;12:476–487.
12. Watanabe Y, Dohke M, Okumura A, et al. Dynamic subtraction contrast-enhanced MR angiography: technique, clinical applications, and pitfalls. *Radiographics* 2000;20:135–152.
13. Westenberg JJ, Wasser MN, van der Geest RJ, et al. Scan optimization of gadolinium-enhanced three-dimensional MRA of peripheral arteries with multiple bolus injections and in vitro validation of stenosis quantification. *Magn Reson Imaging* 1999;17:47–57.

14. Huber A, Heuck A, Bauer A, et al. Dynamic contrast-enhanced MR angiography from the distal aorta to the ankle joint with a step-by-step techniques. *AJR Am J Roentgenol* 2000; 175: 1291–1298.

15. Ho KY, Leiner T, De Haan MW, et al. Peripheral vascular tree stenoses: evaluation with moving-bed infusion-tracking MR angiography. *Radiology* 1998;206:683–692.

16. Wang Y, Lee HM, Khilnani NM, et al. Bolus-chase MR digital subtraction angiography in the lower extremity. *Radiology* 1998;207:263–269.

17. Meaney JF, Ridgway JP, Chakraverty S, et al. Stepping-table gadolinium-enhanced digital subtraction MR angiography of the aorta and lower extremity arteries: preliminary experience. *Radiology* 1999;211:59–67.

18. Alley MT, Grist TM, Swan JS. Development of a phased-array coil for the lower extremities. *Magn Reson Med* 1995; 34:260–267.

19. Leiner T, Nijenhuis RJ, Maki JH, et al. Use of a three-station phased array coil to improve peripheral contrast-enhanced magnetic resonance angiography. *J Magn Reson Imaging* 2004;20:417–425.

20. Sodickson DK, McKenzie CA, Li W, et al. Contrast-enhanced 3D MR angiography with simultaneous acquisition of spatial harmonics: a pilot study. *Radiology* 2000;217:284–289.

21. Weiger M, Pruessmann KP, Kassner A, et al. Contrast-enhanced 3D MRA using SENSE. *J Magn Reson Imaging* 2000;12:671–677.

22. Bezooijen R, van den Bosch HC, Tielbeek AV, et al. Peripheral arterial disease: sensitivity-encoded multiposition MR angiography compared with intraarterial angiography and conventional multiposition MR angiography. *Radiology* 2004;231: 263–271.

23. Binkert CA, Baker PD, Petersen BD, et al. Peripheral vascular disease: blinded study of dedicated calf MR angiography versus standard bolus-chase MR angiography and film hard-copy angiography. *Radiology* 2004;232:860–866.

24. Vogt FM, Ajaj W, Hunold P, et al. Venous compression at high-spatial-resolution three-dimensional MR angiography of peripheral arteries. *Radiology* 2004;233:913–920.

25. Bilecen D, Schulte AC, Bongartz G, et al. Infragenual cuff-compression reduces venous contamination in contrast-enhanced MR angiography of the calf. *J Magn Reson Imaging* 2004;20:347–351.

26. Bilecen D, Jager KA, Aschwanden M, et al. Cuff-compression of the proximal calf to reduce venous contamination in contrast-enhanced stepping-table magnetic resonance angiography. *Acta Radiol* 2004;45:510–515.

27. Mitsuzaki K, Yamashita Y, Onomichi M, et al. Delineation of simulated vascular stenosis with Gd-DTPA-enhanced 3D gradient echo MR angiography: an experimental study. *J Comput Assist Tomogr* 2000;24:77–82.

28. Maki JH, Prince MR, Londy FJ, et al. The effects of time-varying intravascular signal intensity and k-space acquisition order on three-dimensional MR angiography image quality. *J Magn Reson Imaging* 1996;6:642–651.

29. Korosec FR, Mistretta CA. MR angiography: basic principles and theory. *Magn Reson Imaging Clin N Am* 1998;6:223–256.

30. Rubin GD, Schmidt AJ, Logan LJ, et al. Multi-detector row CT angiography of lower extremity arterial inflow and runoff: initial experience. *Radiology* 2001;221:146–158.

31. Martin ML, Tay KH, Flak B, et al. Multidetector CT angiography of the aortoiliac system and lower extremities: a prospective comparison with digital subtraction angiography. *AJR Am J Roentgenol* 2003;180:1085–1091.

32. Rubin GD, Shiau MC, Leung AN, et al. Aorta and iliac arteries: single versus multiple detector-row helical CT angiography. *Radiology* 2000;215:670–676.

33. Catalano C, Fraioli F, Laghi A, et al. Infrarenal aortic and lower-extremity arterial disease: diagnostic performance of multi-detector row CT angiography. *Radiology* 2004;231: 555–563.

34. Ofer A, Nitecki SS, Linn S, et al. Multidetector CT angiography of peripheral vascular disease: a prospective comparison with intraarterial digital subtraction angiography. *AJR Am J Roentgenol* 2003;180:719–724.

35. Heuschmid M, Krieger A, Beierlein W, et al. Assessment of peripheral arterial occlusive disease: comparison of multislice-CT angiography (MS-CTA) and intraarterial digital subtraction angiography (IA-DSA). *Eur J Med Res* 2003;8:389–396.

36. Romano M, Mainenti PP, Imbriaco M, et al. Multidetector row CT angiography of the abdominal aorta and lower extremities in patients with peripheral arterial occlusive disease: diagnostic accuracy and interobserver agreement. *Eur J Radiol* 2004;50: 303–308.

37. Adriaensen ME, Kock MC, Stijnen T, et al. Peripheral arterial disease: therapeutic confidence of CT versus digital subtraction angiography and effects on additional imaging recommendations. *Radiology* 2004;233:385–391.

38. Balzer J. Preinterventional assessment and follow-up of PAOD with a new 16 row multislice CT angiography (MS-CTA). *Eur Radiol* 2003;13:S269.

39. Fleischmann D. Aorto-popliteal bolus transit times in peripheral CT angiography: can fast acquisitions outrun the bolus? *Eur Radiol* 2003;13:S218.

40. Fleischmann D. Present and future trends in multislice detector-row CT applications: CT angiography. *Eur Radiol* 2002;2 Suppl 2:S11–S15.

41. Rofsky NM, Adelman MA. MR angiography in the evaluation of atherosclerotic peripheral vascular disease: what the clinician wants to know. *Radiology* 2000;214:325–338.

42. Kinney TB, Rose SC. Intraarterial pressure measurements during angiographic evaluation of peripheral vascular disease: techniques, interpretation, applications, and limitations. *AJR Am J Roentgenol* 1996;116:277–284.

43. Wasser MN, Westenberg J, van der Hulst VP, et al. Hemodynamic significance of renal artery stenosis: digital subtraction angiography versus systolically gated three-dimensional phase-contrast MR angiography. *Radiology* 1997;202:333–338.

44. Wikstrom J, Holmberg A, Johansson L, et al. Gadolinium-enhanced magnetic resonance angiography, digital subtraction angiography and duplex of the iliac arteries compared with intra-arterial pressure gradient measurements. *Eur J Vasc Endovasc Surg* 2000;19:516–523.

45. Owen RS, Carpenter JP, Baum RA, et al. Magnetic resonance imaging of angiographically occult runoff vessels in peripheral arterial occlusive disease. *N Engl J Med* 1992;326: 1577–1581.

46. Carpenter JP, Owen RS, Baum RA, et al. Magnetic resonance angiography of peripheral vessels. *J Vasc Surg* 1992;16: 807–813.

47. Koelemay MJ, den Hartog D, Prins MH, et al. Diagnosis of arterial disease of the lower extremities with duplex ultrasonography. *Br J Surg* 1996;83:404–409.

48. Legemate DA, Teeuwen C, Hoeneveld H, et al. Value of duplex scanning compared with angiography and pressure measurement in the assessment of aortoiliac arterial lesions. *Br J Surg* 1991;78:1003–1008.

49. Visser K, Hunink MG. Peripheral arterial disease: gadolinium-enhanced MR angiography versus color-guided duplex US—a meta-analysis. *Radiology* 2000;216:67–77.

50. Ruehm SG, Weishaupt D, Debatin JF. Contrast-enhanced MR angiography in patients with aortic occlusion (Leriche syndrome). *J Magn Reson Imaging* 2000;11:401–410.

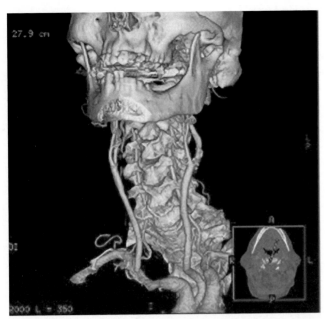

Figure 33.2. Surface-rendered CTA image showing boney landmarks. By separating the enhanced blood density and bone density into separate objects and then displaying the surfaces of the objects in one image, the location of the vessel within the neck may be appreciated. This display is useful for surgical planning.

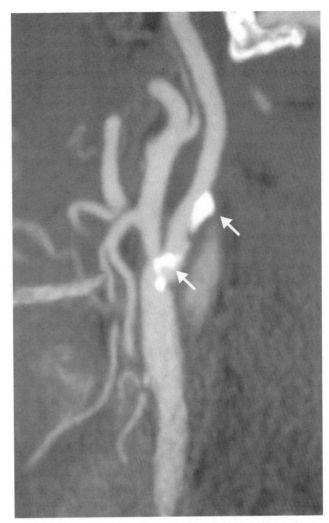

Figure 33.3. Oblique sagittal reformation of the bifurcation in patient with dense mural calcifications (*arrows*) on CTA.

Hounsfield units (HU), and a level of 325, allows differentiation between intravenous contrast and calcified atherosclerotic plaque. However, window settings are often based on individual preference and can be tailored accordingly. In addition, manual windowing at the time of interpretation is frequently performed to better assess specific areas of interest.

Interpretation solely from surface or volume-rendered images is not recommended. On these images, light mural calcifications may be mistaken for enhanced blood. Dense mural calcifications may "bloom" into the lumen and appear too large. The influence of streak or beam hardening artifacts may not be apparent on rendered images, as they are on individual sections.

Motion artifacts of the aortic arch may be recognized by their lack of continuity from one axial section to the next.

Vascular image analysis software may aid in the detection and measurement of carotid stenosis, however, these algorithms are relatively new, and their usefulness is unproven. Initial evaluation of automated stenosis measurement shows that manual corrections must be made to compensate for many interfering factors (10). More work must be done before these techniques can be widely adopted.

MAGNETIC RESONANCE ANGIOGRAPHY TECHNIQUES

ACQUISITION METHODS

The carotid arteries are especially amenable to MRA. Unlike the heart, the neck is stationary during the cardiac and respiratory cycles. High-sensitivity neck imaging coils depict carotid anatomy in great detail. Optimized carotid imaging sequences are widely available. The two common sequences for carotid MRA are time-of-flight (TOF) and contrast-enhanced magnetic resonance angiography (CE-MRA). TOF is an image of the entry of blood into the imaging volume, whereas CE-MRA (11–13) is an image of the distribution of contrast material and not of blood motion per se. TOF may be further categorized as two-dimensional (2D TOF) (14) or three-dimensional (3D TOF) (15), depending on whether the angiogram is constructed from multiple thin sections or from a single thick slab. A hybrid of the 2D and 3D techniques uses multiple overlapping thin slab acquisition (MOTSA) (16). Each of these sequences has been successfully used to measure carotid stenosis. Each has its own strengths and weaknesses.

Two-dimensional Time-of-flight

In 2D TOF one obtains a sequential series of slices transaxial to the neck and extending from the base of the skull to the thoracic inlet. Tissues that remain stationary in a slice are pulsed by radio waves and become dark, whereas blood en-

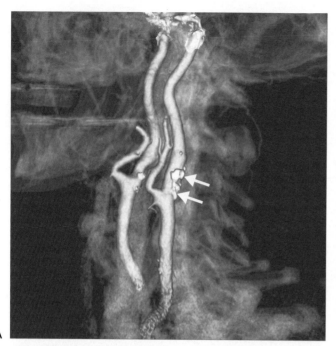 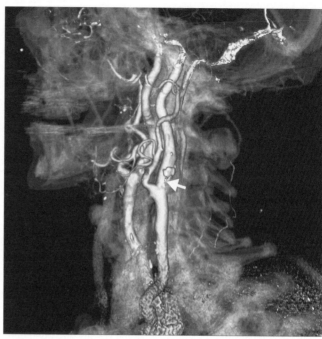

A   B

Figure 33.4. Automated calcium removal from CTA. **(A)** A shaded surface display of the carotid artery shows two prominent clusters of mural calcification (*arrows*). The carotid is superimposed on a volume-rendered, partially transparent, image of the neck to portray anatomic context. **(B)** An automated calcium removal routine has taken away one of the calcifications, revealing a stenosis (*arrow*), but the routine failed to find the second calcification. Interpretation solely from surface displays is not recommended.

tering into the slice between the radiofrequency (RF) pulses has not been pulsed before and is bright. Each slice is fully acquired before moving on to the adjacent slice, so that blood does not have to pass through more than one slice. For adequate resolution, the slices should be 2 mm or less in thickness. If slices this thin cannot be achieved, then they may be overlapped to provide greater apparent resolution. A "walking" or "traveling" saturation band is placed just superior to each slice to remove any signal from the jugular veins. Because the sections in 2D TOF are very thin, they are replaced with inflowing blood, even when the vessel velocity is reduced. Therefore, the technique provides strong blood-to-background signal contrast in slow flow conditions.

Three-dimensional Time-of-flight

In 3D TOF, the bifurcation is acquired by a thick slab obtained transaxial to the neck. The slab is divided into very thin partitions by use of a second phase encoding gradient. The partitions available in 3D TOF are typically 1 mm or less, which is finer than the resolution available from 2D TOF. The 3D method is effective for only relatively fast flow because blood may be pulsed several times and loses its signal before traversing the width of the slab. As in 2D TOF, a saturation band is placed superior and parallel to the acquisition slab to eliminate jugular venous signal.

Multiple Overlapping Thin Slab Acquisition

In MOTSA, the angiogram is built up from many thin slabs. The slabs are acquired sequentially, as in 2D TOF. Each slab is divided into thin partitions, as in 3D TOF. The rela-

tively thin slabs, 1 cm, allow blood to transverse the volume and refresh the signal between RF pulses. Each slab partially overlaps the volume acquired by the prior slab. Only the central partitions of each slab are kept, to improve uniformity of signal. The necessity to overlap volumes results in a relatively inefficient acquisition time of 12 minutes or more.

Contrast-enhanced Magnetic Resonance Angiography

CE-MRA has proven to be very effective for carotid angiography, combining speed of acquisition with an ability to visualize slowly flowing vessels. In addition, the method offers fewer motion artifacts than TOF and is more suitable for patients who cannot remain still. Contrast is injected as a rapid bolus in a peripheral arm vein. Upon arrival of this bolus in the carotid arteries, a fast 3D gradient-echo sequence is acquired. Because the contrast agent remains bright, even when pulsed many times by radio waves, optimizing inflow is not required. The acquisition slab may be oriented in the coronal plane to cover the entire length of the neck to the Circle of Willis. The acquisition is completed in 20 seconds or less, before the jugular vein enhances.

CE-MRA is best done on a modern machine with strong gradients of 20 millitesla per meter (mT/m) or greater. With strong gradients, the acquisition time should be less than 20 seconds. The shorter the acquisition, the less contrast material will need to be injected to sustain enhancement. Typically, 20 to 30 cc of gadolinium is required. Signal intensity, and hence signal-to-noise ratio, improves with greater injection rates. Stronger gradients permit echo times of less than 2 milliseconds, which minimize flow and susceptibility artifacts.

The challenge of CE-MRA is to initiate the brief acquisition at the time of arrival of contrast. The sequence may be initiated by one of several techniques:

1. A 2-mL test bolus may be administered, followed by a 10-mL saline flush. The vessel of interest is repeatedly acquired every second to determine the contrast transit time. The transit time is then used to calculate an imaging delay time for the subsequent full dose injection. Although this technique is time-consuming, it has a low incidence of failure.

2. As with helical computed tomography, some manufacturers have automated the process by programming the machine to initiate a sequence when it senses a signal change in the vessel (17). This avoids a separate test injection. This timing method is often used with centric reordering of the phase encoding steps. Centric reordering ensures that the large echoes are acquired early in the sequence, during peak enhancement, whereas smaller, less important echoes are acquired later in the bolus. Elliptic centric reordering is a further refinement of the technique, in which the smallest echoes are not acquired at all.

3. Following peripheral intravenous contrast injection, the aortic arch may be imaged in real time, using MR fluoroscopy. The fluoroscopy is terminated and the angiogram begun, when contrast is seen entering the aorta (18). As in automated detection, a centrically reordered acquisition is used (19).

4. If the acquisition time is very short, one might simply acquire several angiograms in succession. The angiogram corresponding to peak arterial enhancement is then retained. A more sophisticated implementation of this technique is to acquire only the large central echoes several times during the passage of contrast, while acquiring the smaller echoes just once (20,21). Angiograms so acquired combine strong vessel signal with high resolution.

On CE-MRA, noise may become visible as pixel size is reduced. Using a phase-array neck coil and by increasing the injected volume of contrast material best compensate for this. Another common solution is to acquire lower-resolution data, then calculate a higher-resolution image from that data by interpolation, a practice called "zero-filling." Zero-filling improves apparent resolution but does not provide the same detail as true high-resolution acquisition.

Obtaining two acquisitions in rapid succession following the injection is advisable. The first, which is timed to peak arterial contrast, best demonstrates anatomy. The second acquisition shows late-filling vessels in exceptionally slow flow conditions.

MAGNETIC RESONANCE ANGIOGRAPHY METHODS COMPARED

Resolution

Three-dimensional TOF and CE-MRA provide resolution superior to that of 2D TOF in the slice-selection direction. This lack of resolution may impair the ability of 2D TOF to detect ulcers, small plaques, or fibromuscular dysplasia.

Voxels should be 1 mm^3 or less to permit adequate measurements of lumen width. The diameter of the ICA may be 5 or 6 mm. A pixel width of 1 mm would seem to permit no better than 20% precision in lumen width. In fact, the partial volume of intensities results in higher effective precision when angiograms are interpolated and viewed at higher resolution. However, when measuring the width of a lumen under magnification, the limitations of interpolation become apparent. Use of a 512 image matrix will improve accuracy. The margin of a vessel is more sharply defined on CE-MRA than on 3D TOF because slow flow at the vessel wall is as bright as faster flow in the center of the vessel. This improves the perceived resolution of the gadolinium-enhanced technique (Figs. 33.5 and 33.6).

Near Occlusion

Three-dimensional TOF is not suited to this indication. Two-dimensional TOF is better able to see vessels beyond a high-grade stenosis. Note that the ICA may be atretic when a flow-limiting lesion has been present for a long time, and it may be mistaken for an external carotid artery (ECA) branch. Inspection of the carotid canals may help to differentiate an ascending pharyngeal artery from a small ICA. A congeni-

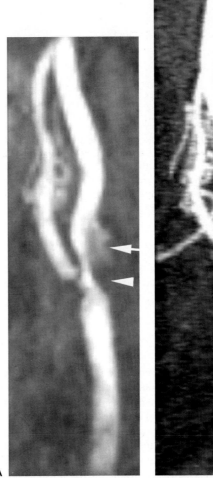

A   B

Figure 33.5. Effect of stagnant blood flow on signal intensity in MOTSA angiography. A moderately stenotic ICA origin is equally apparent by the MOTSA **(A)** and CE-MRA **(B)** technique (*arrowheads*), but the vessel intensity is more uniform on CE-MRA. In particular, blood flowing past the carotid bulb results in relatively stagnant pool within the posterior bulb and weak signal intensity on MOTSA (*arrow*).

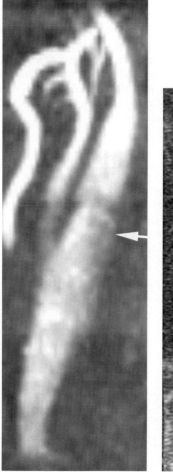
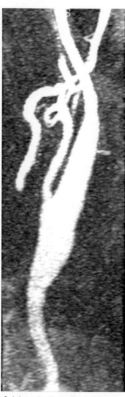

Figure 33.6. Greater uniformity of blood signal on CE-MRA. **(A)** Following endarterectomy, the distal CCA and proximal ICA are patulous, resulting in slower blood flow and weak signal (*arrow*). **(B)** On CE-MRA, the signal intensity is uniform as a result of insensitivity to blood velocity.

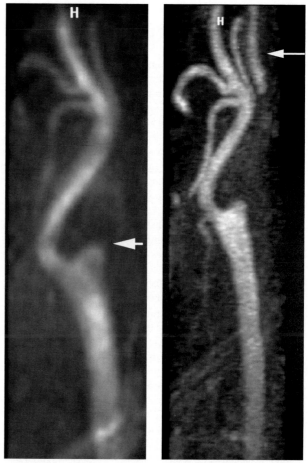

Figure 33.7. ICA reconstitution detected by CE-MRA. **(A)** An apparent occlusion of the ICA (*arrow*) on MOTSA. **(B)** Using CE-MRA, reconstitution of the ICA is noted in the midneck (*arrow*). ICA reconstitution is rare but may often occur from vasa-vasorum collaterals.

tally small ICA may be differentiated from an atretic ICA by the small diameter of the bony canal. CE-MRA in late arterial phase is thought to be the most sensitive sequence for the detection of nearly occluded or reconstituted vessels (Fig. 33.7).

Reversal of Flow

A blood vessel that has reversed its flow direction; for example, the vertebral artery in subclavian steal phenomenon is invisible on TOF because its signal is eliminated by a superior saturation band. If a vessel is not visible on TOF images, the acquisition could be repeated without a saturation band, or with saturation inferior to the acquired volume. Flow that has reversed in a vessel may not be recognized on CE-MRA because the vessel is already bright on the arterial phase image (Fig. 33.8).

Vessel Tortuosity

Horizontal segments of the carotid artery, such as one often encounters in the bulb, or down-going segments, such as

might occur in redundant cervical loops, do not provide inflowing blood to a transaxial 2D TOF section. As a result, horizontal and down-going segments are dark on 2D TOF angiograms. Collateral structures are often incompletely visualized when using this sequence. Furthermore, the vessel intensity may depend upon the angle of incidence of the blood vessel entering the acquired slice. CE-MRA, which is not strongly dependent on blood entry velocity, is uniformly bright in a cervical loop. Furthermore, blood does not loose its signal on CE-MRA as it dwells in the imaging volume.

Phase Dispersion and Stenosis Overestimation

Blood intensity is diminished within the stenotic portion of an arterial lumen. This may result in overestimation of the degree of stenosis. The reason for reduced intensity is twofold. First, the lumen may be smaller than the pixel diameter, in which case there is partial voluming of the signal. Second, there may be phase dispersion within the lumen as a result of a high degree of variability of blood flow velocity and trajectory (22). This mechanism for cancellation of signal is loosely termed "turbulence," although it may not fit the definition of truly turbulent flow. The amount of phase dis-

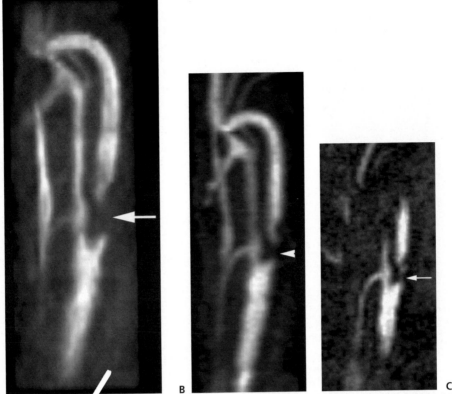

Figure 33.16. Demonstration of the necessity to view both native and projected images when interpreting MRA. **(A)** A gap in proximal ICA signal is present on a MOTSA acquisition (*arrow*). **(B)** In this example, the gap is slightly smaller on the CE-MRA study (*arrowhead*), possibly because some of the signal loss may have resulted from slow flow in the area beyond the plaque. **(C)** The residual lumen is visible on a native partition through the stenosis (*arrow*). Trace residual signal in the lumen was overwhelmed by background signal on MIP.

Shaded surface displays (Fig. 33.17) are visually appealing, but they eliminate a great deal of useful signal information. In calculating these displays, one picks an intensity threshold that defines the margin of the vessel. Because the intensity is reduced within a stenotic lumen, the threshold inevitably exaggerates the degree of stenosis. If the intensity within the residual lumen is less than the threshold, continuity will be lost between the common carotid artery (CCA) and the ICA.

Another common artifact is encountered at a sharp turn in the vessel. Blood velocity is greatest around the outer curve, whereas blood flows more slowly along the inner curve. On 3D TOF sequences, the inner portion of the curve may become saturated, resulting in a false narrowing. This artifact is often encountered where the carotid enters the petrous bone and turns sharply (32). The problem is overcome by CE-MRA.

In a very tight curve, especially within the carotid siphons, the direction of flow may be substantially different during the phase-encoding gradient and frequency-encoding gradient. This results in a mismapping and distortion of the shape of the vessel and the potential for a false stenosis.

Metal susceptibility artifact in the neck may be the result of surgical clips or dental appliances. This artifact is recognized as a dark circular signal void centered outside of the vessel on cross-sectional localizing sequences. As with any type of MR imaging, the artifact is minimized by using a

shorter TE and smaller voxels. CE-MRA, with its very short TE, is the preferred sequence when there is concern for metal artifact (Fig. 33.18).

One should resist the temptation to interpret a study that is compromised by patient motion. Motion may mask a severe stenosis and may generate a false stenosis.

Finally, the interpretation is most useful, if one reports a percent stenosis value, rather than a category or qualitative assessment. A computer workstation with measurement tools or film using a calibrated jeweler's loupe are best options for achieving this.

APPLICATIONS

THE CAROTID ARTERY AND STROKE

Most plaques develop within the bulb of the carotid bifurcation. Atherosclerosis develops at this site because of "flow separation," a blood flow pattern that results in very low velocities along the posterior wall (33,34) (Figs. 33.19 and 33.20). Less common sites of carotid atherosclerosis include the common carotid origin and the internal carotid siphon. Carotid atherosclerosis is a known cause of stroke, but it is not the only etiology. Other causes of stroke are carotid wall dissection (35,36), fibromuscular dysplasia, kinking of a redundant carotid artery as well as cerebral artery thrombosis

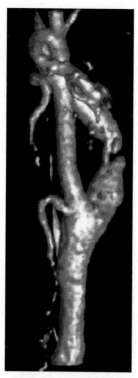

Figure 33.17. A surface-rendered image, derived from a submillimeter-resolution CE-MRA. Although this form of display cleanly eliminates background signal, all nuances of blood flow signal are lost. Variations in signal may be a valuable sign when interpreting MRA.

(37), and emboli arising from the heart (38) or from aortic ulcerations (39).

Carotid atherosclerosis gives rise to stroke by two principal mechanisms: thrombotic stroke, in which the vessel occludes suddenly at a site of stenosis, and embolic stroke, in which material originating at the stenosis occludes intracranial branches. Emboli may be generated when the plaque becomes necrotic and discharges its contents into the vessel lumen (40), when platelets and thrombin collect within an ulceration then break free (41–43), or when thrombin forms within the flow eddies just beyond a stenosis (44). The idea that emboli can form without necrosis of plaque is supported by observations made by transcranial Doppler ultrasound, in which silent emboli are observed with great frequency (45). Yet it is difficult to prove that emboli are the cause of stroke in a specific patient because the emboli are short-lived and may have resolved by the time an angiogram is performed (46). Furthermore, partially resolved emboli may mimic the appearance of an atheroma in an intracranial vessel.

Plaque Morphology and Composition

Investigators have sought to define which morphologic features of atherosclerosis give rise to thrombosis or emboli, so that intervention may be taken before a stroke occurs. One attractive hypothesis is that plaques with a large lipid core and a thin overlying fibrous cap are unstable and may rupture, disgorging their contents. The so-called "vulnerable plaque" has generated much excitement in the coronary artery literature (47,48). Early results with carotid artery

plaque imaging are very promising. In a study of patients with high-grade stenosis, Yuan (49) found that patients with ruptured fibrous caps were 23 times more likely to have a recent transient ischemic attack (TIA) or stroke than were patients with thick fibrous caps. Also, MRA was found to be valuable in monitoring therapy. Corti (50) performed serial volumetric measurements of carotid plaque in human subjects to show that lipid-lowering therapy with simvastatin was associated with significant regression of established atherosclerotic lesions.

CT may visualize the lipid core on the basis of lower density, but there is considerable variability in this finding (51).

The Significance of Carotid Stenosis

The features of plaque that have been most conclusively linked to stroke are the degree of lumen narrowing and the presence of a large ulcer. As stenosis becomes more severe, the risk of stroke increases. Following endarterectomy, the risk of stroke is diminished. This relationship has been confirmed by several well-publicized clinical trials.

The North American Symptomatic Carotid Endarterectomy Trial (NASCET) (52) examined 3,000 patients with recent TIAs and bifurcation stenosis. For those with greater than 70% diameter stenosis, 24% went on to have a stroke within 18 months. Further, the risk of stroke among those with 90% to 99% stenosis was greater than for 80% to 89% stenosis which, in turn, was greater than the risk for 70% to 79% stenosis. If endarterectomy was performed, the rate of stroke fell to 7% in 18 months. Surgery reduced the rate of stroke by 71%, death by 58%.

The European Carotid Surgery Trial (ECST) (53) examined 2,518 symptomatic patients and concluded that endarterectomy for those with greater than 70% stenosis reduced the risk of stroke over 3 years from 21.9% to 12.3%.

The Asymptomatic Carotid Atherosclerosis Study (ACAS) (54) examined 4,465 asymptomatic patients and found that even among this population there was an advantage for endarterectomy, albeit a small one. The risk of stroke within 5 years, among those with stenosis greater than 60%, decreased from 11% to 5.1%.

The advantages of endarterectomy were long-lived. The Veterans Affairs Cooperative Study Group (55) found that over the course of 8 years, 12% of surgical patients had cerebral events, compared with 25% for those who had medical treatment alone.

The surgical consequence of these studies has been that symptomatic patients with at least a 70% diameter stenosis are routinely referred for endarterectomy. In a subsequent publication, the NASCET investigators announced that, upon retrospective restratification of the data, they could recommend endarterectomy for greater than 50% stenosis (56). This practice has not been generally adopted. The appropriate indication for endarterectomy in asymptomatic patients is a matter of debate. A criterion of 60% stenosis, the value used for stratification in the ACAS study, would imply nearly 17 procedures be performed to prevent one stroke in 5 years, or 85 procedures prevent one stroke per year. In practice, many surgeons use a threshold of 80% to 85% for selecting symptomatic candidates for endarterectomy (57).

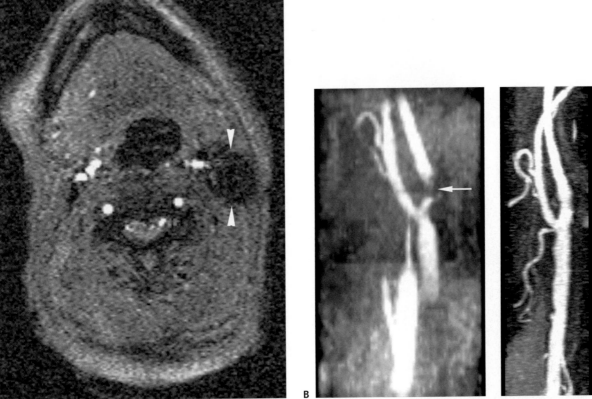

Figure 33.18. Metal clip artifact is minimized on CE-MRA. **(A)** A 2–D-TOF image (TE = 10 milliseconds) shows the prominent dark circle of a metal clip artifact (*arrowhead*). **(B)** The clip generated a false stenosis on 3D TOF (TE = 6 milliseconds) (*arrow*). Note gross rotation of the neck during the study so that the slabs are out of alignment. **(C)** On CE-MRA (TE = 2 milliseconds) the clip artifact is greatly diminished. Metal susceptibility artifact is reduced by short echo times and small voxels.

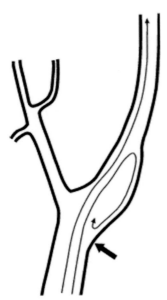

Figure 33.19. The flow separation phenomenon. The blood flow stream separates from the proximal posterior bulb wall *(arrow)*, flowing cephalad in the anterior bulb, and then recirculating to flow caudad in the posterior bulb. The point of flow separation is the common site of plaque formation.

The definition of stenosis grade used in the NASCET and ACAS studies was the narrowest diameter of the ICA at the lesion as a percentage of the diameter of the normal ICA beyond the bulb (Fig. 33.21) (58,59). The decision to use diameter as a measure of stenosis, rather than residual cross-sectional area, was dictated by the choice of conventional catheter angiography (CA), which portrays projectional anatomy.

Validation Studies of Magnetic Resonance Angiography

Publication of the NASCET trial launched a series of validation studies, whose goal was to determine the least costly and most accurate means of differentiating stenosis of greater or less than 70% in severity. Early studies compared 3D TOF or MOTSA with CA (30,60–70). The median sensitivity for a high-grade lesion in these publications was 0.93, whereas the median specificity was 0.88. Studies comparing CE-MRA with CA have showed very similar levels of accuracy (12,71–73). In addition, they demonstrated improved ulcer detection (Fig. 33.22), better depiction of the length of stenosis, and that of slow flow beyond a critical lesion (17). However, the signal-to-noise ratio of CE-MRA images was found to be inferior to MOTSA. This was especially true if the peak arterial enhancement phase was missed by incorrect timing of the acquisition. Use of MOTSA and CE-MRA

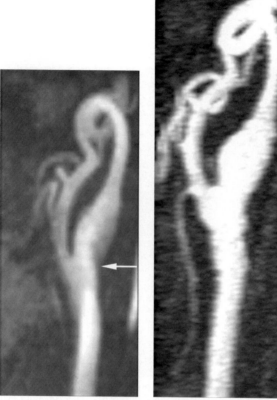

A   B

Figure 33.20. Flow separation. **(A)** A nearly normal carotid bulb is brighter in the anterior bulb than in the posterior on MOTSA. At the entrance to the bulb, a dark line extends from the posterior wall (*arrow*) at the site of flow separation. Carotid plaque most often forms in this location. **(B)** Flow separation is not apparent on CE-MRA, which is less sensitive to blood velocity.

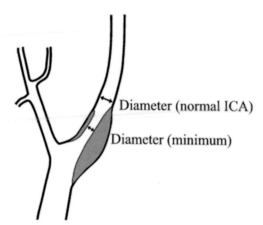

Diameter (normal ICA)

Diameter (minimum)

Figure 33.21. Carotid artery stenosis was measured by the NAS-CET trialists by comparing the smallest residual lumen diameter in the bulb to the normal lumen diameter in the ICA beyond the bulb, using the formula [1−(Diameter[minimum] / Diameter[normal ICA])] × 100.

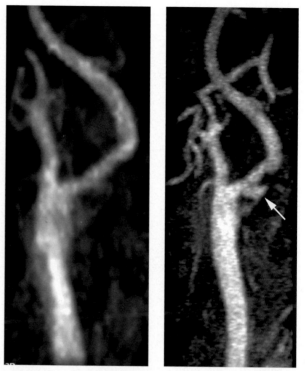

A   B

Figure 33.22. Ulcer detection on CE-MRA. **(A)** On MOTSA, a long segment mild narrowing of the proximal ICA is noted. **(B)** On CE-MRA, an ulcer is visible (*arrow*). The ulcer was not visible on the time-of-flight image as a result of poor inflow into the ulcer cavity.

together resulted in exceptionally high accuracies when compared to CA (25).

Validation studies assume CA to be the gold standard. The problem with this assumption is that any errors in measurement made by CA are counted as errors in MRA. Because the reproducibility of CA itself is no better than 94% (74–76), one can conclude that the actual sensitivities and specificities are better than those reported. In fact, preliminary data suggest that noninvasive imaging may be more sensitive than CA, in some instances (62). A comparison of CA, MRA, and DUS, using surgical specimens rather than CA as the gold standard (77), found that DUS and MRA each correlate better with the endarterectomy specimen than does CA. This finding was also observed in two subsequent trials, which found systematic underestimation of carotid stenosis by CA, when compared to the surgical specimen (78,79). The underestimation was more pronounced with less severe stenosis. These results make one question the popular notion that MRA overestimates stenosis; it is likely that MRA evaluation of carotid stenosis may closely approximate that of surgical specimen. The discrepancy might be attributed to belief that CA often does not appreciate the smallest diameter when the stenosis is elliptical or complex in shape. In fact, the recent availability of rotational angiography, a technique for conventional angiography that acquires images from many orientations following a single catheter injection, has shown that CA may often underestimate the severity of the lesion by not viewing it from the most stenotic direction (80). That is, when comparing MRA to a gold standard of CA, one finds that MRA often overestimates, but when comparing MRA to a gold standard of rotational CA, no tendency to overestimate occurs. The belief that the stenotic lumen is usually noncircular is particularly important when comparing CA and DUS, because Doppler velocities are determined by cross-sectional area rather than by diameter (81).

Information about the shape of the plaque, known by MRA but not by CA, is ignored in the validation studies. The rationale for this approach has been that CA is the only modality known to reduce the incidence of stoke, by virtue of its use in clinical trials. Clinical trials on the scale of NASCET, using MRA rather than CA to quantify stenosis, have never been undertaken. Therefore, MRA and DUS are assumed to be effective to only the degree that they agree with CA diameter measurements.

Validation Studies of Computed Tomography Angiography

In recent years, a new body of literature has arisen, assessing the accuracy of CTA (82,83) and comparing it with MRA (9,84–86). Many of these studies focus on comparison of single-detector helical CTA and 3D TOF MRA, because MDCT was not at first available. Relatively few studies compare directly the accuracy of multidetector CTA and CE-MRA, in comparison with CA.

A consistent finding, and one in concordance with common experience, is that CTA provides better image quality than does 3D TOF (84). However, this subjective observation does not translate into objective improvement in accuracy. In comparing NASCET-style stenosis measurements with CA, single-detector CTA, and MRA, Berg (85) found the modalities to be equivalent and more similar to CA than was DUS. Patel (86) found that single-detector CTA tended to underestimate degree of severity, whereas MRA tended to overestimate, but the differences were relatively small.

Several authors have reported that they use multidetector CTA only for presurgical evaluation (87,88). Although the studies could be faulted for not performing a comparison CA, the authors encountered no unexpected surgical finding or adverse outcome. It is increasingly hard to justify the use of diagnostic catheter angiography in a clinical trial; therefore, this type of uncontrolled study may become more common.

Another trend in the literature is to evaluate the combined accuracy of several noninvasive studies. For example, three publications found that when two modalities agree, there is a very high degree of concordance with CA (25,62,66). Other publications have sought to define the improved accuracy when all three noninvasive modalities—DUS, MRA, and CTA—are available. Patel (86) found that if a third modality is added when two disagree, then the chance of misclassifying a stenosis is substantially reduced. Nonent (9) reported that the improved accuracy of combining noninvasive studies was greatest for the asymptomatic population. In making a pair-wise comparison of CE-MRA, multidetector CTA, and DUS, the investigators found no significant difference in concordance rates when considering all patients. However, for asymptomatic surgical patients, concordance was greatest for the CE-MRA + DUS pair in comparison with the DUS + CTA pair. Furthermore, it was found that CTA alone would misclassify carotid stenosis in 17% of the cases

in the asymptomatic surgical group, compared with 4% for CE-MRA alone and 2% for DUS alone, using surgical findings as the gold standard. The authors cautioned that the finding should be considered preliminary in that there was a lack of standardization of postprocessing and interpretation methodology among the centers contributing data.

Cost-effectiveness

One would expect CTA and MRA to be more cost-effective than CA, as a result of their lower cost and morbidity. Typical costs for these modalities might be $300 (DUS), $600 (CTA), $900 (MRA), and $2,700 (CA); however, these costs vary considerably among medical centers. In a capitated health care program, the target expense for carotid stenosis, including diagnosis, endarterectomy, and follow-up clinic visits, is approximately $15,000. There is little room for a catheter angiogram in this budget.

The frequency of stroke from catheter angiography is between 0.5% and 1% (89–91), whereas the perioperative surgical risk of stroke is 2% to 3% (52,54), so adding CA to the treatment plan substantially increases the overall complication rate. This was clearly demonstrated by the ACAS study, in which the risk of stroke from CA and from endarterectomy was found to be equal (92).

It is not surprising, therefore, that cost-effectiveness calculations have favored noninvasive imaging. These studies have used risk statistics from the NASCET and ACAS trials, together with imaging accuracy statistics from the literature or from local practice, to predict the outcome of a hypothetical or actual cohort of patients, often as a function of the assumed prevalence of disease (66,92–99).

Kent (66) examined the cost-effectiveness of various imaging strategies for a population of symptomatic patients. Use of DUS alone resulted in a quality-adjusted life expectancy (QALE) of 9.619 years. CA alone resulted in 9.632 QALE, with an excessive incremental cost-effectiveness ratio of $99,200 per quality adjusted life year (QALY). The combination of DUS and MRA, followed by CA in the event of disparate results, maximized clinical outcome to 9.639 years, at an incremental cost-effectiveness ratio of just $22,400, and was considered the optimum strategy. MRA alone was nearly identical to CA in outcome (9.631 QALE) but was eliminated by dominance, and its marginal cost was not reported.

This example clearly shows that there is little difference in outcome between the least and most expensive workup algorithm. The inclusion of CA might improve diagnostic accuracy, but it also introduces more complications.

Buskens (98), using actual outcome and diagnostic results for DUS, MRA, and CA of 350 patients presenting with TIA or stroke, concluded that adding MRA to DUS improved diagnostic accuracy and marginally increased the QALY but greatly increased cost. Use of CA, even for confirmation of high-grade stenosis, actually decreased life expectancy as a result of complications.

Obuchowski (99) assumed a 20% prevalence of surgical stenosis in patients who presented with a neck bruit. Three imaging strategies were examined: DUS followed in selected cases by MRA, DUS followed in selected cases by CA, and MRA alone. The QALE of the three strategies was virtually identical, whereas the incremental cost per QALY was

$2,922, $7,470, and $7,700, respectively. DUS alone was not examined. This study again argues for a combined noninvasive approach (100).

When screening asymptomatic patients, the advantages of noninvasive imaging are even stronger. Kuntz (97) concluded that use of CA in this population actually resulted in a greater incident of stroke (7.12% in 5 years) than did DUS alone (6.35%), MRA alone (6.17%), or a combination of DUS and MRA followed by CA, if necessary (6.34%).

Cost-effectiveness of CTA has not been published. Given its equivalent accuracy to MRA, and slightly lower cost, we might expect CTA to be less cost-effective than DUS alone and more cost-effective than MRA as a confirmatory modality.

Limitations of Outcome Studies

The cost-effectiveness calculations assume that CA is precisely accurate, whereas DUS and MRA are miscategorizing about 10% of surgical lesions. If one adopts the more likely assumption that CA, DUS, and MRA are all capable of error, then the cost advantage of noninvasive imaging is even more dramatic.

Furthermore, the models assume that the 70% threshold, when using NASCET risk statistics, and the 60% threshold, when using ACAS risk statistics, represents hard boundaries between individuals with different expected surgical benefits. If the stroke prevalence statistics could be measured as a continuous variable of stenosis degree, then minor differences in measurement of stenosis would be much less important in determining outcome. However, gathering this data would necessitate an impractically large clinical trial.

In one respect, the models may underestimate the effect of imaging accuracy. The models assume proficiency in both DUS and MRA, whereas, in practice, the accuracy of noninvasive imaging is highly variable among medical centers. Howard (101) pointed out this problem when evaluating the DUS data from various centers in the ACAS trial. The NASCET study collected DUS data and showed poor correlation with stroke risk, but there was little uniformity or quality control among the contributors (102,103). The CA data, by comparison, were rigorously specified and read by a single well-trained interpreter (59). One should be cautioned, therefore, that the favorable outcomes predicted by the cost-effectiveness studies only accrue to those centers that perform imaging (and surgery) at a high level of experience (104).

Recommendation for Imaging

The workup of suspected carotid artery stenosis should begin with DUS, performed by an experienced and, preferably, accredited laboratory. If this study is technically adequate, reveals a greater than 70% lesion, and there is no suggestion of a tandem lesion based on the waveform, then the most cost-effective approach is to proceed directly to surgery. Typical technical limitations that might necessitate further imaging include the presence of a shadowing plaque, a deep course of the ICA, discordant gray scale and Doppler measurements, and contralateral disease. Tandem lesions are suggested by the presence of a dampened and delayed waveform (105) or unusually low diastolic velocities.

Although DUS alone is the most cost-effective presurgical imaging algorithm, and one widely used in Europe, a more cautious approach that minimizes unnecessary surgery is to confirm the presence of a surgical lesion with either CTA or MRA.

If patients require further imaging, they should be referred to an experienced CTA or MRA service, which have an ongoing quality assurance program. CTA is the logical choice for the patient with a carotid stent, with metal objects in the neck, or who cannot hold still. MRA is the best choice for the patient who has received contrast within the past 48 hours, who has renal insufficiency, prior contrast reaction, who may have reversed flow, or for whom MRI of the brain is desired. If both DUS and CTA or MRA agree, then there is little or no benefit in obtaining CA.

Use of CA should be minimized in the selection of patients for endarterectomy. It may be argued that performing CA prior to each surgical procedure provides an additional margin of security. In fact, the routine use of CA may worsen the average patient outcome. Furthermore, the quest for a highly precise diameter measurement is meaningless for several reasons. First, lumen shape is highly complex so that a single diameter number does not accurately express any hemodynamic phenomenon. Second, the association between stenosis and stroke is not perfect. Only about one third of strokes result from a surgically accessible stenosis (106), whereas only 25% of those with greater than 70% bifurcation stenosis will suffer a stroke within 18 months (52). Among asymptomatic patients, only 21% with a high-grade lesion will suffer a stroke within 3 years (54). This means that imaging cannot establish the benefit of endarterectomy for a specific individual. Rather, benefit accrues to the surgical population in aggregate. Third, CA subsequent to DUS may occasionally find additional lesions but rarely changes therapy (107–112). Carotid origin disease occurs in only about 2% of patients with significant bifurcation stenosis (112,113), and embolization from this source is unusual (114). Fourth, the 70% surgical threshold is a result of the NASCET study design and does not represent the absolute diameter, below which there is no benefit.

When selecting patients for interventional stenting, it could be argued that CTA and MRA could be removed from the algorithm. The interventional procedure itself confirms the DUS findings. In practice, most interventionalists prefer to obtain three-dimensional imaging before accepting a patient for stenting. MRA is unable to visualize plaque within a stent. Therefore, CTA is the best choice if pre- and postprocedure imaging of the plaque is desired. CTA may confirm the stent location, evaluate complications, and assess for intimal hyperplasia.

CAROTID DISSECTION

Carotid artery dissection (Figs. 33.23 and 33.24) is, most frequently, the result of trauma and presents with headache, neck pain, and sympathetic nerve paresis. The dissection may progress to thrombosis or give rise to an embolus. The dissection consists of a hemorrhage in the media, extending in some cases to the adventitia. The patient is usually treated conservatively with warfarin (Coumadin) for several months as a prophylactic for stroke.

An intimal flap may or may not be apparent. The flap often occurs within or just beyond the bulb and extends up

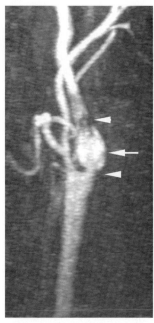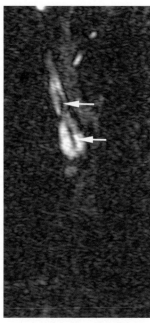

A
B

Figure 33.23. Dissection flap seen on native partitions. **(A)** A CE-MRA of the carotid artery shows an aneurysm of the bulb (*arrowhead*) and focal stenoses (*arrowheads*). **(B)** A dissection flap is noted on a native coronal partition (*arrows*). Intimal flaps are often hidden on maximum intensity projections.

the ICA for a variable distance. On angiography, a narrowing is seen that may be smooth or irregular (35,115). Because not all dissections are stenotic, one must inspect the images for the presence of a mural hematoma. The best choice is spin-echo T1-weighted transverse images, preferably with fat saturation (36). CTA may visualize a flap but may not be able to detect a hematoma. Therefore, MRI with MRA is currently the modality of choice for initial workup and follow-up of craniocervical artery dissection (116).

An important variant of carotid dissection is intramural hematoma. MRI images may be able to demonstrate intramural blood directly, particularly if the hematoma is at least several days old. These images should be augmented with MRA to visualize lumen narrowing.

CAROTID ULCERATION

Detection of ulcerated plaque is clinically significant, because the point of ulceration frequently serves as the site of clot formation. CE-MRA is more sensitive than 3D TOF which, in turn, is more sensitive than 2D TOF in detecting ulcers. CE-MRA and CTA (Fig. 33.25) detect most plaque ulcerations (6,117).

FIBROMUSCULAR DYSPLASIA

Fibromuscular dysplasia (FMD) is a rare idiopathic disease of smooth muscle in which the vessel wall takes on a beaded

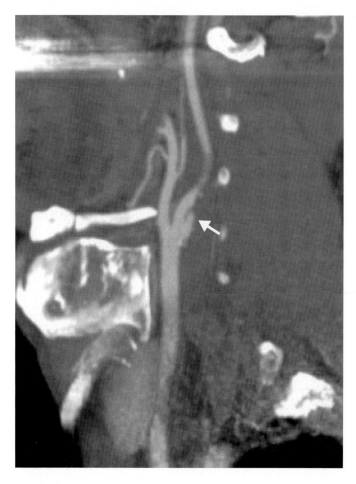

Figure 33.24. Carotid dissection on CTA. In the proximal internal carotid artery near its origin, a conspicuous intimal flap is identified (*arrow*).

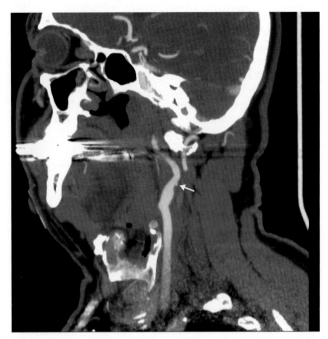

Figure 33.25. Ulcerated plaque on CTA. A 2-mm ulcer is clearly demonstrated (*arrow*). Of note, the streaky artifact along the superior margin of the image is from the patient's denture.

appearance, occurring most common in middle-aged women. The disease may progress to higher grades of stenosis, TIAs, or even stroke. Antiplatelet therapy or dilatations are common therapies. MRA is not as sensitive as CTA for detecting mild cases of FMD. Two-dimensional TOF may often miss FMD because of inadequate resolution. Three-dimensional TOF may miss FMD, if blood flow along the wall is slow, therefore not depicting wall irregularity. CTA should be the first choice in noninvasive FMD detection.

VERTEBROBASILAR INSUFFICIENCY

Vertebrobasilar insufficiency refers to transient ischemic events of the posterior cerebral circulation. This may include loss of consciousness. Hypotension, arrhythmias, anemia, brain tumors, and subclavian steal phenomenon may all be mistaken for vertebral artery stenosis.

Stenosis occurs typically at the proximal vertebral origin, at the intracranial junction of the vertebral arteries, or within the basilar artery. MOTSA is typically used for intracranial posterior circulation imaging but is a laborious technique for the cervical vertebral artery. The vertebral arteries are within the field of view of carotid CE-MRA and are automatically acquired as part of the carotid study. Direction of flow is not often discernible on CE-MRA or on CTA. Subclavian steal must be diagnosed by 2D TOF, acquired with an inferior and then superior saturation band to confirm reversal of vertebral blood flow. DUS can also measure reversal of flow in the vertebral artery. In addition, it can detect early subclavian steal phenomenon with demonstration of type I to IV presteal waveforms. However, DUS requires MRA or CTA to confirm proximal subclavian artery stenosis when vessel origins are not visible.

VERTEBRAL DISSECTION

Vertebral dissections usually occur between the C1 and C2 vertebral posterior elements as a result of twisting of the neck. They present with sudden onset of headache and neck pain as well as ischemic symptoms of the brainstem and cerebellum. Diagnosis is made on the basis of intramural hematoma, pseudoaneurysm, or vessel narrowing, usually performed by MRI with MRA. Subarachnoid hemorrhage is a sign of intracranial dissection.

AORTIC ARCH AND CAROTID ORIGINS

Transcutaneous DUS cannot visualize the aortic arch and carotid origins directly, but proximal disease is implied by a dampened waveform or flow that is reversed in direction. Likewise, an MRA of the carotid bifurcation may suggest the presence of a more proximal lesion when flow is reversed, or when the rate of inflow, and hence the degree of signal saturation on a 3D TOF acquisition, differs between the right and left vessels. A CE-MRA or CTA acquisition of the arch provides a noninvasive alternative to CA. The advent of multidetector CTA with cardiac-gating effectively reduces motion artifacts (118).

The presence of thick aortic plaques or aortic ulcerations is a risk factor for stroke (119). These features are visible on CTA. Mobile, free-floating, plaques may be less visible on MRA than on CTA, as a result of time averaged acquisition.

FUTURE PERSPECTIVE

MRA and CTA continue to push the limits of technology with faster machines. For both MRA and CTA, this means shorter acquisition times with smaller volumes of injected contrast agent but with higher-contrast concentrations. It also means better time-resolved imaging with the ability to complete arterial imaging before veins enhance. For CTA, faster acquisition results in longer fields of view. For MRA, the shorter echo time of high-speed machines helps eliminate both intrinsic and flow-related sources of signal cancellation. This may alleviate the tendency toward overestimation of the degree of stenosis. In addition, as echo times get shorter, and flow artifacts are reduced, MRA contrast agents and blood inflow may no longer be necessary. Angiography may simply become a water-weighted sequence. In that case, the difference between MRI and MRA will disappear. Any number of vessel segments will be acquired in one procedure. Because carotid, coronary, and peripheral arterial diseases are strongly associated, a comprehensive screening study could include all three territories. Ironically, this innovation will bring us full circle to the earliest days of MRA, when blood imaging was attempted using cardiac gated T2-weighted spin-echo sequences.

Another potential approach for whole body vascular imaging is the use of intravascular contrast agents. These agents persist in the blood pool for several hours, allowing prolonged, high-resolution, imaging sequences. Contrast material may be administered before the patient enters the magnet, without the need for a timed injection. Preliminary reports have demonstrated strong image contrast and excellent correspondence with CA (120).

Direct imaging of plaque by MRI is an exciting new capability that might better identify those patients at risk for stroke. The NASCET study considered only diameter stenosis as a predictor of stroke risk but did not consider the plaque directly, its instability, morphology, and effect of blood flow patterns and wall shear. Currently, surgeons must perform five or more procedures before they can change the outcome of a single symptomatic patient. If plaque composition and shape, as determined by high-resolution MRI, could afford a more specific index of those patients in peril of stroke, unnecessary surgery would be greatly reduced. In addition, the ability to measure plaque lipid volume may provide an end point for lipid lowering therapies.

Percutaneous carotid angioplasty and stent placement is a procedure that offers relief of a stenotic lesion, with little or no hospitalization. There remains, however, considerable concern as to whether angioplasty is as safe as surgical endarterectomy. Reviews to date indicate a complication rate that exceeds that of the NASCET trial, however, many of the patients typically treated by angioplasty would not have qualified for the NASCET trial because of their comorbidities (121). If carotid intervention becomes universally accepted, then the usefulness of MRA may be greatly reduced. Patients with stents will no longer be suitable for MRA as a result of RF shielding effects. In addition, some patients will go directly from DUS to the angiography suite for a procedure that will both confirm the findings of Doppler and correct the lesion.

With three capable noninvasive imaging modalities vying for supremacy in carotid imaging, we can expect to see many technical innovations and lively debate in the future.

SUMMARY

CTA and MRA of the carotid artery are common and well-validated imaging procedures that may be used to detect plaque and plaque ulceration, to measure narrowing of the lumen width, to visualize intimal flaps, and to confirm patency. MRA may be advantageous in demonstrating direction of blood flow in locating mural hematomas and is the safer choice for patients with renal insufficiency or prior contrast reaction. CTA may visualize structures within a stent and provides superior images for the patient who cannot remain still.

The two predominant MRA sequences for carotid angiography are MOTSA and CE-MRA. MOTSA does not require the injection of contrast material and so is cheaper and more convenient than CE-MRA, yet CE-MRA is gradually displacing MOTSA as the preferred sequence because of its relative immunity to certain blood flow and motion artifacts. Newer generation MRI machines, with their strong gradients, have improved the quality of MR angiograms. Reliable interpretation of carotid MRA requires an understanding of blood flow patterns in the carotid bulb, and recognition of common signal artifacts, especially the effects of turbulent flow and patient motion. MRA interpretation is improved by a quality control program consisting of routine comparison with other imaging modalities and with surgical observations.

The increasing use of multidetector CTA, capable of up to 64 simultaneous sections, has improved the field of view of these studies, while decreasing the volume of required contrast agent.

Noninvasive imaging of the carotid artery reduces cost, inconvenience, and risk. While the relative roles of DUS, MRA, and CTA are a subject of continuing debate, DUS may be recommended as the preferred screening modality because of its lower expense and risk and high availability. MRA and CTA may be recommended as confirmatory examinations, which obviate the need for nearly all CA.

REFERENCES

1. Kuller LH, Crook LP, Friedman GP. Survey of stroke epidemiology studies. *Stroke* 1972;3:579.
2. Colgan MP, Strode GR, Sommer JD, et al. Prevalence of asymptomatic carotid disease: results of duplex scanning in 348 unselected volunteers. *J Vasc Surg* 1998;8:674–679.
3. Fine-Edelstein JS, Wolf PA, O'Leary DH, et al. Precursors of extracranial carotid atherosclerosis in the Framingham study. *Neurology* 1994;44:1046–1050.
4. Schartz LB, Bridgman AH, Kieffer RW, et al. Asymptomatic carotid artery stenosis and stroke in patients undergoing cardiopulmonary bypass. *J Vasc Surg* 1995;21:146–153.
5. Niwa M. Report on the 89th Scientific Assembly and Annual Meeting of the Radiological Society of North America—balance between the time sensitivity profile and the slice sensitivity profile in multi-slice helical scanning. *Nippon Hoshasen Gijutsu Gakkai Zasshi* 2004;60(12):1666–1667.
6. Beauchamp NJ, Campbell PD. Neuro CTA. In: Fishman EK, Jeffrey RB, eds. *Multi-detector CT.* Philadelphia: Lippincott; 2004:443–462.
7. Rubin GD. Techniques for performing multidetector-row computed tomographic angiography. *Tech Vasc Interv Radiol* 2001;4:2–14.
8. Josephson SA, Bryant SO, Mak HK, et al. Evaluation of carotid stenosis using CT angiography in the initial evaluation of stroke and TIA. *Neurology* 2004;63(3):457–460.
9. Nonent M, Serfaty JM, Nighoghossian N, et al. Concordance rate differences of 3 noninvasive imaging techniques to measure carotid stenosis in clinical routine practice. *Stroke* 2004; 35:682.
10. Zhang Z, Berg MH, Ikonen AE, et al. Carotid artery stenosis: reproducibility of automated 3D CT angiography analysis method. *Eur Radiology* 2004;14(4):665–672.
11. Cloft HJ, Murphy KJ, Prince MR, et al. 3D gadolinium-enhanced MR angiography of the carotid arteries. *Magn Reson Imaging* 1996;14:593–600.
12. Levy R, Prince M. Arterial-phase three-dimensional contrast-enhanced MR angiography of the carotid arteries. *AJR Am J Roentgenol* 1996;67:211–215.
13. Prince M, Chenevert T, Foo T, et al. Contrast-enhanced abdominal MR angiography: optimization of imaging time by automating the detection of contrast arrival time in the aorta. *Radiology* 1997;203:109–114.
14. Keller PJ, Drayer BP, Fram EK, et al. MR angiography with two-dimensional acquisition and three-dimensional display. *Radiology* 1989;173:527–532.
15. Masaryk TJ, Modic MT, Ruggiere PM, et al. Three-dimensional (volume) gradient echo imaging of the carotid bifurcation: preliminary clinical experience. *Radiology* 1989;171: 801–806.

16. Parker DL, Yuan C, Blatter DD. MR angiography by multiple thin slab 3D acquisition. *Magn Reson Med* 1991;17:434–451.

17. DeMarco JK, Schonfeld S, Keller I, et al. Contrast-enhanced carotid MR angiography with commercially available triggering mechanism and elliptic centric phase encoding. *AJR Am J Roentgenol* 2001;176:221–227.

18. Riederer SJ, Bernstein MA, Breen JF, et al. Three-dimensional contrast-enhanced MR angiography with real-time fluoroscopic triggering: design specifications and technical reliability in 330 patient studies. *Radiology* 2000;215:584–593.

19. Huston J, Fain SB, Riederer SJ, et al. Carotid arteries: maximizing arterial to venous contrast in fluoroscopically triggered contrast-enhanced MR angiography with elliptic centric view ordering. *Radiology* 1999;211:265–273.

20. Korosec F, Grist T, Frayne R, et al. Time-resolved contrast-enhanced 3D MR angiography. *Magn Reson Med* 1996;36:345–351.

21. Mistretta CA, Grist TM, Korosec FR, et al. 3D time-resolved contrast-enhanced MR DSA: advantages and tradeoffs. *Magn Reson Med* 1998;40:571–581.

22. Urchuk S, Plewes D. Mechanism of flow induced signal loss in MR angiography. *J Magn Reson Imaging* 1992;2:453–462.

23. Le Bihan, ed. *Diffusion and perfusion magnetic resonance imaging.* Philadelphia: Lippincott-Raven; 1995.

24. Brandt-Zawadski M, Atkinson D, Detrick M, et al. Fluid-attenuated inversion recovery (FLAIR) for assessment of cerebral infarction: clinical experience in 50 patients. *Stroke* 1996;27:1187–1191.

25. Serfaty JM, Chirossel P, Chevallier JM, et al. Accuracy of three-dimensional gadolinium-enhanced MR angiography in the assessment of extracranial carotid artery disease. *AJR Am J Roentgenol* 2000;175:455–463.

26. Prince MR. Body MR angiography with gadolinium contrast agents. *MRI Clin North Am* 1996;4:11–24.

27. Krinsky G, Maya M, Rofsky N, et al. Gadolinium-enhanced 3D MRA of the aortic arch vessels in the detection of atherosclerotic cerebrovascular disease. *JCAT* 1998;22:167–178.

28. Carpenter JP, Holland GA, Golden MA, et al. Magnetic resonance angiography of the aortic arch. *J Vasc Surg* 1997;25:125–151.

29. DeMarco JK, Nesbit GM, Wesbey GE, et al. Prospective evaluation of extracranial carotid stenosis: MR angiography with maximum intensity projections and multiplanar reformation compared with conventional angiography. *AJR Am J Roentgenol* 1994;163:1205–1212.

30. Anderson CM, Lee RL, Levin DL, et al. Measurement of internal carotid artery stenosis from source MR angiograms. *Radiology* 1994;193:219–226.

31. Rossnick S, Laub G, Braeckle R. Three dimensional display of blood vessels in MRI. In: Proceedings of the IEEE computers in cardiology. New York: Institute of Electrical and Electronic Engineers; 1986:193–195.

32. van Tyen R, Saloner D, Jou LD, et al. MR imaging of flow through tortuous vessels: a numerical simulation. *Magn Reson Med* 1994;31:184–195.

33. Zarins C, Giddens D, Balasubramanian L, et al. Carotid plaques localized in regions of low flow velocity and shear stress. *Circulation* 1981;64:44.

34. Shaaban AM, Duerinckx AJ. Wall shear and early atherosclerosis: a review. *AJR Am J Roentgenol* 2000;174:1657–1665.

35. Levy C, Laissy JP, Raveau V, et al. Carotid and vertebral artery dissections: three-dimensional time-of-flight MR angiography and MR imaging versus conventional angiography. *Radiology* 1994;190:97–103.

36. Provenzale JM. Dissection of the internal carotid and vertebral arteries: imaging features. *AJR Am J Roentgenol* 1995;165:1099–1104.

37. Marzewski DJ, Furlan AJ, St. Louis P, et al. Intracranial internal carotid artery stenosis: long-term prognosis. *Stroke* 1981;13:821–824.

38. Castaigne P, Lhermitte F, Gautier J, et al. Internal carotid artery occlusion: a study of 61 instances in 50 patients with post-mortem data. *Brain* 1970;93:321.

39. Amarenco P, Duyckaerts C, Tzourio C, et al. The prevalence of ulcerated plaques in the aortic arch in patients with stroke. *NEJM* 1992;326:221–225.

40. Mohr J, Gautier J, Pessin M. Internal carotid artery disease. In: Barnett H, Mohr J, Stein B, Yatsu F, eds. *Stroke.* New York: Churchill Livingstone; 1992:285–335.

41. Weinberger J, Robbins A. Neurologic symptoms associated with nonobstructive plaque at carotid bifurcation: analysis by real-time B-mode ultrasonography. *Arch Neurol* 1983;40:489–492.

42. Dixon S, Pais S, Raviola C, et al. Natural history of nonstenotic asymptomatic ulcerative lesions of the carotid artery: a further analysis. *Arch Surg* 1982;117:1493.

43. Eliasziw M, Streifler JY, Fox AJ, et al. Significance of plaque ulceration in symptomatic patients with high-grade carotid stenosis. North American Carotid Endarterectomy Trial. *Stroke* 1994;25:304–308.

44. Beal M, Williams R, Richardson E, et al. Cerebral embolism as a cause of transient ischemic attacks and cerebral infarction. *Neurology* 1981;31:860.

45. Akiyama Y, Sakaguchi M, Yoshimoto H, et al. Detection of microemboli in patients with extracranial carotid artery stenosis by transcranial Doppler sonography. *No Shinkei Geka* 1997;25:41–45.

46. Bozzao L, Fantozzi L, Bastianello S, et al. Ischaemic supratentorial stroke: angiographic findings in patients examined in the very early phase. *J Neurol* 1989;236:340.

47. Fayad ZA, Fuster V, Nikolaou K, Becker C. Computed tomography and magnetic resonance imaging for noninvasive coronary angiography and plaque imaging. *Circulation* 2002;106:2026.

48. MacNeill BD, Lowe HC, Takano M, et al. Intravascular modalities for detection of vulnerable plaque: current status. *Arterioscler Thromb Vasc Biol* 2003;23:1333.

49. Yuan C, Zhang S, Polissar N, et al. Identification of fibrous cap rupture with magnetic resonance imaging is highly associated with recent transient ischemic attack or stroke. *Circulation* 2002;105:181.

50. Corti R, Fuster V, Fayad ZA, et al. Lipid lowering by simvastatin induces regression of human atherosclerotic lesions: two years' follow-up by high-resolution noninvasive magnetic resonance imaging. *Circulation* 2002;106:2884.

51. Walker LJ, Ismail A, McMeekin W, et al. Tomography angiography for the evaluation of carotid atherosclerotic plaque correlation with histopathology of endarterectomy specimens. *Stroke* 2002;33:977.

52. Barnett HJ. North American symptomatic carotid trial collaborators. Beneficial effect of carotid endarterectomy in symptomatic patients with high-grade carotid stenosis. *N Engl J Med* 1991;325:445–453.

53. European Carotid Surgery Trialist's Collaborative Group. MRC European carotid surgery trial: interim results for symptomatic patients with severe (70–99%) or with mild (0–29%) carotid stenosis. *Lancet* 1991;337:1235–1243.

54. Executive Committee for the Asymptomatic Carotid Atherosclerosis Study. Endarterectomy for asymptomatic carotid artery stenosis. *JAMA* 1995;273:1421–1428.

55. Hobson RW II, Strandness DE Jr. Carotid artery stenosis: what's in the measurement [Editorial]? *J Vasc Surg* 1993;18:1069–1070.

56. Barnett HJ, Taylor DW, Eliasziw M, et al. Benefit of carotid endarterectomy in patients with symptomatic moderate or severe stenosis. *NEJM* 1998;339:1415–1425.

57. Barnett HJ, Meldrum HE, Eliasziw M. Atherosclerotic disease of the carotid arteries: a medical perspective. In: Barnett HJ, Mohr JP, Stein MB, Yatsu FM, eds. *Stroke.* New York: Churchill Livingstone; 1998:1189–1198.

58. Barnett HJ, Warlow CP. Carotid endarterectomy and the measurement of stenosis [Editorial]. *Stroke* 1993;24:1281–1284.

59. Fox J. How to measure carotid stenosis. *Radiology* 1993;186: 316–318.

60. Korogi Y, Takahashi M, Mabuchi N, et al. Intracranial vascular stenosis and occlusion: diagnostic accuracy of three-dimensional, Fourier transform, time-of-flight MR angiography. *Radiology* 1994;193:187–193.

61. Levi CR, Mitchell A, Fitt G, et al. The accuracy of magnetic resonance angiography in the assessment of extracranial carotid artery occlusive disease: a comparison with digital subtraction angiography using NASCET criteria for stenosis measurement. *Cerebrovasc Dis* 1996;6:231–236.

62. Liberopoulos K, Kaponis A, Kokkinis K, et al. Comparison study of magnetic resonance angiography, digital subtraction angiography, duplex ultrasound examination with surgical and histological findings of atherosclerotic carotid bifurcation disease. *Int Angiol* 1996;15:131–137.

63. Link J, Brinkmann G, Steffens JC, et al. MR angiography of the carotid arteries in 3D TOF technique with sagittal double-slab acquisition using a new head-neck coil. *Rofo Fortschr Geb Rontgenstr Neuen Bildgeb Verfahr* 1996;165:544–550.

64. Vanninen RL, Manninen HI, Partanen PL, et al. Carotid artery stenosis: clinical efficacy of MR phase-contrast flow quantification as an adjunct to MR angiography. *Radiology* 1995; 194:459–467.

65. Vogl TJ, Heinzinger K, Juergens M, et al. Multiple slab MR angiography of the internal carotid artery: a preoperative comparative study. *Rofo Fortschr Geb Rontgenstr Neuen Bildgeb Verfahr* 1995;162:404–411.

66. Kent KC, Kuntz KM, Mahesh RP, et al. Perioperative imaging strategies for carotid endarterectomy: analysis of morbidity and cost-effectiveness in symptomatic patients. *JAMA* 1995;274:888–893.

67. Nicholas GG, Osborne MA, Jaffe JW, et al. Carotid artery stenosis: preoperative noninvasive evaluation in a community hospital. *J Vasc Surg* 1995;22:9–16.

68. Patel MR, Kuntz KM, Roman AK, et al. Preoperative assessment of the carotid bifurcation: can magnetic resonance angiography and duplex ultrasonography replace contrast arteriography? *Stroke* 1995;26:1753–1758.

69. Mittl RL, Broderick M, Carpenter JP, et al. Blinded reader comparison of magnetic resonance angiography and duplex ultrasonography for carotid artery bifurcation stenosis. *Stroke* 1994;25:4–10.

70. Young GR, Humphrey PR, Shaw MD, et al. Comparison of magnetic resonance angiography, duplex ultrasound, and digital subtraction angiography in assessment of extracranial internal carotid artery stenosis. *J Neurol Neurosurg Psychiatry* 1994;57:1466–1478.

71. Willig DS, Turski PA, Frayne R, et al. Contrast-enhanced 3D MR DSA of the carotid artery bifurcation: preliminary study of comparison with unenhanced 2D and 3D time-of-flight MR angiography. *Radiology* 1998;208:447–451.

72. Slosman F, Stolpen AH, Lexa FJ, et al. Extracranial atherosclerotic carotid artery disease: evaluation of non-breath-hold three-dimensional gadolinium-enhanced MR angiography. *AJR Am J Roentgenol* 1998;170:489–495.

73. Enochs WS, Ackerman RH, Kaufman JA, et al. Gadolinium-enhanced MR angiography of the carotid arteries. *J Neuroimaging* 1998;8:185–190.

74. Gagne PJ, Matchett J, MacFarland D, et al. Can the NASCET technique for measuring carotid stenosis be reliably applied outside the trial? *J Vasc Surg* 1996;24:449–455.

75. Young GR, Sandercock PA, Slattery J, et al. Observer variation in the interpretation of intra-arterial angiograms and the risk of inappropriate decisions about carotid endarterectomy. *J Neurol Neurosurg Psychiatry* 1996;60:152–157.

76. Eliasziw M, Fox AJ, Sharpe BL, et al. Carotid artery stenosis: external validity of the North American Symptomatic Carotid Endarterectomy Trial measurement method. *Radiology* 1997; 204:229–233.

77. Pan XM, Saloner D, Reilly LM, et al. Assessment of carotid artery stenosis by ultrasonography, conventional angiography, and magnetic resonance angiography: correlation with ex vivo measurement of plaque stenosis. *J Vasc Surg* 1995; 21:82–88.

78. Benes V, Netuka D, Mandys V, et al. Comparison between degree of carotid stenosis observed at angiography and in histological examination. *Acta Neurochir* 2004;146(7): 671–677.

79. De Monti M, Ghilardi G, Caverni L, et al. Multidetector helical angio CT oblique reconstructions orthogonal to internal carotid artery for preoperative evaluation of stenosis. A prospective study of comparison with color Doppler US, digital subtraction angiography and intraoperative data. *Minerva Cardioangiol* 2003;51(4):373–385.

80. Elgersma OE, Wust AFJ, Buijs PC, et al. Multidirectional depiction of internal carotid artery stenosis: three-dimensional time-of-flight MR angiography versus rotational and conventional digital subtraction angiography. *Radiology* 2000;216:511–516.

81. Prestigiacomo CJ, Connolly ES, Quest DO. Use of carotid ultrasound as a preoperative assessment of extracranial carotid artery blood flow and vascular anatomy. *Neurosurg Clin N Am* 1996;7:577–587.

82. Marcus CD, Ladam-Marcus VJ, Bigot JL, et al. Carotid arterial stenosis: evaluation at CT angiography with the volume-rendering technique. *Radiology* 1999;211:775–780.

83. Anderson GB, Ashforth R, Steinke DE, et al. CT angiography for the detection and characterization of carotid artery bifurcation disease. *Stroke* 2000;31:2168–2174.

84. Berg MH, Manninen HI, Rasanen HT, et al. CT angiography in the assessment of carotid artery atherosclerosis. *Acta Radiol* 2002;43(2):116–124.

85. Binaghi S, Maeder P, Uske A, et al. Three-dimensional computed tomography angiography and magnetic resonance angiography of carotid bifurcation stenosis. *Eur Neurol* 2001; 46(1):25–34.

86. Patel SG, Collie DA, Wardlaw JM, et al. Outcome, observer reliability, and patient preferences if CTA, MRA or Doppler ultrasound were used, individually or together, instead of digital subtraction angiography before carotid endarterectomy. *J Neurol Neurosurg Psychiatry* 2002;73(1):21–28.

87. Katano H, Kato K, Umemura A, et al. Perioperative evaluation of carotid endarterectomy by 3D-CT angiography with refined reconstruction: preliminary experience of CEA without conventional angiography. *Br J Neurosurg* 2004;18(2): 138–148.

88. Hoh BL, Cheung AC, Rabinov JD, et al. Results of a prospective protocol of computed tomographic angiography in place of catheter angiography as the only diagnostic and pretreatment planning study for cerebral aneurysms by a combined neurovascular team. *Neurosurgery* 2004;54(6):1329–1340.

89. Hankey GJ, Warlow CP, Sellar RJ. Cerebral angiographic risk in mild cerebrovascular disease. *Stroke* 1990;21: 209–222.

90. Grzyska U, Freitag J, Zeumer H. Selective arterial intracerebral DSA: complication rate and control of risk factors. *Neuroradiology* 1990;32:296–299.

91. Polak JF. Noninvasive carotid evaluation: carpe diem. *Radiology* 1993;186:329–331.

92. Young B, Moore WS, Robertson JT, et al. An analysis of perioperative surgical mortality and morbidity in the asymptomatic carotid atherosclerosis study. ACAS Investigators. Asymptomatic Carotid Arteriosclerosis Study. *Stroke* 1996; 27:2216–2224.

93. Cronenwett JL, Birkmeyer JD, Nackman GB, et al. Cost-effectiveness of carotid endarterectomy in asymptomatic patients. *J Vasc Surg* 1997;25:298–309.

94. Derdeyn CP, Powers WJ. Cost-effectiveness of screening for asymptomatic carotid atherosclerotic disease. *Stroke* 1996; 27:1944–1950.

95. Lee TT, Solomon NA, Heidenreich PA, et al. Cost-effectiveness of screening for carotid stenosis in asymptomatic persons. *Ann Intern Med* 1997;126:337–346.

96. Vanninen R, Manninen H, Soimakallio S. Imaging of carotid artery stenosis: clinical efficacy and cost-effectiveness. *AJNR Am J Neuroradiol* 1995;16:1875–1883.

97. Kuntz KM, Skillman JJ, Whittemore AD, et al. Carotid endarterectomy in asymptomatic patients—is contrast angiography necessary? A morbidity analysis. *J Vasc Surg* 1995;22: 706–714.

98. Buskens E, Nederkoorn PJ, Buijs-Van Der Woude T, et al. Imaging of carotid arteries in symptomatic patients: cost-effectiveness of diagnostic strategies. *Radiology* 2004;233(1): 101–112.

99. Obuchowski NA, Modic MT, Magdinec M, et al. Assessment of the efficacy of noninvasive screening for patients with asymptomatic neck bruits. *Stroke* 1997;28:1330–1339.

100. Carriero A, Ucchino S, Magarelli N, et al. Carotid bifurcation stenosis: a comparative study between MR angiography and duplex scanning with respect to digital subtraction angiography. *J Neuroradiol* 1995;22:103–111.

101. Howard G, Baker WH, Chambless LE, et al. An approach for the use of Doppler ultrasound as a screening tool for hemodynamically significant stenosis (despite heterogeneity of Doppler performance). A multicenter experience. Asymptomatic Carotid Atherosclerosis Study Investigators. *Stroke* 1996;27:1951–1957.

102. Hobson RW II, Weiss DG, Fields WS, et al. VA Cooperative Trial Efficacy of carotid endarterectomy for asymptomatic carotid stenosis. The Veterans Affairs Cooperative Study Group. *N Engl J Med* 1993;328:221–227.

103. Eliasziw M, Rankin RN, Fox AJ, et al. Accuracy and prognostic consequences of ultrasonography in identifying severe carotid artery stenosis. North American Symptomatic Carotid Endarterectomy Trial (NASCET) Group. *Stroke* 1995;26: 1747–1752.

104. Horrow MM, Stassi J, Shurman A, et al. The limitations of carotid sonography: interpretative and technology-related errors. *AJR Am J Roentgenol* 2000;174:189–194.

105. Kotval PS. Doppler waveforms parvus and tardus: a sign of proximal flow obstruction. *Us Med* 1988;8:435–440.

106. Mohr JP, Caplan LR, Melski JW, et al. The Harvard Cooperative Stroke Registry: a prospective registry. *Neurology* 1978; 28:754.

107. Khaw KT. Does carotid duplex imaging render angiography redundant before carotid endarterectomy? *Br J Radiol* 1997; 70:235–238.

108. Golledge J, Wright R, Pugh N, et al. Colour-coded duplex assessment alone before carotid endarterectomy. *Br J Surg* 1996;83:1234–1237.

109. Ballard JL, Deiparine MK, Bergan JJ, et al. Cost-effective evaluation and treatment for carotid disease. *Arch Surg* 1997; 132:268–271.

110. Hansen F, Bergqvist D, Lindblad B, et al. Accuracy of duplex sonography before carotid endarterectomy—a comparison with angiography. *Eur J Vasc Endovasc Surg* 1996;12:331–336.

111. Jackson MR, Chang AS, Robles HA, et al. Determination of 60% or greater carotid stenosis: a prospective comparison of magnetic resonance angiography and duplex ultrasound with conventional angiography. *Ann Vasc Surg* 1998;12:236–243.

112. Saouaf R, Grassi CJ, Hartnell GG, et al. Complete MR angiography and Doppler ultrasound as the sole imaging modalities prior to carotid endarterectomy. *Clin Radiol* 1998;53: 759–786.

113. Akers D, Markowitz I, Kerstein M, et al. The evaluation of the aortic arch in the evaluation of cerebrovascular insufficiency. *Am J Surg* 1987;154:230.

114. Provan JL. Arteriosclerotic occlusive arterial disease of brachiocephalic and arch vessels. In: Rutherford RB, ed. *Vascular surgery.* Philadelphia: WB Saunders; 1989:822.

115. Djouhri H, Guillon B, Brunereau L, et al. MR angiography for the long-term follow-up of dissection aneurysms of the extracranial internal carotid artery. *AJR Am J Roentgenol* 2000;174:1137–1140.

116. Oelerich M, Stogbauer F, Kurlemann G, et al. Craniocervical artery dissection: MR imaging and MR angiographic findings. *Eur Radiol* 1999;9(7):1385–1391.

117. Randoux B, Marro B, Koskas F, et al. Carotid artery stenosis: prospective comparison of CT, 3D gadolinium-enhanced MR, and conventional angiography. *Radiology* 2001;220: 179–185.

118. Flohr T, Prokop M, Becker C, et al. A retrospectively ECG-gated multislice spiral CT scan and reconstruction technique with suppression of heart pulsation artifacts for cardiothoracic imaging with extended volume coverage. *Eur Radiol* 2002;12(6):1497–1503.

119. The French Study of Aortic Plaques in Stroke Group. Atherosclerotic disease of the aortic arch as a risk factor or recurrent ischemic stroke. *NEJM* 1996;334:1216–1221.

120. Bluemke AB, Stillman AE, Bis KG, et al. Carotid MR angiography: phase II study of safety and efficacy for MS-325. *AJR Am J Roentgenol* 2001;219:114–122.

121. Phatouros CC, Higashida RT, Malek AM, et al. Carotid artery stent placement for atherosclerotic disease: rationale, technique and current status. *Radiology* 2000;217:26–41.

34

Catheter Tracking and Devices

Harald H. Quick

Several attributes make magnetic resonance imaging (MRI) attractive for guidance of intravascular therapeutic procedures, including high soft tissue contrast, imaging in arbitrary oblique planes, lack of ionizing radiation, and the ability to provide functional information, such as flow velocity or flow volume per unit time, in conjunction with morphologic information. For MR guidance of vascular interventions to be safe, the interventionalist must be able to visualize catheters and guidewires relative to the vascular system and surrounding tissues. Several approaches for rendering instruments visible in an MR environment have been developed, including both *passive* and *active* techniques. Passive techniques depend on contrast agents or susceptibil-

ity artifacts that enhance the appearance of the catheter in the image itself, whereas active techniques rely on supplemental hardware built into the catheter, such as a radio frequency (RF) coil. Additionally, the ability to introduce an RF coil mounted on a catheter presents the opportunity to obtain high-resolution images of the vessel wall. These images can provide the capability to distinguish and identify various plaque components. The additional capabilities of MRI could potentially open up new applications within the purview of vascular interventions beyond those currently performed under x-ray fluoroscopic guidance.

This chapter reviews the techniques for instrument visualization, some of the technical requirements for performing interventional cardiovascular MR procedures, and issues of MR safety related to interventional devices visualization.

INTERVENTIONAL DEVICE VISUALIZATION

Prerequisite to the safe and successful performance of vascular interventions with MRI is not only the collection of relevant anatomic information, but also the reliable visualization of catheters and guidewires in relation to the surrounding tissue morphology. In contrast to ultrasound, x-ray fluoroscopy, or computed tomography (CT), visualization of interventional instruments in MR has proven to be difficult.

The technique used to render vascular instruments visible in MR would ideally be characterized by high spatial and temporal resolution. It should also provide a high-contrast instrument signature, making it easy to pick out the instrument in the MR image. Several approaches have been developed for depicting vascular instruments in an MR environment. They can be broadly grouped into two categories: passive and active visualization. The passive techniques are familiar from ultrasound, x-ray fluoroscopy, and CT. The material properties of the instrument are manipulated so that the instrument appears with sufficient contrast in the image itself. No additional hardware or instrument modifications are required. The active techniques rely on additional hardware and postprocessing to achieve instrument localization.

PASSIVE GUIDANCE: CONTRAST AGENTS AND SUSCEPTIBILITY ARTIFACTS

Two approaches to passive catheter guidance exist. The first is to alter the blood signal relative to the catheter signal. This can be achieved with administration of a vascular contrast agent. Gadolinium-diethylenetriaminepentaacetate (DTPA) allows the acquisition of high-resolution MR angiograms that could be used for tracking vascular instruments relative to arterial morphologic background "road maps." However, commercially available contrast agents rapidly leak out of the vascular space, resulting in increased signal in the background tissues. This alters the signal characteristics of the target vessel and potentially reduces catheter visualization. Intravascular MR contrast agents have a prolonged intravascular presence but equally opacify both arteries and veins (1,2). Strategies for reducing venous opacification have been explored by using contrast agents based on superparamagnetic iron oxides with both T1- and T2-shortening effects (3). By filling the catheter with a Gd-based contrast agent, both vascular system and instruments can be visualized separately with a double-echo gradient-echo sequence. The image based on the short echo renders both the vasculature and the catheter bright, whereas the image based on the long-TE echo renders only the catheter bright. The catheter-only image (second echo) can be threshold and overlaid in color on the vascular image (first echo) (3).

The second approach to passive catheter guidance involves altering the catheter signal relative to the blood signal. Instruments can be filled with contrast-doped solution, shortening the relaxation time. Imaging is accomplished by using a short repetition time (TR)/short echo-time (TE) pulse sequence along with a high flip-angle, achieving a catheter image that is bright relative to the background. The slice thickness is generally limited, however, because the instrument rapidly disappears as a result of partial voluming as the thickness is increased (4). Rather than filling the lumen of the catheter with liquid contrast solution, another approach is to treat the surface of the catheter with Gd^{3+} ions (5). As a consequence, the T1 of blood in the immediate vicinity of the catheter is shortened, rendering the catheter visible.

A different approach to achieving adequate catheter contrast is based on enhancing the inherent signal void (i.e., negative contrast) of an instrument as it displaces spins during insertion. Differences in magnetic susceptibility can be used to create large, local losses in signal as a result of intravoxel dephasing (6–8). Unfortunately, these signal losses are most often accompanied by geometric distortion of the underlying vascular anatomy. Additionally, the effect is highly dependent on several factors, including field strength, pulse sequence parameters, and device orientation within the magnetic field. These dependencies prevent a consistent portrayal of instruments. A useful approach has been to incorporate multiple rings of paramagnetic dysprosium oxide (Dy_2O_3) along the catheter tip, allowing the catheter to be consistently visualized independent of orientation (8).

ACTIVE GUIDANCE: RADIO FREQUENCY COIL "TIP-TRACKING" AND "PROFILING"

Several of the active tracking techniques that have been demonstrated to be suitable for vascular interventions involve the incorporation of an RF coil into the instrument itself. MR tracking relies on the incorporation of a miniature solenoidal coil into the instrument (9–13). The coil is connected to the scanner via a thin coaxial cable passing through the catheter and provides a robust signal, identifying the instrument location with high contrast. Early tracking catheter designs incorporated an RF coil on the tip of interventional instruments (Fig. 34.1A,B), thus the tip could be visualized with high contrast and high temporal resolution in three dimensions (10). The actively available three-dimensional (3D) spatial coordinates could also be used to steer the actual imaging plane with the instrument tip, allowing for two-dimensional (2D) imaging updates at the exact location of the coil, with corresponding depiction of the surrounding anatomy. More current setups for catheter tip tracking now combine fast updates of the catheter position with real-time imaging sequences, such that real-time imaging is always performed at the current catheter position (14–16). Up to three tracking coils implemented into the catheter over several centimeters enable to link the slice position and orientation to the distal end of the instrument (14,15). The interventionalist can thus assess the current interventional situation in real time. Practical considerations, however, suggest that the entire instrument needs to be visualized, rather than only the instrument tip.

One way to obtain the curvature information missing with the MR tracking technique is to elongate the RF coil in the instrument. Magnetically coupled antennas with reduced signal penetration depth can be used. These are the traditional looped antennas of MR, familiar from all surface coils: the coils are simply wound very thin and extended over a length of several centimeters (17–19). These antennas generate an outline of very limited extent, which sharply delineates the instrument. The acquisition of a conventional MR image with these antennas leads to an outline or "profile" of the instrument as a result of the localized sensitivity of the coils, thus the designation "MR profiling" (Fig. 34.1C,D) (18,19).

Another group of RF antennas suitable for integration into small diameter vascular instruments are the electrically coupled loopless antennas (dipoles or stubs) (Fig. 34.2) (20,21). Such antennas provide a relatively homogeneous signal profile along the whole instrument. Signal sensitivity here is directed toward the outside of the antenna, providing signal beyond the constraints of the instrument. This might be advantageous for simultaneously displaying the immediate anatomic surrounding when tracking the instrument; however, this signal characteristic hampers sharp delineation of the instrument. Additionally, signal is inherently faint at the antenna tip, which might lead to insufficient instrument tip visibility.

In previous experimental studies that explored the potential for performing MR-guided cardiovascular interventions with actively visualized instruments, the instruments were tracked on preacquired, high-quality contrast-enhanced vascular road maps (12,13,18). With this strategy, the time-

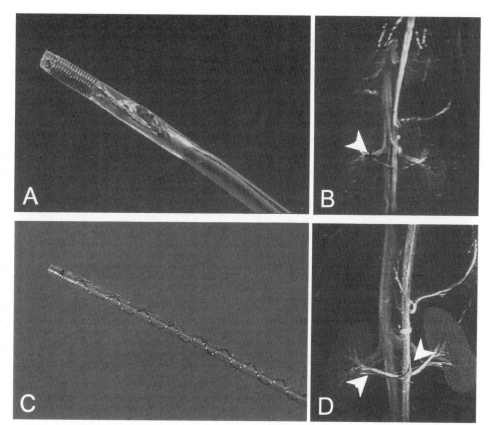

Figure 34.1. Active instrument visualization through implementation of radio frequency (RF) coils into vascular instruments. **(A)** "Tip-tracking" guidewire. The integrated solenoid RF coil at the instrument tip provides localized signal that can be used to superimpose the tip position in color onto a previously acquired road map *(arrow)* or to **(B)** steer the position of the imaging plane in real time, respectively. **(C)** "Profiling" guidewire. The integrated elongated helical wound RF coil provides signal over the distal end of the instrument, resulting in a sharp signal "profile" of the tip and curvature of the instrument **(D)**. **(B,D)** In vivo results in pig experiments.

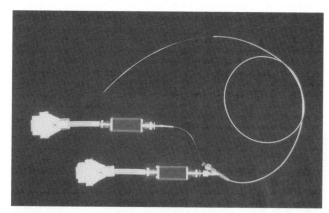

Figure 34.2. Photograph of an active 0.035 "profiling" guidewire and a 6F catheter with integrated dipole antennas. The y-connector at the distal end of the catheter includes the lumen for the guidewire and the RF micro plug for connecting the catheter to the surface coil port of the MR scanner. The antenna tuning, matching, and decoupling for the guidewire and the catheter is housed inside individual RF-shielded boxes at the proximal end of the instruments. The boxes are connected to separate RF receiver channels of the MR scanner. (From Quick HH, Kuehl H, Kaiser G, et al. Interventional MRA using actively visualized catheters, trueFISP, and real-time image fusion. *Magn Reson Med* 2003;49: 129–137, with permission.)

consuming acquisition of vascular road maps could be performed before moving on to the acquisition of real-time updates for continuous display of the instrument position. Although vascular road map and real-time instrument tracking were thus independent from each other, such strategies had obvious drawbacks: the anatomic road map did not always represent the current anatomic situation during the course of an intervention. Gross movements of the patient or cardiac and breathing motion sometimes led to misregistrations between the anatomic road map and the instrument position.

The drawbacks of preinterventional road map acquisition strategies can be overcome by the use of fast imaging techniques with steady state free precession (SSFP), also referred to as TrueFISP, balanced FFE, Fiesta, and so forth. Such sequences, in general, offer high image acquisition speed, signal-to-noise ratio (SNR), contrast-to-noise ratio (CNR), and furthermore, contrast characteristics that render vessels hyperintense, even without the administration of a contrast agent, making them attractive for the guidance of interventional MRA. Current setups for performing MR-guided cardiovascular interventions are based on the combination of actively visualized instruments with real-time TrueFISP imaging (15,22,23). Figures 34.2 through 34.4 show an example of an interventional real-time imaging setup that combines active instrument visualization and TrueFISP imaging to enable real-time image acquisition, reconstruction, fusion, and display with multiple RF receiver channels for the simultaneous and independent display of actively visualized instruments and vascular morphology (22).

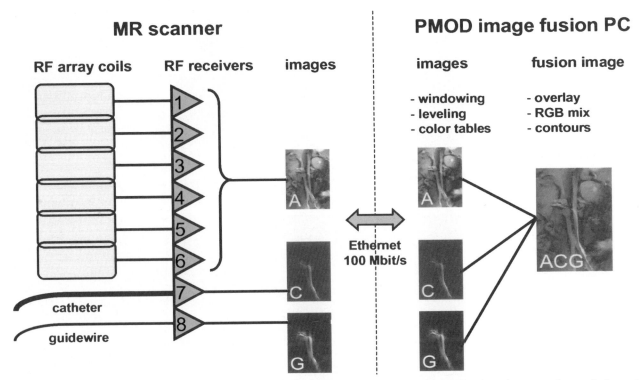

Figure 34.3. Schematic of a setup for real-time instrument visualization. The signals of up to six phased array surface coil elements are fed to separate RF receiver channels. Image reconstruction results in an anatomic image **(A)**. The individual signals of the guidewire and the catheter are fed into separate receiver channels and reconstructed independently (G, guidewire image; C, catheter image). The reconstructed images A, C, and G are transferred via a 100 Mbit per second. Ethernet connection to a stand-alone PC, where a real-time software application enables individual windowing, leveling, and color coding of the individual images. An image fusion function allows the use of an overlay technique, RGB signal mix, or contour visualization in real time. The resulting composite image (ACG) is displayed on an in-room monitor to be viewed by the interventionalist. (From Quick HH, Kuehl H, Kaiser G, et al. Interventional MRA using actively visualized catheters, trueFISP, and real-time image fusion. *Magn Reson Med* 2003;49:129–137, with permission.)

TRACKING OF RESONANT RADIO FREQUENCY MARKERS

Thus far, most of the proposed designs for active instrument visualization in MRI have necessitated some kind of electrically conducting wire connection between the instrument and the MR scanner. This wire connects the RF coil or dipole antenna through the instrument body to remote external tuning, matching, and decoupling electronics. These electronics are typically contained within an RF-shielded box that is connected with an interface plug to the surface coil port of the scanner (Fig. 34.2) (9–23).

An alternative strategy pursues omission of the electrically conducting cable. This strategy is based on self-resonant RF circuits that initially have been successfully used as high-contrast markers for localization purposes in

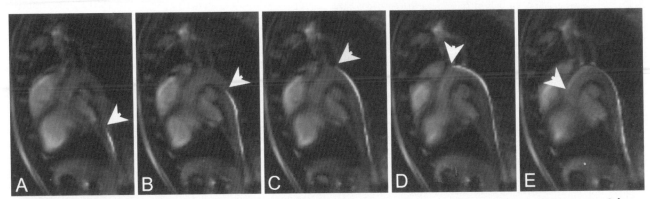

Figure 34.4. Tracking of an active catheter inside the aortic arch. Five out of 120 frames are shown. Image update rate was 3 frames per second. The temporal and spatial resolution of the real-time TrueFISP sequence was sufficient to simultaneously visualize and track the intravascular instrument and anatomy, despite cardiac and respiratory motion. (From Quick HH, Kuehl H, Kaiser G, et al. Interventional MRA using actively visualized catheters, trueFISP, and real-time image fusion. *Magn Reson Med* 2003;49:129–137, with permission.)

MRI (24). Such markers consist of a miniature high-quality RF coil tuned to the Larmor frequency of the scanner and surrounding a small container filled with a short T1 solution. The application of low flip-angle excitation pulses in a fast imaging sequence allows bright depiction of the coil's interior because the effective excitation angle inside the coil is increased as a result of the coil resonance. The background will give relatively little signal at these low excitation angles, resulting in a positive contrast between marker and background. This technique has recently been adapted to instrument tip tracking (25–28), where miniaturized resonant circuits with solenoidal coils have been mounted on vascular catheters. An optical fiber running through the catheter shaft supplies laser light pulses from the scanner to a photodiode at the instrument tip to intermittently tune and detune the resonant circuit. This technique enables high-contrast visibility and thus real-time tracking of the instrument tip (26,27).

WIRELESS ACTIVE CATHETER VISUALIZATION

By omitting the electrically conducting wire connection, potential RF heating issues, associated with long conducting structures exposed to RF fields, can be successfully eliminated with the approach described previously. However, this approach still requires a mechanical connection (laser fiber) between the instrument and the scanner. Such connections (electrical or optical) greatly hamper handling of the interventional instruments. Unlike in conventional x-ray fluoroscopy, instruments cannot be freely manipulated and rotated. Additionally, catheters and other instruments cannot be easily exchanged over an already positioned guidewire, which is a standard maneuver in conventional x-ray fluoroscopy.

The principle of inductive coupling of RF coils (29–33) has recently successfully been applied to catheters to enable a new instrument visualization strategy: wireless active catheter visualization (34). Here, catheters are designed to contain longitudinal single-loop RF resonant circuits. The catheter thus acts as intravascular RF receiver whose signal can be coupled to outside surface coils (Fig. 34.5). This active instrument visualization strategy aims to (a) provide reliable and robust high-contrast visualization of an instrument portion larger than just the tip, (b) avoid an electrically conducting wire connection to avoid RF heating, and (c) avoid hampering instrument handling by eliminating any mechanical (electrical wire or laser fiber) connection. The concept has been evaluated in phantom experiments (Fig. 34.6) and in numerous vascular manipulations performed on pigs (Fig. 34.7). In these interventions, wireless active catheters were guided under real-time visualization into several different arterial segments. Selective, time-resolved contrast-enhanced MR angiography (35–39) has been performed subsequently at each selected location to verify the catheter position (Fig. 34.8).

Inductive coupling of an elongated, resonant structure provides high-contrast visualization of both the instrument tip and the curvature of the distal segment of the catheter body. The method completely eliminates the necessity of a mechanical connection between the catheter and the MR scanner, thereby simplifying instrument handling. Finally, the instrument to background contrast can be influenced by adjusting the flip angle of the guidance sequence. These characteristics make the technique of wireless active catheter visualization an appealing new addition to the palette of available visualization strategies for MR-guided interventions (34).

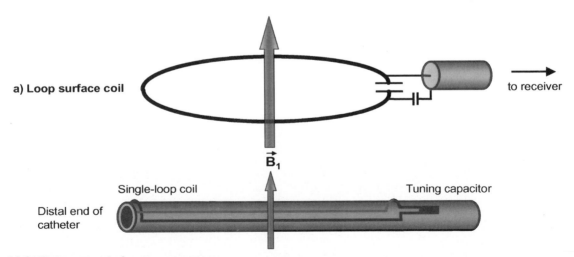

Figure 34.5. Schematic of wireless signal coupling between two RF coils and its application to wireless active catheter visualization. **(A)** Loop surface coil that is connected to the RF receiver of the scanner. **(B)** Distal end of a catheter that is equipped with a closed-loop RF resonator that is tuned to resonance with a capacitor. In body coil (not shown) RF transmit mode, the resonant catheter coil locally multiplies the excitation flip angle. In RF receive mode, the resonant catheter coil picks up the MR signal in its immediate vicinity, resulting in a B_1 field vector that can be inductively coupled to that of the loop surface coil **(A)**. (From Quick HH, Zenge MO, Kuehl H, et al. Interventional MRA with no strings attached: wireless active catheter visualization. *Magn Reson Med* 2005;53:446–455, with permission.)

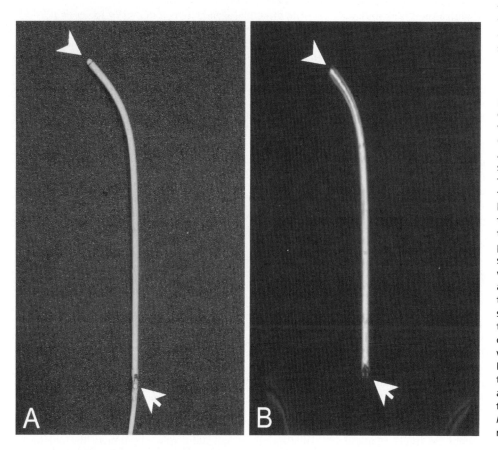

Figure 34.6. **(A)** Photograph of the distal end of a 6F catheter with integrated self-resonant RF circuit, and **(B)** the corresponding signal characteristics in a "high-resolution" TrueFISP image. For MR imaging **(B)**, the catheter was immersed in a 3 L NaCL bottle phantom. A Cartesian TrueFISP sequence with small flip-angle of 5° was used for image acquisition (acquisition time = 0.9 seconds). A 150- × 90-mm image portion is shown. **(B)** Despite the small excitation flip angle, the distal end of the catheter is displayed with high and homogenous signal and thus with high contrast compared to the background. The MR signal profile precisely matches the shape of the catheter up to the very instrument tip. *Arrows* in **(A)** and **(B)** show the position of the tuning capacitor. *Arrowheads* show the distal end of the catheter, where in **(B)**, the NaCL-filled catheter opening can be depicted with excellent detail. (From Quick HH, Zenge MO, Kuehl H, et al. Interventional MRA with no strings attached: wireless active catheter visualization. *Magn Reson Med* 2005;53:446–455, with permission.)

COMBINATION WITH CONVENTIONAL X-RAY FLUOROSCOPY

One approach to bridging the current difficulties with catheter visualization in MR is to combine an MR magnet with an alternative guidance modality, usually an x-ray fluoroscopy system. One system (40,41) couples a conventional C-arm fluoroscopic unit, complete with digital subtraction angiography, road mapping, and so forth, with a cylindrical-bore 1.5 T magnet. The patient is placed on a common table that is both MR-compatible and x-ray transparent. The table can be moved back and forth between the two systems without the need for repositioning the patient. For guidewire and catheter placement, the fluoroscopic system can be used,

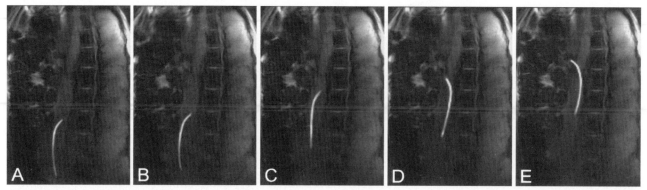

Figure 34.7. Sagittal plane in vivo catheter guidance through the abdominal aorta of a pig into the celiac trunk. Image sequence was a projection reconstruction TrueFISP with a frame rate of 6 frames per second. Five (nonconsecutive) frames out of 120 are shown. Note that the flip angle of 20° allows for bright instrument signal while the background signal remains low, thus allowing for high instrument to background contrast. The position and the curvature of the distal end of the catheter, including the tip, is always exactly determinable. (From Quick HH, Zenge MO, Kuehl H, et al. Interventional MRA with no strings attached: wireless active catheter visualization. *Magn Reson Med* 2005;53:446–455, with permission.)

Figure 34.8. **(A)** Maximum intensity projection (MIP) of an MR angiogram (MRA) acquired in the abdominal aorta of a pig following intravenous contrast injection gives a comprehensive view of the vascular morphology. Images **(B)** and **(C)** show MIPs of selective time-resolved high-resolution 3D FLASH contrast-enhanced MRA of the celiac trunk with the SMA in coronal **(B)** and sagittal **(C)** projections. Contrast agent was administered through the tip of the wireless active catheter, which had been previously tracked into the celiac trunk, as shown in Figure 34.7. The distal active end of the catheter was colored in red. Note excellent correlation between the intravenous MRA in **(A)** and the intra-arterial MRA in **(B)** and **(C)**. (From Quick HH, Zenge MO, Kuehl H, et al. Interventional MRA with no strings attached: wireless active catheter visualization. *Magn Reson Med* 2005;53: 446–455, with permission.)

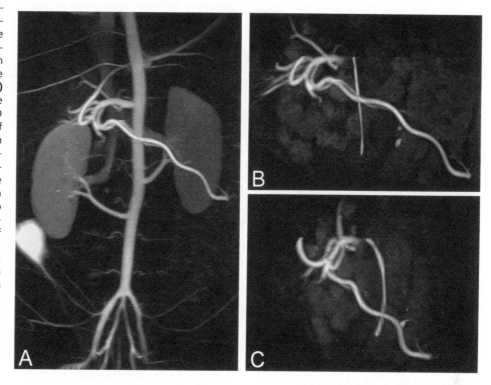

whereas the MR can be used for immediate postdilatation flow measurements. Such combined systems can potentially play an increasingly important role when transferring the MR-guided interventional concepts from preclinical animal studies to human applications.

INTRAVASCULAR MAGNETIC RESONANCE IMAGING

Beyond active catheter visualization for tracking purposes, catheter mounted RF coils potentially offer the ability to acquire high-resolution intravascular MR images of the vessel wall. Because such coils are introduced into and manipulated through the vessels, they can be placed at virtually every vascular region of interest. Such an approach for vessel wall imaging inherently provides very high SNR localized at the lesion of interest, which often outperforms the SNR that surface coils would provide at an identical position (33,42). The concept of intravascular MR imaging has been explored for some time now (43–49). For an intravascular MRI concept to succeed, the design of the imaging coil needs to fulfill various safety and image quality requirements: (a) high local SNR for high-resolution imaging, (b) minimized radial sensitivity falloff for sufficient signal penetration depth into the vessel wall, (c) homogeneous signal response over several centimeters for multislice imaging, and (d) insensitivity to the orientation of the coil, with respect to the main magnetic field B_0. Furthermore, features, such as the suppression of flow artifacts, a small diameter of the RF coil system, and a nonrigid, flexible catheter-based design for easy insertion into small vessels, have to be considered essential prerequisites (48).

A significant number of different coil designs have been developed with the challenging objective to fulfill most of these design requirements that are often conflicting goals and have been evaluated in vitro as well as in vivo animal experiments. Among these intravascular imaging coil designs were opposed solenoid coils (43,44,46,49), flexible single-loop coils for intra-arterial (47,48) and intravenous (50) insertion, balloon-mounted loop coils (Fig. 34.5) (48,51), and "loopless" dipole antennas (21) that inherently provide less SNR in the near-field when compared to conventional looped coils.

Because the placement of such endoluminal coils requires arterial puncture, their use must be coupled with an endovascular intervention and is thus not considered to be purely diagnostic. The outstanding resolution of the intravascular images might be used to characterize various plaque components, thereby providing guidance for choice of the optimal therapeutic strategy to pursue (Fig. 34.9) (52–54). Although intravascular ultrasound can be used currently to characterize plaques, the advantages of MR imaging lie in its superior soft tissue contrast (55), its ability to see behind calcified plaques and the struts of intravascular stents (56), and the ease with which tomographic or 3D data, with a known relation to other anatomic landmarks, can be generated. In a more recent study, the concept of opposed solenoid RF coils has been revisited to combine active catheter tracking with subsequent high-resolution intravascular MRI (Fig. 34.10A) (49). One demonstration revealed that an intravascular RF coil in conjunction with fast TrueFISP sequences can provide sufficient SNR to achieve an in-plane image resolution of around 300 μm within 6 seconds per slice (Fig. 34.10C). Image acquisition speed will be a critical factor when transferring the concept of intravascular MRI to human applications.

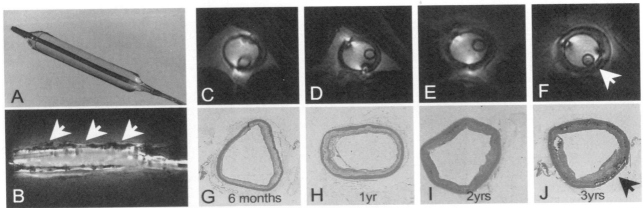

Figure 34.9. **(A)** Close up of the tip of a prototype catheter with a balloon-mounted single-loop RF coil for high-resolution intravascular MR imaging. **(B)** Coronal high-resolution view acquired with the balloon imaging catheter inside an arterial segment. Dark structures inside the vessel wall represent calcifications [*three arrows* in **(B)**]. Images **(C–F)** show in vivo high-resolution (117 × 156 μm) intravascular T2-weighted images, acquired with the balloon mounted intravascular coil inside the abdominal aorta of atherosclerotic Watanabe rabbits. Images **(G–J)** represent histopathologic correlations (hematoxylin-eosin stain) transecting the abdominal aorta of 4 different animals aged 6 **(C,G)**, 12 **(D,H)**, 24 **(E,I)**, and 36 months **(F,J)** in identical locations. Wall thickness and plaque area increase with increasing age. Calcified plaque characterized by reduced signal intensities on MR images (*arrow in* **F**) was confirmed in the histologic hematoxylin-eosin stain [*arrow in* **(J)**]. The 0.035-inch guidewire lumen is visible inside the inflated balloon (*arrow*).

VASCULAR STENTS IN MAGNETIC RESONANCE IMAGING

Many interventional vascular procedures use arterial stents to reduce restenosis rates following angioplasty. A major requirement for such metallic implants to be suited for use in MR-guided procedures is that they are MR compatible. This implies that no hazardous forces or torques that could dislodge the implant occur within the MRI scanner and that the artifacts produced by the implants are acceptable. Many authors have studied the artifacts produced by metallic stents (Fig. 34.11) (57–61), with the conclusion that for the majority of stents a detailed evaluation of the stent lumen is difficult, or even impossible. The extent of the artifact depends

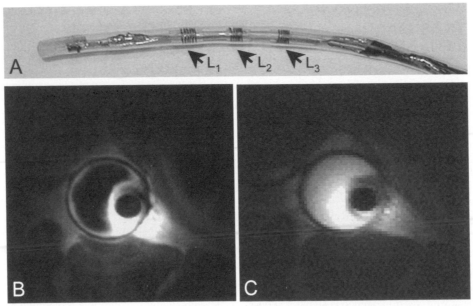

Figure 34.10. Opposed solenoid prototype tracking and intravascular imaging catheter **(A)**. The catheter contains three independent loops (L_1, L_2, L_3) that can be individually connected to independent RF receivers. **(B,C)** Intravascular imaging of the abdominal aorta in a porcine animal model in vivo. Imaging sequence in **(B)** was a double inversion recovery (IR) T2-weighted turbo spin echo with TE 96 milliseconds, TR 2 cardiac cycles, slice thickness 3 mm, in plane resolution 195 × 195 μm and an image acquisition time of 6 minutes per slice. Imaging sequence in **(C)** was a TrueFISP with TE 3.8 milliseconds, TR 7.5 milliseconds, slice thickness 3 mm, in plane resolution 313 × 313 μm. Image acquisition time was 6 seconds per slice only. Although in plane resolution in **(C)** was less than in **(B)**, imaging with the TrueFISP sequence in **(C)** provided enough SNR to significantly reduce the image acquisition time. (Courtesy of Hillenbrand CM and Duerk JL. University Hospitals of Cleveland, Cleveland, OH.)

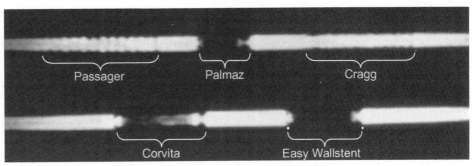

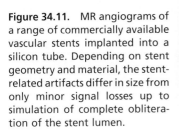

Figure 34.11. MR angiograms of a range of commercially available vascular stents implanted into a silicon tube. Depending on stent geometry and material, the stent-related artifacts differ in size from only minor signal losses up to simulation of complete obliteration of the stent lumen.

on the stent type, the material, the geometry, and the stent orientation to the main magnetic field, B_0. The consequence is that stents that can be used in interventional MRI procedures should preferably be made of so-called low-artifact materials, such as nitinol or tantalum that will not cause extensive susceptibility artifacts. However, even stents that are made of such materials, in general, allow for only qualitative patency assessment but not quantification of in-stent restenosis (61).

ACTIVE STENT VISUALIZATION

To eliminate the above-mentioned MR imaging limitations associated with conventional stents, investigators have pursued the idea to use vascular stents as intravascular RF antennas. In an initial study (62) catheter-mounted self-expandable Wallstents were connected via coaxial cable to tuning and matching electronics. Thus, the stent acted as an active intravascular antenna that provided high signal for MR-guided stent placement. Furthermore, that technique pro-

vided high-resolution imaging of the vessel wall outside the stent and high-resolution imaging inside of the stent lumen. Such a cable-based approach for active stent visualization is invasive and thus is limited to the time of the intervention. Follow-up studies are potentially difficult to achieve, because the approach requires electrical contact between the stent and the MR scanner, and hence repeated invasive access.

A novel study applies the principle of wireless inductive coupling between two RF coils to wireless active visualization of stents (Fig. 34.12) (63,64). Here, the stent mesh itself acts as a closed loop inductor that is tuned with a chip capacitor to resonance. The stent thus functions as an intravascular RF resonator that inductively and thus wireless couples its RF signal to an outside RF surface coil that is connected to the MR scanner. The receive coil system consisting of stent resonator and surface coil performs as an intravascular signal-amplifier and enables high-contrast stent visualization and, furthermore, high-resolution MR imaging of the stent lumen as a result of its high, local signal-to-noise ratio (Figs. 34.13 and 34.14) (64).

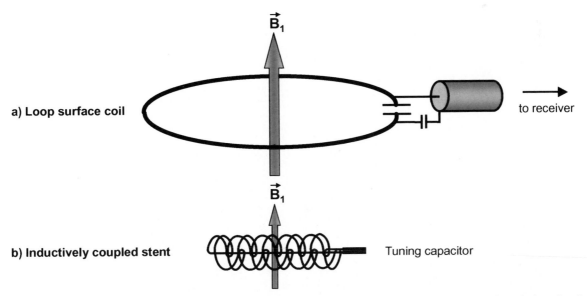

Figure 34.12. Schematic of the principle of inductive coupling between two coils and its application to active wireless visualization of stents. **(A)** Loop surface coil that is connected to the RF receiver of the scanner. **(B)** Schematic of an active stent RF resonator. The mesh of the stent forms a loop coil that is tuned to the Larmor frequency of the MR scanner with a chip tuning capacitor. In body coil (not shown) RF transmit mode, the stent resonator locally multiplies the excitation flip angle. In RF receive mode, the stent resonator picks up the MR signal in its immediate vicinity, resulting in a B_1 field vector that can be inductively coupled to that of the loop surface coil **(A)**. The RF receiver coil system, consisting of implanted stent and surface coil, is thus acting as an intravascular signal amplifier and potentially allows high-resolution MR imaging of deep-sited regions of interest.

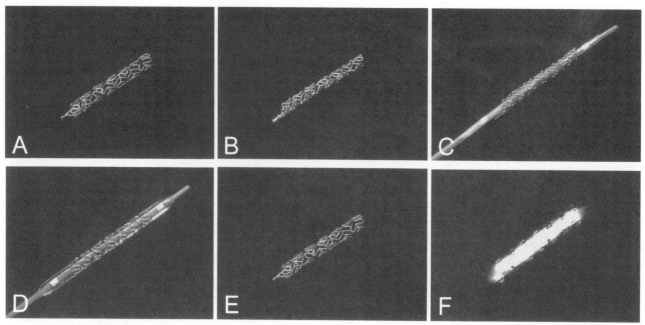

Figure 34.13. Photographs of a balloon-expandable stent resonator prototype, length 28 mm, inner diameter before/after expansion 1.8/4 mm. **(A)** stent resonator in the expanded state, tuned to resonance at 63.8 MHz, **(B)** stent in the folded state, **(C)** folded stent mounted on a 5F balloon catheter (balloon 40 × 4 mm), **(D)** unfolded stent after full inflation of balloon, **(E)** fully deployed stent, and **(F)** MR image acquired with the stent immersed in an NaCl phantom.

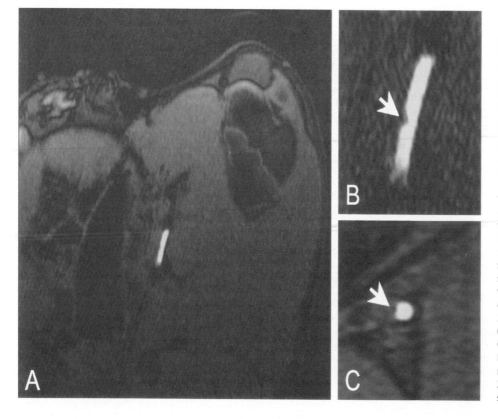

Figure 34.14. In vivo images of a solenoidal stent (length 25 mm, inner diameter 2 mm) implanted into the right iliac artery of a pig. The outside surface receive coil was placed coaxially above the position of the stent. The distance from the middle of the stent to the center of the loop coil was approximately 12 cm. The interior of the stent displays with high signal on the MR image **(A)**. Image parameters were: 2D FLASH, TR/TE 300 per 7 milliseconds, FOV 200 × 200 mm, matrix 256 × 128, slice 2 mm, flip-angle 10°, time 4:18 minutes. Further reduction of the FOV to 100 × 100 mm while maintaining all other imaging parameters enables full assessment of the stent lumen over its full length, parallel **(B)** and orthogonal to the axis of the stent **(C)**. The signal void in the middle of the stent lumen [*arrow in* **(B)** and **(C)**] was identified as thrombus after explantation. Image portions of 30 × 25 mm **(B)** and 25 × 25 mm **(C)** are shown, respectively. (From Quick HH, Kuehl H, Kaiser G, et al. Inductively-coupled stent antennas in MRI. *Magn Reson Med* 2002;48:781–790, with permission.)

By using the stent prototypes as resonant structures in an MR environment, the stent mesh has to fulfill at least two basic requirements (64): the mechanical stent function itself, providing optimal vessel wall support following treatment of the lesion, and the electrical RF antenna function. The latter can be further characterized by the following, often conflicting, goals. For optimal performance, a stent antenna should ideally: (a) resonate at the Larmor frequency of the MR system; (b) provide high, local signal amplification, i.e., provide a high-quality factor, Q, of the resonant circuit; (c) provide high signal homogeneity, both radially and axially inside the stent; (d) function largely independent of orientation relative to the B_1-field of the RF transmit coil; (e) provide optimal coupling to an outside surface coil, with the coupling being largely independent of the stent orientation relative to the surface coil; and (f) be insensitive to different loading conditions once the stent is implanted, i.e., in-stent tissue remodeling, the state of stent expansion, and the radius of stent bending should not influence the resonance frequency or Q. Finally, to facilitate implantation, the stent mesh has to be designed balloon- or self-expandable for catheter-based stent delivery. The proposed method for active stent visualization could provide a powerful diagnostic means for the noninvasive long-term follow-up of stent patency, thereby enhancing the understanding of the mechanisms of in-stent restenosis.

INTERVENTIONAL MAGNETIC RESONANCE SCANNER FEATURES

The transition of MR from a purely diagnostic imaging modality into an imaging platform to guide therapeutic vascular interventions requires realization of more technical features than just instrument and device visualization. For an interventional imaging concept to succeed, the setup must account for imaging flexibility and interactivity to streamline the workflow required for performing image guided interventions. Moving patient tables and flexible, interactive user interfaces with in-room monitors or displays are important prerequisites to successfully perform MR-guided vascular interventions.

MOVING TABLE

So far, MR imaging, in general, and interventional MRA procedures, in particular, have been limited to a single region of interest (ROI). Spatial constraints of the imaging volume, determined by the magnetic field homogeneity and gradient linearity, limit the maximum achievable field of view (FOV) and thus the region to be imaged. Vascular instrument guidance, however, requires the instrument to be imaged from its introduction into the vasculature to the therapeutic region of interest, which often requires the instrument to be advanced beyond the spatial constraints of the imaging volume. To follow the instrument from the "port of first entry" to its final destination (within the vasculature), it is thus mandatory to reposition the patient within the isocenter of the magnet along with any signal-receiving RF surface coils that are placed on top of the patient for enhancing image quality.

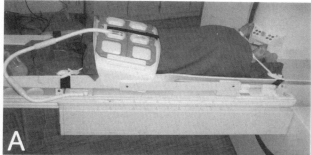
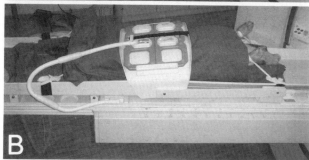
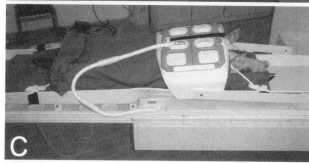

Figure 34.15. The floating *AngioSURF* table (MR-Innovation GmbH, Essen, Germany) allows the fully anesthetized and ventilated pig to be moved manually between the spinal-array surface coil and the phased-array body flex coil that is mounted on the coil glider. **(A–C)** image series demonstrates how the pig is moved to position both surface coils at a new region of interest. For demonstration purposes, photographs were taken outside the bore of the imager. (From Quick HH, Kuehl H, Kaiser G, et al. Interventional MRA with a floating table. *Radiology* 2003;229: 598–602, with permission.)

This procedure is cumbersome, unpractical, as well as time-consuming, and thus limits the overall flexibility of performing MR-guided vascular interventional procedures. Like in conventional x-ray fluoroscopy, a floating table is considered an important feature for future interventional MRI setups (Fig. 34.15) (65). Interventional MRA procedures with a floating table enable the FOV to be moved along with the instrument tip to the region of interest (Fig. 34.16) and thus enhance the usability and flexibility of the interventional MR imaging setup (65).

INTERACTIVE USER INTERFACE

The guidance of vascular interventions with MR imaging requires interactive and flexible adaptation of sequence parameters (e.g., slice position, slice orientation, slice thickness, flip angle, FOV, imaging matrix, and so forth) during

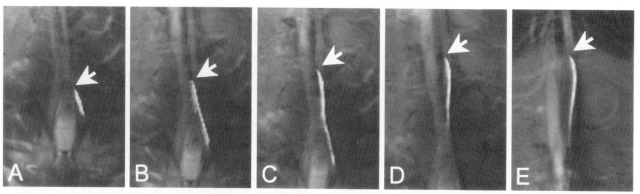

Figure 34.16. Real-time imaging of the advancement of an actively visualized catheter from the iliac artery into the abdominal aorta of a pig. Five out of 180 acquired frames are shown. As soon as the advancing instruments were going to reach the top edge of the FOV **(C)**, the pig on top of the moving table was manually pulled out of the scanner while further advancing the instruments **(D,E)**. This always kept the catheter tip within the visible FOV. Arrows mark the position of the catheter tip advancing inside of the aorta. Imaging frame rate was 4 images per second.

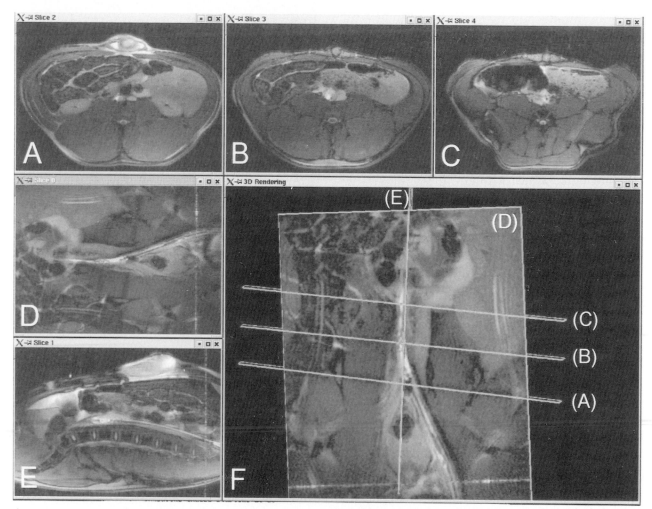

Figure 34.17. Vascular intervention with an actively visualized catheter placed in the aorta of a pig. The interactive multiplanar real-time display in combination with an imaging sequence that allows for fast and interactive multi-planar acquisition of independent imaging slices provides large flexibility for image display. A 3D rendering **(F)** provides a real-time overview of the interventional status and of relative slice positions of the transversal **(A–C)**, coronal **(D)** and sagittal **(E)** real-time slices displayed in the smaller windows. The 3D rendering **(F)** can be interactively tilted and rotated in real time to provide the interventionalist with an adapted overview of the current interventional status. (Courtesy of Raman VK, Guttman MA, Lederman RJ. National Heart, Lung and Blood Institute, Bethesda, Maryland.)

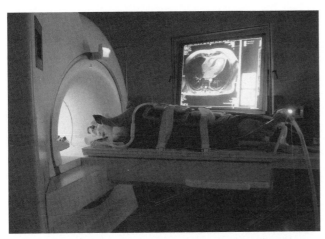

Figure 34.18. High-contrast back projection screen (MR-Innovation GmbH, Essen, Germany) that can be used in the magnet room next to the MR scanner in conjunction with a video projector to provide large in-room display during MR-guided interventional procedures that require instantaneous in-room visual feedback to the interventionalist and rely on real-time guidance of interventional instruments.

continuous real-time data acquisition (15,66). Simultaneous multiplanar data acquisition and display of two or more independent imaging slices facilitates operator orientation and instrument navigation in complex vascular territories (22,66) (Fig. 34.17). The visual information needs to be presented to the interventionalist inside of the scanner room. Large in-room monitors or high-contrast back projection screens, in conjunction with RF-shielded video beamers, have turned out to be a practical and convenient solution (Fig. 34.18).

SAFETY

The primary consideration when performing any intervention is ensuring the safety of the patient. A major concern in interventional MR is the possibility of localized increases in the RF specific absorption rate (SAR) near interventional instruments. The local electric field can be amplified, especially if the instruments are composed of long, conducting structures, making the peak SAR difficult to predict. Most MR tracking, MR profiling, and intravascular imaging techniques currently involve incorporation of a long, electrically conducting cable and a small coil. The small coil, if properly detuned, will not couple significantly with the transmit energy of the body coil. The coupling to the coaxial cable is more difficult to reduce. The cable is basically a long antenna sensitive to the transmit electric field of the body coil. Significant temperature increases have been demonstrated in high-field imagers (1.5 T) near the tips of MR tracking and MR profiling instruments, when using RF-intense imaging sequences, such as fast spin-echo (67,68). This type of heating has also been shown for conventional vascular guidewires with conducting cores (69,70), indicating that the problem is truly related to the long cable not the coil at the tip. Incorporation of coaxial chokes can reduce the electric-field coupling and prevent excessive heating (68,71). Another strategy

is to eliminate the coaxial cable with its potential risk for RF heating, on the basis of the implementation of self-resonant structures into the instruments that are detuned with optical photoresistors driven by optic fibers (25–28) or to completely omit any conducting cable connection, as described in the wireless active catheter visualization section (34).

FUTURE PERSPECTIVE

Interventional cardiovascular MR imaging has the potential to profoundly alter intravascular therapy and is currently a thriving area of research. Beyond duplicating the success of procedures currently performed with x-ray fluoroscopy in an environment free of ionizing radiation, new applications may emerge. Vessel wall characterization has already been demonstrated in proof-of-concept form. Another exciting field of endeavor on the horizon is the transvascular delivery of therapeutic drugs and genes. Magnetic resonance imaging offers a unique opportunity for both guidance of gene delivery and monitoring of gene expression. Beyond the guidance of pure vascular interventions, cardiac interventions benefit from the inherent 2D and 3D natures of MRI and its unique ability to simultaneously visualize cardiac chambers and myocardium, with excellent contrast and sufficient temporal resolution.

In this context, *passive* and *active* instrument visualization techniques both certainly have their right to coexist. Although active techniques offer a broad range of inherent advantages (e.g., high positive instrument contrast, instrument color coding, instrument overlay onto road maps, coordinates available for active steering of the imaging plane, and so forth), their widespread use is currently limited as a result of more complex instrument design and related RF safety issues. Here, the passive instrument visualization techniques are valuable to perform initial basic but safe MR-guided vascular procedures (72,73) and thus to generate confidence into the method. Also, they define the necessary workflow while moving the field from its current research platform with animal feasibility studies into widespread clinical applications for the benefit of patients and investigators. Certainly, these promises warrant further investment in developing this burgeoning field.

REFERENCES

1. Bluemke DA, Stillman AE, Bis KG, et al. Carotid MR angiography: phase II study of safety and efficacy for MS-325. *Radiology* 2001;219:114–122.
2. Grist TM, Korosec FR, Peters DC, et al. Steady-state and dynamic MR angiography with MS-325: initial experience in humans. *Radiology* 1998;207:539–544.
3. Nanz D, Weishaupt D, Quick HH, et al. TE-switched double-contrast enhanced visualization of vascular system and instruments for MR-guided interventions. *Magn Reson Med* 2000; 43:645–648.
4. Unal O, Korosec FR, Frayne R, et al. A rapid 2D time-resolved variable-rate k-space sampling MR technique for passive catheter tracking during endovascular procedures. *Magn Reson Med* 1998;40:356–362.

5. Frayne R, Wehelie A, Yang Z, et al. MR evaluation of signal-emitting coatings. In: Proc., ISMRM, 7th Scientific Meeting and Exhibition. Philadelphia, 1999:580.

6. Rubin DL, Ratner AV, Young SW. Magnetic susceptibility effects and their application in the development of new ferro-magnetic catheters for magnetic resonance imaging. *Invest Radiol* 1990;25:1325–1332.

7. Kochli VD, McKinnon GC, Hofmann E, et al. Vascular interventions guided by ultrafast MR imaging: evaluation of different materials. *Magn Reson Med* 1994;31:309–314.

8. Bakker CJ, Hoogeveen RM, Hurtak WF, et al. MR-guided endovascular interventions: susceptibility-based catheter and near-real-time imaging technique. *Radiology* 1997;202:273–276.

9. Dumoulin CL, Souza SP, Darrow RD. Real-time position monitoring of invasive devices using magnetic resonance. *Magn Reson Med* 1993;29:411–415.

10. Ladd ME, Zimmermann GG, McKinnon GC, et al. Visualization of vascular guidewires using MR tracking. *J Magn Reson Imaging* 1998;8:251–253.

11. Wendt M, Busch M, Wetzler R, et al. Shifted rotated keyhole imaging and active tip-tracking for interventional procedure guidance. *J Magn Reson Imaging* 1998;8:258–261.

12. Leung DA, Debatin JF, Wildermuth S, et al. Intravascular MR tracking catheter: preliminary experimental evaluation. *Am J Roentgenol* 1995;164:1265–1270.

13. Wildermuth S, Debatin JF, Leung DA, et al. MR imaging-guided intravascular procedures: initial demonstration in a pig model. *Radiology* 1997;202:578–583.

14. Zhang Q, Wendt M, Aschoff AJ, et al. A multielement RF coil for MRI guidance of interventional devices. *J Magn Reson Imaging* 2001;14:56–62.

15. Elgort DR, Wong EY, Hillenbrand CM, et al. Real-time catheter tracking and adaptive imaging. *J Magn Reson Imaging* 2003;18:621–626.

16. Zuehlsdorff S, Umathum R, Volz S, et al. MR coil design for simultaneous tip tracking and curvature delineation of a catheter. *Magn Reson Med* 2004;52:214–218.

17. Ladd ME, Erhart P, Debatin JF, et al. Guidewire antennas for MR fluoroscopy. *Magn Reson Med* 1997;37:891–897.

18. Ladd ME, Zimmermann GG, Quick HH, et al. Active MR visualization of a vascular guidewire in vivo. *J Magn Reson Imaging* 1998;8:220–225.

19. Burl M, Coutts GA, Herlihy DJ, et al. Twisted-pair RF coil suitable for locating the track of a catheter. *Magn Reson Med* 1999;41:636–638.

20. McKinnon GC, Debatin JF, Leung DA, et al. Towards active guidewire visualization in interventional magnetic resonance imaging. *MAGMA* 1996;4:13–18.

21. Ocali O, Atalar E. Intravascular magnetic resonance imaging using a loopless catheter antenna. *Magn Reson Med* 1997;37:112–118.

22. Quick HH, Kuehl H, Kaiser G, et al. Interventional MRA using actively visualized catheters, TrueFISP, and real-time image fusion. *Magn Reson Med* 2003;49:129–137.

23. Lederman RJ, Guttman MA, Peters DC, et al. Catheter-based endomyocardial injection with real-time magnetic resonance imaging. *Circulation* 2002;105:1282–1284.

24. Burl M, Coutts GA, Young IA. Tuned fiducial markers to identify body locations with minimal perturbation of tissue magnetization. *Magn Reson Med* 1996;36:491–493.

25. Wong EY, Zhang Q, Duerk JL, et al. An optical system for wireless detuning of parallel resonant circuits. *J Magn Reson Imaging* 2000;12:632–638.

26. Weiss S, Eggers H, Schaeffter T. MR-controlled fast optical switching of a resonant circuit mounted to the tip of a clinical catheter. In: Proceedings of the 9th Annual Meeting of the ISMRM, Glasgow, 2001:544.

27. Weiss S, Kuehne T, Brinkert F, et al. In vivo safe catheter visualization and slice tracking using an optically detunable resonant marker. *Magn Reson Med* 2004;52:860–868.

28. Kuehne T, Fahrig R, Butts K. Pair of resonant fiducial markers for localization of endovascular catheters at all catheter orientations. *J Magn Reson Imaging* 2003;17:620–624.

29. Schnall MD, Barlow C, Subramanian VH, et al. Wireless implanted magnetic resonance probes for in vivo NMR. *J Magn Reson* 1986;68:161–167.

30. Kuhns PL. Inductive coupling and tuning in NMR probes: applications. *J Magn Reson* 1988;78:69–76.

31. Farmer TH, Cofer GP, Johnson GA. Maximizing contrast to noise with inductively coupled implanted coils. *Invest Radiol* 1990;25:552–558.

32. Wirth ED III, Mareci TH, Beck BL, et al. A comparison of an inductively coupled implanted coil with optimized surface coils for in vivo NMR imaging of the spinal cord. *Magn Reson Med* 1993;30:626–633.

33. Arnder LL, Shattuck MD, Black RD. Signal-to-noise ratio comparison between surface coils and implanted coils. *Magn Reson Med* 1996;35:727–733.

34. Quick HH, Zenge MO, Kuehl H, et al. Interventional MR angiography with no strings attached: wireless active catheter visualization. *Magn Reson Med* 2005;53:446–455.

35. Serfaty JM, Atalar E, Declerck J, et al. Real-time projection MR angiography: feasibility study. *Radiology* 2000;217:290–295.

36. Bos C, Smits HF, Bakker CJ, et al. Selective contrast-enhanced MR angiography. *Magn Reson Med* 2000;44:575–582.

37. Serfaty JM, Yang X, Foo TK, et al. MRI-guided coronary catheterization and PTCA: a feasibility study on a dog model. *Magn Reson Med* 2003;49:258–263.

38. Omary RA, Green JD, Schirf BE, et al. Real-time magnetic resonance imaging-guided coronary catheterization in swine. *Circulation* 2003;107:2656–2659.

39. Green JD, Omary RA, Schirf BE, et al. Catheter-directed contrast-enhanced coronary MR angiography in swine using magnetization-prepared True-FISP. *Magn Reson Med* 2003;50:1317–1321.

40. Van Vaals JJ. Interventional MRI with a hybrid high-field system. In: Debatin JF, Adam G, eds. *Interventional magnetic resonance imaging.* Berlin: Springer-Verlag; 1997:19–32.

41. Adam G, Neuerburg J, Bucker A, et al. Interventional magnetic resonance. Initial clinical experience with a 1.5-tesla magnetic resonance system combined with c-arm fluoroscopy. *Invest Radiol* 1997;32:191–197.

42. Ocali O, Atalar E. Ultimate intrinsic signal-to-noise ratio in MRI. *Magn Reson Med* 1998; 39:462–473.

43. Hurst GC, Hua J, Duerk JL, et al. Intravascular (catheter) NMR receiver probe: preliminary design analysis and application to canine iliofemoral imaging. *Magn Reson Med* 1992;24:343–357.

44. Martin AJ, Plewes DB, Henkelman RM. MR imaging of blood vessels with an intravascular coil. *J Magn Reson Imaging* 1992;2:421–429.

45. Kandarpa K, Jakab P, Patz S, et al. Prototype miniature endoluminal MR imaging catheter. *J Vasc Interv Radiol* 1993;4:419–427.

46. Martin AJ, Henkelman RM. Intravascular MR imaging in a porcine animal model. *Magn Reson Med* 1994;32:224–229.

47. Atalar E, Bottomley PA, Ocali O, et al. High resolution intravascular MRI and MRA by using a catheter receiver coil. *Magn Reson Med* 1996;36:596–605.

48. Quick HH, Ladd ME, Zimmermann-Paul GG, et al. Single-loop coil concepts for intravascular MR imaging. *Magn Reson Med* 1999;41:751–758.

49. Hillenbrand CM, Elgort DR, Wong EY, et al. Active device tracking and high-resolution intravascular MRI using a novel

catheter-based, opposed-solenoid phased array coil. *Magn Reson Med* 2004;51:668–675.

50. Martin AJ, McLoughlin RF, Chu KC, et al. An expandable intravenous RF coil for arterial wall imaging. *J Magn Reson Imaging* 1998;8:226–234.

51. Quick HH, Ladd ME, Hilfiker PR, et al. Autoperfused balloon catheter for intravascular MR imaging. *J Magn Reson Imaging* 1999;9:428–434.

52. Zimmermann-Paul GG, Quick HH, Vogt P, et al. High-resolution intravascular magnetic resonance imaging: monitoring of plaque formation in heritable hyperlipidemic rabbits. *Circulation* 1999;99:1054–1061.

53. Martin AJ, Gotlieb AI, Henkelman RM. High-resolution MR imaging of human arteries. *J Magn Reson Imaging* 1995;5:93–100.

54. Correia LC, Atalar E, Kelemen MD, et al. Intravascular magnetic resonance imaging of aortic atherosclerotic plaque composition. *Arterioscler Thromb Vasc Biol* 1997;17:3626–3632.

55. Martin AJ, Ryan LK, Gotlieb AI, et al. Arterial imaging: comparison of high-resolution US and MR imaging with histologic correlation. *Radiographics* 1997;17:189–202.

56. Quick HH, Ladd ME, Nanz D, et al. Vascular stents as RF antennas for intravascular MR guidance and imaging. *Magn Reson Med* 1999;42:738–745.

57. Teitelbaum GP, Bradley WG Jr, Klein BD. MR imaging artifacts, ferromagnetism, and magnetic torque of intravascular filters, stents, and coils. *Radiology* 1988;166:657–664.

58. Hilfiker PR, Quick HH, Debatin JF. Plain and covered stent-grafts: in vitro evaluation of characteristics at three-dimensional MR angiography. *Radiology* 1999;211:693–697.

59. Schurmann K, Vorwerk D, Bucker A, et al. Magnetic resonance angiography of nonferromagnetic iliac artery stents and stent-grafts: a comparative study in sheep. *Cardiovasc Interv Radiol* 1999;22:394–402.

60. Klemm T, Duda S, Machann J, et al. MR imaging in the presence of vascular stents: a systematic assessment of artifacts for various stent orientations, sequence types, and field strengths. *Magn Reson Imaging* 2000;12:606–615.

61. Bartels LW, Smits HF, Bakker CJ, et al. MR imaging of vascular stents: effects of susceptibility, flow, and radio frequency eddy currents. *J Vasc Interv Radiol* 2001;12:365–371.

62. Quick HH, Ladd ME, Nanz D, et al. Vascular stents as RF antennas for intravascular MR guidance and imaging. *Magn Reson Med* 1999;42:738–745.

63. Kivelitz D, Wagner S, Hansel J, et al. The active magnetic resonance imaging stent (AMRIS): initial experimental in vivo results with locally amplified MR angiography and flow measurements. *Invest Radiol* 2001;36:625–631.

64. Quick HH, Kuehl H, Kaiser G, et al. Inductively coupled stent antennas in MRI. *Magn Reson Med* 2002;48:781–790.

65. Quick HH, Kuehl H, Kaiser G, et al. Interventional MR angiography with a floating table. *Radiology* 2003;229:598–602.

66. Guttman MA, Lederman RJ, Sorger JM, et al. Real-time volume rendered MRI for interventional guidance. *J Cardiovasc Magn Reson* 2002;4:431–442.

67. Wildermuth S, Dumoulin CL, Pfammatter T, et al. MR-guided percutaneous angioplasty: assessment of tracking safety, catheter handling and functionality. *Cardiovasc Interv Radiol* 1998;21:404–410.

68. Ladd ME, Quick HH. Reduction of resonant RF heating in intravascular catheters using coaxial chokes. *Magn Reson Med* 2000;43:615–619.

69. Nitz WR, Oppelt A, Renz W, et al. On the heating of linear conductive structures as guide wires and catheters in interventional MRI. *J Magn Reson Imaging* 2001;13:105–114.

70. Konings MK, Bartels LW, Smits HF, et al. Heating around intravascular guidewires by resonating RF waves. *J Magn Reson Imaging* 2000;12:79–85.

71. Atalar E. Safe coaxial cables. In: Proc., ISMRM, 7th Scientific Meeting and Exhibition, 1999. Philadelphia, 1999:1006.

72. Manke C, Nitz WR, Djavidani B, et al. MR imaging-guided stent placement in iliac arterial stenoses: a feasibility study. *Radiology* 2001;219:527–534.

73. Razavi R, Hill DL, Keevil SF, et al. Cardiac catheterisation guided by MRI in children and adults with congenital heart disease. *Lancet* 2003;362:1877–1882.

35

Endovascular Interventional Magnetic Resonance Imaging

Arno Bücker

Magnetic resonance angiography (MRA) is on the verge of supplanting diagnostic x-ray angiography, which was made possible by technical progress on the front of sequence development and through hardware improvement. Although coronary angiography is still a challenge for MRA, the advent of fast gradients with short repetition time (TR) and echo time (TE) enabling breath-held three-dimensional (3D) contrast-enhanced angiography was a break-through for the clinical application of MRA in the region of the aorta, its branches, and even for runoff vessels. The ideal MR sequence for vascular interventions would be the acquisition of a 3D data set with real-time upgrades of the background anatomy and the interventional device. The vascular anatomy and the interventional device would have to be depicted with high-spatial resolution. The application of contrast media should not be necessary to avoid toxic concentrations of commercially available contrast agents in case of multiple injections, as would be necessary by directly applying the technique of diagnostic breath-held 3D MRA. Although the application of blood pool agents can circumvent this problem, the resulting overlap of arterial and venous anatomy is not desirable.

So far, we are struggling to get close to the ideal situation of real-time 3D imaging for vascular MR interventions. The acquisition of 3D data sets is still too slow to allow real-time imaging. But first attempts for vascular interventions have been successfully performed, relying on road maps of 3D data sets in conjunction with real-time projection of a catheter tip onto previously reconstructed maximum intensity projections (MIP) (1). In addition to high temporal, high spatial resolution is also needed to visualize small vessels and interventional instruments. These instruments need to be made of nonferromagnetic material to avoid large artifacts. Furthermore, safety aspects need to be considered, which do not allow the use of metallic devices, like a guidewire, which could act as an antenna (2).

Many of the above-mentioned "challenges" have been, at least partially, met by now, although the ideal solution has not yet been found. Technical developments continue, which will further modify the currently available techniques, before they will be integrated in a clinical routine setup. That almost all of the applications reported have been performed only in animal studies is a reflection of this. Nonetheless, I am convinced that the technical development of real-time

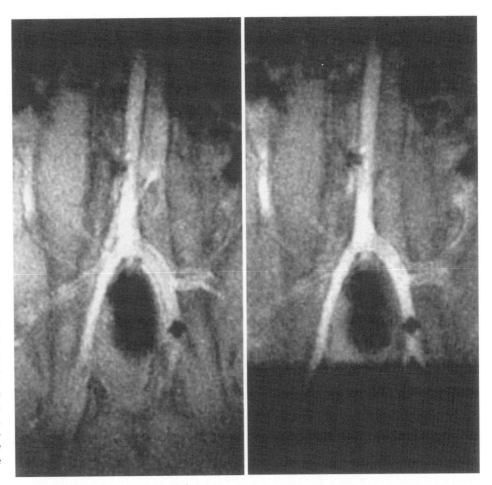

Figure 35.6. Radial scanning of the iliac arteries demonstrates the intrinsic contrast of this gradient-echo technique. For the first image arteries and veins are superimposed. The second image was acquired with a saturation band distally to the imaged area, resulting in a complete suppression of the venous signal, thereby allowing clear depiction of the iliac arteries.

parameters to optimally visualize interventional instruments is not desirable. Furthermore, the tomographic nature of MRI means that a large signal void is advantageous, as long as the instrument is located in a large vessel like the aorta. This will ensure that the device can be localized, even if it is not positioned in the middle of the imaged slice. On the other hand, for smaller vessels large susceptibility artifacts will obscure the vascular anatomy (27). Many dedicated interventional scanners allow "on-the-fly" adaptation of sequence parameters and thereby can, at least, somewhat influence the size of susceptibility markers, but considering reasonable echo times for real-time scanning, the effect is relatively small (Fig. 35.8).

PASSIVE VISUALIZATION WITH THE FIELD INHOMOGENEITY CONCEPT

To be able to change the size of an instrument in the MR image, independently of the sequence parameters, the field inhomogeneity concept was developed (28). A loop of insulated copper wire is wound around the instrument going from the hub to the tip and back (Fig. 35.7). A small energy source is connected to the copper wire loop to allow the flow of a small amount of direct current through the wire. According to the rule of thumb, the flowing current creates a local magnetic field, which causes a local field inhomogeneity and thereby a signal loss. Depending on the strength of the

current, the artifact size can be varied (Fig. 35.9). The signal void can be shaped by different wire configurations. This can produce only local markers at the beginning and end of a balloon or the marking of the whole catheter length. As with the passive method first proposed by Bakker, the wire can be wound to cause signal voids independent of the catheter orientation to B_0 (29). Small currents of up to 150 mA, which were needed to produce sufficiently large areas of signal void during in vivo experiments (30), are too small to be a safety problem. The insulated copper wires can be positioned inside the catheter walls as it is done with standard braiding. Nonetheless, the wires can act as antennas, and, in case of resonance, they could heat up significantly (2). This safety aspect will be discussed in more detail in a later section.

The field inhomogeneity concept has been evaluated in animal experiments showing its advantage for the visualization of the interventional device in vessels of different size (Fig. 35.10) (31). Applying a higher current around 150 mA made it possible to constantly visualize a catheter over its full length in the aorta of a pig. As soon as the catheter was steered into the renal artery the signal void obscured the vascular anatomy. This could be simply changed by switching off the current, while the MR imaging sequence parameters were kept constant (17).

Although the catheter could be visualized in the proximal part of the renal artery, finding the correct imaging plane to depict the full course of the renal artery was difficult. As

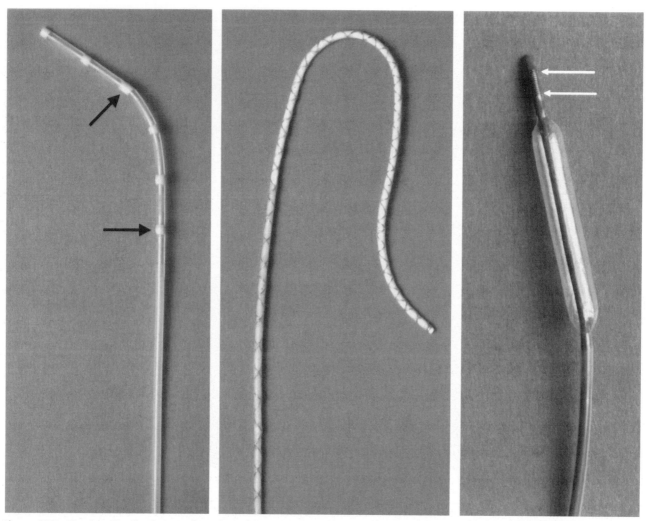

Figure 35.7. Passive visualization can be achieved by susceptibility markers (*left, arrows*) or by the field inhomogeneity principle (*middle*), where a copper wire is forming a loop along the catheter shaft. If wound like double helix, as in this example, a small current send through the insulated copper wire will cause a signal drop around the whole length of the catheter shaft. Active visualization needs a microcoil at the catheter tip to localize its position (*right, arrows*).

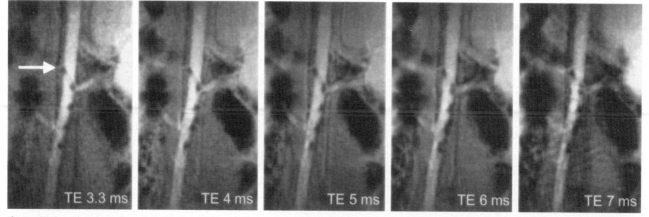

Figure 35.8. The size of passive susceptibility markers can be changed by modifying the echo time. Longer echo times yielding bigger signal voids around the markers, as can be seen on the radial gradient-echo images acquired with increasing TE. Since increasing echo time lengthens the image acquisition and degrades the image quality, there is a limit to the possibility of changing this effect of susceptibility markers.

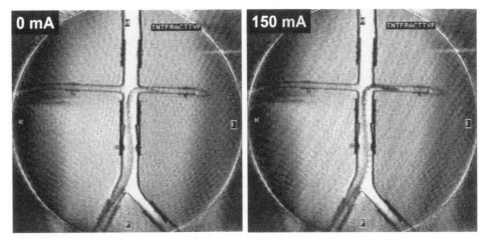

Figure 35.9. A catheter with the field inhomogeneity principle is imaged in a flow phantom by radial scanning. The artifact around the catheter can be increased by sending a current of, for example, 150 mA, through the copper wire running along the catheter shaft.

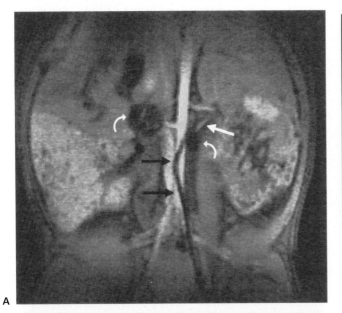

A

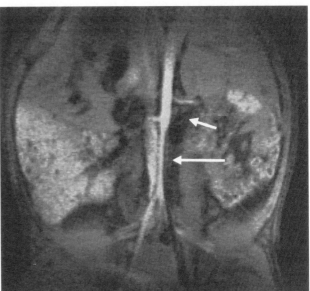

B

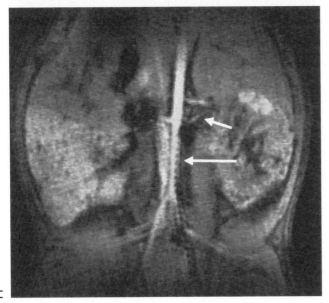

C

Figure 35.10. Real-time radial images of a field inhomogeneity catheter with current switched on (**A,B**) and off (**C**). While the catheter is positioned in the aorta, the proximal part of the left renal artery can be depicted (**A,** *white straight arrow*). Artifacts caused by bowel gas obscures the ostium of the left renal artery and the distal right renal artery (**A,** *curved arrows*). After steering the catheter (**B,** *long arrow*) into the left renal artery, the vessel cannot be seen, with the current switched on (**B,** *short arrow*). Switching the current off allows one to visualize the left renal artery again, although it is still not possible to see the catheter tip on this frozen image. In this image, the contrast of the catheter shaft in the aorta was better, when the current was switched off (**C,** *long arrow*), which is the case, only if the catheter is positioned close to the middle of the imaged slice.

described previously, the tomographic nature of MR is a disadvantage for localizing smaller vessels and/or depicting a tortuous vascular anatomy. Active visualization can help to solve these problems.

ACTIVE VISUALIZATION

Active visualization uses a small microcoil, which is mounted on an instrument (Fig. 35.7). The sensitivity of an MR coil is related to its size. Therefore, a small microcoil used for receiving MR signal yields a signal only in close proximity to the microcoil. Applying an adequate MR sequence, one can use the frequency of this signal to localize the position of the microcoil in two-dimensional (2D) (Fig. 35.11), or even in 3D space (32). If the microcoil is placed on the tip of a catheter, the position of the catheter tip can be calculated and projected onto an MR image (Fig. 35.12) (1,33). Additionally, the knowledge of the position of the microcoil in three-dimensional (3D) space can be exploited to position the MR imaging plane in real time to contain the microcoil, so-called *slice tracking* (34). The number of microcoils can be increased, albeit at the cost of reducing the speed for updating the coil position (35). Furthermore, the shape of the microcoil can be changed to cover the length of an instrument to visualize a longer distance of a guidewire, for example. This technique has been called *MR profiling* (36) and can also be combined with the use of other microcoils.

Initially, the technique of MR tracking was used to superimpose the position of the microcoil onto a previously acquired maximum intensity projection image (1). The 3D data set was acquired in a breath-hold after the bolus application of contrast material. Therefore, a real time update of the background anatomy was not possible, and any movement of the patient or even bending of a vessel as a result of catheter manipulation could lead to the false impression that the microcoil was positioned outside the vascular tree. Nonetheless, balloon occlusion, embolization, and puncture of the portal venous system have been successfully performed with

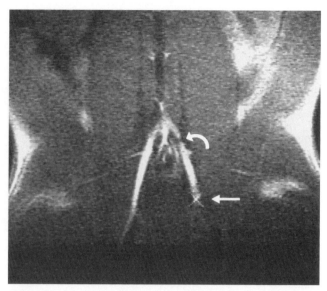

Figure 35.12. The position of an active tip-tracking catheter is projected onto this real-time radial image, being indicated by a blinking cross (*straight arrow*). The plain gradient-echo image demonstrates nicely a stenosis in the proximal iliac artery (*curved arrow*), which could be successfully dilated by real-time tip-tracking of the active balloon catheter.

this technique (1). An in vitro comparison between active MR-catheter tracking and x-ray guided catheter steering showed a similar time needed for both techniques (37). Whether this will hold true for the more complex anatomy of in vivo conditions has yet to be proven. To avoid the above-mentioned movement artifacts for the active tip-tracking technique, real-time imaging of the vascular anatomy and real-time tip tracking is desirable. Simultaneous real-time depiction of the anatomy and the catheter tip was performed applying a 2D radial scanning technique in vitro (34) and in vivo (38). Multiple MR receiver channels are necessary to simultaneously collect the data from the microcoil and from the standard MR coil. For this two-dimensional imaging technique, it is necessary to position the vessel of interest in the imaged slice. This can be ensured by using the slice-tracking technique, which exploits the knowledge of the position of the microcoil to change the position of the imaged slice. The general slice orientation has to be known to ensure that a longer part of the vessel of interest is included in the scan plane. An even more sophisticated technique uses three microcoils mounted on the catheter tip (39). The microcoils are needed to calculate two points near the catheter tip, thereby giving information about the orientation of the interventional instrument. In addition, a software program was developed that could define a point of interest, for example, a stenosis. Those three points could be used to automatically define the optimal imaging plane for an intervention, which contained the instrument tip and the target region. The additional hardware and software modifications and the implementation on a 0.2 T scanner did not allow for real-time imaging. Nonetheless, if this sophisticated approach can be fully automated and combined with a real-time imaging sequence, the whole procedure would be applicable to clinical routine, despite its complexity.

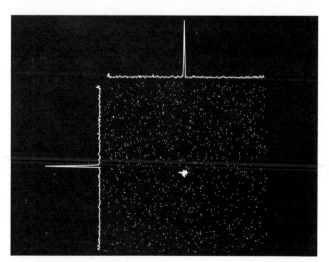

Figure 35.11. A microcoil receives signal only from its very proximity, thereby creating an image that consists of a small, high intensity region. The analysis of this signal allows to calculate the position of the microcoil, which can be projected onto a "standard" MR image.

OTHER TECHNIQUES

The difficulty and complexity of visualizing interventional instruments by fast MR imaging techniques is demonstrated by the number of different approaches. Besides the above-described main categories there are other techniques, which vary greatly concerning their potential imaging speed, the available spatial resolution, and other general advantages and disadvantages. Small tuned antennas at the tip of catheters have been described as fiducial markers (40), electron spin resonance (41), and the Overhauser effect (42) has also been exploited for instrument visualization. Catheters filled with contrast material are used in different imaging strategies (43–45). Intravascular MR imaging was applied for MR-guided dilatation of rabbit aortas (46). This list is far from complete, and the interested reader is referred to the respective literature.

SAFETY ASPECTS

Respecting the general contraindications, MR is a safe examination technique. No ferromagnetic materials can be used near an MR scanner. But even nonferromagnetic metals can cause safety problems as a result of heating (47) or induced electrical currents (48). For interventional instruments the danger lies in that the devices can act as antennas, as soon as a critical length of the instrument is reached. The heating is caused by resonance of the instrument, which leads to a constant feeding of radiofrequency energy into and thereby heating of the device. Like a radio antenna that is tuned in to a radio station, the interventional device may be tuned in (resonant) to the radiofrequency transmitted by the body coil of the MR scanner. The conditions for resonance to occur are difficult to predict under clinical conditions and even impossible to simulate a worst case scenario and measure the maximum heating for one sequence. Besides the position of the instrument inside the magnet bore, its orientation and also the shape of the patient examined play a major role. The amount of radiofrequency energy applied by an MR sequence is also important, but, in the case of resonance, even a sequence with a low specific absorption rate can, in theory, cause significant and potentially harmful heating. First in vitro experiments with an active tip-tracking catheter found no significant heating at 0.5 T but a temperature increase of up to 20°C at 1.5 T (49). Another in vitro study examined guidewires and found only a temperature increase of 15°C at 1.5 T and no significant heating at 0.2 T (50). Experiments performed with guidewires at 1.5 T observed a heating of almost 50°C in 30 seconds, reaching a maximum of 74°C (2). Touching a standard nitinol guidewire did lead to skin burns in one case in this study. During first in vivo animal experiments, we measured a temperature increase of 35°C around the tip of a standard nitinol guidewire placed in the aorta of a living pig. The pig itself was placed as far off center as possible in the magnet bore (Fig. 35.13). Furthermore, we could repeatedly produce sparks at the distal end of the standard nitinol guidewire, simply by bending the distal wire tip to touch the animal (Fig. 35.13) (27).

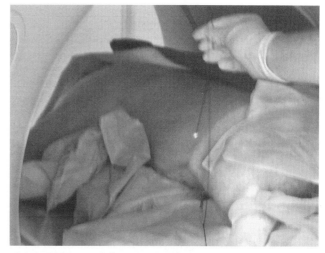

Figure 35.13. A 40-kg pig was placed as far off center in the magnet bore as possible. The tip of the nitinol guidewire is positioned in the aorta and the distal end is bent backward in the magnet to touch, at this time, the dead animal. Sparks, which caused skin burns, could be seen at the distal end of the guidewire.

First steps to solve the safety problems of metallic wires or other metallic instruments have been undertaken. The insertion of chokes along wires has been proposed, and its feasibility to prevent heating has been shown (51). Another method applies photoresistors and photo-optical methods to abolish the need for an electrical connection between the MR scanner and a microcoil, thereby making the occurrence of heating as a result of resonance impossible (52,53). Another approach is the use of a laser fiber to deliver energy to a small coil at the catheter tip, causing intravoxel dephasing, as described by the field inhomogeneity concept but without the need for a conducting wire (54). So far, no commercially available safe MR compatible guidewires are available, which is one of the main reasons why so few MR-guided vascular interventions have been performed clinically.

ENDOVASCULAR APPLICATIONS OF INTERVENTIONAL MAGNETIC RESONANCE IMAGING

Because of the unresolved safety problems for standard metallic instruments, almost all of the MR-guided interventions have been performed in vitro or in animal experiments. The continuously growing number of applications will surely stimulate further research for safe instruments and the commercial production of instruments with the currently available safe techniques.

MAGNETIC RESONANCE–GUIDED PERCUTANEOUS DILATATION

Percutaneous transluminal angioplasties (PTA) were among the first interventions performed under MR-guidance. Initially, active tip-tracking was used projecting the catheter tip onto an MIP of a previously acquired contrast-enhanced 3D data set (1). Despite that this method lacks real-time updates of the vascular anatomy, the technique was successfully applied in one patient in the clinical setup of an open 0.5 T scanner for PTA of an iliac artery. Simultaneous real-time active tip-tracking and real-time visualization of the vascular anatomy was performed to dilate iliac artery stenoses in a pig model (55). Passive visualization was applied for dilatations of the aorta, iliac arteries, and for dialysis shunts (11,13,56). Human studies relied on the visualization of standard nitinol guidewires, stents, and gadolinium-filled balloons for PTA in iliac (13 patients) (57), femoral, and popliteal arteries (3 patients) (58). No side effects because of the use of metallic guidewires were observed during these studies; nonetheless, the risk of heating of nitinol guidewires, especially at high field systems, should not be neglected. Potential radiofrequency heating of guidewires in vitro has been described by several groups (Fig. 35.13) (2,27,50,59,60). Another clinical study involved patients with stenoses of hemodialysis shunts (61). Passive visualization with dysprosium markers was successfully applied in conjunction with a subtraction technique. Also, renal artery dilatation under MR guidance has been performed in an animal model (62).

MAGNETIC RESONANCE–GUIDED STENT PLACEMENT

One drawback of contrast-enhanced 3D MRA is the poor visualization of stent lumina and, consequently, the inability to quantify in stent restenosis (63). Nonetheless, there are stents causing only minor artifacts in the MR images, therefore allowing stent placement under MR guidance (64). First, the feasibility of real-time control of MR-guided stent placement by means of radial scanning and passive visualization of the stents was shown in animal experiments (65). Passive visualization was also applied for the first MR-guided stent placement in humans (66). Real-time MR imaging was not used in this study to perform the intervention. The artifact behavior of stents depends on the type of stent and the imaging sequences applied. Comparing the real-time radial images of ZA stents (67) to the slower standard gradient-echo images of Memotherm stents used in the only clinical study (66), there is a favorable image quality of the real-time images. In vitro comparisons of the artifact behavior of those two stent types indicated a similar artifact behavior. This nicely documents the progress that has been made for real-time image quality (Fig. 35.14), although the hardware and software demands are high (68). Other studies demonstrated this, which exploited active stent visualization for stent placement, having used the stent as a receiver antenna (69) or placed stents in the pulmonary valve and main pulmonary artery (70) or aorta (71) of pigs by passive visualization.

MAGNETIC RESONANCE–GUIDED PLACEMENT OF VENA CAVA FILTERS

The placement of vena cava filters is a relatively simple intervention, which, therefore, could be performed under MR guidance applying relatively slow MR imaging techniques (72–74). All studies were performed relying on pas-

sive visualization of the instruments, including the different vena cava filters. As with stents, the artifact behavior of these filters varies among different filter types and depends on the imaging sequence used. Real-time radial imaging also can be used for vena cava filter placement, being able to show the renal veins and the inferior vena cava allowing for fast and exact positioning of the filter (Fig. 35.15) (75).

MAGNETIC RESONANCE–GUIDED TIPS PROCEDURE

In 1994 MR was used to alleviate the planning of transjugular portosystemic shunts (TIPS) before the procedure itself was performed under x-ray guidance (76). By now there are some reports about MR-guided TIPS procedures (1,77). According to my own experience, MR guidance is helpful for only the puncture of the portal vein. Especially the stent placement is difficult and time-consuming under MR guidance, because the slice has to be oriented along the plane of the TIPS tract (78). In this regard, the tomographic nature of MR is a disadvantage for visualization of the TIPS tract, the portal vein, and the inferior vena cava in one image plane. Special plan scan tools, active tip-tracking and slice-tracking, are needed to allow localization of the ideal MR imaging plane for control of the TIPS procedure in a reasonable time.

MAGNETIC RESONANCE–GUIDED RADIOFREQUENCY ABLATION OF THE HEART

The heart is an especially difficult challenge for MR-guided interventions, because of its constant movement and the complex anatomy. One article claims the possibility for MR-guided catheterization of the coronary arteries, indirectly deducing this possibility from successful steering of a catheter through the aorta (79). Radiofrequency ablation of the heart has been performed under MR guidance by means of passive catheter visualization (80). Besides control of the intervention, MR imaging offered the possibility to directly visualize the success of transmural ablation. The difficulty of defining the correct scan plane, which contains the catheter, was also apparent during this study, and the authors suggested the introduction of active tip-tracking to solve this problem (80).

MAGNETIC RESONANCE–GUIDED COIL EMBOLIZATION

Besides the MR-guided dilatation of renal arteries, coil embolization has been performed in pigs (81). The tortuous anatomy of the renal arteries did hinder the depiction of the whole length of the renal arteries by the applied real-time radial scanning technique. The application of blood pool contrast agents might allow the acquisition of thicker slices while maintaining the vessel-to-background contrast but were not used in this study. The passive visualization of platinum and nitinol coils was possible, allowing their correct placement, and the flow sensitive technique of radial scanning made it possible to directly judge the success of the embolization. But the artifacts of the coils and the relatively low spatial resolution as compared to x-ray angiography made it impossible to exactly visualize the coil shape by real-time MRI.

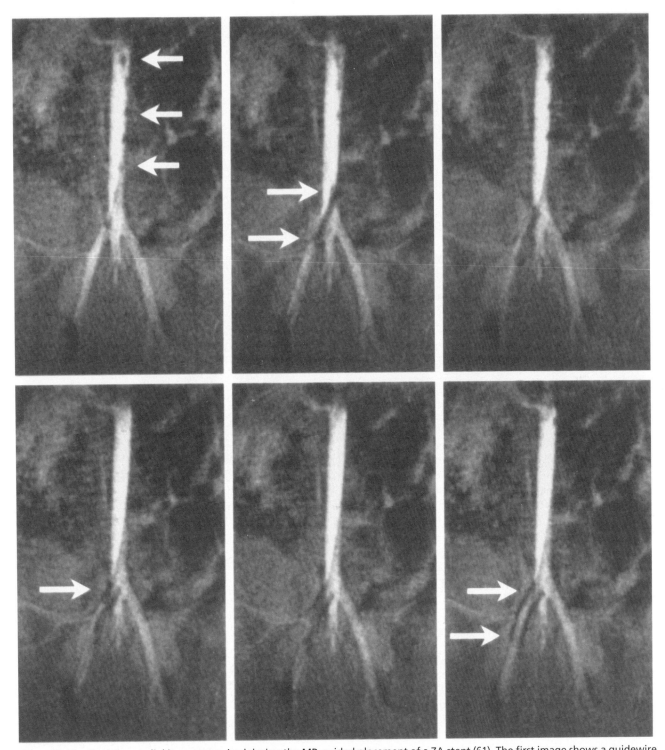

Figure 35.14. Real-time radial images acquired during the MR-guided placement of a ZA stent (61). The first image shows a guidewire with dysprosium markers (*arrows*) in the aorta of a living pig. In the second image the stent is introduced into the aorta (*arrows*). After withdrawing the stent (*third image*) it is partially (*fourth and fifth images*) and then completely deployed (*last image*). (From Smits HF, Bos C, van der Weide R, Bakker CJ. Interventional MR: vascular applications. *Eur Radiol* 1999;9:1488–1495, with permission.)

Successful closure of surgically created canine carotid artery aneurysms was reported applying the superposition of a gadolinium-filled catheter onto MIP of a previously acquired MR angiogram (82). Near real-time visualization (approximately three images per second) was achieved by incorporation of time-resolved imaging contrast kinetics ele-ments and a projection dephaser, but let it suffice to call this technique by its apt abbreviation TRICKS (45). This technique did not allow for direct visualization of the Gu-glielmi detachable coils, which was achieved by repeated acquisition of new MR angiograms and therefore could not be controlled in real time.

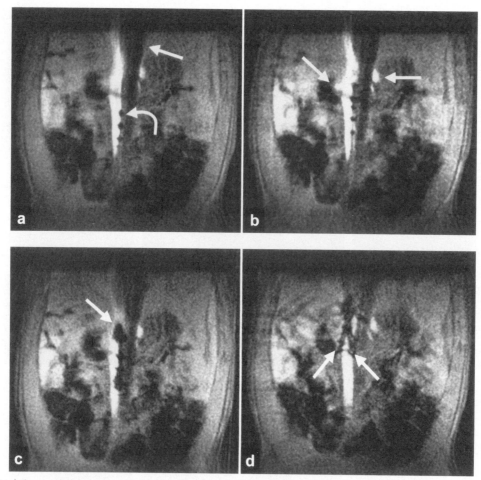

Figure 35.15. Real-time radial images with a cranially positioned saturation slab, yielding a black aorta (**A**, *straight arrow*). The introducer sheath of an inferior vena cava filter is advanced (**A**, *curved arrow*) up to the renal veins (**B**, *arrows*). The filter head (**C**, *arrow*) is positioned at the ostium of the left renal vein. After deployment, the filter legs (**D**, *arrows*) can be seen as well as the position of the filter head.

MAGNETIC RESONANCE–GUIDED CARDIAC INTERVENTIONS

Improved spatial and temporal resolution together with excellent contrast achieved by steady-state imaging has opened MR guidance for different cardiac interventions. Despite their smallness and constant movement, the coronary arteries were catheterized under MR guidance (27,79), and even stent placement was carried out successfully in animal experiments (Fig. 35.16) (83). Placement of atrial septal occluders was performed (84,85) as well as MR-guided radiofrequency ablation (80). The cardiac chambers were successfully negotiated and pressure measurements taken (86). Pulmonary (70) and aortic valve stents (87) were placed under MR guidance. One of the most promising future applications for interventional cardiac MR is the transcatheter delivery of therapeutic solutions into infarcted myocardium. Feasibility studies on intramyocardial injections were done (88,89), and the possibility to correctly demonstrate the distribution of the injected substances by MRI was proven (90).

Because of the lack of safe interventional instruments, all of the above-described cardiac interventions were done in animal experiments only. But a first approach using standard, purely nonmetallic instruments for cardiac catheterization has been made in 16 patients (91). The benefit to children with congenital heart disease is the reduced radiation exposure.

FUTURE PERSPECTIVE

The most obvious advantage of MR is the lack of radiation when compared against x-ray guidance for interventions. In addition to the lack of radiation, there are a number of further potential benefits for MR, including: the ability to visualize vascular anatomy without contrast material and to depict the vessel walls; differentiate between lipid rich and calcified plaques; and the possibility to measure blood flow. These advantages are balanced by difficulties resulting from the tomographic nature of MRI, the problems of using and visualizing standard interventional instruments, the complexity of the MR technique, and the currently still time-consuming acquisition of image data compared to high-resolution real-time x-ray imaging. But all of these still existing problems have been solved or reduced over the last few years. The most important next step will be to develop MR-safe inter-

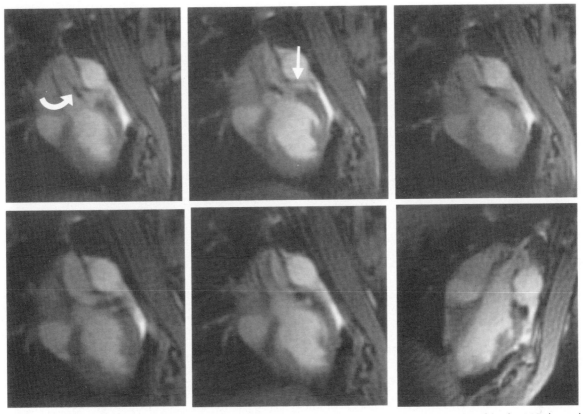

Figure 35.16. Real-time MR radial images showing a stainless steel stent (*curved arrow*), which is placed in the LAD (*arrow*) under MR guidance.

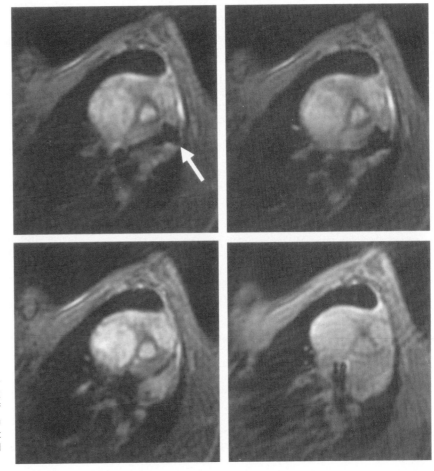

Figure 35.17. MR-compatible occluder placement under real-time spiral MR imaging. After deployment of the first half of the septal occluder in the left atrium (*arrow*), the occluder is withdrawn against the septum, and its second half is deployed in the right atrium.

ventional instruments. The high number of different approaches mirrors the complexity of this task. On the other hand, the manifold applications—successfully performed under MR guidance in animal experiments and a few even in a clinical setting—clearly demonstrate the potential of MR. In the field of pediatric cardiology and radiofrequency ablation, lack of radiation exposure makes it especially worthwhile to explore MR-guided interventions. Furthermore, MR offers unique imaging abilities for the depiction of myocardial infarction and guidance of intramyocardial injections. This might make MR not only an alternative but also the imaging modality of choice for some interventions.

REFERENCES

1. Wildermuth S, Debatin JF, Leung DA, et al. MR imaging-guided intravascular procedures: initial demonstration in a pig model. *Radiology* 1997;202:578–583.
2. Konings MK, Bartels LW, Smits HF, et al. Heating around intravascular guidewires by resonating RF waves. *J Magn Reson Imaging* 2000;12:79–85.
3. Mansfield P. Real-time echo-planar imaging by NMR. *Br Med Bull* 1984;40:187–190.
4. Adam G, Bucker A, Glowinski A, et al. [Interventional MR tomography: equipment concepts]. *Radiologe* 1998;38:168–172.
5. Lewin JS, Duerk JL, Jain VR, et al. Needle localization in MR-guided biopsy and aspiration: effect of field strength, sequence design, and magnetic field orientation. *Am J Roentgenol* 1996;166:1337–1345.
6. Duerk JL, Lewin JS, Wendt M, et al. Remember true FISP? A high SNR, near 1-second imaging method for T2-like contrast in interventional MRI at 0.2 T. *J Magn Reson Imaging* 1998;8:203–208.
7. Busch M, Bornstedt A, Wendt M, et al. Fast "real time" imaging with different k-space update strategies for interventional procedures. *J Magn Reson Imaging* 1998;8:944–954.
8. Adam G, Neuerburg J, Bucker A, et al. Interventional magnetic resonance. Initial clinical experience with a 1.5-tesla magnetic resonance system combined with c-arm fluoroscopy. *Invest Radiol* 1997;32:191–197.
9. Silverman SG, Jolesz FA, Newman RW, et al. Design and implementation of an interventional MR imaging suite. *AJR Am J Roentgenol* 1997;168:1465–1471.
10. Paley M, Mayhew JE, Martindale AJ, et al. Design and initial evaluation of a low-cost 3-tesla research system for combined optical and functional MR imaging with interventional capability. *J Magn Reson Imaging* 2001;13:87–92.
11. Bakker CJ, Smits HF, Bos C, et al. MR-guided balloon angioplasty: in vitro demonstration of the potential of MRI for guiding, monitoring, and evaluating endovascular interventions. *J Magn Reson Imaging* 1998;8:245–250.
12. van der Weide R, Zuiderveld KJ, Bakker CJ, et al. Image guidance of endovascular interventions on a clinical MR scanner. *IEEE Trans Med Imaging* 1998;17:779–785.
13. Smits HF, Bos C, van der Weide R, et al. Endovascular interventional MR: balloon angioplasty in a hemodialysis access flow phantom [corrected] [published erratum appears in *J Vasc Interv Radiol* 1998;9(6):1024]. *J Vasc Interv Radiol* 1998;9:840–845.
14. Spielman DM, Pauly JM, Meyer CH. Magnetic resonance fluoroscopy using spirals with variable sampling densities. *Magn Reson Med* 1995;34:388–394.
15. Pipe JG, Ahunbay E, Menon P. Effects of interleaf order for spiral MRI of dynamic processes. *Magn Reson Med* 1999;41:417–422.
16. Rasche V, de Boer RW, Holz D, et al. Continuous radial data acquisition for dynamic MRI. *Magn Reson Med* 1995;34:754–761.
17. Bucker A, Adam G, Neuerburg JM, et al. [Real-time MRI with radial k-space scanning technique for control of angiographic interventions.] *Rofo Fortschr Geb Rontgenstr Neuen Bildgeb Verfahr* 1998;169:542–546.
18. Peters DC, Korosec FR, Grist TM, et al. Undersampled projection reconstruction applied to MR angiography. *Magn Reson Med* 2000;43:91–101.
19. Riederer SJ, Tasciyan T, Farzaneh F, et al. MR fluoroscopy: technical feasibility. *Magn Reson Med* 1988;8:1–15.
20. Glover GH, Pauly JM. Projection reconstruction techniques for reduction of motion effects in MRI. *Magn Reson Med* 1992;28:275–289.
21. Haage P, Bucker A, Kruger S, et al. [Radial k-scanning for real-time MR imaging of central and peripheral pulmonary vasculature.] *Rofo Fortschr Geb Rontgenstr Neuen Bildgeb Verfahr* 2000;172:203–206.
22. Bakker CJ, Bos C, Weinmann HJ. Passive tracking of catheters and guidewires by contrast-enhanced MR fluoroscopy. *Magn Reson Med* 2001;45:17–23.
23. Guttman MA, Kellman P, Dick AJ, et al. Real-time accelerated interactive MRI with adaptive TSENSE and UNFOLD. *Magn Reson Med* 2003;50:315–321.
24. Rubin DL, Ratner AV, Young SW. Magnetic susceptibility effects and their application in the development of new ferromagnetic catheters for magnetic resonance imaging. *Invest Radiol* 1990;25:1325–1332.
25. Bakker CJ, Hoogeveen RM, Weber J, et al. Visualization of dedicated catheters using fast scanning techniques with potential for MR-guided vascular interventions. *Magn Reson Med* 1996;36:816–820.
26. Bakker CJ, Hoogeveen RM, Hurtak WF, et al. MR-guided endovascular interventions: susceptibility-based catheter and near-real-time imaging technique. *Radiology* 1997;202:273–276.
27. Buecker A, Spuentrup E, Schmitz-Rode T, et al. Use of a nonmetallic guide wire for magnetic resonance-guided coronary artery catheterization. *Invest Radiol* 2004;39:656–660.
28. Glowinski A, Adam G, Bucker A, et al. Catheter visualization using locally induced, actively controlled field inhomogeneities. *Magn Reson Med* 1997;38:253–258.
29. Glowinski A, Kursch J, Adam G, et al. Device visualization for interventional MRI using local magnetic fields: basic theory and its application to catheter visualization. *IEEE Trans Med Imaging* 1998;17:786–793.
30. Adam G, Glowinski A, Neuerburg J, et al. [Catheter visualization in MR-tomography: initial experimental results with field-inhomogeneity catheters.] *Rofo Fortschr Geb Rontgenstr Neuen Bildgeb Verfahr* 1997;166:324–328.
31. Adam G, Glowinski A, Neuerburg J, et al. Visualization of MR-compatible catheters by electrically induced local field inhomogeneities: evaluation in vivo. *J Magn Reson Imaging* 1998;8:209–213.
32. Ackerman JL, Offutt MC, Buxton RB, et al. Rapid 3-D tracking of small RF coils. In: *Proc SMRM 5th Annual Meeting, Montreal, Canada*; 1986:1131.
33. Dumoulin CL, Souza SP, Darrow RD. Real time position monitoring of invasive devices using magnetic resonance imaging. *Magn Reson Med* 1993;29:411–415.
34. Rasche V, Holz D, Kohler J, et al. Catheter tracking using continuous radial MRI. *Magn Reson Med* 1997;37:963–968.
35. Ladd ME, Zimmermann GG, McKinnon GC, et al. Visualization of vascular guidewires using MR tracking. *J Magn Reson Imaging* 1998;8:251–253.

36. Ladd ME, Erhart P, Debatin JF, et al. Guidewire antennas for MR fluoroscopy. *Magn Reson* Med 1997;37:891–897.

37. Zimmermann-Paul GG, Ladd ME, Pfammatter T, et al. MR versus fluoroscopic guidance of a catheter/guidewire system: in vitro comparison of steerability. *J Magn Reson Imaging* 1998;8:1177–1181.

38. Buecker A, Adam G, Neuerburg JM, et al. Simultaneous real-time visualization of the catheter tip and vascular anatomy for MR-guided PTA of iliac arteries in an animal model. *J Magn Reson Imaging* 2002;16:201–208.

39. Zhang Q, Wendt M, Aschoff AJ, et al. Active MR guidance of interventional devices with target-navigation. *Magn Reson Med* 2000;44:56–65.

40. Coutts GA, Gilderdale DJ, Chui M, et al. Integrated and interactive position tracking and imaging of interventional tools and internal devices using small fiducial receiver coils. *Magn Reson Med* 1998;40:908–913.

41. Ehnholm GJ, Vahala ET, Kinnunen J, et al. Electron spin resonance (ESR) probe for interventional MRI instrument localization. *J Magn Reson Imaging* 1999;10:216–219.

42. Joensuu RP, Sepponen RE, Lamminen AE, et al. A shielded Overhauser marker for MR tracking of interventional devices. *Magn Reson Med* 2000;43:139–145.

43. Nanz D, Weishaupt D, Quick HH, et al. TE-switched double-contrast enhanced visualization of vascular system and instruments for MR-guided interventions. *Magn Reson Med* 2000; 43:645–648.

44. Omary RA, Unal O, Koscielski DS, et al. Real-time MR imaging-guided passive catheter tracking with use of gadolinium-filled catheters. *J Vasc Interv Radiol* 2000;11:1079–1085.

45. Unal O, Korosec FR, Frayne R, et al. A rapid 2D time-resolved variable-rate k-space sampling MR technique for passive catheter tracking during endovascular procedures. *Magn Reson Med* 1998;40:356–362.

46. Yang X, Atalar E. Intravascular MR imaging-guided balloon angioplasty with an MR imaging guide wire: feasibility study in rabbits. *Radiology* 2000;217:501–506.

47. Buchli R, Boesiger P, Meier D. Heating effects of metallic implants by MRI examinations. *Magn Reson Med* 1988;7: 255–261.

48. Peden CJ, Collins AG, Butson PC, et al. Induction of microcurrents in critically ill patients in magnetic resonance systems. *Crit Care Med* 1993;21:1923–1928.

49. Wildermuth S, Erhart P, Leung DA, et al. [Active instrumental guidance in interventional MR tomography: introduction to a new concept.] *Rofo Fortschr Geb Rontgenstr Neuen Bildgeb Verfahr* 1998;169:77–84.

50. Liu CY, Farahani K, Lu DS, et al. Safety of MRI-guided endovascular guidewire applications. *J Magn Reson Imaging* 2000; 12:75–78.

51. Ladd ME, Quick HH. Reduction of resonant RF heating in intravascular catheters using coaxial chokes. *Magn Reson Med* 2000;43:615–619.

52. Wong ME, Zhang Ph DQ, Duerk Ph DJ, et al. An optical system for wireless detuning of parallel resonant circuits. *J Magn Reson Imaging* 2000;12:632–638.

53. Weiss S, Kuehne T, Brinkert F, et al. In-vivo safe catheter visualization and slice tracking using an optically detunable resonant marker. *Magn Reson Med* 2004;52:860–868.

54. Konings MK, Bartels LW, van Swol CF, et al. Development of an MR-safe tracking catheter with a laser-driven tip coil. *J Magn Reson Imaging* 2001;13:131–135.

55. Buecker A, Adam G, Neuerburg J, et al. MR-guided PTA applying radial k-space filling and active tip tracking: simultaneous real-time visualization of the catheter tip and the anatomy. *Proc Int Soc Magn Reson Med* 1999:575.

56. Godart F, Beregi JP, Nicol L, et al. MR-guided balloon angioplasty of stenosed aorta: in vivo evaluation using near-standard instruments and a passive tracking technique. *J Magn Reson Imaging* 2000;12:639–644.

57. Manke C, Nitz WR, Djavidani B, et al. MR imaging-guided stent placement in iliac arterial stenoses: a feasibility study. *Radiology* 2001;219:527–534.

58. Paetzel C, Zorger N, Bachthaler M, et al. Feasibility of MR-guided angioplasty of femoral artery stenoses using real-time imaging and intra-arterial contrast-enhanced MR angiography. *Rofo* 2004;176:1232–1236.

59. Nitz WR, Oppelt A, Renz W, et al. On the heating of linear conductive structures as guide wires and catheters in interventional MRI. *J Magn Reson Imaging* 2001;13:105–114.

60. Wildermuth S, Dumoulin CL, Pfammatter T, et al. MR-guided percutaneous angioplasty: assessment of tracking safety, catheter handling and functionality. *Cardiovasc Interv Radiol* 1998; 21:404–410.

61. Smits HF, Bos C, van der Weide R, et al. Interventional MR: vascular applications. *Eur Radiol* 1999;9:1488–1495.

62. Omary RA, Frayne R, Unal O, et al. MR-guided angioplasty of renal artery stenosis in a pig model: a feasibility study. *J Vasc Interv Radiol* 2000;11:373–381.

63. Meyer JM, Buecker A, Schuermann K, et al. MR evaluation of stent patency: in vitro tests of 22 metallic stents and the possibility of determining their patency by MR angiography. *Invest Radiol* 2000;35:739–746.

64. Manke C, Nitz WR, Lenhart M, et al. Magnetic resonance monitoring of stent deployment: in vitro evaluation of different stent designs and stent delivery systems. *Invest Radiol* 2000; 35:343–351.

65. Bucker A, Neuerburg JM, Adam G, et al. [Stent placement with real time MRI guidance: initial animal experiment experiences.] *Rofo Fortschr Geb Rontgenstr Neuen Bildgeb Verfahr* 1998;169:655–657.

66. Manke C, Nitz WR, Lenhart M, et al. [Stent angioplasty of pelvic artery stenosis with MRI control: initial clinical results.] *Rofo Fortschr Geb Rontgenstr Neuen Bildgeb Verfahr* 2000; 172:92–97.

67. Buecker A, Neuerburg JM, Adam GB, et al. Real-time MR fluoroscopy for MR-guided iliac artery stent placement. *J Magn Reson Imaging* 2000;12:616–622.

68. Bucker A, Adam G, Neuerburg JM, et al. [Interventional magnetic resonance imaging—non-invasive imaging for interventions.] *Rofo Fortschr Geb Rontgenstr Neuen Bildgeb Verfahr* 2000;172:105–114.

69. Quick HH, Ladd ME, Nanz D, et al. Vascular stents as RF antennas for intravascular MR guidance and imaging. *Magn Reson Med* 1999;42:738–745.

70. Kuehne T, Saeed M, Higgins CB, et al. Endovascular stents in pulmonary valve and artery in swine: feasibility study of MR imaging-guided deployment and postinterventional assessment. *Radiology* 2003;226:475–481.

71. Mahnken AH, Chalabi K, Jalali F, et al. Magnetic resonance-guided placement of aortic stents grafts: feasibility with real-time magnetic resonance fluoroscopy. *J Vasc Interv Radiol* 2004;15:189–195.

72. Neuerburg J, Bücker A, Adam G, et al. Kavafilterimplantation unter MRT-kontrolle: experimentelle in vitro- und in vivo-untersuchungen. *Fortschr Röntgenstr* 1997;167:418–424.

73. Bartels LW, Bos C, van Der Weide R, et al. Placement of an inferior vena cava filter in a pig guided by high-resolution MR fluoroscopy at 1.5 T. *J Magn Reson Imaging* 2000;12: 599–605.

74. Frahm C, Gehl HB, Lorch H, et al. MR-guided placement of a temporary vena cava filter: technique and feasibility. *J Magn Reson Imaging* 1998;8:105–109.

75. Buecker A, Neuerburg JM, Adam G, et al. Real-time MR guidance for inferior vena cava filter placement. *J Vasc Interv Radiol* 2001;12:753–756.

76. Muller MF, Siewert B, Stokes KR, et al. MR angiographic guidance for transjugular intrahepatic portosystemic shunt procedures. *J Magn Reson Imaging* 1994;4:145–150.

77. Kee ST, Rhee JS, Butts K, et al. MR-guided transjugular portosystemic shunt placement in a swine model. *J Vasc Interv Radiol* 1999;10:529–535.

78. Bücker A, Neuerburg JM, Adam GB, et al. MR-guidance of TIPS procedures performed at 1.5 T. *Eur Radiol* 2000; 10(Suppl 1):171.

79. Serfaty JM, Yang X, Aksit P, et al. Toward MRI-guided coronary catheterization: visualization of guiding catheters, guidewires, and anatomy in real time. *J Magn Reson Imaging* 2000; 12:590–594.

80. Lardo AC, McVeigh ER, Jumrussirikul P, et al. Visualization and temporal/spatial characterization of cardiac radiofrequency ablation lesions using magnetic resonance imaging. *Circulation* 2000;102:698–705.

81. Bücker A, Neuerburg JM, Adam G, et al. MR-gesteurte spiralembolisation von nierenarterien in einem tiermodell. *Rofo Fortschr Geb Rontgenstr Neuen Bildgeb Verfahr*, 2003.

82. Strother CM, Unal O, Frayne R, et al. Endovascular treatment of experimental canine aneurysms: feasibility with MR imaging guidance. *Radiology* 2000;215:516–519.

83. Spuentrup E, Ruebben A, Schaeffter T, et al. MR-guided coronary stent placement in a pig model. *Circulation* 2002;105: 874–879.

84. Buecker A, Spuentrup E, Grabitz R, et al. Magnetic resonance-guided placement of atrial septal closure device in animal model of patent foramen ovale. *Circulation* 2002;106: 511–515.

85. Rickers C, Jerosch-Herold M, Hu X, et al. Magnetic resonance image-guided transcatheter closure of atrial septal defects. *Circulation* 2003;107:132–138.

86. Schalla S, Saeed M, Higgins CB, et al. Magnetic resonance-guided cardiac catheterization in a swine model of atrial septal defect. *Circulation* 2003;108:1865–1870.

87. Kuehne T, Yilmaz S, Meinus C, et al. Magnetic resonance imaging-guided transcatheter implantation of a prosthetic valve in aortic valve position: feasibility study in swine. *J Am Coll Cardiol* 2004;44:2247–2249.

88. Lederman RJ, Guttman MA, Peters DC, et al. Catheter-based endomyocardial injection with real-time magnetic resonance imaging. *Circulation* 2002;105:1282–1284.

89. Saeed M, Lee R, Martin A, et al. Transendocardial delivery of extracellular myocardial markers by using combination x-ray/MR fluoroscopic guidance: feasibility study in dogs. *Radiology* 2004;231:689–696.

90. Krombach GA, Baireuther R, Higgins CB, et al. Distribution of intramyocardially injected extracellular MR contrast medium: effects of concentration and volume. *Eur Radiol* 2004;14: 334–340.

91. Razavi R, Hill DL, Keevil SF, et al. Cardiac catheterisation guided by MRI in children and adults with congenital heart disease. *Lancet* 2003;362:1877–1882.

36

Endovascular Interventions— Congenital Heart Disease

Titus Kuehne and Peter Ewert

The ability of magnetic resonance imaging (MRI) to acquire images with detailed information about anatomy and function has set new diagnostic standards for the assessment of patients with congenital heart disease. During the past few years, fast imaging techniques have emerged that have extended MRI from a purely diagnostic to a dynamic modality that is suited to guide endovascular interventions and to provide immediate information about the physiologic response to pharmacologic or catheter-based treatment.

The desire to replace x-ray fluoroscopy by alternative imaging modalities for the guidance of catheter-based intervention is motivated by the association of x-ray with significant exposure to ionizing radiation (1) and contrast media and also its lack of soft-tissue visualization and functional data acquisition. As an alternative to x-ray, transesophageal echocardiography (TEE) was recently introduced for transcatheter closure of atrial septal defects (ASD) and evolved in a short time into an important tool that can completely substitute fluoroscopy (2). The capability of MRI, however, to acquire at any arbitrary orientation in three-dimensional (3D) space real-time images with high soft-tissue contrast, makes this technique attractive for technically even more demanding procedures. In addition, MRI allows accurate preinterventional and immediate postinterventional assessment of cardiovascular morphology and function and thus may simplify catheter-based procedures.

Mortality rates in patients with congenital heart disease have decreased significantly over the past decades. Therefore, in the future the work of clinicians caring for such patients is likely to focus more on maintaining higher quality of life. This requires the development of optimized diagnostic tools to better guide therapy, the establishment of nonionizing and less invasive interventional methods, and the progressive replacement of surgical by transcatheter techniques. Interventional MRI has the potential to make important steps toward these goals. However, several important barriers remain, such as MRI compatible and safe devices and reliable catheter tracking methods. This chapter describes the major developments in MR hardware, imaging techniques, devices, and interventional procedures, with a focus on congenital heart diseases.

593

TECHNIQUES

INTERVENTIONAL MAGNETIC RESONANCE IMAGING UNIT: GENERAL CONSIDERATIONS AND SAFETY ASPECTS

To date clinical MRI scanners are available with field strengths of 0.5, 1.5, and 3.0 tesla (T). The first open 0.5 tesla scanners were developed to improve patient access. However, imaging with low gradient systems does not meet the criteria in terms of spatial and temporal resolutions that are required to perform endovascular interventions. Currently, considerable efforts are being undertaken to design open MR scanners with higher field strength (1.0 T), which may provide good patient access in conjunction with fair spatial and temporal resolution. As an alternative to open MRI systems, 1.5-T short bore scanners have been propagated, and these currently provide the most extensive experience in sequence design for cardiac and real-time imaging. In addition, the short bore allows reasonable access to the groin or neck of the patient, although catheter manipulation can be difficult in small infants or children. To further improve imaging speed and spatial resolution, scanners with 3.0 T were recently released (3). So far, little clinical experience exists with such high field systems. In addition, it must be considered that imaging at high magnetic field strengths is very susceptible to field inhomogeneities that can amplify problems with image distortion associated with catheters, guidewires, and devices (4).

Currently, x-ray fluoroscopy is used for almost all endovascular interventions, as a result of excellent spatial and temporal resolutions in combination with high contrast between vessels and background. Recent developments, such as contrast-enhanced 3D rotational angiography, exploit these features further and open up new possibilities. However, x-ray is still limited in terms of soft-tissue visualization and acquisition of quantitative functional parameters. Combined x-ray/MRI units were proposed to take advantage of both imaging modalities. Fahrig et al (5) reported simultaneous x-ray and MRI imaging by integrating an x-ray camera into an open 0.5-T scanner. A different strategy is to connect the MRI scanner over a mobile table with C-arms or even fully equipped x-ray angiography laboratories (6,7). The use of such combined units makes sense, until MRI catheter tracking techniques have reached a higher standard in terms of reliability and safety. Until then an x-ray safety backup system should be available. In addition, catheter guidance can be accomplished under x-ray fluoroscopy, whereas functional imaging or acquisition of images that require high soft-tissue contrast can be performed using MRI (6,7). However, the use of such combined x-ray/MRI units often interrupts work flow, is time-consuming, and costly, and therefore will be used as a temporary bridge until MRI catheter tracking methods are optimized.

MRI-compatible equipment for anesthesia and monitoring vital parameters are offered by an increasing number of manufacturers. In-room display monitors and operation consoles allow image acquisition by an interventionalist and imaging expert standing alongside. However, the monitors currently provided by the manufacturers of MR scanners are still too small. Larger displays or screen projectors have been successfully implemented in some laboratories and are now commercially available. A further aspect that must be considered when performing MRI-guided intervention is high noise levels during imaging. However, our experience shows that communication can be well adapted to intermittent noise by some training or by the use of headphones with voice transmission.

Safety aspects for the use of an interventional MRI unit require that general contraindications for MRI of patients are respected. In addition, the use of interventional instruments must be chosen with their interaction with the static and rotational magnetic field in mind (4,8–10). Metallic materials that yield significant magnetic torque, such as introducer needles or wires, must not be brought into close proximity to the magnetic field. In addition, all elongated electrical conductors, metallic or not, are prone to heating effects if they reach the critical length of 20 cm at 1.5 T (8–12). Therefore, such interventional instruments must be excluded from endovascular manipulation. Further details on the MRI-compatibility of catheters, guidewires, and medical implants are provided in other chapters.

REAL-TIME AND FAST IMAGING TECHNIQUES FOR MAGNETIC RESONANCE IMAGING-GUIDED INTERVENTION

Real-time 3D imaging is a task that remains to be realized. However, MRI already offers an exceptional variety of 2D real-time and ultra-fast acquisition modalities for the assessment of anatomy and function. Up-to-date high gradient systems provide the short repetition time (TR) and echo time (TE) needed for fast imaging with steady-state free precession (SSFP). This acquisition technique in conjunction with spiral or radial filling of the k-space is currently considered one of the most reliable tools for high quality and robust real-time imaging (13,14).

Nevertheless, during real-time MRI the interventionalist has to find a compromise between temporal and spatial resolutions or signal-to-noise ratio (SNR). In-plane resolutions of 1 mm can be obtained, if lower acquisition rates of approximately 5 frames per second are accepted. In contrast, at lower spatial resolutions frame rates of up to 20 per second can be achieved. Importantly, phase duration should not exceed the limit of approximately 200 milliseconds to avoid extensive blurring as a result of cardiac and respiratory motion.

Important to note is that x-ray fluoroscopic frame rates of less than 10 frames per second are often applied to minimize the radiation exposure of the patient. In addition, MRI allows interleaved high resolution imaging if needed. The rationale for MRI would be the transition between different imaging sequences that provide either high-spatial/low-temporal or low-spatial/high-temporal resolution.

Accurate assessment of cardiovascular morphology prior to the intervention can facilitate the procedure and reduce its duration. Acquisition of high resolution navigator-based

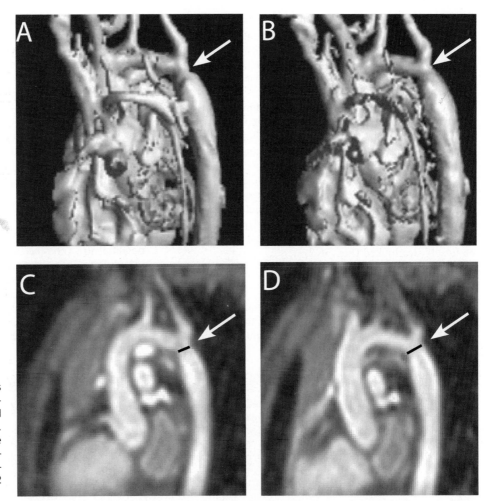

Figure 36.1. Whole heart images of a patient with aortic coarctation (*arrows*) before **(A,C)** and after **(B,D)** balloon angioplasty. Images are shown with 3D volume rendering **(A,B)** and 2D reformatting. Images have high resolution with voxel dimensions of 1.2 × 1.2 × 1.2 mm.

whole heart imaging can be helpful to plan MRI-guided intervention. Such a set of high-quality images provides detailed 3D information about anatomy, allows images to be interactively reformatted in any arbitrary 2D plane, and can provide high resolution images with voxel dimensions of only 1 mm^3 (Fig. 36.1) (15).

Another characteristic of MRI-guided endovascular interventions is the ability to determine immediately quantitative parameters of cardiovascular function. Pulse sequences that integrate parallel imaging (SENSE), kt-blast factors, or echo-planar imaging techniques are capable of acquiring a full set of multiphase-multislice images of the heart or phasic blood flow within only one breath-hold or even at real-time (16–18). In fact, the combination of the 3D, real-time, and functional capabilities of MRI is what makes this technique so attractive for the guidance of endovascular procedures.

MAGNETIC RESONANCE IMAGING CHARACTERISTICS OF MEDICAL IMPLANTS

To date most medical implants used in cardiovascular medicine comprise, at least in part, metal alloys that can cause artifacts on MR images. Such devices include endovascular stents or stent-prostheses, septal or duct occluders, embolization coils, and prosthetic heart valves. These implants are generally not a contraindication for MRI studies; they yield only minor magnetic torque and heating and therefore can be considered MRI-compatible in terms of patient safety (8,12,19,20). However, susceptibility artifacts of the metallic device can cause pitfalls or even make assessment of cardiovascular morphology and function impossible (20).

The extent of imaging artifacts depends mainly on the paramagnetic properties of the device and the field strength of the magnet. Less important factors are material thickness, the orientation of metallic struts toward the B_0 field direction, and the sequence parameters used during MRI.

Metals with weak paramagnetic properties, such as nitinol, yield susceptibility values that are relatively close to those of human tissue and therefore cause only slight local imaging artifacts (8,21–23). By contrast, metals with strong paramagnetic properties, such as stainless steel, produce severe image distortion (8,21–23). Furthermore, the extent of susceptibility is directly related to the magnetic field strength. MR scanners with high field strengths cause more susceptibility artifacts than scanners with low-field strengths (4,24). Finally, parallel alignment of a metallic strut to the B_0 field direction causes fewer artifacts than orthogonal alignment (24–26). However, the orientation of a metallic implant toward the field direction is obviously difficult to predict in the clinical setting.

The MR artifact behavior of endovascular stents is further complicated by radiofrequency (RF) shielding effects.

Shielding effects are caused by eddy currents on the surface of the stent that prevent RF pulses from fully penetrating the wire mesh. This results in decreased signal intensities within the lumen of the stent. The obscured lumen can be misinterpreted as in-stent stenosis or obstruction (21,25, 27,28).

The impact of pulse sequences for minimizing susceptibility or RF shielding was investigated in several studies (23,26,27,29,30). Short TE and read recording direction parallel to B_0 were reported to reduce dephasing and thus susceptibility (27,31). A further, effective sequence implement is 180-degree refocusing pulses, as used in spin-echo imaging. However, artifacts on spin echo images must be carefully interpreted because remaining RF shielding and residual susceptibility artifacts cannot be easily differentiated from the dark blood pool, and thus in-stent stenosis could be falsely overlooked (Fig. 36.2).

Endovascular Stents

MRI has been proven to be an effective noninvasive tool to assess vascular stenosis (32,33). However, the evaluation of in-stent stenosis, a frequently encountered problem, is difficult using MRI because of susceptibility artifacts and RF shielding effects of the stent.

Several in-vitro and in-vivo studies have investigated the artifact behavior of clinically available stents and aimed to grade them in terms of their MRI suitability (21,22, 24,26,28,34,35). Although several findings of these studies were not congruent, all studies demonstrated that stainless steel stents are generally not suited for MRI examination because of severe susceptibility artifacts. In terms of susceptibility, platinum and tantalum stents showed intermediate results, and nitinol stents showed positive results. In addition, the degree of observed RF shielding varied greatly between different stent types because specific design properties can either favor or reduce eddy currents and thus RF shielding.

In some circumstances MR flow measurements have the potential to overcome, at least in part, the problem of RF shielding for the assessment of stent lumen patency, because phase images do not depend on the amplitude of flip-angle excitation (36–39). Therefore, stenosed stents will not contain any phase information in areas with tissue ingrowth or thrombus formation. However, phase images are very sensitive to susceptibility effects and, therefore, this technique

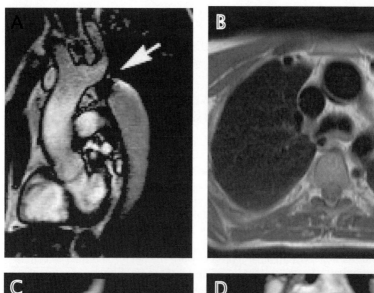

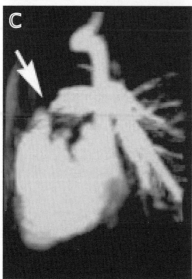

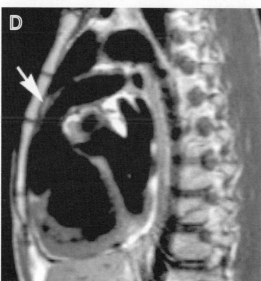

Figure 36.2. Cine steady-state free precession, contrast media enhanced angiogram **(A,C)**, and spin-echo images **(B,D)** of patients with a Palmatz stent in the aortic isthmus (*arrows, upper panels*) and CP stent in the pulmonary artery (*arrows, lower panels*). Note severe signal void as a result of susceptibility and radiofrequency shielding. Susceptibility is substantially reduced on spin-echo images. However, assessment of the stent lumen is still problematic because remaining radiofrequency shielding effects cannot be properly differentiated from the black blood pool.

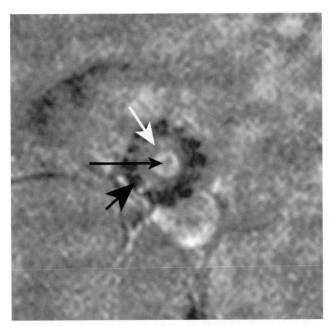

Figure 36.3. Cross-sectional MR image of a nitinol stent (diameter, 8 mm) with in-stent stenosis in the iliac artery of a pig. The design of the stent minimizes radiofrequency shielding effects and allows excellent visualization of the stent lumen. Note the patent vascular blood pool (*long small arrow*) that can be differentiated from tissue ingrowth (*white arrow*). The borders of the stent are delineated by local susceptibility artifacts (*short black arrow*).

requires stents with both low paramagnetic properties and relatively larger diameter. Although accurate quantification of blood flow within the lumen of stents was shown, this technique still needs to be validated for accurate quantification of vascular stenosis within the lumen of stents (36–39).

Other studies have focused on new design concepts for metallic stents to overcome the problem of susceptibility and RF shielding (40–47). Resonating stents have been described, which produce local signal enhancement as a result of small tip excitation and enhanced signal intensity within the lumen of stents (44–47). Another report suggested woven balloon expandable stents made from a metal alloy that contains copper and produce no MR artifacts (42,43,48). Copper is a metal with very low susceptibility values, and the woven design of the stent minimizes eddy currents. At

our institution we are currently investigating self-expanding nitinol stents with specific design properties for reduction of RF shielding. In an animal model of iliac artery stenosis we were able to demonstrate that susceptibility and RF artifacts are negligible and that excellent visualization of the lumen of stents can be achieved. The use of inflow sequences even enabled good differentiation between tissue ingrowth and the surface area of the patent vessel (Fig. 36.3). First results are promising, but each of these three concepts for MRI-compatible stent design needs further evaluation, including safety testing, before they may become available for clinical use.

Embolization Coils and Duct Occluders

Most embolization coils are made of platinum or nitinol alloys that produce only slight local susceptibility artifacts (20). On the other hand, some occluders for the closure of patent ductus arteriosus contain stainless steel components that can severely distort MR images as a result of susceptibility and make assessment of the adjacent pulmonary arteries and thoracic aorta problematic (Fig. 36.4).

Atrial and Ventricular Septal Occluders

Metallic components of atrial and ventricular septal occluders are generally manufactured from a nitinol mesh that produces only moderate susceptibility artifacts (49,50). Because of the relatively large size of the device, the artifact can sometimes extend to the adjacent anatomy and make analysis of atrial or ventricular volumes problematic. In contrast, the magnetic torque on such devices is minor, and patients can be safely examined with MRI (Fig. 36.5).

Mechanical Heart Valve Prostheses

Only few mechanical heart valves are known to have contraindication for MRI, including some early models of the Starr-Edwards and Jomed Monodisc prosthesis (51). Other mechanical valves are safe with MRI, however, morphologic and, to some extent, functional assessment is difficult because of susceptibility artifacts (52).

MAGNETIC RESONANCE IMAGING TRACKING OF ENDOVASCULAR CATHETERS AND GUIDEWIRES

There are a broad range of catheters that are manufactured for specific cardiovascular applications. Some of these cath-

Figure 36.4. Axial steady-state free precession (*left panel*) and spin-echo image (*right panel*) of a patient with a Cook coil in a patent ductus arteriosus (*arrows*). Note severe image distortion as a result of susceptibility artifacts. Spin-echo refocusing pulses reduce, but do not fully eliminate, susceptibility artifacts.

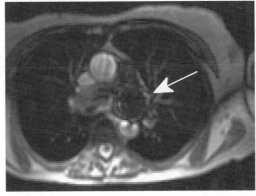
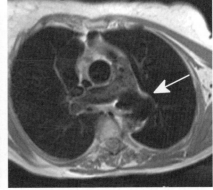

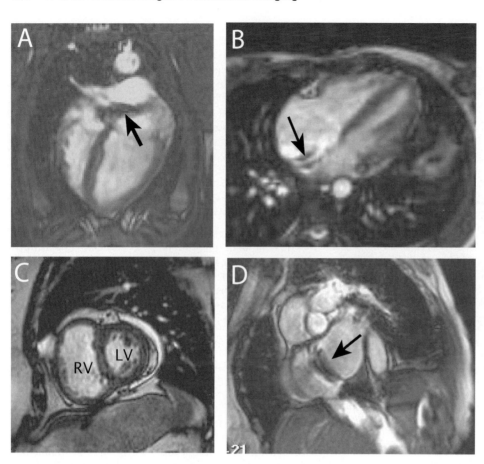

Figure 36.5. Pseudo four-chamber view of the heart (pig) with the commercially available delivery system of an Amplatzer septal occluder placed across the atrial septum (**A**, *arrow*). The metallic components of the release system cause image distortion as a result of susceptibility (**B–D**). Images of the heart of an elderly patient with restrictive left ventricular (LV) function as a result of atrial septal defect (ASD). Note the small LV in **C** compared to enlarged right ventricle. Cardiac function was conditioned prior to the transcatheter closure of the ASD to improve LV function. Function was assessed by simulating ASD closure by transitory occlusion of the septal defect with a balloon catheter filled with CO_2 (**D**). In **B** the Amplatzer septal occluder is shown immediately after its release. In contrast to the delivery system the occluder itself does not yield high susceptibility, and MRI even allows visualization of both discs of the occluder.

eters are braided with iron oxides or wire meshes to make them radiopaque or to add flexibility. Such catheters are generally not suited for use during MRI because they can produce severe image distortion as a result of susceptibility. On the other hand, catheters made from polyesters only do not generate any signal at all and are therefore invisible during MRI. However, appropriate catheter tracking methods are essential to perform successful MRI-guided endovascular procedures. Ideally, tracking methods generate high contrast between the catheter and the background anatomy and readily allow automated slice and tip detection. In addition, the method should visualize both the tip of the catheter and its shaft to be able to identify possible looping of the catheter. The development of catheter tracking methods is currently an area of research that has resulted in several approaches that can be classified as active, passive, and hybrid-tracking. Each of these methods has distinctive advantages and disadvantages, and their application can be chosen in view of the interventional procedure to be performed.

Active Tracking

Active tracking is commonly accomplished by incorporating a small receiver coil into the tip of a device (53–55). The coil picks up signal during slice excitation and generates frequency-encoded recall echoes. These echoes can be detected in 3D space in real time and at a spatial resolution of approximately 1 mm. However, the drawback of this technique is that simultaneous imaging of the device and its background anatomy is technically difficult. The use of active tracking is problematic in regions of interest that are prone to motion. In addition, there is still controversy regarding its safety because of potential heating effects of the signal transmitting lines (9,12,56). Coaxial chokes were reported to divide the transmitting line into small segments (57). They reduce substantially tip heating, however, cause resonance and, in turn, heating at the level of the interpolated segments. In a different approach, transformers were used to segment the transmission line, and no significant heating was noted at any site of the line (58). This approach has great potential to overcome safety issues of active tracking and might allow in the near future its application in the human.

Passive Tracking

Passive tracking techniques aim to directly visualize the interventional instrument within the imaging plane and therefore do not require any additional data postprocessing. Passive techniques are based either on local signal voids as a result of field inhomogeneities/susceptibility or signal enhancement by the use of specific MRI contrast media (59–62). A broad variety of passive markers has been reported for the visualization of catheters that generally consists of metal alloys or dysprosium oxide (Fig. 36.6). In addition, carbon dioxide (CO_2), iron oxide, or gadolinium-based contrast media has been used for the visualization of

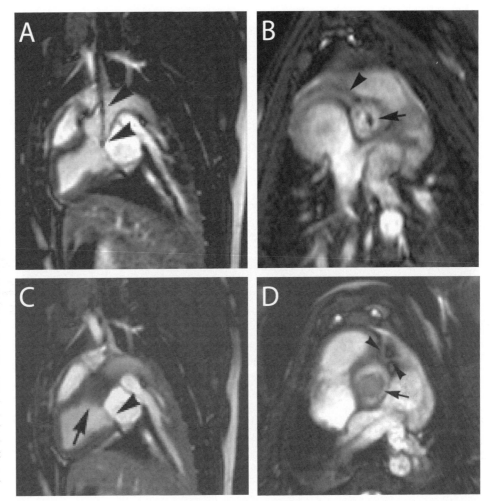

Figure 36.6. MRI-guided transcatheter placement of a valved stent in the aortic valve position in swine. MRI enables continuous visualization of anatomy and interventional instruments. Passive catheter tracking of the delivery system is achieved by the use of two small susceptibility markers that are positioned at the distal and proximal ends of the loaded valved stent (**A,B**, *arrows,*). Important anatomic landmarks can be identified during MRI, including the coronary arteries or mitral valve leaflet (*arrowheads* on **B–D**). The position of the implanted valved stent can be clearly identified by slight local susceptibility artifacts and radiofrequency shielding. (**D**) The prosthetic valve leaflets within the valved stent (*arrow*), the unobstructed orifice, and first segments of the left coronary artery (*arrowheads*).

balloon-tipped catheters (60,61,63–65). Whereas CO_2 or iron oxide contrast media again produce susceptibility, a solution of 10% gadolinium-diethylenetriamine pentaacetic acid (Gd-DTPA) offers maximum T1 enhancement on T1-weighted images (Figs. 36.5–36.8) (60,61,63,65,66).

Common to all of these passive catheter tracking methods is the problem that they either generate only slight and often insufficient signal-contrast between the device and its background anatomy or generate too much signal void that distorts the adjacent anatomic structures. However, passive

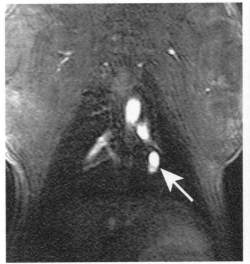

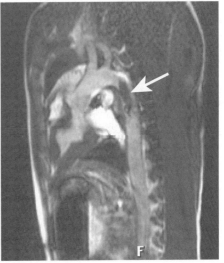

Figure 36.7. *Left panel* shows a coronal T1-weighted turbo field-echo image of the pulmonary artery (swine) with a balloon catheter filled with 10% gadolinium solution (*arrow*). Note the bright signal enhancement of the balloon but poor visualization of the blood pool. *Right panel* shows sagittal T2/T2* weighted steady-state free precession image of the aortic isthmus (swine) with a balloon catheter filled with 1% Resovist (*arrow*). Note the local susceptibility-based signal void of the balloon and bright visualization of the vascular blood pool.

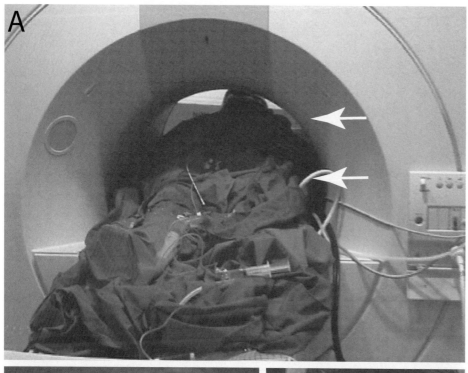

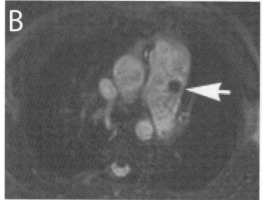

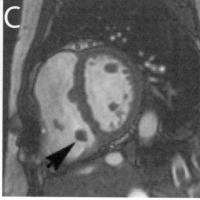

Figure 36.8. MRI-guided cardiac catheterization of a patient with pulmonary hypertension **(A)**. The vascular access to the patient positioned within a 1.5 tesla short bore scanner **(B,C)**. The balloon of a flow directed catheter (*arrows*) within the main pulmonary artery **(B)** and the right ventricle **(C)**. The balloon is filled with CO_2 for susceptibility-based visualization during MRI.

catheter tracking methods are, if carefully chosen in respect to the requirements of an interventional procedure, well suited for various applications and are readily available and relatively inexpensive.

Hybrid Tracking

Small, wireless resonance circuits (RC) were recently proposed as fiducial markers of endovascular catheters (39,67–69). This hybrid of active and passive tracking techniques generates an intense local signal enhancement that is readily perceptible to the observer, allows automated slice tracking, and is safe for the patient because no elongated conductors are used (Fig. 36.9) (70). RCs are based on small copper coils that are tuned to the Larmor frequency. Single or multiple coils mounted on endovascular catheters can serve for catheter tip and shaft detection or placed on stent delivery systems to mark the distal and proximal margin of the loaded stent (Fig. 36.9) (39). However, RCs are techni-

cally difficult to manufacture and are therefore, currently, not readily available.

Tracking of Guidewires

Although there are many promising new concepts for improving catheter tracking, the use of metallic guidewires remains problematic. Although good visualization of the shaft of guidewires can be achieved by the concept of loopless antennas, visualization of the tip of the antenna is ambiguous because of significant signal decreases toward its ends (71,72). Even more important are unsolved safety issues (9,56,73,74). All electrical conductors, metallic or not, are prone to heating effects, and, therefore, currently available metallic guidewires should not be used in humans. In fact, the development of MRI-compatible guidewires that are bioelectrically safe but have all the qualities needed for technically demanding endovascular interventions is one of the key problems that must be solved for the success of interventional MRI.

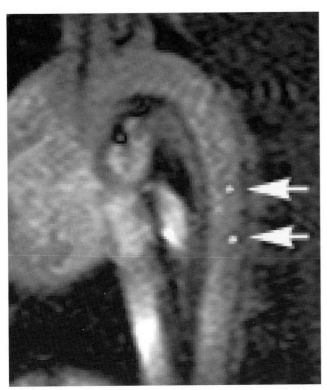

Figure 36.9. Sagittal real-time steady-state free precession image of the heart and the aorta (swine). The image shows a stent delivery system that is advanced through the isthmus of the aorta. Two resonance circuits mark the borders of a loaded stent on the delivery system. The resonance circuits produce a bright local signal enhancement (*arrows*) that enables fast position monitoring of the delivery system.

APPLICATIONS

MAGNETIC RESONANCE IMAGING-GUIDED CARDIAC CATHETERIZATION

One important characteristic of MRI is its ability to assess both cardiovascular anatomy and function. To date MRI is widely considered the gold standard for quantification of ventricular volumes and blood flow. Measurements have been demonstrated to be accurate and reproducible and to have relatively low interobserver variability (75–77). In addition, the advent of fast imaging techniques enables a full set of data to be acquired in short imaging times. Fast imaging methods allow ventricular volumes to be determined within only one breath-hold period and blood flow to be measured even in real time (17,18,78).

Whereas conventional x-ray angiography is limited in the quantitation of ventricular volumes and vascular blood flow, MRI is restricted in its ability to determine cardiovascular pressures. However, increased understanding and experience in the field of real-time imaging and catheter tracking has enabled successful MRI-guided cardiac catheterization studies in patients with congenital heart disease (7,66,79). In these studies invasive pressures were measured in the right heart and pulmonary artery by use of flow directional cathe-

ters. The balloon at the catheter tip was visualized during MRI by susceptibility as a result of CO_2 inflation (Fig. 36.8). The contrast generated between the inflated balloon and the bright blood pool of the heart chambers and the main segments of the pulmonary arterial system was sufficient to safely control catheter advancement.

Measurement of pressures was realized by connecting the liquid-filled catheters to conventional pressure transducers (66,79). However, in the MRI environment the transducer has to be effectively shielded to avoid electromagnetic interaction with the RF pulses. Recording of pressure data can be accomplished by some commercially available MRI-compatible monitoring equipment. However, to date the manufacturers do not offer a solution for transferring the recorded data in digital form for further data processing. As an alternative to liquid-filled catheters, MRI-compatible pressure tipped micromanometer catheters are available but are not suited for human application because of safety issues as a result of potential heating effects.

The combined assessment of cardiovascular pressures and quantitative ventricular volumes or blood flow is an important requirement to improve current diagnostic standards in various congenital heart diseases. From these data the pressure-volume relation can be constructed that might increase insight into the complex physiology of the right heart and the pulmonary vascular system (66). Pressure-volume relations allow determination of load independent parameters of myocardial contractility, ventricular-arterial coupling, and pulmonary vascular resistance, among other parameters (Figs. 36.10 and 36.11) (66,80–82).

In the clinical setting there are several important advantages of MRI over other available methods for the assessment of ventricular pressure-volume relations or the measurement of pulmonary vascular resistance. MRI-guided catheterization is technically easy to perform, measurements are very reproducible, and data acquisition can be accomplished in short imaging times (66,79,83). In contrast, combined pressure-conductance catheter techniques are more complicated and often require multiple catheter manipulation (84). Furthermore, thermodilution and the Fick methods for deriving pulmonary vascular resistance are susceptible to several sources of error, particularly in the presence of intracardiac shunts or right ventricular dysfunction, and are thus associated with high variability of measurements (85).

With the advent of MRI-guided cardiac catheterization and the progress made with ultra-fast and even real-time imaging of ventricular volumes or blood flow, many future applications may be envisaged that would extend current diagnostic capabilities. In conjunction with the well-known ability of MRI to assess even complex anatomy, this technique may, in future, become the method of choice for diagnostic cardiac catheterization of patients with congenital heart disease.

MAGNETIC RESONANCE IMAGING-GUIDED CATHETER-BASED INTERVENTION

The desire to replace x-ray fluoroscopy and angiography by alternative imaging methods for the guidance of endovascular intervention was fueled by the disadvantages of repeated exposure to often significant doses of ionizing radiation in

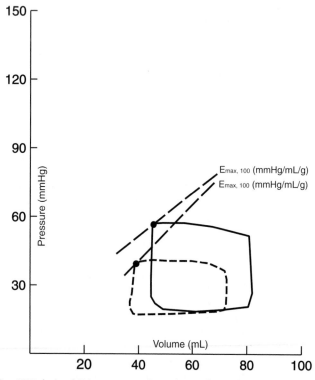

Figure 36.10. MRI-derived RV pressure-volume loop of a patient before (*solid line*) and after (*dashed line*) surgical replacement of a stenotic and insufficient pulmonary valve. Note increased end systolic and end diastolic RV volumes as well as decreased slope of the end systolic pressure-volume relation ($E_{max, 100}$) in the pressure-volume overloaded RV before surgery.

infants and children (1), possible renal dysfunction as a result of considerable quantities of contrast media, and the lack of soft-tissue visualization and incomplete functional data. Although MRI has considerable potential for monitoring endovascular interventions, most MRI-guided procedures described in the literature are still performed in animal models, mainly because of unsolved safety or compatibility issues in connection with the currently available implants, catheters, or delivery systems. A further limiting factor is that more experience needs to be accumulated to make the move to an entirely new environment of interventional MRI units, with their limited patient access, high noise levels, and tomographic images. Finally, the costs of MRI-guided procedures have to be weighed against the potential advantages and benefits. Therefore, in future it seems to be important to define specific applications that emphasize the strengths of MRI rather than attempting to transfer one-to-one interventional procedures from x-ray to MRI. MRI-guided intervention would add considerable benefit for procedures that rely on good visualization of soft-tissue anatomy or immediate

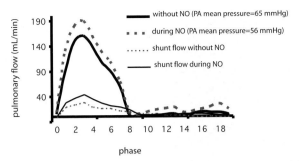

Figure 36.11. Pulmonary flow volumes in a young patient with secondary pulmonary arterial (*PA*) hypertension as a result of a ventricular septal defect. Note increased PA flow volumes during inhalation of nitric oxide (*NO*). Simultaneous recording of invasive PA pressures also reveals a decrease of PA pressures during NO inhalation (from 65 to 56 mm Hg) and, in turn, decreased PA resistance, indicative of a reactive pulmonary vascular system. However, lower PA resistance during NO inhalation causes an increase in left-to-right shunt flow through the septal defect.

preinterventional and postinterventional assessment of physiologic parameters of cardiovascular function.

Transcatheter Closure of Septal Defects and Patent Ductus Arteriosus

Over the past decade transcatheter closure of ASD has became a routine procedure and is carried out in many clinical centers under guidance with TEE (2). Several animal and first human reports have been published that describe successful MRI-guided transcatheter closure of ASD (7,49,50,86). Septal closure devices that are manufactured from nitinol mesh are not prone to significant magnetic torque or susceptibility (Fig. 36.5). Therefore, the devices can be considered safe and suited for the use within the MRI environments. In contrast, commercially available delivery systems for ASD closure devices are generally not suited for MRI, because their release system either contains ferromagnetic materials that cause significant susceptibility artifacts and/or they comprise elongated conductors that are prone to heating effects (Fig. 36.5).

Noninvasive sizing of ASD would be desirable. However, similar to the findings of echocardiography studies, sizing with MRI is described as difficult (2,49,87). Nevertheless, MRI-guided transcatheter closure of ASD is of potential clinical interest because there would be no need to sedate the patient, as for closure under TEE guidance.

Another application of clinical interest would be the one-stop assessment and treatment of elderly patients with ASD. These patients are at risk of developing pulmonary edema after ASD closure because of left ventricle (LV) diastolic dysfunction (88). Conditioning these patients with diuretics and positive inotropic medication can help to prevent the onset of diastolic and systolic LV dysfunction. At our institution we assess biventricular function with MRI during transient balloon occlusion of the ASD to monitor the effectiveness of medical conditioning prior to final ASD closure (Fig. 36.5).

To our knowledge no reports have yet been published of successful MRI-guided transcatheter closure of ventricular septal defects or patent ductus arteriosus. Coil embolization was described for the renal arteries in pigs (89). Coils manufactured from platinum or nitinol produce only slight susceptibility artifacts. The final coil position and its shape cannot be defined after delivery with MRI because of too small device artifacts and limited spatial resolution of MRI compared to x-ray fluoroscopy (26,90).

Balloon Angioplasty for Treatment of Aortic Coarctation and Pulmonary Stenosis

MRI-guided percutaneous balloon angioplasty is a promising technique for the treatment of various congenital heart disease. MR-guided angioplasty of the pulmonary, iliac, and renal arteries and the aorta have been conducted in animals (91–94). A first human study of angioplasty of the iliac artery has been reported, but safety issues were raised because metallic guidewires caused hazards to the patients as a result of potential heating (95).

MRI can provide detailed information on 3D anatomy and blood flow profiles and insight into the morphology of the vascular wall. This information is beneficial in planning the intervention, monitoring its success, and keeping catheter manipulation limited. However, the performance of balloon angioplasty under MRI control poses two specific problems. First, the balloon has to be inflated with contrast media that are suited for MRI. The use of saline solution with approximately 10% gadolinium was proposed to use the maximum T1 effect in T1-weighted pulse sequences (96). Inflation of the balloon produces a bright signal that is easily perceptible to the observer (Fig. 36.7). However, in general, signal-to-noise ratios and visualization of anatomy show lower quality in T1-weighted real-time images than in T2/T2*-weighted SSFP (Fig. 36.7). As an alternative to gadolinium, an iron oxide based MR contrast media Resovist (Schering AG, Berlin, Germany) was evaluated. Resovist yields 500 mmol Fe + per mL, which produces a susceptibility effect on SSFP images. The intensity of the T2* effect can be modulated by diluting the contrast media with saline solution. In an animal study and a first human trial in patients with aortic coarctation we found that 1% Resovist solution produced good contrast between the inflated balloon and the surrounding bright blood pool of the aorta (Figs. 36.1 and 36.12). In addition, the inflated balloon produced only slight and local susceptibility artifacts that did not extend to the adjacent anatomy and allowed accurate determination of the size of the balloon (Fig. 36.12).

The second problem associated with MRI-guided balloon angioplasty is that no metallic guidewires can be used because of safety issues. To guide and stabilize the balloon catheter during angioplasty, we are currently testing custom-made guidewires manufactured from polyesters in conjunction with long sheaths that splint the shaft of the balloon catheter (Fig. 36.12). First results are promising, although further evaluation of this technique is needed.

Endovascular Stent Placement

Modern stents are characterized by high radial strength and surface properties that minimize tissue ingrowth and thrombus formation (97). In addition, low profiles and minimal

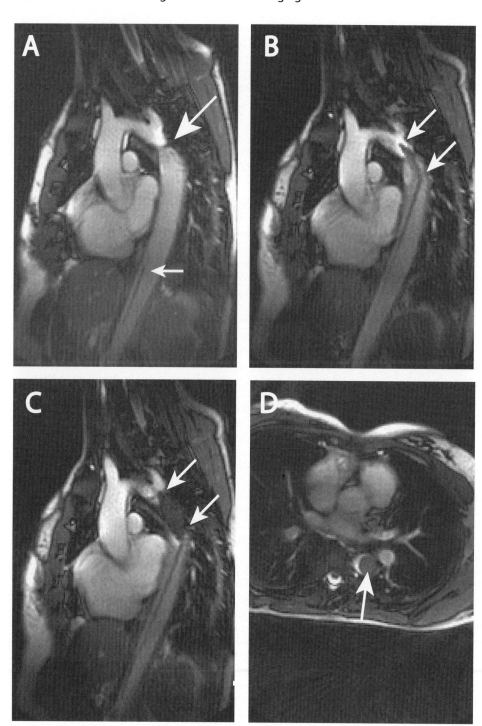

Figure 36.12. Interactive real-time images of a patient with aortic coarctation (**A**, *large arrow*). A balloon angioplasty catheter is advanced from the ascending aorta through the coarctation (**A,B**, *small arrows*). Angioplasty is performed with an iron oxide based contrast media. The process is monitored with MRI in a parasagittal and axial plane (**C,D**, *arrows*). The contrast medium produces good contrast between the catheter shaft and balloon and the blood pool of the aorta.

shortening enables the stents to be deployed from small delivery systems with high precision (97–99). There are several studies that aimed to add MRI-compatible properties to stents to enable MR assessment of in-stent stenosis (40,42). Such stents must be either nonmetallic or made from metal alloys with low paramagnetic properties and only minor RF shielding.

The use of MRI-compatible stents is a basic requirement for MRI-guided stent placement. Several studies, mostly in animal models, reported that MRI-guided endovascular

stenting is feasible. In these studies the stents of different manufacturers were positioned in the aorta and pulmonary arteries and in the peripheral vasculature, including the carotid, renal, and iliac arteries (Fig. 36.13) (39,64,100,101). However, the results of these studies demonstrate that stents have to be carefully selected in terms of their MRI artifact behavior to guarantee that stent position and the patency of the stented vessel can be assessed after their deployment. Misplacement or migration of the stent and residual stenosis, thrombus formation, or vascular injury cannot be assessed

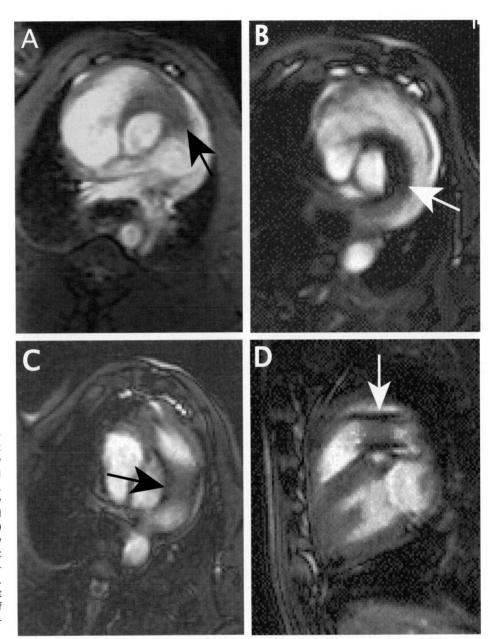

Figure 36.13. Real-time MRI-guided transcatheter placement of a nitinol stent in the outflow tract of the right ventricle and the main pulmonary artery **(A)**. The advancement of the delivery system using susceptibility-based passive catheter tracking *(arrow)* **(B)**. The nitinol stent during early expansion *(arrow)* **(C,D)**. The stent after deployment in axial and sagittal views, respectively *(arrows)*. Note that the position of the stent is easy to determine because of slight susceptibility and radiofrequency shielding artifacts.

when using stents without good MRI artifact characteristics (Fig. 36.2).

To maintain the high precision of stent implantation that is currently achieved under x-ray fluoroscopy, MRI catheter tracking modalities with automated slice and tip detection are needed (54). This would allow continuous visualization of both the site of vascular stenosis and the delivery system. Patient-safe resonance circuits were demonstrated to serve as fiducial markers on stent delivery systems (39). In addition, they allow automated tip tracking and slice detection (70). Therefore, the use of active receiver coils or resonance circuits has the potential to perform high-precision MRI-guided stent placement. In addition, the local signal enhancement of resonance circuits can enable—similarly to active receiver coils—high resolution imaging of the vascular wall, including plaque characterization (102–104). Better insight into the morphology of vascular stenosis may be important information in selecting the optimal stent types.

Valved Stent Placement

Over the past few years percutaneous transcatheter placement of valved stents has become possible (105). Different concepts of valved stents were proposed for application in the pulmonary, aortic, and atrioventricular valve position (106–109). However, transcatheter placement of valved stents is a technically demanding procedure, and misplacement can cause life-threatening situations. The lack of soft-tissue visualization is a major drawback of x-ray fluoroscopy, limiting accurate placement of valved stents, particularly in the aortic and atrioventricular valve position. In addition, x-ray fluoroscopy methods do not provide quantitative information on the function of the implemented prosthetic valve. Against this background, the capabilities of MRI open up new horizons for the transcatheter placement of valved stents. Successful MRI-guided implantation of a valved stent in aortic position was recently described (110).

In this animal study, MRI enabled visualization of important anatomic landmarks in 3D space, including the coronary arteries and the mitral and aortic valve leaflets (Fig. 36.6). In addition, continuous imaging of both the anatomy and the application system allowed accurate delivery of the valved stent, without malpositioning of the stent across the mitral valve or the ostia of the coronary arteries (Fig. 36.6). Furthermore, the carrier stent used in this study produced only minor susceptibility artifacts and RF shielding. This allowed immediate postinterventional assessment of the position of the stent (Fig. 36.6), quantitative assessment of valvular regurgitation, and the exclusion of paravalvular leakage. This study demonstrates the potential strengths of interventional MRI techniques. However, more research is indicated to evaluate whether this technique can provide definite benefits over conventional x-ray fluoroscopy for transcatheter placement of valved stents.

MAGNETIC RESONANCE IMAGING-GUIDED ELECTROPHYSIOLOGY AND CATHETER ABLATION

MR imaging for the guidance of catheter ablation offers several specific advantages over x-ray fluoroscopy techniques. Exposure of the patient and the physician to high doses of ionizing radiation can be eliminated. In addition, MRI allows direct visualization of the electrode-endocardial tissue interface and lesion formation. Finally, changes in atrial and ventricular functions can be determined immediately after ablation to evaluate its hemodynamic impact.

Developments in MRI-guided catheter ablation are promising but are still at an early stage (111–115). Lardo et al (116,117) described a first electrophysiologic system and demonstrated the feasibility of radiofrequency ablation in an animal study. This group was able to acquire intracardiac electrograms and to monitor lesion formation using fast T1- and T2-weighted imaging (117).

The dimension and location of the lesions as determined during MRI agreed well with the results of postmortem examination (117).

FUTURE PERSPECTIVE

Methods of MRI-guided cardiac catheterization and endovascular interventions are in the process of transition from a purely experimental stage of research to their first introduction in the clinical setting. Indeed the continued refinements of endovascular catheters, medical implants, and their delivery systems may soon extend the use of interventional MRI to a larger variety of clinical applications. However, much more research is needed to improve these hardware components, and this will certainly remain one of the major challenges within the next few years. Already recent advances have fueled increasing industrial interest in intensified collaboration with basic scientists and clinicians.

The promise and potential applications of interventional MRI are plentiful. The substantial successes of cardiac surgery necessitate more comprehensive management of patients with congenital heart disease over their lifetime to guarantee a higher quality of life. In this setting, the continuous improvement of MR imaging techniques, in conjunction with more sophisticated methods for performing endovascular interventions, forms a new basis to refine current diagnostic and therapeutic standards. Interventional MRI techniques combine high-quality anatomic and functional imaging and will likely be important in the future management of patients with congenital heart disease.

Acknowledgments

I would like to thank Anne M. Gale, ELS, of the Deutsches Herzzentrum, Berlin, for editorial assistance. The work presented in this chapter was funded in part by the BMBF, Germany.

REFERENCES

1. Modan B, Keinan L, Blumstein T. Cancer following cardiac catheterization in childhood. *Int J Epidemiol* 2000;29: 424–428.
2. Ewert P, Berger F, Daehnert I, et al. Transcatheter closure of atrial septal defects without fluoroscopy: feasibility of a new method. *Circulation* 2000;8:847–849.
3. McGee KP, Debbins JP, Boskamp EB, et al. Cardiac magnetic resonance parallel imaging at 3.0 tesla: technical feasibility and advantages. *J Magn Reson Imaging* 2004;19(3):291–297.
4. Shellock FG. Biomedical implants and devices: assessment of magnetic field interactions with a 3.0-tesla MR system. *J Magn Reson Imaging* 2002;16(6):721–732.
5. Fahrig R, Butts K, Wen Z, et al. Truly hybrid interventional MR/X-ray system: investigation of in vivo applications. *Acad Radiol* 2001;8(12):1200–1207.
6. Saeed M, Lee R, Martin A, et al. Transendocardial delivery of extracellular myocardial markers by using combination x-Ray/MR fluoroscopic guidance: feasibility study in dogs. *Radiology* 2004;231(3):689–696.
7. Razavi R, Hill D, Keevil S, et al. Cardiac catheterisation guided by MRI in children and adults with congenital heart disease. *Lancet* 2003;362:1877–1882.
8. Schenck J. The role of magnetic susceptibility in magnetic resonance imaging: MRI magnetic compatibility of the first and second kind. *Med Phys* 1996;23:815–850.
9. Yeung CJ, Susil RC, Atalar E. RF safety of wires in interventional MRI: using a safety index. *Magn Reson Med* 2002; 47(1):187–193.
10. Ordidge RJ, Shellock FG, Kanal E. A Y2000 update of current safety issues related to MRI. *J Magn Reson Imaging* 2000; 12(1):1.
11. Nitz WR, Oppelt A, Renz W, et al. On the heating of linear conductive structures as guide wires and catheters in interventional MRI. *J Magn Reson Imaging* 2001;13(1):105–114.
12. Shellock FG. Radiofrequency energy-induced heating during MR procedures: a review. *J Magn Reson Imaging* 2000;12(1): 30–36.
13. Martin AJ, Weber OM, Saeed M, et al. Steady-state imaging for visualization of endovascular interventions. *Magn Reson Med* 2003;50(2):434–438.
14. Spuentrup E, Schroeder J, Mahnken AH, et al. Quantitative assessment of left ventricular function with interactive real-time spiral and radial MR imaging. *Radiology* 2003;227(3): 870–876.
15. Sorensen TS, Korperich H, Greil GF, et al. Operator-independent isotropic three-dimensional magnetic resonance imaging

for morphology in congenital heart disease: a validation study. *Circulation* 2004;110(2):163–169.

16. Pruessmann K, Weiger M, Scheidegger M, et al. SENSE: Sensitivity encoding for fast MRl. *Magn Reson Med* 1999; 42:952–962.

17. Korperich H, Gieseke J, Barth P, et al. Flow volume and shunt quantification in pediatric congenital heart disease by real-time magnetic resonance velocity mapping: a validation study. *Circulation* 2004;109(16):1987–1993.

18. Kozerke S, Tsao J, Razavi R, et al. Accelerating cardiac cine 3D imaging using k-t BLAST. *Magn Reson Med* 2004;52(1): 19–26.

19. Shellock FG, Shellock VJ. Metallic stents: evaluation of MR imaging safety. *AJR Am J Roentgenol* 1999;173(3):543–547.

20. Teitelbaum GP, Bradley WG Jr, Klein BD. MR imaging artifacts, ferromagnetism, and magnetic torque of intravascular filters, stents, and coils. *Radiology* 1988;166(3):657–664.

21. Wang Y, Truong TN, Yen C, et al. Quantitative evaluation of susceptibility and shielding effects of nitinol, platinum, cobalt-alloy, and stainless steel stents. *Magn Reson Med* 2003;49(5):972–976.

22. Meyer J, Buecker A, Schuermann K, et al. MR evaluation of stent patency: in vitro test of 22 metallic stents and the possibility of determining their patency by MR angiography. *Invest Radiol* 2000;35:739–746.

23. Lenhart M, Volk M, Manke C, et al. Stent appearance at contrast-enhanced MR angiography: in vitro examination with 14 stents. *Radiology* 2000;217:173–178.

24. Klemm T, Duda S, Machnan J, et al. MR imaging in the presence of vascular stents: a systematic assessment of artifacts for various stent orientations, stent types, and field strengths. *J Magn Reson Imaging* 2000;12:606–615.

25. Bartels LW, Smits HF, Bakker CJ, et al. MR imaging of vascular stents: effects of susceptibility, flow, and radiofrequency eddy currents. *J Vasc Interv Radiol* 2001;12(3): 365–371.

26. Graf H, Klemm T, Lauer UA, et al. [Systematics of imaging artifacts in MRT caused by metallic vascular implants (stents).] *Rofo* 2003;175(12):1711–1719.

27. Bartels LW, Bakker CJ, Viergever MA. Improved lumen visualization in metallic vascular implants by reducing RF artifacts. *Magn Reson Med* 2002;47(1):171–180.

28. Schuermann K, Vorwerk D, Buecker A. Magnetic resonance angiography of nonferromagnetic iliac artery stents and stent grafts: a comparative study in sheep. *Cardiovasc Interv Radiol* 1999;22:394–402.

29. Meyer JM, Buecker A, Spuentrup E, et al. Improved in-stent magnetic resonance angiography with high flip angle excitation. *Invest Radiol* 2001;36(11):677–681.

30. Kuehne T, Saeed M, Moore P, et al. Influence of blood-pool contrast media on MR imaging and flow measurements in the presence of pulmonary arterial stents in swine. *Radiology* 2002;223(2):439–445.

31. Meyer J, Bruecker A, Spuentrup E, et al. Improved in-stent magnetic resonance angiography with high flip angle excitation. *Invest Radiol* 2001;36:677–681.

32. Loewe C, Schillinger M, Haumer M, et al. MRA versus DSA in the assessment of occlusive disease in the aortic arch vessels: accuracy in detecting the severity, number, and length of stenoses. *J Endovasc Ther* 2004;11(2):152–160.

33. Sundgren PC, Sunden P, Lindgren A, et al. Carotid artery stenosis: contrast-enhanced MR angiography with two different scan times compared with digital subtraction angiography. *Neuroradiology* 2002;44(7):592–599.

34. Maintz D, Kugel H, Schellhammer F, et al. In vitro evaluation of intravascular stent artifacts in three-dimensional MR angiography. *Invest Radiol* 2001;36(4):218–224.

35. Manke C, Nitz WR, Lenhart M, et al. Magnetic resonance monitoring of stent deployment: in vitro evaluation of different stent designs and stent delivery systems. *Invest Radiol* 2000;35(6):343–351.

36. van Holten J, Kunz P, Mulder PG, et al. MR-velocity mapping in vascular stents to assess peak systolic velocity. In vitro comparison of various stent designs made of stainless steel and nitinol. *Magma* 2002;15(1–3):52–57.

37. Lethimonnier F, Bouligand B, Thouveny F, et al. Error assessment due to coronary stents in flow-encoded phase contrast MR angiography: a phantom study. *J Magn Reson Imaging* 1999;10(5):899–902.

38. Kuehne T, Saeed M, Reddy G, et al. Sequential magnetic resonance monitoring of pulmonary flow with endovascular stents placed across the pulmonary valve in growing swine. *Circulation* 2001;104(19):2363–2368.

39. Kuehne T, Weiss S, Brinkert F, et al. Catheter visualization with resonant markers at MR imaging-guided deployment of endovascular stents in swine. *Radiology* 2004;233(3):774–780.

40. van Dijk LC, van Holten J, van Dijk BP, et al. A precious metal alloy for construction of MR imaging-compatible balloon-expandable vascular stents. *Radiology* 2001;219(1): 284–287.

41. Hietala EM, Maasilta P, Stahls A, et al. Magnetic resonance evaluation of luminal patency after polylactide stent implantation: an experimental study in a rabbit aorta model. *Eur Radiol* 2003;13(5):1025–1032.

42. Buecker A, Spuentrup E, Ruebben A, et al. Artifact-free in-stent lumen visualization by standard magnetic resonance imaging stent. *Circulation* 2002;105:1772–1775.

43. Buecker A, Spuentrup E, Ruebben A, et al. New metallic MR stents for artifact-free coronary MR angiography: feasibility study in a swine model. *Invest Radiol* 2004;39(5):250–253.

44. Kivelitz D, Wagner S, Hansel J, et al. The active magnetic resonance imaging stent: initial experimental in vivo results with locally amplified MR angiography and flow measurement. *Invest Radiol* 2001;36:625–631.

45. Kivelitz D, Wagner S, Schnorr J, et al. A vascular stent as an active component for locally enhanced magnetic resonance imaging. *Invest Radiol* 2003;38:147–152.

46. Quick H, Kuehl H, Kaiser G, et al. Inductively coupled stent antennas in MRI. *Magn Reson Med* 2002;48(5):781–791.

47. Quick H, Ladd M, Nanz D, et al. Vascular stents as RF antennas for intravascular MR guidance and imaging. *Magn Reson Med* 1999;42:738–745.

48. Spuentrup E, Ruebben A, Stuber M, et al. Metallic renal artery MR imaging stent: artifact-free lumen visualization with projection and standard renal MR angiography. *Radiology* 2003; 227:897–902.

49. Rickers C, Jerosch-Herold M, Hu X, et al. Magnetic resonance image-guided transcatheter closure of atrial septal defects. *Circulation* 2003;107:132–138.

50. Schalla S, Saeed M, Higgins C, et al. Magnetic resonance-guided cardiac catheterization in a swine model of atrial septal defects. *Circulation* 2003;108:1865–1870.

51. Hassler M, Le Bas JF, Wolf JE, et al. [Effects of the magnetic field in magnetic resonance imaging on 15 tested cardiac valve prostheses]. *J Radiol* 1986;67(10):661–666.

52. Edwards MB, Taylor KM, Shellock FG. Prosthetic heart valves: evaluation of magnetic field interactions, heating, and artifacts at 1.5 T. *J Magn Reson Imaging* 2000;12(2): 363–369.

53. Bock M, Volz S, Zühlsdorff S, et al. MR-guided intravascular procedures: real-time parameter control and automated slice positioning with active tracking coils. *J Magn Reson Imaging* 2004;19:580–589.

54. Hillenbrand CM, Elgort DR, Wong EY, et al. Active device tracking and high-resolution intravascular MRI using a novel catheter-based, opposed-solenoid phased array coil. *Magn Reson Med* 2004;51(4):668–675.

55. Zhang Q, Wendt M, Aschoff A, et al. Active MR guidance of interventional devices with target-navigation. *J Magn Reson Med* 2000;44:56–65.

56. Yang X, Yeung CJ, Ji H, et al. Thermal effect of intravascular MR imaging using an MR imaging-guidewire: an in vivo laboratory and histopathological evaluation. *Med Sci Monit* 2002;8(7):MT113–MT117.

57. Ladd ME, Quick HH. Reduction of resonant RF heating in intravascular catheters using coaxial chokes. *Magn Reson Med* 2000;43(4):615–619.

58. Weiss P, Vernickel T, Schaeffter T, et al. A safe transmission line for interventional devices. Interventional MRI Symposium, Boston, Massachusetts. October 15–16, 2004.

59. Bakker CJ, Hoogeveen RM, Weber J, et al. Visualization of dedicated catheters using fast scanning techniques with potential for MR-guided vascular interventions. *Magn Reson Med* 1996;36(6):816–820.

60. Wacker F, Reither K, Ebert W, et al. MR image-guided endovascular procedures with the ultrasmall superparamagnetic iron oxide SH U 555 C as an intravascular contrast agent: study in pigs. *Radiology* 2003;226(2):459–464.

61. Wacker FK, Maes RM, Jesberger JA, et al. MR imaging-guided vascular procedures using CO2 as a contrast agent. *AJR Am J Roentgenol* 2003;181(2):485–489.

62. Glowinski A, Adam G, Brucker A, et al. Catheter visualization using locally induced, actively controlled field inhomogeneities. *Magn Reson Med* 1997;38:253–258.

63. Miquel ME, Hegde S, Muthurangu V, et al. Visualization and tracking of an inflatable balloon catheter using SSFP in a flow phantom and in the heart and great vessels of patients. *Magn Reson Med* 2004;51(5):988–995.

64. Kuehne T, Saeed M, Higgins CB, et al. Endovascular stents in pulmonary valve and artery in swine: feasibility study of MR imaging-guided deployment and postinterventional assessment. *Radiology* 2003;226(2):475–481.

65. Omary R, Unal O, Koscielski D, et al. Real-time MR imaging-guided passive catheter tracking with use of gadolinium-filled catheters. *J Vasc Interv Radiol* 2000;11(8):1079–1085.

66. Kuehne T, Yilmaz S, Steendijk P, et al. Magnetic resonance imaging analysis of right ventricular pressure-volume loops: in vivo validation and clinical application in patients with pulmonary hypertension. *Circulation* 2004;110(14):2010–2016.

67. Kuehne T, Fahrig R, Butts K. Pair of resonant fiducial markers for localization of endovascular catheters at all catheter orientations. *J Magn Reson Imaging* 2003;17(5):620–624.

68. Flask C, Elgort D, Wong E, et al. A method for fast 3D tracking using tuned fiducial markers and a limited projection reconstruction FISP (LPR-FISP) sequence. *J Magn Reson Imaging* 2001;14(5):617–627.

69. Burl M, Coutts GA, Young IR. Tuned fiducial markers to identify body locations with minimal perturbation of tissue magnetization. *Magn Reson Med* 1996;36(3):491–493.

70. Weiss S, Kuehne T, Brinkert F, et al. In vivo safe catheter visualization and slice tracking using an optically detunable resonant marker. *Magn Reson Med* 2004;52(4):860–868.

71. Ladd ME, Erhart P, Debatin JF, et al. Guidewire antennas for MR fluoroscopy. *Magn Reson Med* 1997;37(6):891–897.

72. Ocali O, Atalar E. Intravascular magnetic resonance imaging using a loopless catheter antenna. *Magn Reson Med* 1997;37(1):112–118.

73. Ladd M, Zimmermann G, McKinnon G, et al. Visualization of vascular guidewires using MR tracking. *Magn Reson Imaging* 1998;8:251–253.

74. Liu CY, Farahani K, Lu DS, et al. Safety of MRI-guided endovascular guidewire applications. *J Magn Reson Imaging* 2000;12(1):75–78.

75. Grothues F, Moon JC, Bellenger NG, et al. Interstudy reproducibility of right ventricular volumes, function, and mass with cardiovascular magnetic resonance. *Am Heart J* 2004; 147(2):218–223.

76. Beerbaum P, Korperich H, Barth P, et al. Noninvasive quantification of left-to-right shunt in pediatric patients: phase-contrast cine magnetic resonance imaging compared with invasive oximetry. *Circulation* 2001;103(20):2476–2482.

77. Rominger MB, Bachmann GF, Pabst W, et al. Right ventricular volumes and ejection fraction with fast cine MR imaging in breath-hold technique: applicability, normal values from 52 volunteers, and evaluation of 325 adult cardiac patients. *J Magn Reson Imaging* 1999;10(6):908–918.

78. Thompson RB, McVeigh ER. Real-time volumetric flow measurements with complex-difference MRI. *Magn Reson Med* 2003;50(6):1248–1255.

79. Kuehne T. *Heart,* 2005. In press.

80. Baan J, van der Velde E, Steendijk P. Ventricular pressure-volume relations in vivo. *Eur Heart J* 1992;13(Suppl E):2–6.

81. Burkhoff D, Sagawa K. Ventricular efficiency predicted by an analytical model. *Am J Physiol* 1986;250(6 Pt 2): R1021–R1027.

82. Kuehne T, Saeed M, Gleason K, et al. Effects of pulmonary insufficiency on biventricular function in the developing heart of growing swine. *Circulation* 2003;108(16):2007–2013.

83. Muthurangu V, Taylor A, Andriantsimiavona R, et al. Novel method of quantifying vascular resistance by use of simultaneous invasive pressure monitoring and phase-contrast magnetic resonance flow. *Circulation* 2004;110(7):826–834.

84. Bishop A, White P, Oldershaw P, et al. Clinical application of the conductance catheter technique in the adult human right ventricle. *Int J Cardiol* 1997;58(3):211–221.

85. Hillis L, Firth B, Winniford M. Variability of right-sided cardiac oxygen saturations in adults with and without left-to-right intracardiac shunting. *Am J Cardiol* 1986;58(1): 129–132.

86. Buecker A, Spuentrup E, Grabitz R, et al. Magnetic resonance-guided placement of atrial septal closure device in animal model of patent foramen ovale. *Circulation* 2002;106(4): 511–515.

87. Beerbaum P, Korperich H, Esdorn H, et al. Atrial septal defects in pediatric patients: noninvasive sizing with cardiovascular MR imaging. *Radiology* 2003;228(2):361–369.

88. Ewert P, Berger F, Nagdyman N, et al. Masked left ventricular restriction in elderly patients with atrial septal defects: a contraindication for closure? *Catheter Cardiovasc Interv* 2001; 52(2):177–180.

89. Bucker A, Neuerburg JM, Adam G, et al. [MR-guided coil embolisation of renal arteries in an animal model.] *Rofo* 2003; 175(2):271–274.

90. Marshall MW, Teitelbaum GP, Kim HS, et al. Ferromagnetism and magnetic resonance artifacts of platinum embolization microcoils. *Cardiovasc Interv Radiol* 1991;14(3):163–166.

91. Yang X, Atalar E. Intravascular MR imaging-guided balloon angioplasty with an MR imaging guide wire: feasibility study in rabbits. *Radiology* 2000;217(2):501–506.

92. Yang X, Bolster BD Jr, Kraitchman DL, et al. Intravascular MR-monitored balloon angioplasty: an in vivo feasibility study. *J Vasc Interv Radiol* 1998;9(6):953–959.

93. Rickers C, Seethamraju R, Jerosch-Herold M, et al. Magnetic resonance imaging guided cardiovascular interventions in congenital heart diseases. *J Interv Cardiol* 2003;161:143–147.

of investigating the pathophysiology of pulmonary vascular compliance and impedance, as well as ventricular pressure volume loops and the parameters that can be derived from the measurements for assessment of load independent ventricular function (e.g., end-systolic elastance) (Fig. 37.2).

BETTER CATHETER GUIDANCE AND REDUCED RISKS

Guidance of catheter guidewires and devices through the heart and great vessels of patients, especially with complex congenital heart disease, can be challenging. During x-ray fluoroscopy, only the catheters or devices are normally visualized, and the heart and vessels are not seen. It can, for example, be difficult to differentiate between a catheter pointing anteriorly or posteriorly when looking from the anterior–posterior (AP) view. In more difficult cases, or with a less experienced operator, there is a risk of perforating the heart or vessel, especially in infants and young children. Although previous x-ray angiographic images may help the understanding of the anatomy, the inability to visualize the surrounding anatomy during catheter/device manipulation remains a real problem. MR-guided cardiac catheterization allows visualization of the anatomy during catheter guidance and so has the potential to make more difficult cases safer as well as easier and quicker to perform.

BETTER INFORMATION AND MORE DIFFICULT INTERVENTIONAL PROCEDURES

Over the last few years, many procedures that were previously performed surgically have been carried out with interventional cardiac catheterization in patients with congenital heart disease. In some centers most cases of atrial septal defects (ASDs), branch pulmonary narrowing, and recoarctation or coarctation in older children and adults are treated with interventional cardiac catheterization. More recently, some ventricular septal defect (21,22) and pulmonary valve replacement (23) procedures have been performed by interventional cardiac catheterization, though there remain a siza-

ble percentage of these cases that are still repaired surgically. To be able to perform these more challenging cases under cardiac catheterization, the ability to visualize 3D anatomy during device placement would be helpful. For example, for complex aortic coarctation with transverse arch narrowing, stent positioning needs to be accurate to avoid obstruction of the brachiocephalic vessels. In the future, if transcatheter aortic valve replacement becomes a reality, accurate positioning of the aortic valve to avoid the coronary ostia and anterior leaflet of the mitral valve will be necessary. Such accurate placement of devices can be difficult with x-ray fluoroscopy alone, whereas MR guidance has the potential to help with these procedures and make them possible. The advantages of visualization of anatomy with MR for interventional cases also apply to difficult cases of RF ablation of arrhythmias. In particular, during ablation of atrial arrhythmias via the pulmonary veins, it can be difficult to judge the exact position of the RF ablation catheter, without superimposed 3D anatomic data.

MAGNETIC RESONANCE-GUIDED INTERVENTION AND MAGNETIC RESONANCE-GUIDED CARDIAC CATHETERIZATION

Performing procedures under MR guidance to take advantage of the precise anatomic and functional information has been the subject of extensive research and development over the last 10 years. Originally, it was thought that open, low-field systems would be the way forward, because they provide easy access to the patient (24). However, this is at the expense of the better quality and faster imaging obtained on higher field-strength (1.5 T) systems.

Significant progress has been made with both low-field and high-field systems in MR-guided intervention in the field of neurosurgery (25,26). However, other applications, such as vascular and cardiac imaging, which would also benefit from MR guidance, have been much slower to develop. Several recent developments are making MR-guided vascular and cardiac procedures possible. First, it is now possible is to acquire reasonable quality (spatial resolution) images very quickly (high temporal resolution) (27). From clinical experience and experimental data, MR catheter guidance requires a temporal resolution of at least 10 images per second. Second, to interactively move the imaging plane of the catheter is possible, because it is manipulated in real time (28). The temporal and spatial resolution required for this is only possible in a 1.5-T MR scanner. Visualization of cardiac catheters, guidewires, and devices under MR guidance has also been an area of active research for several years.

The two main methods of active (29–31) and passive visualization (32,33) have distinct advantages and drawbacks. A third method, semiactive visualization, consists of a microcoil without the wire connections seen in active visualization (34). Although a great deal of phantom and animal experimental work has been carried out, this work has only recently been translated to humans.

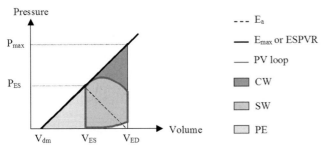

Figure 37.2. Schematic plot of right ventricular single-beat pressure volume loop. Such loops offer the potential to measure load-independent parameters of ventricular function. Ea, arterial elastance; ESPVR (Emax), end-systolic pressure-volume relation; CW, cardiac work; SW, stroke work; PE, potential energy; PES, end-systolic pressure; VES, end-systolic volume; VED, end-diastolic volume; PV loop, pressure-volume loop.

PASSIVE CATHETER TRACKING

Passive catheter visualization relies on either increased signal or, more usually, signal void/artifact for tracking. Unlike active tracking, no external connections go to the MR scanner or source of electrical energy, and therefore passive tracking does not have the same safety concerns as active tracking. The signal void is secondary to (a) displacement of fluid and hence water protons by the catheter or device and (b) differing magnetic susceptibilities between the materials used for passive tracking (dysprosium oxide, gadolinium, or, in our clinical experience, carbon dioxide filled balloon); the surrounding tissues cause field inhomogeneity and thus shortening of T2 (Fig. 37.3) (32). Both factors lead to loss of local signal and provide negative contrast within a vessel imaged with "bright blood" sequences, such as b-SSFP. The susceptibility artifact produced by these passive catheter methods is dependent on device shape, orientation to the magnetic field, and the phase-encode and readout directions. Most catheters used in routine x-ray catheterization are metal braided for extra torque and are therefore not MR-compatible. They are not only moved by the MR scanner's magnetic field, but also have the potential to induce current within them and so can experience a temperature rise within the MR scanner. Currently, available guidewires also are not safe to use in the MR environment. Even nonferrous guidewires (e.g., those made from nitinol) can have current induced in them and heat up to over 70°C (35–37). Much work has been carried out on passive catheter tracking from several groups. In particular, the group at University Hospital, Utrecht, has demonstrated that conventional, nonbraided catheters marked with dysprosium rings along their length can be visualized using fast, real-time imaging sequences when the catheter is moved in the vessels in phantoms and experimental animals (32). Although nitinol guidewires, similarly marked with dysprosium, have also been visualized with passive tracking, safety concerns have precluded their use in humans. Passive catheter tracking, using increased signal from the catheter, has been more difficult to establish, despite good, early work with catheters filled with diluted (4% to 6%) gadolinium (33). The main reason is because modern, fast, real-time imaging techniques use bright-blood b-SSFP, and so a signal void (negative contrast) from the catheter is easier to visualize. Recently, the use of saturation pulses to reduce background signal has made dilute gadolinium-filled catheter visualization more realistic. However, this has the disadvantage of masking the image of the heart and vessels, one of the main motivations of MR-guided cardiac catheterization. In the x-ray/magnetic resonance (XMR) imaging unit at Guy's Hospital, London, we performed several phantom experiments with both high-signal and signal-void passive catheter visualization techniques with several different sequences and parameters in a flow phantom setting. We found that optimum passive tracking was achieved using nonbraided routine balloon angiographic catheters. By filling the distal balloon with carbon dioxide, we were able to visualize the signal void at the catheter tip when manipulating the catheter in phantoms and subsequently in human subjects (Fig. 37.4).

ACTIVE CATHETER TRACKING

An active catheter is one that contains a device that is electronically connected to the scanner. One type of active catheter tracking uses the field inhomogeneity caused by running a small amount of DC current in wires running along the length of the catheter (38). This then provides a susceptibility artifact similar to that seen in passive tracking with dysprosium oxide. More typical types of active catheters contain a coil or antenna, which receives the signal from tissue in its immediate vicinity. These devices do not transmit signal into the patient but rely on the body coil to transmit to the patient. The signal received by these coils can then be used to either pinpoint their position or image local tissue or both (39). Two important types of these active catheters are (a) those based on small coils positioned, for example, at the end of a catheter and (b) those based on a loopless antenna that can run along the catheter or be made into a guidewire. The great advantage of these active systems is that the location of the catheter is unambiguous. Charles DeMoulin of GE Medical Systems is widely credited with inventing this approach. He showed that the location of a small resonant coil at the tip of a catheter could be identified by a series of three, 1D projections along each axis (40). This can be done quickly (in three repetition times) and therefore repeated for very fast update of the catheter position, allowing real-time tracking of the catheter. The position of the catheter can then be projected over a previously acquired road map. Similar techniques have been combined with fast, real-time

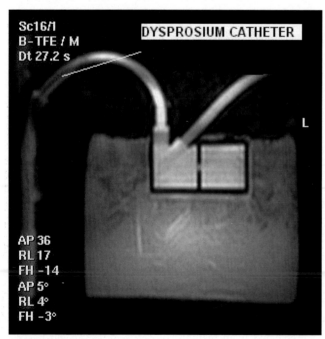

Figure 37.3. Dysprosium catheter. A dysprosium oxide-impregnated catheter is seen within a static phantom. The catheter is clearly visualized along its full length, despite being orientated along B0 (worst case visualization conditions for susceptibility techniques). Fast field echo image: TR 23 milliseconds, TE 7.8 milliseconds, flip angle 50 degrees, rectangular FOV 35%, slice thickness 3 mm, matrix 1,024 × 1,024.

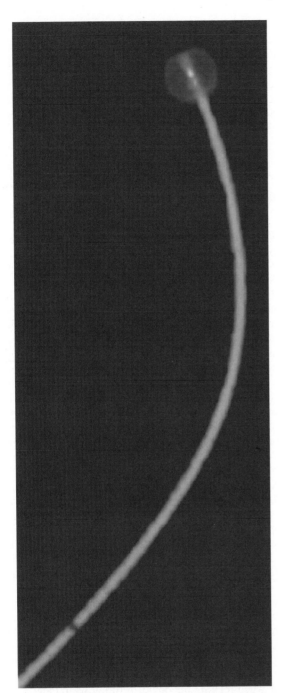

Figure 37.4. Photograph of a balloon angiographic Berman catheter (Arrow International, Reading, PA) filled with 0.8 mL CO_2.

through-plane when only one imaging plane is visualized (41). This technique has been used to great effect in animal experiments demonstrating the potential of MR-guided cardiac catheterization in targeted intramyocardial injection of progenitor stem cells in myocardial infarction, where the position of the delivery device was visualized using active catheter tracking (42). Active visualization has great potential, because it allows the whole length of the catheter or guidewire to be visualized, the imaging plane to be automatically adapted to the moving catheter, and potentially the ability to acquire high-resolution images of small areas of interest adjacent to the coil, when the coil or antenna is used in its imaging mode (e.g., vessel wall plaque). However, the main disadvantage of active devices is concerns over safety. These devices use intravascular coils as RF antennas that are connected to the external circuits via a long wire, which can possibly induce electrical current and heating within the MR static field. Developments to overcome these risks are electrical decoupling of loopless antennas (30,43) and the use of optical coupling and long fiber optic connections (44,45). However, further safety testing is required for both active guidewire and the optically coupled system.

SEMIACTIVE CATHETER TRACKING

Semiactive devices incorporate tuned coils, which have no direct connection to the scanner. These devices can be incorporated into fiducial markers by surrounding a small cell containing a short T1 solution surrounded by tuned windings (Fig. 37.5). These semiactive devices can also be used to enhance externally applied RF pulses and hence produce a high signal intensity using "flip-angle amplification." The

imaging of the heart or vessels using surface coils, and the combined (interleaved) sequence has allowed simultaneous localization of the catheter as well as imaging of the surrounding tissues. Further adaptation of these sequences has allowed automatic imaging plane manipulation to keep track of changes in catheter position (Philips, Hamburg catheter tracking software). More recently, the group at the National Institutes of Health (NIH), USA, has developed a technique that allows real-time visualization of two simultaneously acquired planes, as well as the catheter or device position, thus overcoming the major problem of the catheter moving

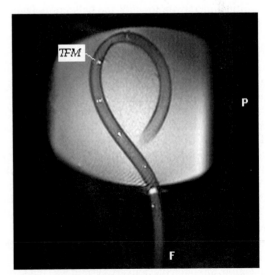

Figure 37.5. Real-time SSFP image (TR 3.2 milliseconds, TE 1.6 milliseconds, slice thickness 15 mm, flip angle 10 degrees) of a 5-Fr balloon angiographic catheter (*arrow, reading,* **A**) with six "quadrature" tuned fiducial markers within a flow phantom. These markers are orientation-independent, and, by using novel imaging sequences which allow for interleaving high and low flip angles, reliable catheter tracking is possible.

main disadvantage of semiactive devices is that the signal produced is dependent on the device orientation to the main magnetic field, *B*0. Recently, these tuned coils have been used in pairs at an angle to each other (quadrature) to overcome this problem and therefore produce signal enhancement for any catheter orientation (34). This technique looks promising, especially if several coils are attached along the length of the catheter so that a longer segment of the catheter can be visualized. Semiactive devices do not have the same safety implications as active devices, because no long conductors are attached to them. A further advantage is the potential for automatic tracking and slice-plane following, in a similar fashion to active catheter tracking. However, before these devices can be used in patients, further miniaturization of the capacitors and coils to make the catheters a reasonable diameter, while maintaining the catheter's flexibility and maneuverability, is necessary. Also important is to have a fault-proof system of securing the capacitors and coils to the catheter so that there is no risk of embolization of the small coils.

EXPERIENCE OF MAGNETIC RESONANCE-GUIDED CARDIAC CATHETERIZATION IN ANIMALS

Over the last few years, there have been several studies performed demonstrating the possibility of MR-guided cardiac catheterization in animal models. These include work from centers in San Francisco and Aachen, both of which have XMR (combined MR and x-ray catheterization suites; see Chaps. 35 and 36) cardiac catheterization laboratories. The group in San Francisco, led by Professor Charles Higgins, has manipulated a homemade pulmonary valve stent into the pulmonary valve of a pig under MR guidance (46). They used a nitinol guidewire to guide the balloon-mounted stent into position. The pulmonary valve stent was successfully inserted by using passive visualization and interactive/real-time b-SSFP to guide the stent into position. This study also demonstrated that phase contrast through plane flow in the pulmonary trunk was useful for quantifying the amount of pulmonary incompetence seen before and after device placement. Higgins et al (47) have also shown the benefits of active catheter tracking, using an active catheter manufactured by Cordis and Philips Medical Systems. Again in an animal model, they have demonstrated that the catheter can be guided to the different chambers of the heart, while the automatic catheter tracking software shows the position of the coil at the tip of the catheter and also automatically changes the imaging plane to keep pace with the catheter position. The group in Aachen has demonstrated that atrial septal defects can be closed using a homemade device and delivery system in a swine model (48). They used passive visualization, although the delivery system was made of nitinol, which is not safe for use in patients. A similar demonstration of ASD closure using a commercially available Amplatzer device has also been performed (49). However, again, the guidewire used for the delivery device is not safe for patient use. The group in Aachen has also published studies demonstrating coronary stent implantation using pas-

sive visualization (50), as well as balloon dilation of iliac stenosis in swine models (51). As mentioned previously, the group at NIH has performed a number of studies demonstrating how active catheters can be used to guide myocardial injection of stem cells (42). None of the previously mentioned studies can currently be translated directly to patients, because there remain safety concerns about guidewires and active devices.

INTRODUCTION TO COMBINED X-RAY/ MAGNETIC RESONANCE (XMR)

XMR is the term used to indicate the potential for MR and x-ray imaging to be used in the same facility, with easy transfer between the two imaging modalities. Although the potential for MR-guided cardiac catheterization is great, currently, it remains crucial to have x-ray angiography available as an adjunct. The main reason is because the nonbraided catheters available for MR guidance have less torque, and, in some instances, a guidewire and/or a braided catheter is required for catheter manipulation. In these cases, the availability of x-ray fluoroscopy and angiography is essential, with easy and safe transfer of patients between the two imaging modalities, even when anesthetized. As we gain more experience with MR-guided cardiac catheterization, and especially with the introduction of more MR-compatible catheters and, most importantly, guidewires, it may become possible to perform cardiac catheterization under MR guidance alone in the future. Over the next few years it will be desirable, both practically and ethically, to have two imaging modalities side-by-side.

Importantly, for several indications, MR and x-ray act as complementary tools, for example, for performing interventional cardiac catheterization and RF ablation procedures, because none of the catheters or delivery mechanisms used for these procedures are MR-compatible. However, the 3D MR anatomic data are useful for planning and carrying out the procedures. By using registration methods, anatomic information from MR can be combined with the x-ray images of the catheters and devices, so that the exact position of these is visualized in relation to the anatomy (52). This gives some of the advantages of MR without having to compromise the catheters and devices being used. Also, instances occur when relating the device position seen under x-ray to the same anatomic MR coordinates is useful. An example is relating the position of electrophysiologic catheters and thus the electrical map of the heart to the same anatomic coordinates of myocardial motion measured by MR tagging techniques. In these instances, it appears that XMR has added advantages over x-ray or MR systems in isolation.

MAGNETIC RESONANCE HAZARDS AND SAFETY ISSUES OF X-RAY/ MAGNETIC RESONANCE

A great deal of literature is available on MR hazards and safety issues, and a comprehensive review and discussion of the subject is outside the scope of this chapter (53–57). However, this area is probably one of the most important considerations in setting up a program of MR-guided cardiac catheterization, and we have spent a great deal of time and effort to insure that we minimized the hazards related to the MR scanner, to maintain very high safety standards in our own facility. Any ferromagnetic object that comes within the MR scanner's magnetic field will be attracted to the scanner. For modern MR scanners, with active shielding, the field is reduced peripherally, thus allowing safe use of ferromagnetic material at distance; however, there is a dramatic increase in this magnetic field over a short distance at close proximity to the magnet bore. Thus, ferromagnetic objects that feel easily controllable at distance can suddenly be pulled with irresistible force into magnets and act as uncontrollable projectiles, which can potentially cause damage, injury, or even death. All catheterizations are therefore done beyond the 5-gauss line. Several safety issues need to be addressed with regard to catheters and devices used during MR-guided cardiac catheterization. Any object that can potentially conduct electricity, and that includes all metals (including nonferromagnetic metals, such as nitinol or platinum), can have current induced within it in the MR scanner and can therefore potentially act as an electrical and/or heating hazard. This does not preclude the use of all metals in the MR environment, because, of course, the imaging coils and wires connecting the electrocardiogram (ECG) signal from patient to the scanner have metal components. However, such leads have been designed to be safe and, if used in the correct manner, do not provide a significant safety risk. Similarly, devices that are implanted into the patient during cardiac catheterization, such as ASD closure devices and stents, are made from metal and have been found to be safe in the MR environment. When we plan to use any catheters or devices that are a potential safety hazard, we perform extensive testing for hazards before using them in patients. *Thus, we always err on the side of caution and ensure that nothing is introduced beyond the 5-gauss line that has the slightest potential to be a hazard.*

PLANNING OF AN X-RAY/MAGNETIC RESONANCE FACILITY

The room design of the XMR facility at Guy's Hospital, London, is outlined in Figure 37.6. Many design features make this room different from standard MRI facilities. The facility is designed so that half of the room is outside the 5-gauss line (Fig. 37.6) of the magnet, permitting use of traditional instruments and devices, as well as transesophageal echocardiography (TEE) and RF ablation equipment when required. A moveable tabletop allows patients to be easily moved between modalities in less than 60 seconds. The paramount factor in the design, build, and operation of an XMR facility is safety, and a comprehensive safety protocol has been drawn up to minimize possible hazards. The safety features of our XMR facility include:

1. All staff who are involved in XMR procedures undergo compulsory MR safety training prior to performing an XMR case on a patient.
2. Clear demarcation of the ferromagnetic safe and unsafe areas by different color floor covering and a moveable barrier.
3. Restricted entrance to the facility during an XMR procedure, with two entrances into the room. The large entrance directly into the room is used only to bring large pieces of equipment (such as anesthetic equipment) into the room before proceeding and for transporting the patient into and out of the room at the beginning and end of the procedure. This entrance is otherwise closed, and access to the room during the procedure is via the control room, through the scrub room. This entrance is constantly monitored, and admittance is limited to staff who have undergone the appropriate safety training and wear specially designed clothes without pockets, to prevent accidentally carrying unsafe material into the room.
4. Ferromagnetic equipment is tethered to the walls as an added safety precaution.
5. A designated safety officer in the room throughout the procedure to ensure that the safety protocols are adhered to, especially at

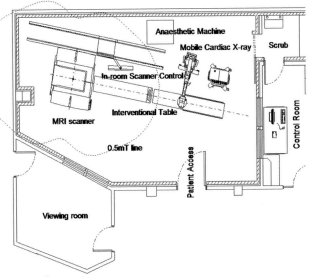

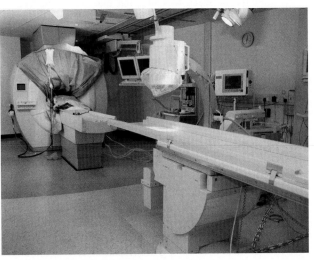

A **B**

Figure 37.6. **(A)** Schematic room plan of our XMR facility. **(B)** Photographs of the room.

the time of patient transfer. All ferromagnetic equipment used is monitored and logged. Prior to transfer of the patient beyond the 5-gauss line, a double check is performed to ensure that all ferromagnetic equipment is accounted for.

6. A written log is kept of all safety infringements, no matter how minor, and is discussed weekly, with the safety protocol being adapted as necessary.

Traditionally, MR scans are planned and run from the control room away from the magnet and the patient. However, during MR-guided cardiac catheterization, there exists a need for real-time changes to the scanning-sequence parameters to follow catheter manipulation in the heart and great vessels. Also, the imager needs to have a clear view of the MR images while performing the procedure. Therefore, a fully functional set of ceiling-mounted, moveable screens and scanner controls within the MR scanner room is available, that can be placed at either end of the bore of the scanner in close proximity to the patient.

The XMR suite includes appropriate MR-compatible anesthetic equipment and monitoring equipment for invasive pressure monitoring via the catheter. A great deal of thought has been given to safety of patients under anesthetic, especially during the transfer between the x-ray and MR tables. All of the anesthetic and monitoring tubing and lines are designed with extra length and are secured to the moveable tabletop to ensure smooth patient transfer. The ECG and invasive pressure data are sent from the MR-compatible monitoring equipment via an optical network to a computer in the control room, where the cardiac technician is stationed. The appropriate measurement and recording of the data are made in the usual way. The technician has access to monitors, which show the appropriate x-ray or MR images of the procedure. The imagers in the room can view the MR images and any monitoring data (i.e., ECG, invasive pressure data). Blood samples taken during the procedure are labeled in the room and passed to the technician in the control room via a waveguide. Another complication of performing cardiac catheterization under MR guidance is the noise generated during scanning. A headphone and microphone system in the room reduces the noise but allows staff to communicate with each other in both the scanner and control rooms. Some MR coils have x–ray-visible components and would need to be removed between MR imaging and x-ray imaging of patients. Therefore, specifically designed coils that are sufficiently radio-translucent are necessary to be left in place during x-ray imaging without any deterioration of image quality. We use these coils in our procedures so that the patients do not have to be disturbed when moving from one imaging modality to the other. The XMR suite has positive-pressure air handling and filtration appropriate for a catheterization laboratory. A scrub room, which is also RF and x-ray shielded, can be accessed from both the XMR suite and control room. The scrub room acts as an RF lock, allowing access to the XMR suite during MR scanning.

From the previous discussion, clearly, some parts of an MR-guided catheterization will have to be performed under x-ray guidance because the appropriate MR-compatible catheters and devices are still not available. However, often useful is to have anatomic and functional information from MR images available during x-ray fluoroscopy. Similarly, knowledge of the position of a catheter under x-ray, such as

the tip of an ablation catheter following successful RF ablation of an accessory pathway, would be useful in subsequent MR imaging of the results of the ablation. We, therefore, have developed a method of registering and overlaying the MR and x-ray images. This requires the tracking of the x-ray table and x-ray C-arm by an optical tracking system, which is positioned at the x-ray end of the room (Fig. 37.7).

RELIABLE ELECTROCARDIOGRAM

Reliable and accurate ECG synchronization is essential for cardiovascular MRI and, in particular, MR-guided cardiac catheterization. When manipulating catheters in the heart, a potential exists for causing arrhythmias (tachyarrhythmias and/or heart block). Therefore, performing accurate monitoring of the cardiac rhythm at all times during XMR catheterization is important. Obtaining a reliable ECG in the magnet, particularly during some MR sequences, can be difficult. The magnetohydrodynamic effect and gradient noise can seriously disturb the ECG signal (58). This interference can reduce trigger signal reliability to less than 40%. Vector electrocardiogram (VCG) is a quantronic resonance system (QRS) detection algorithm, which automatically adjusts to the actual electrical axis of the patient's heart and the specific multidimensional QRS waveform. In our experience, this greatly improves reliability of R-wave detection to nearly 100%. A reliable R wave, with the P and T waves that are also always clearly seen with the VCG, allows detection of nearly all arrhythmias. Unfortunately, no ECG systems can reliably provide ST segment or T-wave morphologic information. In the future, using signal processing techniques, it may be possible to obtain ECG during MRI scanning that reliably provides ST- and T-wave information.

TECHNIQUES USED IN MAGNETIC RESONANCE-GUIDED CARDIAC CATHETERIZATION

The majority of MR sequences used during an MR-guided cardiac catheterization have been covered elsewhere in this book; however, two specific sequences—3D volume b-SSFP and interactive/real time—are very useful for MR-guided cardiac catheterization, and they will be described in detail in this section.

Three-dimensional Volume-balanced SSFP

We have recently described a new 3D b-SSFP sequence in combination with parallel imaging (SENSE factor 2) that allows rapid acquisition of the entire cardiac volume (59). Cardiovascular MR provides the capability of imaging in any plane. This distinguishes it from echocardiography, which is limited by acoustic windows and x-ray angiography, which only provides projectional imaging. Unfortunately, the 3D nature of some congenital cardiac defects is difficult to demonstrate with 2D imaging. Acquiring 3D anatomic information plays a particularly important part in MR-guided cardiac catheterization in congenital heart disease, because it complements the invasive pressure and physiologic measures, such as pulmonary blood flow. Gadolinium-enhanced MR

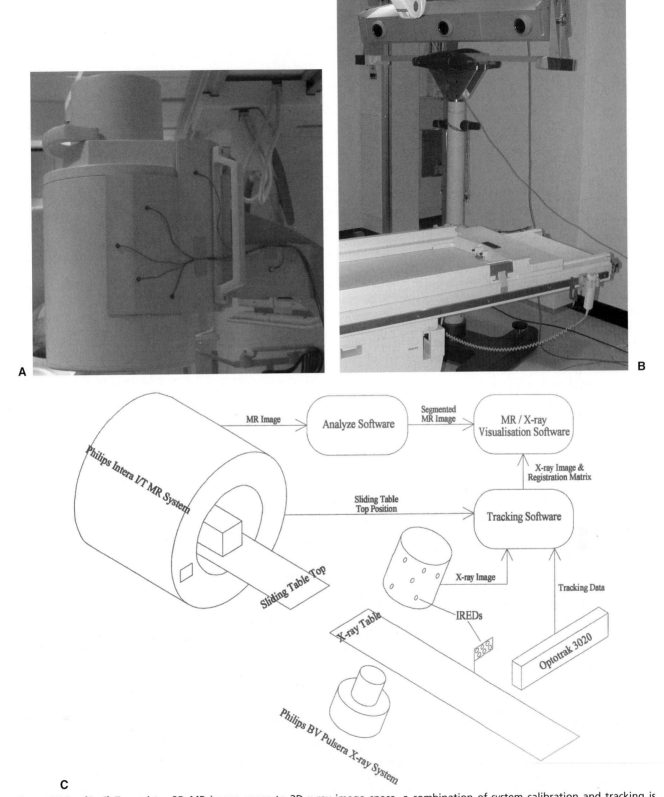

Figure 37.7. **(A–C)** To register 3D MR image space to 2D x-ray image space, a combination of system calibration and tracking is required. Tracking the moving components of the MR system is necessary. These comprise the x-ray C-arm **(A)** and the x-ray table **(B)**, each of which has six affixed infrared-emitting diodes (IREDS). These are tracked by a Northern Digital Optotrak 3020 system (NDI, Ontario, Canada). The tabletop is automatically tracked by the MR scanner when docked with the MR table. The relationship between these coordinate systems is shown **(C)**.

angiography is an accurate 3D imaging technique that allows assessment of congenital malformation of vessels, such as the aorta, pulmonary arteries, and veins (Fig. 37.8). However, the lack of cardiac synchronization leads to blurring of the image as a result of cardiac motion, which is particularly problematic when assessing intracardiac anatomy. The 3D b-SSFP sequence has the advantage of providing clear intracardiac images at different points in the cardiac cycle, with good contrast and resolution. These 3D data sets are more amenable to visualization techniques based on thresholding, rather than the time-consuming manual segmentation required for older gradient-echo techniques (60). Three-dimensional b-SSFP scans are acquired, using a multichunk, multi-breath–hold, multiphase technique [repetition time (TR) 4 milliseconds; echo time (TE) 2 milliseconds; field of view (FOV) 300 to 350 mm; image matrix 192×256 pixels]. Because imaging the whole cardiac volume is not possible in 1 breath-hold, the scan is divided into 8 to 12 smaller chunks. Each chunk is acquired as a single breath-hold of 8 to 15 seconds. The acquisition time for the whole sequence is between 6 to 10 minutes. The scan is acquired in the axial plane and therefore requires no complex planning. High-resolution images are reconstructed with a resolution of approximately 1 mm in all three directions. Typically, one volume scan yields 80 to 144 slices (Fig. 37.9A–D). Each volume is also acquired in multiple phases of the cardiac cycle. In most cases, delineation of anatomy is the most important consideration and, to keep scan times to a minimum, only three to seven phases of the cardiac cycle are acquired. However, up to 10 cardiac phases can be obtained, each acquired in approximately 8% of the cardiac cycle to give information about cardiac motion and sharp systolic images. This leads to an increase in scan time of 25 to 30 seconds per breath-hold. Because the great majority of our patients undergoing MR-guided cardiac catheterization are ventilated, breath-holds are achieved through suspension of ventilation. Therefore, the position of the heart is uniformly maintained between chunks, preventing misregistration of volume data. Images are analyzed offline on a commercial image- analysis workstation (View Forum 4.2, Philips Medical Systems, Best, The Netherlands). As well as looking through the volume in the original axial slices, one can use multiplanar reformatting, which allows viewing of the volume in any plane. Volume rendering of the blood pool can also be performed, using an automated segmentation technique in which the user sets a threshold and seeds the structures of interest by clicking on them with the mouse. This enables different structures of the heart to be segmented separately and given different colors in the rendering process (Fig. 37.9E). A rendering of the image is generated on the same workstation and can be visualized from any direction, and movies of the heart rotating can also be generated. In most patients, only the end-diastolic images are segmented, but with a clinical interest, the systolic volume can also be rendered. The segmentation and rendering process takes normally between 5 and 10 minutes.

Interactive/Real-time Magnetic Resonance Imaging

One of the major recent developments that has made MR-guided cardiac catheterization possible is the introduction of

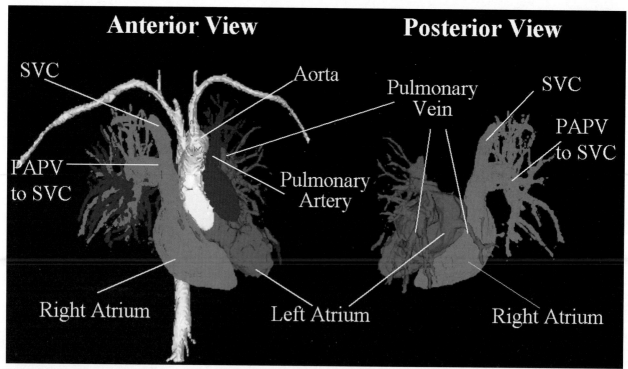

Figure 37.8. Three-dimensional volume-rendered reconstructions from gadolinium-enhanced MR angiograms in a 46-year-old who presented with shortness of breath on exercise and intermittent atrial tachycardia. The images show partial anomalous pulmonary venous drainage of the right upper and middle lobes into the superior vena cava (SVC), with the smaller right lower lobe pulmonary vein draining into the left atrium.

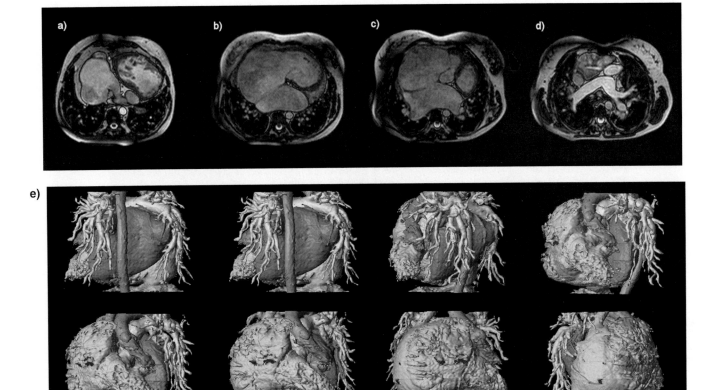

Figure 37.9. **(A–E)** Multichunk, multi-breath–hold 3D steady-state free precession (SSFP) axial images (selected images). The images show atrioventricular and ventricular-arterial discordance, tricuspid atresia, and right ventricular hypoplasia. **(A)** Coronary sinus entering right atrium. **(B)** Right atrium to left ventricle and with left atrium and right ventricle separated by atretic tricuspid valve. **(C)** Atrial septal defect. **(D)** Posterior pulmonary arteries and anterior aorta. **(E)** Three-dimensional volume-rendered images created from the multichunk, multi-breath–hold 3D balanced-SSFP axial images. Three-dimensional volume rotating from posterior to left lateral projection (*top row, left to right*), and from left lateral to anterior projection (*bottom row, left to right*). Massively dilated right atrium connects to left ventricle, connects to pulmonary trunk; left atrium. Hypoplastic right ventricle connects to aorta.

fast b-SSFP sequences that allow acquisition, rapid reconstruction, and visualization of a slice through the heart and great vessels in around 100 milliseconds (27). Because of the speed of these sequences, ECG gating is not needed, with dynamic real-time images acquired at approximately 10 frames per cardiac cycle, depending on heart rate. The ability to perform what is, in effect, MR fluoroscopy means that rapidly changing images of the moving catheter can be seen with very little latency and immediate feedback to the operator who is manipulating the catheter. The interactive sequence has a number of added functionalities that allow changes in scan geometry and parameters, such as slice thickness, field of view, and fold-over (readout) direction on the fly. There are also four viewing windows so that up to three previously acquired images can be seen as well as the active imaging window. This allows the relationship of the active imaging window to the three predetermined imaging planes to be visualized in real time, with the active imaging plane depicted as a line overlaid on the stored images (Fig. 37.10). The geometry of the active imaging plane can be manipulated in several different ways:

1. A line in any direction can be drawn on any of the three saved images to determine the active imaging plane.

2. The three lines on the three stored images can be moved in any direction to change the geometry of the active imaging plane.
3. The active imaging plane can be "pulled" or "pushed" and therefore shifted in parallel to the imaging plane by any predetermined amount (as little as 1 mm).

Both the image and the geometry of the active imaging plane can be stored for later reference. The one drawback of this technique is that, because such a large number of images are acquired (more than 1,000 every 2 minutes), images cannot be automatically saved and so specific images of interest have to be saved by the click of the mouse. We have implemented a local solution with a separate computer that grabs the images from the MR console screen, enabling storage of the interactive images as movies. The parameters for the interactive sequence are TR, 2.8 milliseconds; TE, 1.4 milliseconds; flip angle, 50 degrees; image matrix, 128×128; and a 75% scan percentage. Other parameters, including rectangular field of view, are adjusted for each patient. The minimum frame rate (depending on rectangular field of view) is at least 10 frames per second. The interactive sequence is used both in determining the likely planes of interest before the MR-guided cardiac catheterization procedure and for catheter tracking during the procedure.

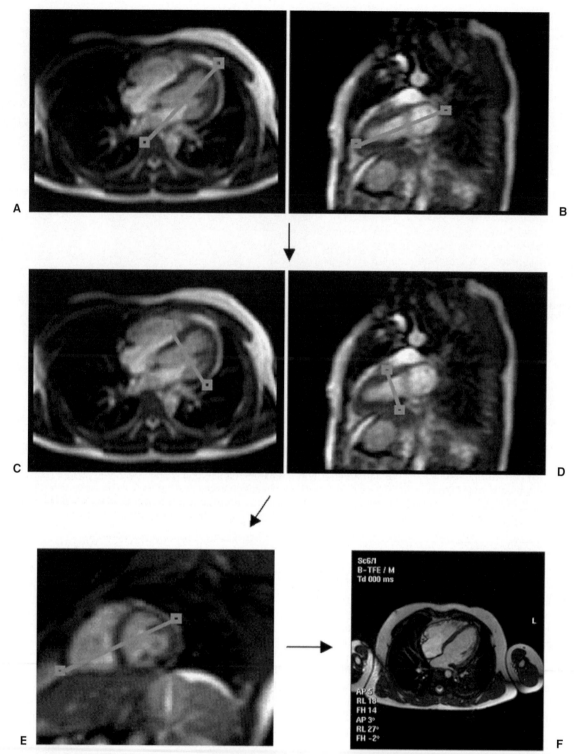

Figure 37.10. (A–F) Real-time interactive images: TR 2.9 milliseconds, TE 1.45 milliseconds, flip angle 45 degrees, matrix 128×128, FOV 250–350, temporal resolution of 10–14 frames per second. (A) Axial image, with alignment of the vertical long-axis (VLA) through the mitral valve and left ventricular apex to give (B) short-axis plane planned on the axial (C) and VLA (D) images to give (E) mid-ventricular short-axis slice. The four-chamber view is then planned from (E) to yield (F). (F) High-resolution four-chamber view (diastolic frame of a b-SSFP cine image).

PERFORMING A TYPICAL CASE

A typical MR-guided catheter case is described in the following section (61). Following induction of anesthesia, the patient is transferred to the MR end of the XMR facility and positioned on the MR scanner tabletop (Fig. 37.11A). The monitoring and anesthetic equipment are attached. The patient monitoring includes a three-lead ECG, separate from the VCG used for ECG triggering/monitoring during MR scanning. The VCG electrodes are placed on the subcostal margin outside the x-ray field of view. An MR-compatible pulse oximeter and noninvasive blood pressure monitoring are also attached. The exhaled anesthetic gases are monitored for end-tidal carbon dioxide as well as the concentration of the volatile anesthetic agents. Flexible phase array coils are used. These coils are relatively x-ray lucent and thus do not need to be removed between MR and x-ray imaging. The patient is then placed in the MR scanner, and a multi-breath–hold 3D SSFP scan of the heart and great vessels (1.1 mm × 1.1 mm × 1 mm resolution) is obtained (59). Using an interactive SSFP sequence (10 frames per second), with real-time manipulation of scan parameters, the likely imaging planes needed for subsequent catheter tracking, ventricular function, and flow quantification are stored.

The patient is then transferred to the x-ray end of the room. Draping and vascular access are carried out as per routine cardiac catheterization (Fig. 37.11B). A second large drape is placed over the patient. Following safety checks, including an operating theater-style "ticking off" of all metallic objects on the catheterization trolley or given to the operators, the patient is transferred back to the MR scanner. The second drape is lifted up and taped to the top of the magnet—in effect providing sterile draping of the bore and sides of the magnet (Fig. 37.11C). An end hole, or side-holes balloon angiographic catheter (4F–7F) is placed in the sheath and, with the balloon inflated with CO_2 (Fig. 37.4), the catheter tip is passively visualized, using the interactive sequences described earlier. The previously stored imaging planes are used, and, when necessary, using the interactive positioning, the imaging plane is changed to track the catheter. Because only the tip of the catheter is visualized, care is taken not to push the catheter too fast and thus beyond the MR imaging plane. This also ensures that the catheter does not accidentally form loops and possible knots. During catheter manipulation, the duplicate MR control console is positioned next to the bore of the magnet so that the interactive window can be easily visualized while the catheter is manipulated (Fig. 37.12). This requires two operators: one to move the catheter and one to alter the MR imaging planes to ensure that the

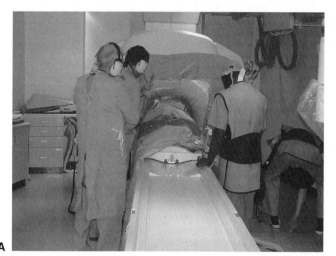

A

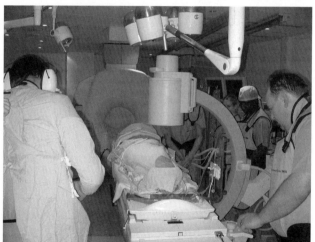

B

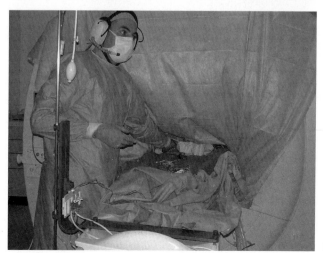

C

Figure 37.11. **(A–C)** Photographs of XMR facility. **(A)** Patient being placed on MR tabletop. **(B)** Patient slid across to the x-ray half of the room for sheath insertion. **(C)** Passive catheter manipulation under MR guidance.

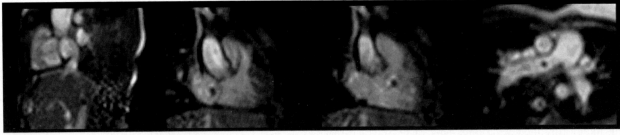

A,B   C,D

Figure 37.12. **(A–D)** Manipulation of carbon dioxide-filled balloon catheter from inferior vena cava to right pulmonary artery, using solely MR guidance. Real-time interactive images: TR 2.9 milliseconds, TE 1.45 milliseconds, flip angle 45 degrees, matrix 128×128, FOV 250–350, temporal resolution of 10–14 frames per second. **(A)** Sagittal plane—balloon in IVC. **(B)** Coronal plane—balloon in right atrium, about to cross the tricuspid valve. **(C)** Coronal plane—balloon in right ventricular outflow tract. **(D)** Axial plane—balloon in right pulmonary artery.

catheter tip is tracked, using the real-time interactive sequence. Once the catheter is positioned in the desired vessel or chamber, the appropriated pressure data and saturation/blood gas samples are obtained as for a routine cardiac catheterization. If necessary, ventricular function (short-axis b-SSFP) and flow (phase contrast) scans can be performed using the appropriate previously stored imaging planes. If it is not possible to position the catheter into a particular heart chamber or vessel using MR guidance alone, the patient is transferred back to the x-ray end of the room, where the catheterization can be continued under x-ray fluoroscopy (e.g., to use a guidewire or a non–MRI-compatible catheter). Once the catheter is correctly positioned, the patient can be transferred back to the MR scanner for further MR measurements. In cases where an interventional cardiac catheter or RF ablation of arrhythmias is performed, the main part of the procedure is performed under x-ray fluoroscopy, because the ablation catheters and delivery devices are not MR compatible. Thus, MR imaging is performed at the beginning of the procedure for planning and use in guiding the procedure, and at the end of the procedure for evaluation of the outcome. At the end of the procedure, the vascular sheaths are removed and the patient transferred to the recovery area.

INITIAL EXPERIENCE IN PATIENTS

DIAGNOSTIC X-RAY/MAGNETIC RESONANCE CARDIAC CATHETERIZATION

We have performed 40 diagnostic cardiac catheterizations under XMR guidance at Guy's Hospital in London. Patients ranged in age from 1 month to 42 years (61). We performed 12 of these cases without the need for x-ray imaging, and in all other patients a significant portion of the procedures was performed under MR guidance. For all patients, the overall x-ray dose for the XMR procedure was significantly less than for control cases performed under standard x-ray guidance (5.5×10 Gycm^2 versus 35.4×36.7 Gycm^2, respectively). In some cases, we performed selective contrast-enhanced (CE) MRA through an injection in the catheter (61). Pulmonary vascular resistance was also assessed in the majority of patients, as described in the next section.

ASSESSMENT OF PULMONARY VASCULAR RESISTANCE USING X-RAY/MAGNETIC RESONANCE

We have used XMR to measure PVR in 24 patients. MR-guided cardiac catheterization was used to acquire simultaneous measurement of invasive pressures and MR flow data. The results were compared with conventional PVR measurements acquired using the Fick calculation, performed during the same procedure (Fig. 37.13). In this study, we demonstrated moderate/good agreement between Fick and phase contrast-derived PVR at baseline. This corroborates several studies that have shown reasonable agreement between phase-contrast MR flow and invasive methods of flow quantification (e.g., Fick) (16,17). However, in the presence of nitric oxide (NO), used to assess pulmonary vasoreactivity, there was less agreement between the two methods. In the presence of 100% oxygen and NO, there was not only worsening agreement, but also a large bias. The Fick principle is known to be inaccurate and imprecise in the presence of high pulmonary blood flow and high concentrations of oxygen (62). We also demonstrated the in vitro accuracy and precision of phase-contrast MR in our facility, using a flow phantom that replicates in vivo conditions more closely than previous studies (63). In addition, the oxygen content of pulmonary arterial blood at 100% oxygen is similar to the oxygen content of aortic blood at baseline, where it has been shown that phase-contrast MR is accurate (17). We therefore believe that the worsening agreement between the two methods in response to pulmonary vasodilatation is a result of errors in the Fick method rather than phase-contrast MR, and that the Fick method underestimates PVR in the presence of 100% oxygen and 20 prediction by partial matching (PPM) of NO. This has important implications for patient management, because response to vasodilators is integral to the assessment of patients with pulmonary hypertension. Overall, this study demonstrates the feasibility of combining invasive pressure measurements and MR flow data to quantify PVR in humans (63). This technique raises the possibility of a more accurate method of PVR quantification, leading to better management of patients with pulmonary hypertension. In addition, this technique is straightforward to carry out, leads to reduced exposure to ionizing radiation, and can be combined with other MR techniques, allowing comprehensive cardiac assessment.

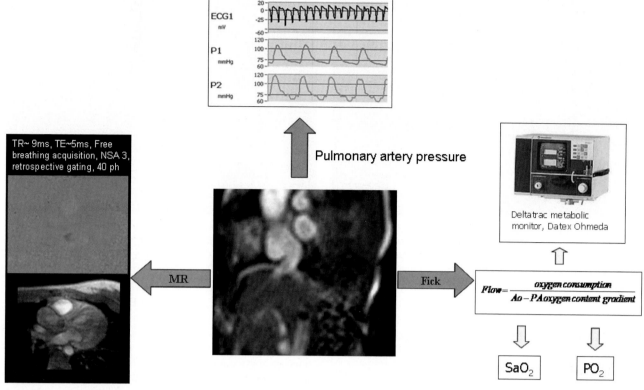

Figure 37.13. Assessment of pulmonary vascular resistance, using MR-guided catheterization, comparison of MR method, and conventional Fick method. The *middle panel* shows the CO_2-filled angiographic balloon catheter tip in the pulmonary artery. The *right panel* shows the MR flow measurement. The *left panel* shows the equipment used to measure blood oxygen content to calculate flow using the Fick principle. The *upper panel* shows the simultaneous pressure data recorded in the right pulmonary artery (*bottom*) and the aorta (*middle*; catheter not shown).

PLANNING AND MONITORING DEVICE INSERTION USING X-RAY/MAGNETIC RESONANCE

We performed MR-guided interventional cardiac catheterization on a few patients: ASD device closure (Fig. 37.14), dilatation of a right pulmonary artery stent, and stent implantation of coarctation (Fig. 37.15). In all of these cases, some catheter manipulation was done under MR guidance, but the interventional procedures were performed under x-ray fluoroscopy. The reason for this was the MR-incompatible nature of the catheters and devices. In all cases, MR imaging was helpful at the beginning of the procedure for planning the intervention and, at the end of the procedure, for evaluating the outcome. For the aortic coarctation patient, the stent was deployed in the correct position, using both the fluoroscopic images overlaid with the 3D MR-derived images of the aorta. This additional information was found to be helpful in positioning the stent, particularly in this anatomically difficult case (Fig. 37.15). These cases demonstrate the feasibility of performing interventional cardiac catheterization procedures under XMR guidance. However, we will have to perform this in a larger number of patients and compare it to procedures performed in the standard x-ray cardiac catheterization laboratory to prove the efficacy and benefits of this technique.

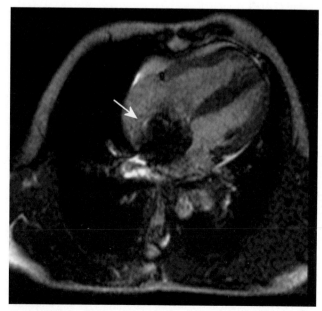

Figure 37.14. Amplatzer atrial septal defect (ASD) device after implantation in a 7-year-old patient. A diastolic frame of four-chambers.

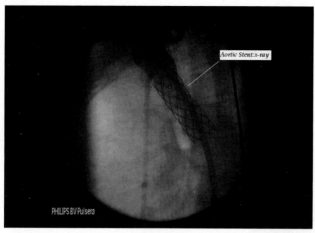

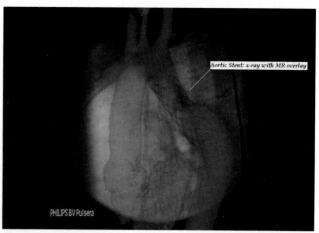

A   B

Figure 37.15. **(A,B)** MR angiography image superimposed onto the x-ray cardiac catheter image during stent implantation. The combined images show that the implanted open stent lies in a satisfactory position, distal to the origin of the left subclavian artery and across the coarctation narrowing. **(A)** Stent and guidewire across the coarctation site under x-ray. **(B)** Inflated stent. Note that stent implantation was performed in the x-ray half of the XMR facility. MRI was used prior to stent insertion to acquire the 3D MRA images and after the procedure (guidewires removed) to confirm no aortic obstruction and satisfactory position of the stent.

ELECTROPHYSIOLOGIC STUDIES AND RADIOFREQUENCY ABLATION USING X-RAY/MAGNETIC RESONANCE

We performed several cases of electrophysiologic study and RF ablation in the Guy's XMR facility. Most of the cases involved RF ablation in the pulmonary veins for patients with atrial fibrillation. Initially, a CE-MRA was performed to acquire the 3D pulmonary venous anatomy. The patients were then returned to the x-ray fluoroscopic area, where a needle atrial septostomy was performed under x-ray guidance. We used the combined MR-derived surface and x-ray fluoroscopic images to guide the ablation catheter and steerable long sheath into each pulmonary vein. Iodine-contrast x-ray angiograms were also performed to visualize the pulmonary veins, and this allowed a comparison between the MR and x-ray anatomies. We found in all cases that there was good registration when comparing the x-ray angiograms to the MR surface-rendered images, taking into account different breath-hold positions at the beginning of the case. Once the long sheath was placed into the appropriate pulmonary vein, a T-flex helical ablation catheter (Cardima and Freemont, CA) was deployed and positioned so that it sat at the proximal end of the pulmonary vein (Fig. 37.16). This initial work needs to be extended to see the true added value of this technique.

SUMMARY

In this chapter we have described the feasibility of performing cardiac catheterizations under XMR guidance. In our experience, XMR is a safe technique with several benefits and potential benefits over standard x-ray–guided cardiac catheterization and great potential for the future. However, several issues still need to be addressed before MR-guided cardiac catheterization becomes routine practice. These include practical issues, such as noise management and communications, improved access to the patient, and improved safety procedures. Most importantly, catheter and device manufacturers need to produce tools specifically for MR-guided cardiac catheterization. However, even in this early stage, there have been a number of important gains from this new technique. They include the reduction of x-ray dose, accurate assessment of pulmonary vascular resistance, better visualization of complex anatomy for both diagnostic cardiac catheterization and interventional cardiac catheterization, and radiofrequency ablation of arrhythmias, using XMR images.

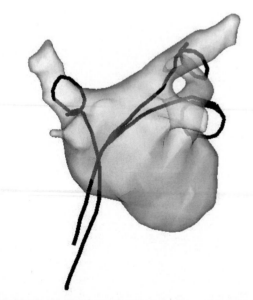

Figure 37.16. Pulmonary vein ablation. Three-dimensional MRA images and T-flex helical catheters superimposed on each other, showing the position of the catheters within the pulmonary vein orifices.

In the future, with better catheter visualization and tracking techniques, it should be possible to reduce, and even eliminate, the x-radiation dose in diagnostic cardiac catheterization and provide more accurate and varied pathophysiologic information. Applying the x-ray and MR image registration technique in a larger group of patients should allow the potential benefits of XMR over standard x–ray-guided cardiac catheterization to be established. This may make MR guidance the method of choice for diagnostic cardiac catheterization in congenital heart disease patients and an important tool in interventional cardiac catheterization and RF ablation of arrhythmias in the future.

Acknowledgments

The work described in this chapter was performed at Guy's Hospital, London, UK, by a team of academic and clinical staff. As well as the authors, particular acknowledgment, in the Division of Imaging Sciences, is due to Vivek Muthurangu, Sanjeet Hegde, Derek Hill, Steve Keevil, Marc Miquel, Kawal Rhode, Rado Andriantsimiavona, Redha Boubertakh, Maxime Sermesant, and David Hawkes; and, in the Departments of Paediatric and Adult Cardiology, Shakeel Qureshi, Jas Gill, Eric Rosenthal, Robert Tulloh, and Edward Baker. We would also like to acknowledge Michael Barnet and other members of the Anaesthetic Department; and John Spence, Stephen Sinclear, Rebecca Lund, and other staff from the Radiology Department who have provided considerable support.

REFERENCES

1. Pihkala J, Nykanen D, Freedom RM, et al. Interventional cardiac catheterization. *Pediatr Clin North Am* 1999;46:441–464.
2. Silverman NH, Schiller NB. Apex echocardiography. A two-dimensional technique for evaluating congenital heart disease. *Circulation* 1978;57:503–511.
3. Razavi R, Baker E. Magnetic resonance imaging comes of age. *Cardiol Young* 1999;9:529–538.
4. Magni G, Hijazi ZM, Pandian NG, et al. Two- and three-dimensional transesophageal echocardiography in patient selection and assessment of atrial septal defect closure by the new DAS-Angel Wings device: initial clinical experience. *Circulation* 1997;96:1722–1728.
5. Koenig PR, Abdulla RI, Cao QL, et al. Use of intracardiac echocardiography to guide catheter closure of atrial communications. *Echocardiography* 2003;20:781–787.
6. Modan B, Keinan L, Blumstein T, et al. Cancer following cardiac catheterization in childhood. *Int J Epidemiol* 2000;29:424–428.
7. Berrington de Gonzalez A, Darby S. Risk of cancer from diagnostic x-rays: estimates for the UK and 14 other countries. *Lancet* 2004;363:345–351.
8. Faulkner K, Love HG, Sweeney JK, et al. Radiation doses and somatic risk to patients during cardiac radiological procedures. *Br J Radiol* 1986;59:359–363.
9. Kovoor P, Ricciardello M, Collins L, et al. Risk to patients from radiation associated with radiofrequency ablation for supraventricular tachycardia. *Circulation* 1998;98:1534–1540.
10. National Radiation Protection Board (NRPB). Guidelines on patient dose to promote the optimization of protection for diagnostic medical exposures. *NRPB* 1999;10:1.
11. International Commission on Radiological Protection (ICRP). Recommendations of the International Commission on Radiological Protection. *ICRP 60. Ann ICRP* 1990;21:1–3.
12. Hillis LD, Winniford MD, Jackson JA, et al. Measurements of left-to-right intracardiac shunting in adults: oximetric versus indicator dilution techniques. *Cathet Cardiovasc Diagn* 1985a;11:467–472.
13. Cigarroa RG, Lange RA, Hillis LD. Oximetric quantitation of intracardiac left-to-right shunting: limitations of the Qp/Qs ratio. *Am J Cardiol* 1989;64:246–247.
14. Dhingra VK, Fenwick JC, Walley KR, et al. Lack of agreement between thermodilution and Fick cardiac output in critically ill patients. *Chest* 2002;122:990–997.
15. Razavi RS, Baker A, Qureshi SA, et al. Hemodynamic response to continuous infusion of dobutamine in Alagille's syndrome. *Transplantation* 2001;72:823–828.
16. Hundley WG, Li HF, Hillis LD, et al. Quantitation of cardiac output with velocity-encoded, phase-difference magnetic resonance imaging. *Am J Cardiol* 1995;75:1250–1255.
17. Beerbaum P, Korperich H, Barth P, et al. Noninvasive quantification of left-to-right shunt in pediatric patients: phase-contrast cine magnetic resonance imaging compared with invasive oximetry. *Circulation* 2001;103:2476–2482.
18. Robertson MB, Kohler U, Hoskins PR, et al. Quantitative analysis of PC MRI velocity maps: pulsatile flow in cylindrical vessels. *Magn Reson Imaging* 2001;19:685–695.
19. Bellenger NG, Marcus NJ, Rajappan K, et al. Comparison of techniques for the measurement of left ventricular function following cardiac transplantation. *J Cardiovasc Magn Reson* 2002;4:255–263.
20. Helbing WA, Rebergen SA, Maliepaard C, et al. Quantification of right ventricular function with magnetic resonance imaging in children with normal hearts and with congenital heart disease. *Am Heart J* 1995;130:828–837.
21. Hijazi ZM, Hakim F, Haweleh AA, et al. Catheter closure of perimembranous ventricular septal defects using the new Amplatzer membranous VSD occluder: initial clinical experience. *Catheter Cardiovasc Interv* 2002;56:508–515.
22. Holzer R, Balzer D, Cao QL, et al. Device closure of muscular ventricular septal defects using the Amplatzer muscular ventricular septal defect occluder: immediate and mid-term results of a U.S. registry. *J Am Coll Cardiol* 2004;43:1257–1263.
23. Bonhoeffer P, Boudjemline Y, Qureshi SA, et al. Percutaneous insertion of the pulmonary valve. *J Am Coll Cardiol* 2002;39:1664–1669.
24. Fahrig R, Butts K, Wen Z, et al. Truly hybrid interventional MR/x-ray system: investigation of in vivo applications. *Acad Radiol* 2001;8:1200–1207.
25. Liu H, Hall WA, Martin AJ, et al. MR-guided and MR-monitored neurosurgical procedures at 1.5 T. *J Comput Assist Tomogr* 2000;24:909–918.
26. Fahrig R, Heit G, Wen Z, et al. First use of a truly hybrid x-ray/MR imaging system for guidance of brain biopsy. *Acta Neurochir (Wien)* 2003;145:995–997; discussion 997.
27. Bakker CJ, Hoogeveen RM, Weber J, et al. Visualization of dedicated catheters using fast scanning techniques with potential for MR-guided vascular interventions. *Magn Reson Med* 1996;36:816–820.
28. Miquel ME, Hegde S, Muthurangu V, et al. Visualization and tracking of an inflatable balloon catheter using SSFP in a flow phantom and in the heart and great vessels of patients. *Magn Reson Med* 2004;51:988–995.
29. Leung DA, Debatin JF, Wildermuth S, et al. Intravascular MR tracking catheter: preliminary experimental evaluation. *Am J Roentgenol* 1995;164:1265–1270.
30. Ocali O, Atalar E. Intravascular magnetic resonance imaging using a loopless catheter antenna. *Magn Reson Med* 1997;37:112–118.

31. Ladd ME, Zimmermann GG, Quick HH, et al. Active MR visualization of a vascular guide wire in vivo. *J Magn Reson Imaging* 1998a;8:220–225.

32. Bakker CJ, Hoogeveen RM, Hurtak WF, et al. MR-guided endovascular interventions: susceptibility-based catheter and near-real-time imaging technique. *Radiology* 1997;202:273–276.

33. Omary RA, Unal O, Koscielski DS, et al. Real-time MR imaging-guided passive catheter tracking with use of gadolinium-filled catheters. *J Vasc Interv Radiol* 200;11:1079–1085

34. Kuehne T, Fahrig R, Butts K. Pair of resonant fiducial markers for localization of endovascular catheters at all catheter orientations. *J Magn Reson Imaging* 2003;17:620–624.

35. Konings MK, Bartels LW, Smits HF, et al. Heating around intravascular guide wires by resonating RF waves. *J Magn Reson Imaging* 2000;12:79–85.

36. Nitz WR, Oppelt A, Renz W, et al. On the heating of linear conductive structures as guide wires and catheters 538 R. Razavi et al. in interventional MRI. *J Magn Reson Imaging* 2001;13:105–114.

37. Yeung CJ, Susil RC, Atalar E. RF safety of wires in interventional MRI: using a safety index. *Magn Reson Med* 2002;47:187–193.

38. Glowinski A, Adam G, Bucker A, et al. Catheter visualization using locally induced, actively controlled field inhomogeneities. *Magn Reson Med* 1997;38:253–258.

39. Ladd ME, Erhart P, Debatin JF, et al. Guide wire antennas for MR fluoroscopy. *Magn Reson Med* 1997;37:891–897.

40. Leung DA, Debatin JF, Wildermuth S, et al. Intravascular MR tracking catheter: preliminary experimental evaluation. *Am J Roentgenol* 1995;164:1265–1270.

41. Guttman MA, Lederman RJ, Sorger JM, et al. Real-time volume rendered MRI for interventional guidance. *J Cardiovasc Magn Reson* 2002;4:431–442; erratum: *J Cardiovasc Magn Reson* 2003;5:407.

42. Hill JM, Dick AJ, Raman VK, et al. Serial cardiac magnetic resonance imaging of injected mesenchymal stem cells. *Circulation* 2003;108:1009–1014. Epub August 11, 2003.

43. Serfaty JM, Yang X, Aksit P, et al. Toward MRI-guided coronary catheterization: visualization of guiding catheters, guide wires, and anatomy in real time. *J Magn Reson Imaging* 2000;12:590–594.

44. Wong EY, Zhang Q, Duerk JL, et al. An optical system for wireless detuning of parallel resonant circuits. *J Magn Reson Imaging* 2000;12:632–638.

45. Eggers H, Weiss S, Boernert P, et al. Image-based tracking of optically detonable parallel resonant circuits. *Magn Reson Med* 2003;49:1163–1174.

46. Kuehne T, Saeed M, Higgins CB, et al. Endovascular stents in pulmonary valve and artery in swine: feasibility study of MR imaging-guided deployment and postinterventional assessment. *Radiology* 2003b;226:475–481.

47. Schalla S, Saeed M, Higgins CB, et al. Magnetic resonance-guided cardiac catheterization in a swine model of atrial septal defect. *Circulation* 2003;108:1865–1870.

48. Buecker A, Spuentrup E, Grabitz R, et al. Real-time MR guidance for placement of a self-made fully MR-compatible atrial septal occluder: in vitro test. *Rofo* 2002;174:283–285.

49. Rickers C, Seethamraju RT, Jerosch-Herold M, et al. Magnetic resonance imaging guided cardiovascular interventions in congenital heart diseases. *J Interv Cardiol* 2003;16:143–147.

50. Spuentrup E, Ruebben A, Schaeffter T, et al. Magnetic resonance-guided coronary artery stent placement in a swine model. *Circulation* 2002;105:874–879.

51. Buecker A, Neuerburg JM, Adam GB, et al. Real-time MR fluoroscopy for MR-guided iliac artery stent placement. *J Magn Reson Imaging* 2000;12:616–622.

52. Rhode KS, Hill DL, Edwards PJ, et al. Registration and tracking to integrate x-ray and MR images in an XMR facility. *IEEE Trans Med Imaging* 2003;22:1369–1378.

53. Shellock FG. Biological effects and safety aspects of magnetic resonance imaging. *Magn Reson Q* 1989;5:243–261.

54. Shellock FG, Kanal E. Policies, guidelines, and recommendations for MR imaging safety and patient management. SMRI Safety Committee. *J Magn Reson Imaging* 1991;1:97–101.

55. Shellock FG, Kanal E. Burns associated with the use of monitoring equipment during MR procedures. *J Magn Reson Imaging* 1996;6:271–272.

56. Shellock FG, Shellock VJ. Cardiovascular catheters and accessories: ex vivo testing of ferromagnetism, heating, and artifacts associated with MRI. *J Magn Reson Imaging* 1998;8:1338–1342.

57. Shellock FG, Shellock VJ. Metallic stents: evaluation of MR imaging safety. *Am J Roentgenol* 1999;173:543–547.

58. Dimick RN, Hedlund LW, Herfkens RJ, et al. Optimizing electrocardiograph electrode placement for cardiac-gated magnetic resonance imaging. *Invest Radiol* 1987;22:17–22.

59. Razavi RS, Hill DL, Muthurangu V, et al. Three-dimensional magnetic resonance imaging of congenital cardiac anomalies. *Cardiol Young* 2003;13:461–465.

60. Miquel ME, Hill DL, Baker EJ, et al. Three- and four-dimensional reconstruction of intra-cardiac anatomy from two-dimensional magnetic resonance images. *Int J Cardiovasc Imaging* 2003;19:239–254; discussion 255–256.

61. Razavi R, Hill DL, Keevil SF, et al. Cardiac catheterization guided by MRI in children and adults with congenital heart disease. *Lancet* 2003;362:1877–1882.

62. Hillis LD, Firth BG, Winniford MD. Analysis of factors affecting the variability of Fick versus indicator dilution measurements of cardiac output. *Am J Cardiol* 1985;56:764–768.

63. Muthurangu V, Taylor AM, Andriantsimiavona R, et al. A novel method of quantifying pulmonary vascular resistance utilizing simultaneous invasive pressure monitoring and phase-contrast MR flow. *Circulation,* 2004. In press.

38

Endovascular Delivery of Gene and Stem Cell Therapy

Dara L. Kraitchman

Most preclinical studies of the efficacy of gene and stem cell therapies have relied on validation by postmortem tissue analysis using techniques, such as immunohistochemistry or polymerase chain reaction. These techniques can provide high spatial resolution information, which is microscopic, and, when used in combination with serial animal sacrifice, the distribution of stem cells or longevity of gene expression can also be obtained. However, clinical trials will require methodologies that can be used to noninvasively, serially assess the presence of stem cells or gene expression to determine the safety and the efficacy of these therapies. Thus, the introduction of magnetic resonance imaging (MRI) scanners with real-time imaging capabilities has expanded MRI from a diagnostic imaging tool to interventional applications directed at gene and cellular therapeutic delivery.

MR delivery of endovascular and transmyocardial therapies offers four major advantages over other imaging modalities: (a) the ability to acquire full three-dimensional (3D) images of the cardiovascular system with soft-tissue detail; (b) the lack of ionizing radiation for the interventionalist and the patient; (c) the lack of iodinated contrast agents that are often poorly tolerated by patients with cardiac or renal compromise; and (d) the ability to better target the therapeutic whether it be to determine viable myocardium using delayed contrast-enhanced MRI for stem cell targeting or vulnerable atherosclerotic plaques by MR vessel wall imaging for gene therapy targeting. In addition, the development of MR-visible labeling techniques offers a method to view targeted delivery and track the fate of these therapeutics over weeks to months.

Although computed tomography (CT) is emerging as a new technology for whole body screening and rapid determination of stenotic coronary vessels and global left ventricular function, CT alone does not lend itself to endovascular delivery procedures. Nonetheless, the recent development of hybrid x-ray/MRI systems is an obvious extension that enables reductions in radiation dose while deriving the benefits of MRI along with the high temporal resolution and angiographic capabilities of x-ray imaging. As multislice CT scanners are developed, it is likely that hybrid MRI/CT systems will be developed akin to hybrid single photon emission computed tomography/computed tomography (SPECT/CT) and positron emission tomography/computed tomography (PET/CT) systems and, perhaps, be used for interventional procedures.

ENDOVASCULAR MAGNETIC RESONANCE IMAGING DELIVERY DEVICES

In concert with the development of MR scanner with real-time acquisition capabilities, another obvious hurdle is the development of delivery devices that are MR-compatible. In the simplest form, a conventional x-ray delivery catheter could be redesigned using nonmagnetic materials. However, often these MR-compatible devices either create large magnetic susceptibility artifacts or signal voids that either limit or prevent passive tracking of the device. At the other extreme, nonmetallic materials, such as nitinol guide-wires or platinum stents, are essentially MR-invisible (Fig. 38.1), making passive tracking of these devices difficult (1).

Several mechanisms for improving the passive visualization of these devices have been developed. A simple approach is to visualize a catheter lumen during injection of MR contrast agents similar to an x-ray angiogram (2–4). Another approach is to incorporate markers or coatings of paramagnetic or superparamagnetic iron oxide contrast agents in the devices (5–8) that can be tracked. Similarly, current-controlled susceptibility artifacts have also been used historically for tracking (9,10).

Active tracking approaches incorporate small MR receiver coil(s) into the device to receive the MR signal (11–14). In the simplest approach, a guidewire is used as a receiver coil or loopless antenna for imaging (15–17). The advantage of the active tracking approaches is the ability to obtain high resolution imaging from the miniaturized coils and the ability to perform catheter or catheter tip localization by triangulation of several of these small coils (11,18,19). The cost of this improved resolution and localization is the increased complexity of both device manufacture and image acquisition control. In addition, increases in device diameter to accommodate the wiring from multiple coils and the increase risk of localized heating of the device have limited their use to preclinical animal studies. Currently, only MR imaging guidewires have been safety tested and used in human clinical trials in transesophageal and transvenous approaches (Fig. 38.2) (20,21).

Specialized devices for the injection of stem cell therapies using MRI are currently under development. A modified injection catheter system (Boston Scientific, Inc.), developed for transmyocardial delivery of gene and stem cells consisting of a curved guide catheter and spring-loaded injection needle, has been used for active catheter tracking and delivery in relevant large animal models of stem cell delivery for cardiac regeneration (22,23). A prototype steerable catheter with a nitinol needle for endovascular injections (Bioheart,

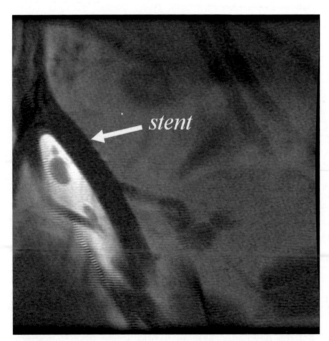

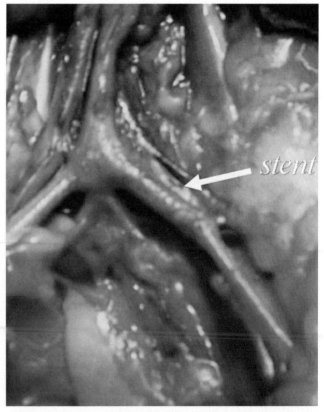

Figure 38.1. Transvenous T_1-weighted MR coronal image (*left*) of a platinum stent (Omniflex, Angiodynamics), placed under x-ray fluoroscopy in the iliac artery, in a normal pig obtained using an MR imaging guidewire placed in the iliac vein. Notice that the stent is virtually invisible in the MRI using a double inversion fast spin-echo sequence (612 milliseconds repetition time, 11 milliseconds echo time, 6 signal averages, 0.19 mm² in plane resolution). Placement of the stent is demonstrated in pathology (*right*). (Images courtesy of Lawrence V. Hofmann, MD.)

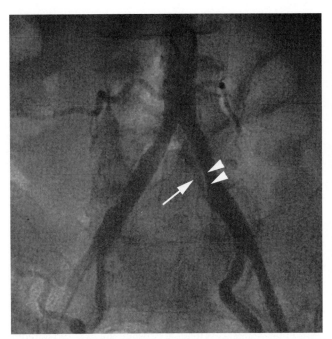

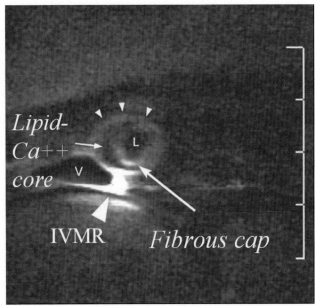

Figure 38.2. X-ray angiogram (*left*) obtained in a 61-year-old patient with claudication demonstrates a large plaque (*arrows, arrowhead*) in the common iliac artery. An axial MRI image (*right*) shows the imaging guidewire (IVMR) in the common iliac vein (V) and the bright fibrous cap with the hypointense lipid calcium in the iliac artery. L, lumen. (Images courtesy of Lawrence V. Hofmann, MD.)

Inc.) has been coated with gadolinium oxide markers for visualization under a hybrid x-ray/MR scanner (8). Using this hybrid imaging system, cardiac catheterization can be performed under x-ray guidance with accurate targeting to infarcted myocardium using MRI. A custom injection catheter has also been developed for stem cell therapeutic delivery with MR fluoroscopy (24) that enables access to all portions of the left ventricle because of a flexible steerable and bendable distal portion (Fig. 38.3).

INTERVENTIONAL MAGNETIC RESONANCE IMAGING TECHNIQUES

In addition to developing MR-compatible devices, a suite of imaging platforms is emerging to enable real-time interventional MR imaging of gene and stem cell delivery, using active delivery devices. Thus, in-room imaging displays and

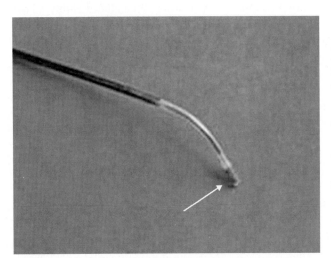

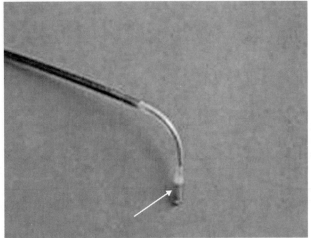

Figure 38.3. The distal tip of a custom MR-compatible loopless antenna for transendocardial injection of genetic and cellular therapeutics will appear as a bright signal at the distal tip (*arrow*) on MR images. The mechanical properties for steering and flexibility to reach all portions of the left ventricular endocardium are incorporated into a pull-wire. Approximately 25% (*left*) and 50% (*right*) deflection of the catheter tip are demonstrated. (From Karmarkar PV, Kraitchman DL, Izbudak I, et al. MR-trackable intramyocardial injection catheter. *Mag Reson Med* 2004;51:1163–1172, with permission.)

monitoring capabilities, which were originally developed for biopsy and neurointerventional procedures, are rapidly being adapted for cardiovascular applications. The inclusion of track balls and keyboards to enable full scanner operation within the scan room has now been implemented by all major MR vendors. Feedback systems to automatically adapt the imaging planes based on catheter position or velocity are now available (25). Graphic user interfaces that allow rapid plane manipulation and table motion are becoming more common (26). Multiple approaches have been developed to fuse the signal from the catheter coils with body coil images to fuse higher spatial resolution data from road maps, with images acquired at a high temporal resolution to track motion.

However, many hurdles still remain to the widespread acceptance of interventional MRI. The implementation of methods to rapidly adjust imaging parameters "on the fly" are still limited. Although techniques, such as SENSE (27) and SMASH (28), have enabled increases in the temporal resolution of interventional MRI, even at the highest frame rates, the temporal and spatial resolutions are much lower than x-ray fluoroscopy, making precise targeting difficult in a moving heart. In addition, the high noise level of the MR suite requires specialized systems for communications within the interventionalist team.

GENE TRANSFER GUIDED MAGNETIC RESONANCE IMAGING

The explosion of potential uses of gene therapy in clinical medicine, along with the initiation of the first human clinical trials in the United States in the 1990s, has brought forth the importance of not only interventional techniques to deliver genetic materials but also imaging methods to monitor the efficacy of gene transfection and expression. Endovascular delivery of gene products offers a method to apply high concentration of vectors in a localized region as compared to systemic intravenous administration. Besides using gene therapy to replace defective or missing genes, genes may be introduced to (a) up-regulate or inhibit expression, as in vascular endothelial growth factor (VEGF) production, to enhance angiogenesis in a stenotic vessel (29) or phospholamban inhibition of SERCA2a to enhance contractility in heart failure (30); (b) deliver genes that may produce a toxic product or cause cell suicide, as in the use of herpes simplex virus thymidine kinase/ganciclovir (HSV-tk/GCV) systems (31); or (c) act as reporter gene either to monitor the life span of a transfected cell or to image an event, such as cell differentiation that causes production of a new protein, enzyme product, or cell receptor.

There are two primary methods to transfect cells with genes. Nonviral transfection methods use either naked plasmid DNA alone or in combination with substances called transfection agents, like cationic liposomes. Viral transfection methods include retroviral, adenoviral, adeno-associated viral, lentiviral, and herpes (simplex) viral vectors to transfer genetic material to the cell. The primary advantage of viral transfection methods is their more efficient transfection rate than nonviral transfection techniques. The negative

aspect of this higher transfection efficiency is the tendency for these techniques to be immunogenic and the inability to cause stable, long-term transfection and expression.

CONTRAST AGENTS FOR GENE TRACKING AND CELL LABELING

Because of the low background signal, labeling techniques with radionuclides for radionuclide imaging are exquisitely sensitive to an extremely low number of molecular targets. MR or CT methods would require 10- to 100-fold large amplification of these targets for detection. In addition, cellular labeling for x-ray imaging would require an iodinated contrast agent load that is incompatible with maintaining normal cellular function and viability. However, using techniques largely adapted from monoclonal antibody techniques of radionuclide imaging, cellular, and genetic labeling strategies for MR imaging have been developed using conventional MR contrast agents. The inherent advantage of labeling with MR contrast agents is that the cells are not exposed to radioactive species that can become especially cytotoxic when internalized.

MR contrast agents can be divided into two major classes of agents: the paramagnetic and superparamagnetic iron oxide contrast agents. Gadolinium chelates, which form the most widely used clinically approved MR contrast agents, are in the paramagnetic class of agents. The adoption of gadolinium-based MR contrast agents for noncellular imaging is largely a result of the ability of these agents to decrease the T_1 relaxation time at low doses. This decrease in T_1 results in an increase signal intensity (i.e., hyperintense signal) of tissues exposed to the contrast agent using T_1-weighted imaging sequences. However, because of the high toxicity of free gadolinium, chelation of gadolinium is paramount. Concerns about dechelation of the gadolinium compounds in applications for genetic and cellular labeling have largely limited the development of these agents for these purposes. More problematic is the reduced ability of paramagnetic compounds when internalized to affect extracellular water, and, hence, the ability to alter signal intensity is greatly reduced.

The superparamagnetic iron oxide (SPIO) particles were developed shortly after the gadolinium-based contrast agents (32,33). The large magnetic moments, which are more than three orders of magnitude greater than paramagnetic-based contrast agents, of SPIO particles cause a greater effect on T_2 relaxation and a smaller effect on T_1 relaxation. Thus, on T_2^*-weighted images, SPIO particles appear hypointense and create a much larger signal change or contrast per unit of metal particle than paramagnetic contrast agents. Thus, small quantities of SPIO particles can be used for gene or cellular labeling, yet with a much larger amplification effect than paramagnetic compounds. Importantly, less agent must be internalized to create image contrast, thereby limiting cellular toxicity. Moreover, if the SPIO is degraded, the free iron that is released does not appreciably expand the native iron pool and, thus, can be degraded along normal iron recycling pathways. Most commercially available forms of SPIOs and ultrasmall SPIOs (USPIOS) have coatings to prevent particle aggregation. One of the most common USPIO coatings is dextran, which is a convenient surface for binding ligands and other functional groups for labeling.

IMAGING GENE DELIVERY

As stated previously, MR imaging for gene detection is largely inferior to radionuclide imaging techniques because of the adherently lower sensitivity for detecting genetic targets. Until amplification strategies to increase MR sensitivity are more fully developed, the ability to harness the high spatial resolution and interventional capabilities of MRI for cardiac gene therapies will not be recognized.

In an early attempt to apply these techniques for cardiovascular gene delivery, Gao et al (34) developed a novel MR gene delivery system that was validated in a swine model on a clinical MR scanner. A gene delivery catheter was combined with an MR imaging guidewire, and a lentiviral vector carrying green fluorescent protein (GFP) mixed with 6% gadolinium contrast agent was delivered intra-arterially and monitored in real time (Fig. 38.4). Radiofrequency (RF) heating of imaging guidewires, which is a concern of active catheter systems, has been exploited in this application by this group to enhance transfection rates. In a similar study to visualize gene delivery, Barbash et al (35) used a percutaneous approach in a rat infarction model to deliver an adenoviral LacZ reporter gene mixed with gadolinium via a 22-gauge needle.

A more sophisticated method to monitor sustained release of a gene would be to encapsulate the gene and paramagnetic contrast agent in a biodegradable sphere. Faranesh et al (36) have developed a poly(DL-lactic-co-glycolic acid) (PLGA)

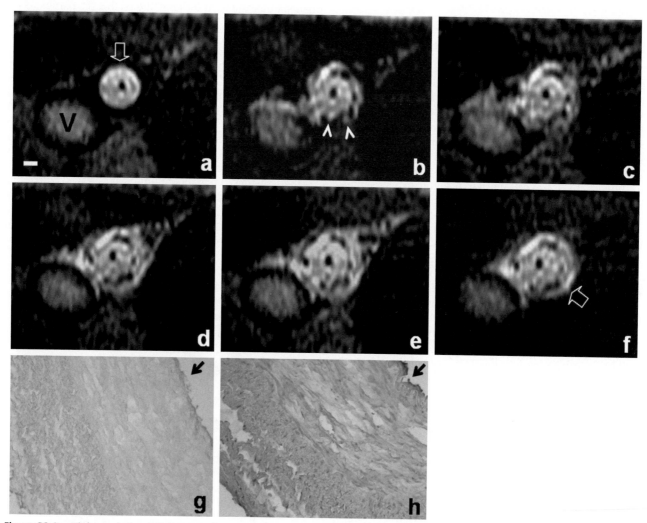

Figure 38.4.   High-resolution MR images of the gadolinium/GFP-lentivirus transfer in the iliac artery of a pig. **(A)** Before gadolinium/GFP-lentivirus infusion, the balloon is inflated with 3% Magnevist. The *open arrow* indicates the artery. **(B–F)** During gadolinium/GFP-lentivirus infusion from minute 3 to minute 15 (at 3-minute intervals), the arterial wall is enhanced by the gadolinium coming from the gene infusion channels (*arrowheads* in **B**) of the gene delivery catheter. At minute 15, the arterial wall is enhanced as a ring (*arrow* in **F**). **(G,H)** Corresponding immunohistochemistry in both control **(G)** and GFP-targeted **(H)** arteries. **(H)** GFP is detected as brown-colored precipitates through all layers of the intima (*arrows*) and media as well as the adventitia. Original magnification, 200X. V, vein. Scale = 1 mm. (Reprinted from Yang X, Atalar E, Li D, et al. Magnetic resonance imaging permits in vivo monitoring of catheter-based vascular gene delivery. *Circulation* 2001;104:1588–1590, with permission.)

microsphere containing VEGF and gadolinium diethyl-enetriamine pentaacetic acid (Gd-DTPA), which releases the gene and contrast agent over 6 weeks that can be noninvasively imaged as hyperenhancement on T_1-weighted MRI. Microsphere systems, such as this system, enable a sustained release of the gene product over many weeks to assist with higher or sustained transfection rates. But what is unlikely is that the kinetics of Gd-DTPA and VEGF release from the microsphere are equivalent, such that absolute quantitation of gene release from MRI can be obtained using this delivery technique.

Another area in which MR delivery may be useful is in combination with ultrasonography. High frequency ultrasound has been used to increase vascular permeability and also rupture ultrasound microbubbles (37,38). MR paramagnetic agents encapsulated in liposomes could be combined with naked DNA to enable high resolution localization of the genes followed by enhanced transfection using high frequency ultrasound.

IMAGING GENE EXPRESSION

Several groups have been able to develop amplification systems to visualize gene expression using MRI. In particular, Weissleder et al (39) and Ichikawa et al (40) have transfected tumor cells with an engineered transferrin receptor (Tfr). Monocrystalline iron oxides (MION) can be conjugated to transferrin (Tf), the natural ligand of Tfr. After systemic injection, the MION-Tf will be taken up preferentially by the tumor cells overexpressing Tfr, resulting in a hypointensity on T_2^*-weighted images of the tumors. In this model system, amplification has been achieved in two ways: (a) the overexpression of the receptor and (b) the ability of superparamagnetic iron oxide particles with high magnetic moments to cause large dephasing of local protons, resulting in a dramatic shortening of T_2 far beyond what could be achieved by conventional gadolinium chelates.

In a similar strategy, the up-regulation of the enzyme tyrosinase in melanomas results in increased melanin production. Like Tfr, melanin has a high affinity for iron, and gene expression can thus be probed using exogenous administration of MION (41,42). Internalization of the MION results in a bright signal in T_1-weighted MRI.

The potential also exists for the development of smart MR contrast agents, which either act as substrates that are cleaved by specific enzymatic activity to expose the magnetic nanoparticle or are assembled into larger polypeptides when specific enzymes or proteases are present to amplify the magnetic signal. In essence, the magnetic relaxation of the particle can be changed as a result of the increased size of the magnetic particle resulting from cross linking as multiple ligands are bound to multiple targets. Perez et al (43–46), Bogdanov et al (47), and Josephson et al (48) have developed several of these enzyme-sensing particles that cluster in the presence of peroxidases. In particular, Perez et al (46) have developed a superparamagnetic nanoparticle in this class, which, in the presence of myeloperoxidase (MPO), assemble to cause decreases in spin-spin relaxation times that can be detected by MRI. Although gadolinium substrates lack the amplification of iron oxide nanoparticles, this same group

has designed a nanoparticle particle probe with gadolinium substrates that polymerize in the presence of MPO (49). Myeloperoxidase, which is produced by activated macrophages, has been implicated in inflammation and, particularly, atherosclerotic plaques. Thus, the vulnerable atherosclerotic plaque could be detected, or the response of the plaque to genetic modification could be performed using this targeted MPO agent. Particles in this class can also be used as MR switches to sense that assembly and dispersal of the particles, as occurs in the presence of restriction endonucleases during DNA cleavage (50). However, none of these particles has yet been tested in vivo.

Lanza et al (51) and Yu et al (52) have developed a targeted nanoparticle containing a liquid perfluorocarbon core with chelated gadolinium (Gd) complexes incorporated into the outer surface. They have overcome the amplification problem with gadolinium-based agents by two means: (a) numerous Gd molecules can be bound to the surface of the nanoparticle; and (b) antibody receptor complexes on the nanoparticle are used for targeting so that the particle is not internalized, which would reduce T_1 relaxivity (Fig. 38.5). Thus, changes in T_1 relaxation can be achieved in vivo. In addition, therapeutics can be incorporated into the surface of the nanoparticle for drug delivery (53). By modifying the antibody receptor complex, targeting of this agent has been performed to fibrin (i.e., thrombus) for cardiovascular applications (54,55). To decrease the potential toxicity of the gadolinium chelate, several paramagnetic formulations have been explored, which have also increased the relaxivity of the agent resulting in enhanced signal enhancement after injection (55). The most exciting cardiovascular application is the targeting to markers of angiogenesis (i.e., $\alpha_v \beta_3$ integrins) using this agent (Fig. 38.6) (56,57). The fluorine signal of the nanoparticle can also be detected with MR spectroscopy, providing an independent method for validating the bright Gd signal detected in proton imaging. In addition,

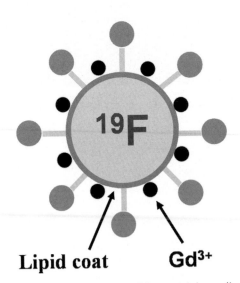

Figure 38.5. A targeted nanoparticle containing a liquid perfluorocarbon core with chelated gadolinium (Gd^{3+}) complexes incorporated into the outer surface. Monoclonal antibodies or targeted therapeutics can be placed on the surface of the nanoparticle. (Image courtesy of Samuel Wickline, MD, and Greg Lanza, MD, PhD.)

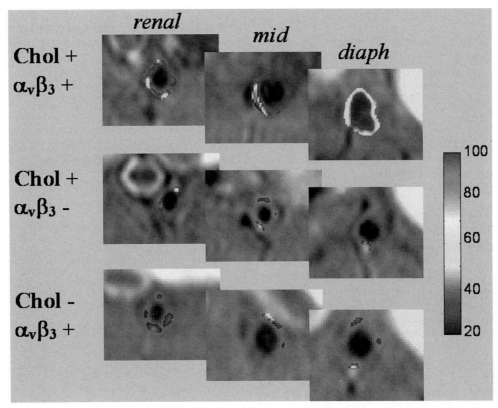

Figure 38.6.   Percent enhancement maps created from MR axial images from individual aortic segments at renal artery (*renal*), mid-aorta (*mid*), and diaphragm (*diaph*) 2 hours after treatment with $\alpha_v\beta_3$-targeted paramagnetic nanoparticles in cholesterol-fed rabbit (*top*), with $\alpha_v\beta_3$-targeted nonparamagnetic nanoparticles in cholesterol-fed rabbit (*middle*), and with $\alpha_v\beta_3$-targeted paramagnetic nanoparticles in rabbit on a normal diet (*bottom*). The induction of angiogenesis in the vasa vasorum seen as increased signal enhancement is evident in the cholesterol fed rabbit receiving the targeted gadolinium nanoparticle (*top*). (Adapted from Winter PM, Morawski AM, Caruthers SD, et al. Molecular imaging of angiogenesis in early-stage atherosclerosis with alpha(v)beta3-integrin-targeted nanoparticles. *Circulation* 2003;108:2270–2274, with permission.)

the introduction of higher field strength magnets for clinical imaging may overcome the signal-to-noise ratio issues associated with ^{19}F spectroscopy and imaging.

The potential to measure gene expression has also been demonstrated with ^{19}F spectroscopy in a tumor model (58). In this model, genetically modified tumor cells expressing cytosine deaminase from yeast were implanted in mice. The concept of gene-directed proenzyme therapy is to introduce a nonmammalian enzyme into tumor cells that efficiently converts a nontoxic prodrug into a cytotoxic metabolite. In this case, yeast cytosine deaminase efficiently converts 5-fluorocytosine into 5-fluorouracil (5-FU), thereby limiting the dose of the widely used chemotherapeutic agent 5-FU to the solid tumor. From the MR spectra, the pharmacokinetics of the 5-FC metabolites can be determined and, hence, the gene expression in the tumor. It can be envisioned that gene-directed proenzyme therapy for atherosclerosis could be monitored in a similar manner.

CELLULAR LABELING STRATEGIES

As with gene therapy, most of the stem cell labeling strategies have been directed toward labeling with iron oxide com-

pounds. Unlike gene therapy applications, surface labeling for stem cells is not preferred because the label may become detached and transferred to other cells. Thus, most stem cell labeling techniques have been developed to optimize internalization of the label. A few individuals have been developing techniques with paramagnetic compounds, but the focus at present has been on neurologic applications or have not yet been tested in vivo for cardiovascular applications. Modo et al (59) have developed a gadolinium-based compound linked to dextran and a fluorescent dye, rhodamine, that can be taken up by stem cells in vitro for intracellular labeling. These exogenously labeled stem cells have been implanted in a rat stroke model, and the migration has been tracked in vivo by MRI and validated by detection of the fluorescent label by histology (60). Using a calcium phosphate transfection technique, Rudelius et al (61) performed intracellular labeling of neuronal and embryonic stem cells with Gd-DTPA. Using this labeling technique Daldrup-Link et al (62) were able to achieve intracellular labeling of hematopoietic progenitor cells that resulted in significant lengthening of R_1 such that detection of 500,000 cells or greater should be possible. However, as stated previously, the internalization of these Gd particles will greatly reduce the potential contrast enhancement imparted by these agents. Thus, because of amplification problems and toxicity concerns, iron oxide compounds remain the preferred agents for cellular labeling.

Cardiovascular applications of MR imaging with iron oxide compounds were first implemented because of the recognition of the rapid uptake of these compounds by macrophages after systemic administration. Monocyte recruitment by the atherosclerotic plaque has been demonstrated using MRI and accumulation of SPIOs in the hyperlipidemic rabbit and apoE knockout mice models (63–66). Subsequently, retrospective and prospective patient studies with USPIOs to identify atheromas vulnerable to rupture have been undertaken (67,68). Similarly, SPIO uptake by macrophages during allogeneic cardiac transplant rejection has been demonstrated in the rat (69).

As with MR labeling for gene therapy, the initial methods for cellular MR labeling with iron oxides were based on radionuclide monoclonal antibody (MoAb) techniques. Using the dextran coating of iron oxides, immunoglobulins could be covalently linked using a periodate oxidation/borohydrides reduction method in which the lysine groups of the monoclonal antibodies are joined to the alcohol groups of the dextrans (70). Using this technique, MION has been conjugated to an antimyosin MoAb for detection of infarcted myocardium in the rat (71). Although there are many other alternate methods to attach MoAbs to magnetic nanoparticles, the lack of species cross reactivity for many MoAbs requires that separate formulations be developed for animal validation and human studies.

Meldrum et al (72) attempted to circumvent the species specificity problem by developing an iron oxide encapsulated with a ferritin protein shell called *magnetoferritin*. Ferritin is highly conserved across species, and, thus, this agent has the potential for molecular imaging and cellular labeling. However, in vivo studies with magnetoferritin showed a rapid clearance of the agent from the vascular pool that was unrelated to ferritin receptor binding (73), suggesting a limited use for this agent.

Because dedrimers offer an efficient method to transfect cells (74–76), the development of dedrimer-encapsulated SPIOs or "magnetodedrimers" offered another nonspecies specific agent that could be used for cellular labeling. One formulation of magnetodedrimers, MD-100, consists of iron oxide nanoparticles coated with a generation 4.5 carboxylated dedrimer (77). These highly charged polymers bind to the cell membrane, induce membrane binding and endocytosis. Many different cell types from many different animal species cultured in vitro for 24 to 48 hours with MD-100 show a consistent, low iron concentration (10 to 25 μg Fe/mL) with the agent stably maintained within endosomes (77–79). Importantly, cell viability and proliferation was not affected by labeling with MD-100.

Billotey et al (80) and Wilhelm et al (81) have developed an anionic magnetic nanoparticle for cellular labeling that is also maintained within endosomes. However, one major disadvantage of these particles, as well as magnetodedrimers, is that they do not use commercially available agents and are costly to produce with limited availability. Recently, a magnetic labeling method, based on commercially available SPIO/USPIOs (e.g., Feridex or Combidex), has been developed. The USPIOs are mixed with commonly used transfection agents (e.g., SuperFect, poly-L-lysine, Lipofectin, FuGENE, and so forth) that result in complexes via elec-

trostatic interactions of the two agents (82,83). The concentration of both agents must be carefully titrated to ensure good cellular uptake without the formation of precipitates of the complex. Currently, poly-L-lysine (PLL) has become the preferred transfection agent, because it is inexpensive and available through several manufacturers. The complex is then incubated with the cells in culture media for 24 to 48 hours, resulting in a consistent endosomal iron uptake of 10 to 20 pg Fe per cell in a wide variety of cell lines without species specificity (Fig. 38.7) (84–91). Although Feridex-PLL labeling of human mesenchymal stem cells (MSCs) does not affect cell proliferation or viability, chondrogenic differentiation assays performed in vitro were inhibited, whereas osteogenic and adipogenic differentiations were not impaired (92,93). Interestingly, the inhibition of chondro-

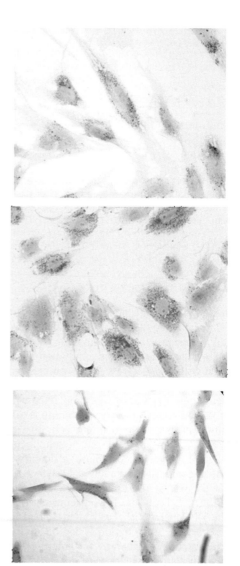

Figure 38.7. Magnetic labeling of mesenchymal stem cells (MSCs), using superparamagnetic iron oxide particles (Feridex) coated with a transfection agent (poly-L-lysine, PLL). Cells were labeled for 48 hours (*top, middle*) or 24 hours (*bottom*), with 25 mg Fe/mL Feridex and 375 ng/mL PLL. Prussian blue staining of labeled human (*top*), porcine (*middle*), and canine (*bottom*) MSCs shows an efficient intracellular uptake of particles into endosomes that is nonspecific across species.

genesis was not mediated by the PLL but by the Feridex, suggesting some interaction of iron with cellular signaling. Arbab et al (94) have reported, when using protamine sulfate instead of PLL for Feridex labeled, that Collagen X was still formed. These studies emphasize the need for more detailed examination of the possible biologic effects of labeling schemes in stem cells prior to initiating clinical trials. Nonetheless, protamine sulfate has the advantage over PLL of being an approved drug by the U.S. Food and Drug Administration (FDA) and thereby has less barriers to FDA approval of this labeling method.

Another approach for cellular labeling has been developed using large styrene/divinyl benzene-coated magnetic microspheres (Bang Laboratories) (23,95). However, the biocompatibility of these large spheres, because the degradation pathway is unknown, will probably limit their clinical applicability. Nonetheless, these iron oxide particles are so large that a single particle can be detected by MRI as a hypointense spot (95–97).

CELLULAR DETECTION LIMITS

Estimates of the required amount of iron oxide per cell to detect a single cell at the spatial resolution of 100 $\times 100 \times 200$ μm range from 1.4 to 3.0 pg Fe per cell. Fortunately, this range is approximately 10 pg Fe/cell range seen with USPIO cellular labeling (98). Indeed, imaging of single cells has been performed using both USPIO (98) and Bang particles (95–97) at both 1.5 T and higher field strengths. However, with cell division, the label is diluted and detection may not be possible beyond several cell divisions, depending on the initial labeling concentration. Short-term studies of stem cells injected intramyocardially in animal models of myocardial infarction have demonstrated persistence beyond 3 weeks of injection (23,87) and as long as 8 weeks postinjection (99), perhaps reflecting the low division rate of these cells.

Another problem with iron oxide labeling is that any cells or genetic material that are degraded can potentially release the iron oxide, which may be incorporated by adjacent phagocytic cells. Thus, hypointense artifacts in images at later time points after injection may represent cells other than the original exogenously labeled cells or cells that do not contain the transfected gene. Therefore, strict quantification of cell numbers based on the change in the volume of the hypointense artifact will be difficult to determine.

IMAGING STEM CELL DELIVERY

Many of the in vivo studies of cell trafficking and migration using SPIO labeled stem cells were originally performed in neurovascular and oncologic applications (77,100–103). Cardiovascular applications have recently been explored following advances in interventional MRI techniques, devices, and labeling methodologies. Because of the limited regenerative capacity of the heart, the exogenous administration of stem cells holds promise as a method to repair or regenerate cardiac tissue after an ischemic event. Hematopoietic bone-marrow derived stem cells, endothelial progenitor cells, multipotent adult progenitor cells (MAPCs), mesenchymal stem cells (MSCs), and skeletal myoblasts are all thought to be potential candidates to provide stromal support, angiogenesis, and/or new cardiomyocytes. Several European stem cell clinical trials for ischemic heart disease are already under way (104–108). Modest improvements in left ventricular function by MRI after stem cell therapy have been demonstrated in several trials (105–108). But it is difficult to determine whether further improvements in left ventricular function could be gained by administering different doses or dosing intervals of the stem cells because of the inability to determine whether the stem cells persist in the myocardium and, if so, the extent of engraftment. Thus, MRI methods to monitor delivery and track the persistence of engraftment using labeled stem cells appear poised to answer some of these questions.

Numerous MR studies of magnetically labeled MSCs have been performed for cardiac applications in the last few years. Lederman et al (109) were the first to demonstrate using a real-time imaging platform and prototype device proof of principle using transendocardial injections of contrast agent under MR fluoroscopy on a clinical 1.5-T scanner. This study as well as subsequent studies with stem cells used fast gradient-echo and steady-state free precession techniques to monitor real-time delivery.

Subsequently, Kraitchman et al (87) demonstrated the ability to track the migration of SPIO-PLL-labeled allogeneic MSCs as hypointense artifacts on T_2*-weighted images in a clinically relevant swine model of acute myocardial infarction (MI). Follow-up MRI at several weeks after MSC showed changes in signal intensity and volume of the hypoenhancing artifact indicative of migration of the MSC within the myocardial infarction (Fig. 38.8). Delivery of the magnetically labeled MSCs was performed under x-ray fluoroscopy with only about 70% of the injections visualized by MRI. Thus, the potential for enhanced injection success rate could be envisioned using MR delivery of magnetically labeled stem. In an effort to more precisely target cells to the infarcted tissue, Garot et al (88) used electromechanical mapping of iron oxide labeled myogenic progenitor cells in an acute swine MI. Within 2 hours after injection, MRI was used to determine the location of the magnetically labeled cells.

Subsequently, Dick et al (22), using the Bang particle labeled MSCs in a swine MI model, were able to precisely target the magnetically labeled MSCs to the infarct with a 100% success rate using MR fluoroscopic delivery. Furthermore, Hill et al (23), in this same magnetically labeled MSC swine MI model, showed that as few as 10^5 cells could be detected. In a dosing study in a canine model of myocardial infarction, Bulte et al (99) were able to demonstrate that 10^5 autologous SPIO-PLL labeled MSCs injected under MR fluoroscopy were still visible by MRI at 2 months postinjection as well as precise targeting to the peri-infarction region (Fig. 38.9). Thus, magnetically labeled stem cells can be successfully delivered noninvasively using MR fluoroscopy with noninvasive serial follow-up of the persistence, and hence engraftment of the MSCs.

The advantage of all of these large animal MI models, such as pigs and dogs, is that the devices used for endocardial

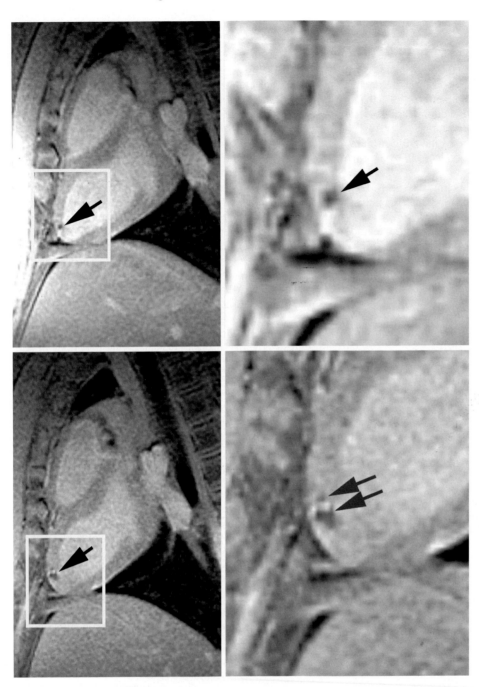

Figure 38.8. Long-axis MRIs acquired with a high resolution, breath-hold ECG-gated fast gradient echo pulse ($500 \times 500 \times 5000$ μm^3 resolution) sequence show hypointense lesions (*arrows*) caused by Feridex-PLL-labeled mesenchymal stem cells acquired within 24 hours (*top*) and 1 week (*bottom*) of injection in a pig with a myocardial infarction. The inset (*right*) shows a magnified view demonstrating expansion of lesion over 1 week and a change in the shape of the hypointense lesion from an ovid shape to a shape with more irregular borders, suggesting migration of the MSCs. (Adapted from Kraitchman DL, Heldman AW, Atalar E, et al. In vivo magnetic resonance imaging of mesenchymal stem cells in myocardial infarction. *Circulation* 2003; 107:2290–2293, with permission.)

injection of stem cells are similar to those that would be used in human trials. In addition, the large animal closed-chest models of myocardial infarction are minimally invasive and, thus, more comparable to human MI pathology than open-chest rodent procedures. Moreover, the imaging protocols developed are typically performed on 1.5 T MR clinical scanners and, therefore, demonstrate the feasibility for future human trials. Furthermore, it can be expected that many of these studies with magnetically labeled stem cells will soon present results of regional changes in infarction size, perfusion, global, and regional function using the inherent advantages of the high spatial resolution and noninvasiveness of techniques. In a dog model of chronic MI, Rickers et al (110) have used MRI in this manner to assess

improvements in myocardial perfusion reserve and regional myocardial function in animals that received unlabeled stem cells, for example, MAPCs, when compared to control animals that received sham intramyocardial injections via a surgical approach.

Finally, the tracking of systemic delivery of magnetically labeled stem cells will be highly dependent on the sensitivity of the imaging technique. Cahill et al (111) have shown repeatable T_2 measurements in murine skeletal muscle that imply that extremely small numbers of SPIO labeled cells can be detected. Furthermore, this group has shown that after intra-arterial delivery of SPIO-PLL labeled immortalized muscle cells in a rabbit model the dynamic removal of the cells can be followed by MRI (111). Similarly, Bos et al

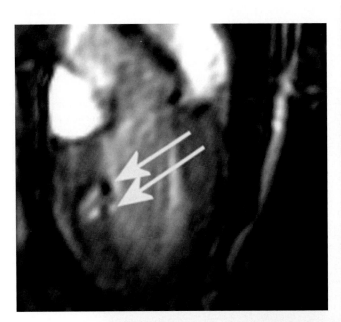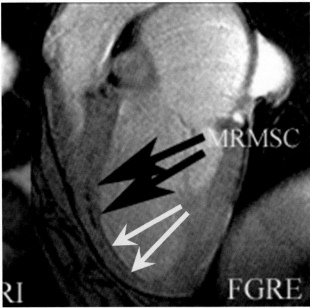

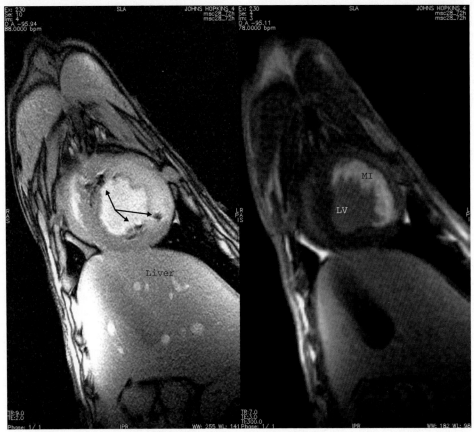

Figure 38.9. Injection of Feridex-PLL-labeled autologous canine mesenchymal stem cells (MSCs) in a dog myocardial infarct model. Still frame long-axis view from real-time MRI (*top left*) demonstrating Feridex-labeled MSCs as hypoenhancing artifacts (*arrows*) after initial two injections at 3 days postinfarction (*MI*). *Top* lesion is 7×10^6 Feridex-labeled MSCs; *bottom* lesion is 3×10^6 labeled MSC with 4×10^6 unlabeled MSCs. At 8 weeks after injection, initial two injections (*top right, upper arrows*) are still visible, as well as additional injections (*top right, lower arrows*), with as low as 1×10^5 labeled MSCs at initial injection in fast gradient echo images (FGRE). Hypoenhancing artifacts change from round lesions to linear lesions by 8 weeks. Targeting of the labeled MSCs (*arrows, bottom left*) to the peri-infarction region using MR fluoroscopic delivery can be guided by delayed contrast-enhanced short-axis MRI, which shows infarcted myocardium (*bottom right, MI*). Stem cell placement was validated on high resolution FGRE short-axis images (*bottom left*). (Adapted from Bulte JW, Kraitchman DL. Monitoring cell therapy using iron oxide MR contrast agents. *Curr Pharm Biotechnol* 2004;5:567–584, with permission.)

(112) have also watched the distribution kinetics of intra-arterial and intravenous injection of SPIO-PLL labeled rat MSCs as long as 7 to 11 days postinjection. Thus, stem cell therapies for patients with peripheral artery disease that may be more amenable to intravenous delivery of stem cells could be monitored dynamically by MRI. But methods to detect small numbers of cells will still be needed. However, recently, techniques based on the methods of Seppenwoolde et al (113) for white marker tracking of passive devices have been adapted for imaging of the hypointense susceptibility artifacts caused by iron oxide labeled stem cells (114,115). These new techniques lend promise to the ability to image even smaller numbers of magnetically labeled stem cells that can often be confused with other hypointense image artifacts.

SUMMARY

Gene and stem cell therapeutics for the heart have been advancing rapidly in the last few years. In concert, MR imaging methods and devices have been rapidly evolving to keep pace. Although CT offers many benefits in terms of cost and rapid image acquisition, MR techniques for tracking gene expression and cellular labeling will provide noninvasive means to determine the success of these therapies as we move into clinical trials.

REFERENCES

1. Spuentrup E, Ruebben A, Schaeffter T, et al. Magnetic resonance—guided coronary artery stent placement in a swine model. *Circulation* 2002;105:874–879.
2. Omary RA, Unal O, Koscielski DS, et al. Real-time MR imaging-guided passive catheter tracking with use of gadolinium-filled catheters. *J Vasc Interv Radiol* 2000;11:1079–1085.
3. Strother CM, Unal O, Frayne R, et al. Endovascular treatment of experimental canine aneurysms: feasibility with MR imaging guidance. *Radiology* 2000;215:516–519.
4. Bakker CJ, Bos C, Weinmann HJ. Passive tracking of catheters and guidewires by contrast-enhanced MR fluoroscopy. *Magn Reson Med* 2001;45:17–23.
5. Buecker A, Spuentrup E, Schmitz-Rode T, et al. Use of a nonmetallic guidewire for magnetic resonance-guided coronary artery catheterization. *Invest Radiol* 2004;39:656–660.
6. Wacker FK, Reither K, Ebert W, et al. MR image-guided endovascular procedures with the ultrasmall superparamagnetic iron oxide SH U 555 C as an intravascular contrast agent: study in pigs. *Radiology* 2003;226:459–464.
7. Bakker CJ, Smits HF, Bos C, et al. MR-guided balloon angioplasty: in vitro demonstration of the potential of MRI for guiding, monitoring, and evaluating endovascular interventions. *J Magn Reson Imaging* 1998;8:245–250.
8. Saeed M, Lee R, Martin A, et al. Transendocardial delivery of extracellular myocardial markers by using combination x-ray/MR fluoroscopic guidance: feasibility study in dogs. *Radiology* 2004;231:689–696.
9. Glowinski A, Adam G, Bucker A, et al. Catheter visualization using locally induced, actively controlled field inhomogeneities. *Magn Reson Med* 1997;38:253–258.
10. Adam G, Glowinski A, Neuerburg J, et al. Visualization of MR-compatible catheters by electrically induced local field inhomogeneities: evaluation in vivo. *J Magn Reson Imaging* 1998;8:209–213.
11. Dumoulin CL, Souza SP, Darrow RD. Real-time position monitoring of invasive devices using magnetic resonance. *Magn Reson Med* 1993;29:411–415.
12. Leung DA, Debatin JF, Wildermuth S, et al. Intravascular MR tracking catheter: preliminary experimental evaluation. *AJR Am J Roentgenol* 1995;164:1265–1270.
13. Worthley SG, Helft G, Fuster V, et al. A novel nonobstructive intravascular MRI coil: in vivo imaging of experimental atherosclerosis. *Arterioscler Thromb Vasc Biol* 2003;23:346–350.
14. Hillenbrand CM, Elgort DR, Wong EY, et al. Active device tracking and high-resolution intravascular MRI using a novel catheter-based, opposed-solenoid phased array coil. *Magn Reson Med* 2004;51:668–675.
15. Ladd ME, Zimmermann GG, Quick HH, et al. Active MR visualization of a vascular guidewire in vivo. *J Magn Reson Imaging* 1998;8:220–225.
16. Ladd ME, Zimmermann GG, McKinnon GC, et al. Visualization of vascular guidewires using MR tracking. *J Magn Reson Imaging* 1998;8:251–253.
17. Ocali O, Atalar E. Intravascular magnetic resonance imaging using a loopless catheter antenna. *Magn Reson Med* 1997;37:112–118.
18. Elgort DR, Wong EY, Hillenbrand CM, et al. Real-time catheter tracking and adaptive imaging. *J Magn Reson Imaging* 2003;18:621–626.
19. Omary RA, Green JD, Fang WS, et al. Use of internal coils for independent and direct MR imaging-guided endovascular device tracking. *J Vasc Interv Radiol* 2003;14:247–254.
20. Shunk KA, Atalar E, Lima JA. Possibilities of transesophageal MRI for assessment of aortic disease: a review. *Int J Cardiovasc Imaging* 2001;17:179–185.
21. Hofmann L, Liddell R, Eng J, et al. Human peripheral arteries: feasibility of transvenous intravascular MR imaging of the arterial wall. *Radiology* 2005;235(2):617–622.
22. Dick AJ, Guttman MA, Raman VK, et al. Magnetic resonance fluoroscopy allows targeted delivery of mesenchymal stem cells to infarct borders in swine. *Circulation* 2003;108:2899–2904.
23. Hill JM, Dick AJ, Raman VK, et al. Serial cardiac magnetic resonance imaging of injected mesenchymal stem cells. *Circulation* 2003;11:11.
24. Karmarkar PV, Kraitchman DL, Izbudak I, et al. MR-trackable intramyocardial injection catheter. *Mag Reson Med* 2004;51:1163–1172.
25. Wacker FK, Elgort D, Hillenbrand CM, et al. The catheter-driven MRI scanner: a new approach to intravascular catheter tracking and imaging-parameter adjustment for interventional MRI. *AJR Am J Roentgenol* 2004;183:391–395.
26. Guttman MA, Kellman P, Dick AJ, et al. Real-time accelerated interactive MRI with adaptive TSENSE and UNFOLD. *Magn Reson Med* 2003;50:315–321.
27. Pruessmann KP, Weiger M, Scheidegger MB, et al. SENSE: sensitivity encoding for fast MRI. *Magn Reson Med* 1999;42:952–962.
28. Sodickson DK, Manning WJ. Simultaneous acquisition of spatial harmonics (SMASH): fast imaging with radiofrequency coil arrays. *Magn Reson Med* 1997;38:591–603.
29. Isner JM, Walsh K, Symes J, et al. Arterial gene therapy for therapeutic angiogenesis in patients with peripheral artery disease. *Circulation* 1995;91:2687–2692.
30. del Monte F, Harding SE, Dec GW, et al. Targeting phospholamban by gene transfer in human heart failure. *Circulation* 2002;105:904–907.

31. Moolten FL. Tumor chemosensitivity conferred by inserted herpes thymidine kinase genes: paradigm for a prospective cancer control strategy. *Cancer Res* 1986;46:5276–5281.

32. Mendonca Dias MH, Lauterbur PC. Ferromagnetic particles as contrast agents for magnetic resonance imaging of liver and spleen. *Magn Reson Med* 1986;3:328–330.

33. Renshaw PF, Owen CS, McLaughlin AC, et al. Ferromagnetic contrast agents: a new approach. *Magn Reson Med* 1986;3:217–225.

34. Gao F, Qui B, Kar S, et al. Intravascular MR/RF-enhanced VEFG gene therapy of atherosclerotic in-stent restenosis. *Proc Int Soc Magn Reson Med* 2004:377.

35. Barbash IM, Leor J, Feinberg MS, et al. Interventional magnetic resonance imaging for guiding gene and cell transfer in the heart. *Heart* 2004;90:87–91.

36. Faranesh AZ, Nastley MT, Perez de la Cruz C, et al. In vitro release of vascular endothelial growth factor from gadolinium-doped biodegradable microspheres. *Magn Reson Med* 2004;51:1265–1271.

37. Lawrie A, Brisken AF, Francis SE, et al. Microbubble-enhanced ultrasound for vascular gene delivery. *Gene Ther* 2000;7:2023–2027.

38. Unger EC, McCreery TP, Sweitzer RH. Ultrasound enhances gene expression of liposomal transfection. *Invest Radiol* 1997;32:723–727.

39. Weissleder R, Moore A, Mahmood U, et al. In vivo magnetic resonance imaging of transgene expression. *Nat Med* 2000;6:351–355.

40. Ichikawa T, Hogemann D, Saeki Y, et al. MRI of transgene expression: correlation to therapeutic gene expression. *Neoplasia* 2002;4:523–530.

41. Enochs WS, Petherick P, Bogdanova A, et al. Paramagnetic metal scavenging by melanin: MR imaging. *Radiology* 1997;204:417–423.

42. Weissleder R, Cheng HC, Bogdanova A, et al. Magnetically labeled cells can be detected by MR imaging. *J Magn Reson Imaging* 1997;7:258–263.

43. Perez JM, Josephson L, Weissleder R. Use of magnetic nanoparticles as nanosensors to probe for molecular interactions. *Chembiochem* 2004;5:261–264.

44. Perez JM, Josephson L, O'Loughlin T, et al. Magnetic relaxation switches capable of sensing molecular interactions. *Nat Biotechnol* 2002;20:816–820.

45. Perez JM, Simeone FJ, Saeki Y, et al. Viral-induced self-assembly of magnetic nanoparticles allows the detection of viral particles in biological media. *J Am Chem Soc* 2003;125:10192–10193.

46. Perez JM, Simeone FJ, Tsourkas A, et al. Peroxidase substrate nanosensors for MR imaging. *Nano Lett* 2004;4:119–122.

47. Bogdanov A Jr, Matuszewski L, Bremer C, et al. Oligomerization of paramagnetic substrates result in signal amplification and can be used for MR imaging of molecular targets. *Mol Imaging* 2002;1:16–23.

48. Josephson L, Tung CH, Moore A, et al. High-efficiency intracellular magnetic labeling with novel superparamagnetic-Tat peptide conjugates. *Bioconjug Chem* 1999;10:186–191.

49. Chen JW, Parm W, Weissleder R, et al. Molecular imaging of human myeloperoxidase: a potential target for imaging unstable plaques in atherosclerosis. In: *90th Scientific Assembly and Annual Meeting of the Radiology Society of North America*. Chicago: 2004:614.

50. Perez JM, O'Loughin T, Simeone FJ, et al. DNA-based magnetic nanoparticle assembly acts as a magnetic relaxation nano switch allowing screening of DNA-cleaving agents. *J Am Chem Soc* 2002;124:2856–2857.

51. Lanza GM, Lorenz CH, Fischer SE, et al. Enhanced detection of thrombi with a novel fibrin-targeted magnetic resonance imaging agent. *Acad Radiol* 1998;5(Suppl 1):S173–S176; discussion S183–S184.

52. Yu X, Song SK, Chen J, et al. High-resolution MRI characterization of human thrombus using a novel fibrin-targeted paramagnetic nanoparticle contrast agent. *Magn Reson Med* 2000;44:867–872.

53. Winter PM, Morawski AM, Caruthers SD, et al. Molecular imaging of angiogenesis in early-stage atherosclerosis with alpha(v)beta3-integrin-targeted nanoparticles. *Circulation* 2003;108:2270–2274.

54. Flacke S, Fischer S, Scott MJ, et al. Novel MRI contrast agent for molecular imaging of fibrin: implications for detecting vulnerable plaques. *Circulation* 2001;104:1280–1285.

55. Lanza GM, Yu X, Winter PM, et al. Targeted antiproliferative drug delivery to vascular smooth muscle cells with an MRI nanoparticle contrast agent: implications for rational therapy of restenosis. *Circulation* 2002;106:2842–2847.

56. Anderson SA, Rader RK, Westlin WF, et al. Magnetic resonance contrast enhancement of neovasculature with alpha(v)beta(3)-targeted nanoparticles. *Magn Reson Med* 2000;44:433–439.

57. Winter PM, Morawski AM, Caruthers SD, et al. Molecular imaging of angiogenesis in early-stage atherosclerosis with alpha (v) beta3-integrin-targeted nanoparticles. *Circulation* 2003;108:2270–2274.

58. Stegman LD, Rehemtulla A, Beattie B, et al. Noninvasive quantitation of cytosine deaminase transgene expression in human tumor xenografts in vivo magnetic resonance spectroscopy. *Proc Natl Acad Sci U S A* 1999;96:9821–9826.

59. Modo M, Cash D, Mellodew K, et al. Tracking transplanted stem cell migration using bifunctional, contrast agent-enhanced, magnetic resonance imaging. *Neuroimage* 2002;17:803–811.

60. Modo M, Roberts TJ, Sandhu JK, et al. In vivo monitoring of cellular transplants by magnetic resonance imaging and positron emission tomography. *Expert Opin Biol Ther* 2004;4:145–155.

61. Rudelius M, Daldrup-Link HE, Heinzmann U, et al. Highly efficient paramagnetic labeling of embryonic and neuronal stem cells. *Eur J Nucl Med Mol Imaging* 2003;30:1038–1044.

62. Daldrup-Link HE, Rudelius M, Oostendorp RA, et al. Targeting of hematopoietic progenitor cells with MR contrast agents. *Radiology* 2003;228:760–767.

63. Schmitz SA, Taupitz M, Wagner S, et al. Iron-oxide-enhanced magnetic resonance imaging of atherosclerotic plaques: postmortem analysis of accuracy, inter-observer agreement, and pitfalls. *Invest Radiol* 2002;37:405–411.

64. Schmitz SA, Coupland SE, Gust R, et al. Superparamagnetic iron oxide-enhanced MRI of atherosclerotic plaques in Watanabe hereditable hyperlipidemic rabbits. *Invest Radiol* 2000;35:460–471.

65. Ruehm SG, Corot C, Vogt P, et al. Magnetic resonance imaging of atherosclerotic plaque with ultrasmall superparamagnetic particles of iron oxide in hyperlipidemic rabbits. *Circulation* 2001;103:415–422.

66. Litovsky S, Madjid M, Zarrabi A, et al. Superparamagnetic iron oxide-based method for quantifying recruitment of monocytes to mouse atherosclerotic lesions in vivo: enhancement by tissue necrosis factor-alpha, interleukin-1beta, and interferon-gamma. *Circulation* 2003;107:1545–1549.

67. Schmitz SA, Taupitz M, Wagner S, et al. Magnetic resonance imaging of atherosclerotic plaques using superparamagnetic iron oxide particles. *J Magn Reson Imaging* 2001;14:355–361.

68. Kooi ME, Cappendijk VC, Cleutjens KB, et al. Accumulation of ultrasmall superparamagnetic particles of iron oxide in

human atherosclerotic plaques can be detected by in vivo magnetic resonance imaging. *Circulation* 2003;107:2453–2458.

69. Kanno S, Wu YJ, Lee PC, et al. Macrophage accumulation associated with rat cardiac allograft rejection detected by magnetic resonance imaging with ultrasmall superparamagnetic iron oxide particles. *Circulation* 2001;104:934–938.

70. Sanderson CJ, Wilson DV. Methods for coupling protein or polysaccharide to red cells by periodate oxidation. *Immunochemistry* 1971;8:163–168.

71. Weissleder R, Lee AS, Khaw BA, et al. Antimyosin-labeled monocrystalline iron oxide allows detection of myocardial infarct: MR antibody imaging. *Radiology* 1992;182:381–385.

72. Meldrum FC, Heywood BR, Mann S. Magnetoferritin: in vitro synthesis of a novel magnetic protein. *Science* 1992;257:522–523.

73. Bulte JW, Douglas T, Mann S, et al. Initial assessment of magnetoferritin biokinetics and proton relaxation enhancement in rats. *Acad Radiol* 1995;2:871–878.

74. Kukowska-Latallo JF, Bielinska AU, Johnson J, et al. Efficient transfer of genetic material into mammalian cells using Starburst polyamidoamine dendrimers. *Proc Natl Acad Sci U S A* 1996;93:4897–4902.

75. Tang MX, Redemann CT, Szoka FC Jr. In vitro gene delivery by degraded polyamidoamine dendrimers. *Bioconjug Chem* 1996;7:703–714.

76. Delong R, Stephenson K, Loftus T, et al. Characterization of complexes of oligonucleotides with polyamidoamine Starburst dendrimers and effects on intracellular delivery. *J Pharm Sci* 1997;86:762–764.

77. Bulte JW, Douglas T, Witwer B, et al. Magnetodendrimers allow endosomal magnetic labeling and in vivo tracking of stem cells. *Nat Biotechnol* 2001;19:1141–1147.

78. Hakumaki JM, Savitt JM, Gearhart JD, et al. MRI detection of labeled neural progenitor cells in a mouse model of Parkinson's disease. *Brain Res Dev Brain Res* 2001;132:A43–A44.

79. Walter GA, Cahill KS, Huard J, et al. Noninvasive monitoring of stem cell transfer for muscle disorders. *Magn Reson Med* 2004;51:273–277.

80. Billotey C, Wilhelm C, Devaud M, et al. Cell internalization of anionic maghemite nanoparticles: quantitative effect on magnetic resonance imaging. *Magn Reson Med* 2003;49:646–654.

81. Wilhelm C, Billotey C, Roger J, et al. Intracellular uptake of anionic superparamagnetic nanoparticles as a function of their surface coating. *Biomaterials* 2003;24:1001–1011.

82. Frank JA, Zywicke H, Jordan EK, et al. Magnetic intracellular labeling of mammalian cells by combining (FDA-approved) superparamagnetic iron oxide MR contrast agents and commonly used transfection agents. *Acad Radiol* 2002;9(Suppl 2):S484–S487.

83. Frank JA, Miller BR, Arbab AS, et al. Clinically applicable labeling of mammalian and stem cells by combining superparamagnetic iron oxides and transfection agents. *Radiology* 2003;228:480–487.

84. Arbab AS, Yocum GT, Wilson LB, et al. Comparison of transfection agents in forming complexes with ferumoxides, cell labeling efficiency, and cellular viability. *Mol Imaging* 2004;3:24–32.

85. Arbab AS, Bashaw LA, Miller BR, et al. Characterization of biophysical and metabolic properties of cells labeled with superparamagnetic iron oxide nanoparticles and transfection agent for cellular MR imaging. *Radiology* 2003;229:838–846.

86. Arbab AS, Bashaw LA, Miller BR, et al. Intracytoplasmic tagging of cells with ferumoxides and transfection agent for cellular magnetic resonance imaging after cell transplantation: methods and techniques. *Transplantation* 2003;76:1123–1130.

87. Kraitchman DL, Heldman AW, Atalar E, et al. In vivo magnetic resonance imaging of mesenchymal stem cells in myocardial infarction. *Circulation* 2003;107:2290–2293.

88. Garot J, Unterseeh T, Teiger E, et al. Magnetic resonance imaging of targeted catheter-based implantation of myogenic precursor cells into infarcted left ventricular myocardium. *J Am Coll Cardiol* 2003;41:1841–1846.

89. Walter GA, Cahill KS, Huard J, et al. Noninvasive monitoring of stem cell transfer for muscle disorders. *Magn Reson Med* 2004;51:273–277.

90. Anderson SA, Glod J, Arbab AS, et al. Noninvasive MR imaging of magnetically labeled stem cells to directly identify neovasculature in a glioma model. *Blood* 2005;105:420–425.

91. Arbab AS, Jordan EK, Wilson LB, et al. In vivo trafficking and targeted delivery of magnetically labeled stem cells. *Hum Gene Ther* 2004;15:351–360.

92. Kostura L, Kraitchman DL, Mackay AM, et al. Feridex labeling of mesenchymal stem cells inhibits chondrogenesis but not adipogenesis or osteogenesis. *NMR Biomed* 2004;17:513–517.

93. Bulte JW, Kraitchman DL, Mackay AM, et al. Chondrogenic differentiation of mesenchymal stem cells is inhibited after magnetic labeling with ferumoxides. *Blood* 2004;104:3410–3413.

94. Arbab AS, Yocum GT, Kalish H, et al. Efficient magnetic cell labeling with protamine sulfate complexed to ferumoxides for cellular MRI. *Blood* 2004;104:1217–1223.

95. Hinds KA, Hill JM, Shapiro EM, et al. Highly efficient endosomal labeling of progenitor and stem cells with large magnetic particles allows magnetic resonance imaging of single cells. *Blood* 2003;102:867–872.

96. Dodd SJ, Williams M, Suhan JP, et al. Detection of single mammalian cells by high-resolution magnetic resonance imaging. *Biophys J* 1999;76:103–109.

97. Shapiro EM, Skrtic S, Sharer K, et al. MRI detection of single particles for cellular imaging. *Proc Natl Acad Sci U S A* 2004;101:10901–10906.

98. Foster-Gareau P, Heyn C, Alejski A, et al. Imaging single mammalian cells with a 1.5 T clinical MRI scanner. *Magn Reson Med* 2003;49:968–971.

99. Bulte JW, Kraitchman DL. Monitoring cell therapy using iron oxide MR contrast agents. *Curr Pharm Biotechnol* 2004;5:567–584.

100. Bulte JW, Zhang S, van Gelderen P, et al. Neurotransplantation of magnetically labeled oligodendrocyte progenitors: magnetic resonance tracking of cell migration and myelination. *Proc Natl Acad Sci U S A* 1999;96:15256–15261.

101. Hoehn M, Kustermann E, Blunk J, et al. Monitoring of implanted stem cell migration in vivo: a highly resolved in vivo magnetic resonance imaging investigation of experimental stroke in rat. *Proc Natl Acad Sci U S A* 2002;99:16267–16272.

102. Jendelova P, Herynek V, deCroos J, et al. Imaging the fate of implanted bone marrow stromal cells labeled with superparamagnetic nanoparticles. *Magn Reson Med* 2003;50:767–776.

103. Yeh TC, Zhang W, Ildstad ST, et al. In vivo dynamic MRI tracking of rat T-cells labeled with superparamagnetic iron-oxide particles. *Magn Reson Med* 1995;33:200–208.

104. Strauer BE, Brehm M, Zeus T, et al. Repair of infarcted myocardium by autologous intracoronary mononuclear bone marrow cell transplantation in humans. *Circulation* 2002;106:1913–1918.

105. Assmus B, Schachinger V, Teupe C, et al. Transplantation of progenitor cells and regeneration enhancement in acute

myocardial infarction (TOPCARE-AMI). *Circulation* 2002; 106:3009–3017.

106. Schachinger V, Assmus B, Britten MB, et al. Transplantation of progenitor cells and regeneration enhancement in acute myocardial infarction: final one-year results of the TOPC-ARE-AMI trial. *J Am Coll Cardiol* 2004;44:1690–1699.

107. Wollert KC, Meyer GP, Lotz J, et al. Intracoronary autologous bone-marrow cell transfer after myocardial infarction: the BOOST randomised controlled clinical trial. *Lancet* 2004; 364:141–148.

108. Smits PC, van Geuns RJ, Poldermans D, et al. Catheter-based intramyocardial injection of autologous skeletal myoblasts as a primary treatment of ischemic heart failure: clinical experience with six-month follow-up. *J Am Coll Cardiol* 2003;42: 2063–2069.

109. Lederman RJ, Guttman MA, Peters DC, et al. Catheter-based endomyocardial injection with real-time magnetic resonance imaging. *Circulation* 2002;105:1282–1284.

110. Rickers C, Gallegos R, Seethamraju RT, et al. Applications of magnetic resonance imaging for cardiac stem cell therapy. *J Interv Cardiol* 2004;17:37–46.

111. Cahill KS, Gaidosh G, Huard J, et al. Noninvasive monitoring and tracking of muscle stem cell transplants. *Transplantation* 2004;78:1626–1633.

112. Bos C, Delmas Y, Desmouliere A, et al. In vivo MR imaging of intravascularly injected magnetically labeled mesenchymal stem cells in rat kidney and liver. *Radiology* 2004;233: 781–789.

113. Seppenwoolde JH, Viergever MA, Bakker CJ. Passive tracking exploiting local signal conservation: the white marker phenomenon. *Magn Reson Med* 2003;50:784–790.

114. Cunningham CH, Arai T, Terashima M, et al. Positive contrast MRI of cells labeled with magnetic nanoparticles. In: *The society for molecular imaging*. St Louis: 2004:170.

115. Coristine AJ, Foster P, Deoni SC, et al. Positive contrast labeling of SPIO loaded cells in cell samples and spinal cord injury. In: *Proc ISMRM*. Kyoto, Japan: 2004:163.

INDEX

Page numbers set in *italics* denote figures; those followed by a *t* denote tables